LIBRARY

Silica and Silica-Induced Lung Diseases

Edited by
Vincent Castranova
Val Vallyathan
William E. Wallace

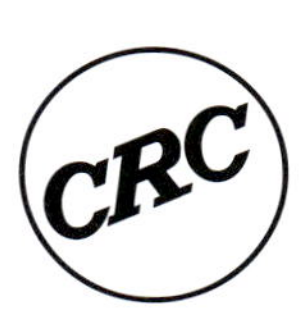

CRC Press
Boca Raton New York London Tokyo
1996

Library of Congress Cataloging-in-Publication Data

Silica and silica-induced lung diseases / edited by Vincent
Castranova, Val Vallyathan, William E. Wallace.
p. cm.
Includes bibliographical references and index.
ISBN 0-8493-4709-2
1. Silicosis. I. Castranova, Vincent. II. Vallyathan, Val.
III. Wallace, William E., 1942– .
[DNLM: 1. Lung Diseases--chemically induced. 2. Lung Neoplasms-
-chemically induced. 3. Silicon Dioxide--adverse effects.
4. Silicosis--etiology. 5. Occupational Exposure. WF 600 S583
1995]
RC774.S52 1995
616.2′44--dc20
DNLM/DLC
for Library of Congress 95-6538
CIP

International Standard Book Number 0-8493-4709-2
Library of Congress Card Number 95-6538
Printed in the United States of America 1 2 3 4 5 6 7 8 9 0
Printed on acid-free paper

THE EDITORS

Vincent Castranova, Ph.D., is the Chief of the Biochemistry Section in the Division of Respiratory Disease Studies of the National Institute for Occupational Safety and Health, Morgantown, West Virginia. He is also an adjunct professor in the Department of Physiology at West Virginia University, Morgantown, West Virginia. He is a member of the American Physiological Society, the Society of Toxicology, Sigma Xi, Beta Beta Beta, the Red Cell Club, and the Allegheny-Erie Chapter of SOT.

Vincent Castranova received a B.S. in Biology from Mount Saint Mary's College, Emmitsburgh, Maryland in 1970 and obtained a Ph.D. in Physiology and Biophysics in 1974 under Dr. Philip R. Miles, Professor of Physiology, West Virginia University, Morgantown, West Virginia. His graduate research concerned the pharmacological modification and characterization of cation pathways in the plasma membrane of erythrocytes.

After completion of his graduate studies, Dr. Castranova was an NIH fellow and research faculty member in the laboratory of Dr. Joseph F. Hoffman, Professor of Physiology, Yale University, New Haven, Connecticut. His research at Yale involved characterization and isolation of the anion exchange pathway in erythrocytes. He also was involved in the measurement of anion transport properties in red blood cells from patients with various diseases and the use of fluorescent probes to monitor membrane potential in red blood cells.

In 1977, Dr. Castranova received a research staff position at the National Institute for Occupational Safety and Health and an adjunct faculty position at West Virginia University, Morgantown, West Virginia. He has served at these institutions since that time.

Since 1977, Dr. Castranova's research interests have concentrated on three cell types, i.e., alveolar macrophages, polymorphonuclear leukocytes, and alveolar type II epithelial cells. Studies with alveolar macrophages have involved investigation of the phagocytotic process. These studies have included measurement of resting and stimulant-activated chemiluminescence (CL), oxygen consumption, superoxide generation, hydrogen peroxide secretion, lysosomal enzyme release, cytokine production, and glycolysis as well as particulate uptake. The effects of exposure of alveolar macrophages to various occupational and environmental pollutants on these processes have also been investigated. Pollutants of interest include coal dust, diesel particulate, heavy metals, silica, organic solvents, asbestos, cotton dust, and grain dust. In addition, changes in membrane permeability and transmembrane potential associated with activation of alveolar macrophages have also been investigated. Studies with polymorphonuclear leukocytes have included purification by centrifugal elutriation, measurement of ionic transport and membrane potential changes involved in the stimulus-secretion process, measurement of respiratory burst activity and myeloperoxidase release, studies of defects associated with chronic granulomatous disease, and the effect of platelet-activating factor as an inflammatory mediator. Studies with alveolar type II cells have involved purification by centrifugal elutriation, measurement of transmembrane potential and identification of an electrogenic Na^+-Ka^+ pump, characterization of volume regulation mechanisms, measurement of surfactant synthesis, characterization of xenobiotic metabolism, interferon production, and identification of amino acid-Na^+ coupled transport.

In collaboration with numerous colleagues, *in vitro* and *in vivo* investigations concerning mechanisms involved in the development and progression of silicosis have included: measurement of the direct toxicity of silica on lung cells, characterization of the stimulatory effects of silica on the production of oxidant species (such as superoxide anion, hydrogen peroxide, and nitric oxide) and the secretion of cytokines, and quantitation of the effects of silica exposure on fibrosis. Studies on the antifibrotic effects of tetrandrine and protection by organosilane coatings have been conducted as well as characterization of the unique surface properties and toxicity of freshly fractured silica.

Val Vallyathan, Ph.D., is a Research Pathologist of the Pathology Section in the Division of Respiratory Disease Studies of the National Institute for Occupational Safety and Health, Morgantown, West Virginia. He is also a Professor of Pathology in the Department of Pathology, West Virginia University, Morgantown, West Virginia and a member of several international scientific societies.

Val Vallyathan received a B.Sc. (Honors) in Biology in 1957 and a M.Sc. in Physiology in 1959 from University of Baroda, India. He subsequently obtained a Ph.D. in Physiology in 1964 under Dr. John C. George, Professor of Zoology, University of Baroda, India. His graduate research concerned the morphologic, metabolic, and biochemical adaptation of muscle and blood during exercise and disuse atrophy.

After completion of his graduate studies, Dr. Vallyathan worked as a post-doctoral fellow on a muscular dystrophy scheme at the University of Baroda, India. His research involved characterization of micromolecular and enzymatic changes in disuse muscular atrophy. In 1964, he was appointed as an Assistant Professor at the University of Baroda. He was involved in teaching physiology, anatomy, and histochemistry at the undergraduate and graduate levels.

In 1968, Dr. Vallyathan was awarded a National Research Council post-doctoral fellowship at the University of Guelph, Ontario, Canada. His research at the University of Guelph involved the characterization of adaptational changes in seals and migratory birds. These studies involved cellular changes and lipid metabolic alterations.

In 1971, Dr. Vallyathan was appointed as a Senior Scientist at the Institute for Muscle Disease, New York. There he was involved in studies on Duchenne muscular dystrophy and investigations on the effects of therapeutic modalities.

In 1974, Dr. Vallyathan was appointed at the University of Vermont as a research associate and assistant professor in the Department of Pathology. As a member of the research group with John Craighead, M.D., Professor of Pathology, Dr. Vallyathan received extensive training into investigations of pneumoconiosis, cigarette smoke-induced pulmonary emphysema, and other pulmonary diseases.

In 1979, Dr. Vallyathan was appointed as a Research Pathologist at the National Institute for Occupational Safety and Health. He was also appointed as Professor of Pathology at West Virginia University, Pathology Department, Morgantown, West Virginia. He has continued to serve at these institutions since that time pursuing an active research agenda in occupational lung diseases and teaching graduate and undergraduate students.

At the National Institute for Occupational Safety and Health and at the West Virginia University, Dr. Vallyathan's research interests have been focused on several disciplines. The major areas of research included pathogenesis of occupational lung diseases, occupational lung cancers, emphysema, oxygen radical-induced lung injury, microchemical changes in lung and lung fluids, cytotoxicity of minerals, smoking and health effects, and the role of inflammatory cytokines in the development of occupational lung disease. His research interests have concentrated in the last several years on the generation of oxygen radicals in the lung and pulmonary phagocytes and their potential role in the cell injury and disease processes. His studies in these areas have included stimulation, secretion, detection, and kinetic studies of oxygen species and several antioxidant enzymes in the lung and isolated phagocytes during respiratory burst reactions. These studies utilized state-of-the-art techniques including electron spin resonance spectometry, spin trapping *in vivo* electron spin imaging, electron microscopy with energy dispersive X-ray analysis, selected area electron diffraction, and quantitative morphometry.

Dr. Vallyathan participated in several advisory committees and study panels. He was a panel member for the development of standards for "Asbestos-Associated Diseases" and "Diseases Associated With Exposure to Silica and Nonfibrous Silicate Minerals." His studies concerning the mechanisms and development of silica inhalation-associated diseases include: characterization and identification of surface free radicals on freshly fractured silica, generation of hydroxyl radicals from freshly fractured silica, enhanced cytotoxicity and pathogenicity of freshly fractured silica *in vitro* and *in vivo*, identification and characterization of oxygen radicals in the pathogenesis of acute silicolipoproteinosis, and detection of early markers in lung injury.

William E. Wallace, Ph.D., is the leader of the Aerosol Research Team in the Division of Respiratory Disease Studies of the National Institute for Occupational Safety and Health (NIOSH), Morgantown, West Virginia. He is an adjunct professor of Chemical Engineering and is a member of the Graduate Faculty of West Virginia University.

William Wallace received his Ph.D. in physics from West Virginia University in 1969 under Dr. William E. Vehse. His graduate research concerned the investigation of the Fermi surface of lithium using nuclear magnetic resonance analyses of the spin-lattice relaxation time of lithium-magnesium alloys.

After completion of his dissertation, Dr. Wallace accepted a National Research Council Postdoctoral Research Associateship with the U.S. Bureau of Mines. In that capacity and subsequently as a research physicist for the U.S. Bureau of Mines, he developed and mathematically modeled pulsed nuclear magnetic resonance sequences to speed the acquisition of spectra and of relaxation time measurements. As a result of the Farmington, West Virginia, mine disaster, he also began to analyze the interactions of pulmonary surfactant phospholipid with respirable mineral dusts. He became an Assistant Director of the

U.S. Department of Energy — Morgantown Energy Technology Center, developing the Fossil Energy Advanced Environmental Control Technology Program and building the Center's Analytical and Supporting Research Division. In 1980, he joined NIOSH as a research physicist and soon began adjunct teaching and research activities at West Virginia University. His activities at NIOSH include serving as a National Research Council-Postdoctoral Research Advisor. He has participated as a member of an International Agency for Research on Cancer (IARC) working group and on a National Research Council working group on synthetic fuels facilities safety.

Dr. Wallace is pursuing research on the properties which affect the cytotoxic and genotoxic activities of respirable mineral and organic particles, fibers, and complex respirable particulate materials. This has included measurement of the specific adsorption of phospholipid components of pulmonary surfactant by respirable quartz and clay dusts and spectroscopic analyses of the adsorbed state, measurement of the effect of surfactant coverage on mineral membranolysis and *in vitro* cytotoxicity, and measurement and mathematical modeling of the kinetics of enzymatic digestive removal of surfactant and consequent modification of cytotoxicity. Heterogeneous surface composition of workplace respirable dusts is being studied by a NIOSH-patented method using multiple electron accelerating voltages for scanning electron microscopy — energy dispersive X-ray analysis. The *in vitro* genotoxicity of diesel soot and complex mineral-organic respirable particles and fibers is being investigated using the finding that respirable soot particles express mutagenic, clastogenic, and DNA-damaging activities as intact particles when dispersed in components of pulmonary surfactant. This research is carried out in collaboration with researchers across NIOSH and at several universities and other U.S. government agencies. Support has been provided for this research performed at NIOSH by the U.S. Department of Interior and the U.S. Department of Energy.

DISCLAIMER

CONTRIBUTORS

James M. Antonini, Ph.D.
Research Associate
Department of Environmental Health
Harvard School of Public Health
Boston, Massachusetts

Michael D. Attfield, Ph.D.
Epidemiologist
Epidemiological Investigations Branch
National Institute for Occupational Safety and Health
Morgantown, West Virginia

Daniel E. Banks, M.D.
N. LeRoy Lapp Professor of Medicine and Chief
Section of Pulmonary and Critical Care Medicine
West Virginia University
School of Medicine
Morgantown, West Virginia

Peter Bitterman, M.D.
Professor and Chief
Pulmonary Medicine and Critical Care
Department of Medicine
University of Minnesota
Minneapolis, Minnesota

Peter P. Bolsaitis, Ph.D.
Research Scientist
Energy Laboratory
Massachusetts Institute of Technology
Cambridge, Massachusetts

Joseph D. Brain, S.D. in Hyg.
Chair
Department of Environmental Health
Harvard School of Public Health
Boston, Massachusetts

Patricia S. Brower, M.S.
Statistician
Epidemiological Investigations Branch
National Institute for Occupational Safety and Health
Morgantown, West Virginia

Geraldine M. Brown, Ph.D.
Scientist
Astra Clinical Research Unit
Edinburgh, Scotland

Vincent Castranova, Ph.D.
Professor
Department of Physiology
Robert C. Byrd Health Sciences Center
West Virginia University
and
Chief Biochemistry Section
National Institute for Occupational Safety and Health
Morgantown, West Virginia

De-Hwa Chao, Ph.D.
Research Associate
School of Pharmacy
Robert C. Byrd Health Sciences Center — North
West Virginia University
Morgantown, West Virginia

Leslie Couch, M.D.
Assistant Professor of Medicine
University of Texas
Health Center at Tyler
Tyler, Texas

John Craighead, M.D.
Professor
University of Vermont
Colchester Research Facility
Colchester, Vermont

Nar S. Dalal, Ph.D.
Professor
Department of Chemistry
West Virginia University
Morgantown, West Virginia

Lambert N. Daniel, M.D.
Senior Staff Fellow
Laboratory of Experimental Pathology
National Cancer Institute
Bethesda, Maryland

Kenneth Donaldson, Ph.D.
Reader
Department of Biological Sciences
Napier University
Merchiston Campus
Edinburgh, Scotland

Kevin E. Driscoll, Ph.D.
Principal Scientist
Miami Valley Laboratories
Procter and Gamble Company
Cincinnati, Ohio

R. Larry Grayson, Ph.D.
Professor of Mining Engineering
College of Engineering and Mineral Resources
West Virginia University
Morgantown, West Virginia

Francis H. Y. Green, M.D.
Professor
Department of Pathology
Faculty of Medicine
University of Calgary
Calgary, Alberta, Canada

Zu-Wei Gu, M.D., Ph.D.
Professor
Shanghai Institute of Labour Hygiene and Occupational Diseases
Shanghai, People's Republic of China

Jaime Gutierrez, M.S., M.D.
Department of Pharmacology and Toxicology
Robert C. Byrd Health Sciences Center
West Virginia University
Morgantown, West Virginia

Russell A. Harley, M.D.
Professor
Department of Pathology
Medical University of South Carolina
Charleston, South Carolina

Joel C. Harrison, B.S.
Physical Scientist
Environmental Investigations Branch
National Institute for Occupational Safety and Health
Morgantown, West Virginia

Frank J. Hearl, P.E.
Chief
Environmental Investigations Branch
National Institute for Occupational Safety and Health
Morgantown, West Virginia

Andrij Holian, Ph.D.
Associate Professor
Pulmonary Division/Internal Medicine
University of Texas
Houston, Texas

Gary E. R. Hook, Ph.D., D.Sc.
National Institute of Environmental Health Sciences
Research Triangle Park, North Carolina

Ann Hubbs, DVM, Ph.D.
Toxicologist
National Institute for Occupational Safety and Health
Morgantown, West Virginia

Rashi Iyer, M.S.
Scientist
Pulmonary Division/Internal Medicine
University of Texas
Houston, Texas

Abdullah J. Jabbour, Ph.D.
Scientist
Pulmonary Division/Internal Medicine
University of Texas
Houston, Texas

M. Edward Kaighn, Ph.D.
Scientist
Experimental Pathology
National Cancer Institute
Bethesda, Maryland

Agnes B. Kane, M.D., Ph.D.
Professor
Department of Pathology & Lab Medicine
Brown University
Providence, Rhode Island

Michael J. Keane, M.S.
Research Chemist
Environmental Investigations Branch
National Institute for Occupational Safety and Health
Morgantown, West Virginia

Shixuan Lu, M.D.
Professor, Head,
National Panel of Pneumoconioses Diagnosis
Institute of Occupational Medicine
Chinese Academy of Preventive Medicine
Beijing, People's Republic of China

Xirong Lu, M.D.
Professor
Institute of Occupational Medicine
Chinese Academy of Preventive Medicine
Beijing, People's Republic of China

Jane Y. C. Ma, Ph.D.
Research Chemist, Biochemistry Section
National Institute for Occupational Safety and Health
Morgantown, West Virginia

Joseph K. H. Ma, Ph.D.
Professor
School of Pharmacy
Robert C. Byrd Health Sciences Center - North
West Virginia University
Morgantown, West Virginia

Gretchen Mandel, Ph.D.
Associate Professor
Medical College of Wisconsin
Zablocki VA Medical Center
Milwaukee, Wisconsin

Neil Mandel, Ph.D.
Professor
Medical College of Wisconsin
Zablocki VA Medical Center
Milwaukee, Wisconsin

Yan Mao, Ph.D.
Biotechnology Fellow
Laboratory of Experimental Pathology
National Cancer Institute
Bethesda, Maryland

J. Corbett McDonald, M.D.
Professor
National Heart and Lung Institute
London, United Kingdom

Tong-man Ong, Ph.D.
Professor
Division of Plant and Soil Sciences
West Virginia University
and
Chief, Microbiology Section
National Institute for Occupational Safety and Health
Morgantown, West Virginia

Mark Reasor, Ph.D.
Professor
Department of Pharmacology and Toxicology
Robert C. Byrd Health Sciences Center - North
West Virginia University
Morgantown, West Virginia

Yongyut Rojanasakul, Ph.D.
Associate Professor
School of Pharmacy
Robert C. Byrd Health Sciences Center
West Virginia University
Morgantown, West Virginia

Umberto Saffiotti, M.D.
Chief
Laboratory of Experimental Pathology
National Cancer Institute
Bethesda, Maryland

Ronald K. Scheule, Ph.D.
Senior Scientist
Genzyme Corporation
Framingham, Massachusetts

Xianglin Shi, Ph.D.
Scientist
Experimental Pathology
National Cancer Institute
Bethesda, Maryland

James W. Stephens, Ph.D.
Research Physical Chemist
Environmental Investigations Branch
National Institute for Occupational Safety and Health
Morgantown, West Virginia

Theresa Sweeney, Ph.D.
Scientist
Pharmaceutical R & D
Genentech, Inc.
South San Francisco, California

Val Vallyathan, Ph.D.
Professor
Department of Pathology
Robert C. Byrd Health Sciences Center
West Virginia University
and
Research Pathologist
National Institute for Occupational Safety and Health
Morgantown, West Virginia

Chris Van Dyke, B.S.E.E.
Department of Pharmacology and Toxicology
Robert C. Byrd Health Sciences Center
West Virginia University
Morgantown, West Virginia

Knox Van Dyke, Ph.D.
Professor
Department of Pharmacology and Toxicology
Robert C. Byrd Health Sciences Center - North
West Virginia University
Morgantown, West Virginia

Charles J. Viviano, Ph.D.
Scientist
Yale University
Medical School
New Haven, Connecticut

William E. Wallace, Ph.D.
Professor
College of Engineering
West Virginia University
and
Research Physicist
National Institute for Occupational Safety and Health
Morgantown, West Virginia

A. Olufemi Williams, Ph.D.
Scientist
Experimental Pathology
National Cancer Institute
Bethesda, Maryland

Lixin Wu, M.S.
Department of Pharmacology and Toxicology
Robert C. Byrd Health Sciences Center
West Virginia University
Morgantown, West Virginia

Changqi Zou, M.D.
Professor of Pathology
Department of Pneumoconiosis
Director
Institute of Occupational Medicine
Chinese Academy of Preventive Medicine
Beijing, People's Republic of China

CONTENTS

Section I
Background and Definitions

Section I
Chapter 1

PATHOGENIC CONSIDERATIONS REGARDING DISEASE RELATED TO SILICA DUST EXPOSURE

John Craighead

CONTENTS

I. UNRESOLVED QUESTIONS

Although silicosis has long been recognized as a significant pneumoconiosis, it now can be prevented by environmental dust control. Nonetheless, diseases resulting from exposure to silica in the workplace continues to occur sporadically on a worldwide basis. The prevention of silicosis is now a problem for education and public health risk management rather than one that can be resolved by future basic research. Yet the study of the body's response to silica dust and the mechanisms whereby disease develops continues to provide stimulating insights into pathogenesis. Despite our current remarkable appreciation of the pathobiology of mineral dust disease, many key questions regarding the body's response to silica particulates remain to be answered. Resolution of these issues could provide opportunities for disease prophylaxis that are not yet envisioned by the scientific and medical community. Ultimately, this could make it possible for humans to work in a dusty environment without adverse health effects. More realistically, understanding the pathogenesis of silicosis will also provide us with a broader appreciation of disease mechanisms. In considering the less well-understood phenomenology of silicosis, I envision the following questions to be relevant, but yet unresolved.

A. IS THE VARIABILITY IN DISEASE DEVELOPMENT AMONG MEMBERS OF A POPULATION EXPOSED TO COMPARABLE AMOUNTS OF SILICA A REFLECTION OF INDIVIDUAL HOST SUSCEPTIBILITY?

Increasingly, issues of host susceptibility arise in considering pathogeneic mechanisms. I know of no significant biologic information in the literature on mineral lung diseases which allows one to answer this

0-8493-4709-2/96/$0.00+$.50

question. Intriguing possibilities exist that should be the subject of future research. If oxidant injury is intrinsic to the development of silica lesions, as contemporary research suggests, then we must ask if there is variability in the individual tissue response to exposure. Differences in the intrinsic antioxidant capacities of individuals no doubt exist, possibly on a hereditary basis, but they can also be due to such factors as adaptation to stress or the dietary consumption of antioxidants. If oxidants and antioxidants are as critical to the response to dust as the current evidence suggests, then their role in individual susceptibility is implicit. Similar questions might be posed with regard to cytokine generation by immunologically activated cells in the dust-exposed tissue and the elaboration of growth factors which, without a doubt, play a role in the development of the unique silicotic lesion. As the reader will appreciate, several of these key issues have been addressed in this book.

The availability of transgenic and "knockout" strains of mice should make it possible to explore, in animal models, the role of oxidants and antioxidants as well as cytokines and growth factors in the development of disease in controlled, experimental situations. Similarly, studies in selected strains of animals having unique patterns of immunologic responsivity could provide opportunities to explore, in the future, the role of the immune system in the pathogenesis of the silicotic nodule. This work builds naturally on the abundant experimental studies with silica that have already been conducted in laboratories worldwide.

B. THE NODULAR LESION OF SILICOSIS IS A UNIQUE PATHOLOGIC ENTITY. WHAT IS THE MECHANISM OF ITS PATHOGENESIS?

This question is one of the most obvious of the unresolved issues related to the pathogenesis of silicosis. No other organic or inorganic particulate cause of disease in humans produces a lesion comparable to the silicotic nodule. The nodule is comprised of whirled bundles of dense, hyalinized acellular fibrous tissue arranged in a concentric pattern. That silica dust is the central actor in the picture is clear, for the particles appear to be sequestered in the approximate center of the nodule. Silicotic nodules symmetrically enlarge with the passage of time, as was shown in systematic studies conducted years ago. Thus, it is a progressive lesion, but what is the mechanism of progression in this set of circumstances? It is highly probable that cytokines and growth factors are involved, but which ones and in what manner? If this is so, it seems probable that these humoral factors are generated by the presence of the dust for extended periods of time as the lesion progresses. Could this be a reflection of an immune-mediated process? If so, what cells are the major actors? Is it exclusively the domain of the macrophage as current dogma implies? If it were possible to identify the key elements in lesion development, it would then be possible to interfere with their generation and, thus, prevent the development of the lesion. Modern experimental cell and molecular biologic approaches for identifying sites of gene activation and expression in tissue, such as fluorescence *in situ* hybridization, offer opportunities for exploring these questions. The availability of monoclonal antibodies and antisense molecules potentially makes it possible for the investigator to focus "magic bullets" on specific active elements involved in the development of lesions.

C. WHAT FEATURES OF THE SILICA PARTICLE ACCOUNT FOR ITS PATHOGENICITY AND WHY ARE THE POLYMORPHS, CRISTOBALITE AND TRIDYMITE, MORE PATHOGENIC THAN ALPHA QUARTZ? WHY DO THE SILICA PARTICLES DIFFER SO STRIKINGLY FROM CRYSTALLINE GLASS, AMORPHOUS SILICONE AND THE SILICATES WHICH SHARE COMMON CHARACTERISTICS WITH SILICA PARTICULATES?

These are some of the most intriguing questions of the pathobiology of the mineral lung diseases, yet our intrinsic understanding is limited. The crystallography of silica and silicates have been exhaustively explored, but questions related to pathogenesis are largely the subjects of descriptive research. The lucid, detailed description of silica crystallography by Mandel and Mandel in Section II, Chapter 1 provides a sound, state-of-the-art discussion of the topic. We now have available experimental tools to explore the responsivity of cell membranes and other organelles of the cell to silica dust particulates.

Intriguing observations exist that require further biological elucidation. It is now recognized that freshly fractured particles of silica are more pathogenic than weathered particles of comparable size and makeup. What are the surface properties of the particles that account for this finding? On the other hand, contaminating silicates have the capacity to attenuate the pathogenicity of silica particles in mixed dust exposures. How do we account for this observation?

D. IS SILICA DUST A CARCINOGEN, AND IF SO, IS IT AN INITIATOR OR A PROMOTER SUBSTANCE?

As considered in Section V Chapter 2, McDonald now believes, on the basis of epidemiological studies, that it no longer seems reasonable to dismiss the positive evidence supporting an association between silica exposure and bronchogenic carcinoma. However, the discrepancies and the outcomes of various epidemiological studies in different human populations have not been explained satisfactorily.

Compelling evidence documents the carcinogenicity of silica dust in rats (but not in mice, hamsters, and guinea pigs). However, numerous questions remain to be resolved. For example, is silica a genotoxic carcinogen in rats and, if so, by what mechanism and why not in other rodent species? One could envision, for example, oxidant generation by the silica-exposed cell as the key mechanism involved and, if so, could this question be resolved by the experimental use of antioxidants in prophylaxis? It would be interesting to explore the role of nutrients in this process, for we now know the carotenoids and vitamin A analogues have prophylactic properties in tobacco smoke-related lung cancer. Alternatively, one can picture silica playing a role in carcinogenesis through the mechanisms of pulmonary fibrosis. Under such circumstances, it could serve as a nongenotoxic promoter substance enhancing the effects of cigarette smoke or other, still unidentified, initiators. Although the concept of scar carcinogenesis has long been accepted as one of the possible pathogenic mechanisms in bronchogenic carcinoma, we have not explained the phenomena satisfactorily.

The development of models of silica carcinogenesis has been restricted to only a few laboratories, and this work was largely undertaken to resolve pragmatic problems of risk assessment. We are now in a position to explore these questions mechanistically in the context of the human experience. Thus, insightful animal experiments may contribute to our understanding.

The human questions will be more difficult to resolve. Not only do the epidemiologic observations conflict, but the circumstances under which silica might cause lung cancer remain to be resolved. The lack of human tissue from cases of possible silica-related cancer is one obvious problem at the outset, but what questions should be asked if the tissue becomes available? Recent studies of human lung cancers have shown that amplification of the *myc* gene occurs in some, *ras* gene mutations and overexpression in others, and overall, there is a striking prevalence of tumors with altered *p53* suppressor gene expression due to specific mutations or deletions. Can these observations be fit into a formula that will provide insights into the pathogenesis of silica-related lung cancer? For example, does silica and the tissue response to its presence result in mutations of oncogenes or suppressor genes? Recent evidence suggests that exposures of specific types may result in "fingerprint" mutational changes in the *p53* gene which would allow the investigator to pinpoint the exposure that has resulted in loss of tumor suppression. If so, would it then be possible to relate, on a molecular basis, a patient's cancer to silica? While the problems related to research of this type are imposing, reliance on epidemiologic evidence of questionable merit, or historical information of alleged exposure in individual patients, is too tenuous a basis for establishing "cause and effect" relationships.

E. DOES THE EVOLVING CONCERN REGARDING MAMMARY SILICONE IMPLANTS PROVIDE INSIGHTS INTO THE MECHANISMS WHEREBY SILICA CAUSES DISEASE?

Silicone-containing mammary prostheses have provoked increasing concern as allegations of disease complications continue to be voiced. What have we learned about silica that applies to the health problems believed by some to be associated with implants, and can understanding that evolves from the study of breast prostheses provide insights into the mechanisms involved in the generation of lesions related to silica dust exposure? First, it should be emphasized that the crystals of silica have little physical commonality with noncrystalline silica formulated into silicone products. Yet both substances can provoke a luxuriant tissue response involving macrophages as key elements. Whether the silicone breast implant recipient develops specific antibodies to silicone (as claimed), is an unresolved question. But, it is well-known that silicotic patients with pulmonary fibrosis exhibit increases in serum polyclonal immunoglobulins, often accompanied by elevated concentrations of circulating rheumatoid factor, antinuclear antibodies and immune complexes. Is there a commonality to these responses, and do they provide insight into tissue reactions to silicon dioxide containing materials?

Scleroderma (systemic sclerosis) occurs sporadically among those who are exposed to silica dust occupationally, as well as in members of the mammary implant community. Unfortunately, no meaningful prevalence data has accumulated on the occurrence of this complication and there are those that deny an association. Caplan's lesion (so-called rheumatoid pneumoconiosis) is an interesting, but unexplained, condition that occasionally occurs in those with heavy silica dust exposures who have rheumatoid arthritis. Microscopically, the pulmonary lesions exhibit features reminiscent of the rheumatoid granuloma observed in those with severe, active rheumatoid arthritis. One must ask whether a comparable tissue response occurs in the silicone implant recipient who develops rheumatic complaints. Clearly, these immunopathologic phenomena require further insightful inquiry.

F. WHAT ARE THE MECHANISMS OF LYMPHATIC PARTICLE TRANSPORT AND THE FACTORS WHICH INFLUENCE SITES OF PARTICLE DEPOSITION IN THE LUNG AND THE SUBSEQUENT DEVELOPMENT OF LESIONS?

Silicosis and silicatosis, in contrast to asbestosis, are diseases which are generated by particle deposition along the lymphatic routes of transport of these particulates from the air spaces to the hilar and mediastinal lymph nodes. Interestingly enough, some individuals develop the localized so-called "candle wax" lesions in the pleura, whereas others do not, despite exposure to comparable amounts of dust. Still other individuals develop lesions only in the hilar lymph nodes while some form nodules sporadically in the parenchyma of the lungs. We know very little about the kinetics of dust transport over the course of the lymphatics and the factors that influence its deposition at sites in these channels and the perilymphatic interstitium. Are the particles transported in macrophages or free in the lymph? Does the phenomena relate to differences in particle size and concentration or to variability in host responsiveness to particles in transit in the lymphatics? In my view, physiologists have yet to adequately focus on these problems that surely can be answered by contemporary experimental tools.

II. CONCLUDING REMARKS

Remarkable progress has been made in our understanding of the health impacts of silica dust exposure. Worldwide, the problem is of critical public health importance and is not likely to abate in the foreseeable future. The editors of this book have insightfully assembled an outstanding, timely, and comprehensive compilation of chapters which represents our understanding of this rapidly evolving area of contemporary environmental and occupational health science.

Section I
Chapter 2

HISTORY OF SILICOSIS

Russell A. Harley and Val Vallyathan

CONTENTS

I. INTRODUCTION

Silicosis is a debilitating lung disease caused by the inhalation of crystalline silica. Despite several decades of intensive research and effective (frequently unenforced) environmental dust control measures, silicosis, a disease of historical importance, continues to be a problem in our workplaces. It is important to emphasize and recapitulate the history of silicosis because in the past it was believed that the disease was a reflection of an individual's peculiar, social, personal, hereditary, and economic circumstances. The disease was considered to occur as a result of the special relationship between an individual and a complex, highly peculiarized environment. In the past, silicosis and other pneumoconioses were diseases of the poor, of slaves, or of prisoners forced to work. The rampant tuberculosis prevalent in the 18th and 19th centuries made a significant impact on the concomitant increased mortality of people with silicosis. Roentgenographic examination of the chest was not available as a diagnostic tool until 1885, i.e., long after the recognition of silicosis.

II. PREHISTORIC EVIDENCE

Silica dust as a cause of pulmonary disease (silicosis) is one of civilization's first examples of understanding the etiology of an occupational lung disease. It was certainly the oldest pneumoconiosis recognized to be associated with specific occupations such as stone cutting, quarrying, and mining. Silicosis was described to have existed in neolithic men, who were engaged in shaping flints for arrow heads, spearheads, and other weapons of defense.[1] Anthracosis has been seen in the lungs of Egyptian mummies.[2]

Mining activities which may have caused silicosis in workers were started in China, India, and along the Nile in Egypt between 4000 and 3000 B.C.[3] Hippocrates described clinical lung disease in miners (pneumoconiosis) in approximately 400 B.C.[3] He described the metal digger as a man who breathes with difficulty, which was suggestive of the presence of pneumoconiosis among the miners.

Pliny (A.D. 23–79) advocated the use of protective masks for miners to prevent the inhalation of "fatal dust" produced in the mines. Pliny's description of protective devices to avoid dust inhalation clearly points to the dangers of dust-induced lung disease known to the Romans during these early times.[4] Galen (A.D. 131–201) was the first to describe the pulmonary disease symptoms of silicosis which developed in gypsum miners.[3]

III. EUROPEAN EXPERIENCE

In 1556, Georgius Agricola[5] published a book entitled *De Re Metallica*. In it, he described mining, metallurgy, and the lung diseases of miners in Bohemia. Agricola stated that the "mines produced asthma, and some mines are so dry that they are entirely devoid of water, and this dryness causes workmen even greater harm, for the dust which is stirred and beaten up by digging penetrates into the windpipe and lungs and produces difficulty in breathing and disease. If the dust was corrosive, it ulcerated the lungs and caused consumption." Agricola's statements concerning lung disease in miners are considered as one of the earliest and best, if not the first, descriptions of this dust-induced pulmonary clinical condition and its pathologic effect on lungs.

In 1567, Paracelsus, a Swiss physician and alchemist, wrote the first monograph on the diseases of miners entitled "Von der Bergsucht und anderen Bergkrankheiten." In this monograph, the mineralogy of the mines as well as the pathology and etiology of the miners' diseases are discussed in detail. He attributed the origin of miners' lung diseases to the mine air. This monograph greatly influenced the study of occupational lung diseases.[3]

In the Carpathian mines of Poland, Czechoslovakia, and Rumania, the mining tools were called "widow-makers" by the miners.[3,5] In the mining communities, records exist of women who married seven or more husbands, "all of whom this terrible consumption has carried away."[3] Van Diemerbrock, in 1649, described the lungs of stone cutters in Netherlands (who had died of "asthma") as having "piles of sand" in the lungs at autopsy.[6]

Bernardino Ramazzini's book *De Morbis Artficum Diatriba* (Padua, 1700) described the diseases of stone cutters and many other occupations.[7] He described in detail the special hazards involved in each occupation, including dust diseases and their related pulmonary lesions. He described lungs of stone cutters that were "found to be stuffed with small stones."[7] The stone cutters, sculptors, quarrymen, and marble cutters were described as "breathing the rough, sharp, jagged splinters that glance off while making statues and other objects and hence they are usually troubled with cough, and some of them contract asthmatic affections and become consumptive."[7]

In Sheffield, England, young needlepointers and cutlery workers suffered high mortality due to silicosis in the 1790s.[8] During this time flint was powdered dry and used as grinding powder in the manufacture of grindstones and in cutlery polishing. Thomas Benson was first granted patents for wet grinding of flint in 1726 and again in 1732, which reduced the dust levels in grinding operations in England. This wet grinding of flint greatly reduced the incidence of silicosis and the high rate of grindstone workers dying at the early ages of 28–32, as evident from the writings of Arnold Knight.[3]

Charles Thackrah was credited as the first to compare, on an epidemiologic basis, the life expectancy of British workers in different trades and occupations.[9] He correlated the mortality of workers with dust exposure. His conclusion was that workers in sandstone quarries died at an early age (less than 40 years) because of the large dust clouds produced at work sites. He found no evidence of lung disease among brick and limestone workers because these mines had vertical fissures which allowed water to percolate through their roofs, thus decreasing the dust exposure. He described the benefits of this process: "particles are laid as they are formed, by the continuous oozing, dropping and splashing of the insinuated water." This concept of continuously wetting mining areas is considered the "basis of the modern practice of infusing the working face in a mine with water."[9]

T.B. Peacock was the first to distinguish the differences between miners' phthisis and pulmonary tuberculosis.[10] Phthisis, a descriptive term coined by the Greeks, meaning "to waste away," was also called consumption. The clinical and pathological descriptions of autopsied stoneworkers by E.H. Greenhow[11] include deposits and drifts of sand in the lung tissue and its isolation for quantitative measurements. He was able to isolate about 30 gm of so-called sand from the lungs of one stone cutter. Greenhow is credited as the first to use polarized light microscopy to demonstrate silica particles in the lungs.[11]

In 1866, Friedrich von Zenker studied the pathology of lung disease caused by the inhalation of iron dust.[12] He described the disease as "iron lung: sclerosis pulmonum," and stated that iron dust was the "injurious agent which is the essential cause of the entire disease."[12] To group all the diseases of identical cause, he coined the term "pneumonokoniosis." This was derived from the term "konis," meaning dust. The term "silicosis," (Latin, silex, flint) was originally used by Visconti in Italy in 1870.[13]

Allison and Hugh Miller in 1869 observed that stone drillers appear to suffer more from the rapid onset of the disease silicosis than other miners.[14] From their studies it was evident that hard-stone work seriously affected the health of workers, while the soft-stone workers seem to have a less severe lung disease.

Silicosis was recognized as a distinct disease entity by the late 19th century in Europe. The introduction of the pneumatic hammer drill in 1897 by John Leyner generated large amounts of fine dust and contributed to an abnormal increase in the incidence and mortality of silicosis.[3,8] In the operation of the pneumatic hammer drill, air is blown through the drill to remove rock particles. This produced excessive amounts of dust, and once again the term "widow maker" was ascribed to a mining tool due to the short life span of the drillers. By 1898, water was commingled with air to suppress the dust in rock cutting using pneumatic drills.[8] Sandblasting was introduced in 1904 as a specialized method for the cleaning, polishing, and abrasion of surfaces.[8] This has resulted in countless numbers of silicosis cases.

In 1902, John Haldane reported that "primary injury of the lungs is solely caused by the inhalation of stone dust and that this injury also predisposes enormously to tuberculosis."[15] Silicosis, as an industrial hazard in sandstone workers of South Africa, was established by Haldane et al. in 1904.[15] In Witwatersrand, South Africa about one sixth of the rock drillers were found to have died from silicosis prior to the Boer War. In 1914, Haldane presented significant evidence on the dangerous effect of silica in the lungs before a Royal Commission, which greatly influenced the passing of the Workman's Compensation Act for silicosis in Great Britain.[16,17] After chest x-rays became increasingly popular in the medical diagnosis of lung diseases, Sutherland and Bryson found radiographic evidence of silicosis in 25% of the sandstone workers examined in 1929.[18] Sutherland et al., in a later study of granite workers, found x-ray changes consistent with silicosis in approximately 54% of the cases.[19]

IV. NORTH AMERICAN EXPERIENCE

Although several cases of silicosis were reported in North American literature during the 1800s,[20–22] awareness of the health importance of silica dust was apparently very minimal until the early 19th century. Case reports of silicosis were found occasionally in physicians' reports of lung diseases with suspected occupational involvement. The first case report on a stove foundry worker in Poughkeepsie, NY, was considered a true documentation of silicosis.[20] In 1887, another report on 34 cutlery factory workers described a chronic airway disease and stated that 23 workers died of silicosis.[21] Around 1900, another report appeared in Utah, which described 30 men dying after only 1 to 2 years of dust exposure from crushing quartz ore in a gold assaying mill in Nevada.[22]

Silicosis emerged as a major industrial scourge to the American workers with the industrial revolution and technological innovations. David Rosener and Gerald Markowitz described the awareness of this disease and its political, social, and economic impact in a book, *Deadly Dust, Silicosis and the Politics of Occupational Disease in Twentieth-century America*.[23] The introduction of power equipment in the mines, mills, factories, and other work places significantly increased a widespread hazard because of the generation of greater quantities of fine dust in confined spaces of worksites. This led to the re-emergence of silicosis as a major occupational threat in North America with the complicating companion disease, tuberculosis.[24]

Dust produced at work sites was well recognized as a problem for hard-rock miners, sandblasters, potters, foundry workers, and cutters. Nonetheless, silicosis was not considered a major health hazard in America until the U.S. Bureau of Mines and the U.S. Public Health Service, in the early 19th century, documented the widespread occurrence of silicosis in various worker groups.[25–28] The first major effort in this regard was undertaken from 1913 to 1915 in the lead and zinc mining industry of Joplin, MO, by these two agencies.[25] In a study of 720 miners, 46% were found to have silicosis, with another 14% exhibiting silicosis complicated by tuberculosis. In a report to the "Committee on Mortality from Tuberculosis in Dusty Trades," as quoted by Hosey et al.,[29] it is stated that 93% of the workers examined in the Vermont granite industry in 1920 were affected with silicosis. This was followed by the studies of 427 granite workers in Barre, VT, from 1924 to 1926 by local physicians and the U.S. Public Health Service. In these studies, all Vermont granite workers exposed to high concentrations of dust were found to have silicosis, tuberculosis, or silico-tuberculosis.[24,26] In 1928, Smith reported silicosis in 57% of the 208 workers employed in rock tunneling in New York.[27] There were several other studies conducted in metal grinding, cement processing, porcelain enameling, sandstone grinding, and abrasive grinding in which evidence of silicosis was documented as high as 67%, which provided incriminating evidence of a widespread silicosis hazard and the dire need for dust control.[30]

V. SIGNIFICANT EVENTS IN U.S. HISTORY OF SILICOSIS

In the 1930s, public health awareness grew and silicosis was well recognized as a serious health hazard in North America. This public health awareness and the economic depression precipitated a large number of lawsuits based on both legitimate and spurious claims. Sappington[31] estimated that approximately $100 million in damage suits were outstanding for settlement in 1933. This public awareness was further galvanized by the Gauley Bridge disaster in West Virginia, which initiated a congressional hearing in 1936. This incident, described in detail by Martin Cherniack in his book *The Hawk's Nest Incident,* was America's worst industrial disaster in silicosis. Within two years, 476 workers died of acute silicosis, while an additional 1500 suffered impairment from lung disease they contracted while digging a rock tunnel to divert water to a hydroelectric plant from 1932 to 1934.[32,33] This disaster provided an impetus for industrial health reform in the U.S. from 1936 to 1939, several states passed compensation laws and industrial hygiene dust control standards. In the Vermont granite industry, dust concentrations were regulated to 10 million particles per cubic foot of air sampled (mppcf) from a previous average dust level of 60 mppcf.[30]

Almost 25 years after the first report of silicosis in Joplin, MO, Alice Hamilton wrote "A Mid-American Tragedy," an article on lead and zinc mining.[34] A preliminary survey of industries in 1940 by the U.S. Public Health Service established a silica exposed population of 1.5 to 2 million.[35] Cummings, at the Fourth Saranac Laboratory Symposium on Silicosis, presented estimates of about 50,000 workers having definite silicosis.[36] Uncontrolled dust exposures and silicosis incidence continued to occur in isolated industries. The implementation of dust control measures was impaired since ventilation equipment was scarce due to World War II between 1941 and 1945. As a result, inadequate dust control measures were common in several North American industrial workplaces. For example, in Georgia it was revealed that the granite industry exceeded recommended limits for silica exposure many-fold.[37]

After World War II, widespread mechanization and technological advances for new uses of crystalline silica increased the possibility of several new dusty operations. So the mounting concern of silicosis as a continuing problem led to a second Congressional hearing on silicosis as an occupational hazard in 1956.[38]

In the U.S., during 1950 to 1956, approximately 2000 deaths were recorded due to occupational pneumoconioses.[39] About 60% of these deaths were attributed to silicosis and 28% to silicosis combined with tuberculosis.[39] In a 1958 study of Vermont granite industries, Trasko reported that silicosis was a continuing problem with a substantial increase in silicosis and anthracosilicosis in spite of appreciable declines in tuberculosis since 1949.[30] Although changes in the international coding of disease were partially responsible for this increase in deaths attributed to silicosis, the steady rate at which silicosis occurred was very evident. Follow-up studies of the Vermont granite industry by the Public Health Service and the Vermont Industrial Hygiene Division documented a high degree of success achieved in controlling dust levels and a low incidence of silicosis in workers. Hosey et al.[39] documented the prevalence of silicosis in a group of 1112 workers who began employment in the industry before 1937 and compared this to 1134 workers employed after dust control measures were instituted. The prevalence of silicosis, as determined by chest radiographic survey, had decreased to 15% from a pre-1937 prevalence of 45% in workers with comparable work histories. In 1964, Ashe and Bergstrom[40] re-evaluated chest x-rays of 1478 granite workers and confirmed earlier findings of Hosey et al.[39] showing a decline in the prevalence of silicosis. Data from these studies suggest that dust control measures implemented in 1937 had successfully reduced the exposure to granite dust and decreased the rate of silicosis in workers exposed to granite dust for up to 26 years.

VI. CURRENT STATUS OF SILICOSIS IN U.S.

In 1937, one of the first recommendations for upper limits of exposure to quartz-containing industrial dusts was made by Russell for the Vermont granite industry. Russell based his recommendation on the

TABLE 1
Significant Events in the History of Silicosis

Hippocrates	Described clinical Pneumoconiosis	400 B.C.
Pliny	Described "Fatal Dust"	70 A.D.
Agricola	Described lung disease	1556
Ramazzini	Described dust lung diseases and lesions	1700
Benson	Granted patent for wet grinding	1726
Knight	Described silicosis	1830
Greenhow	Demonstrated silica (polarized light) in lungs	1865
Visconti	Used the term silicosis	1885
Canedy	Case reports of silicosis in U.S.	1887
Leyner	Introduced the pneumatic drill	1897
Haldane	Worker's Compensation Act, U.K.	1918
West Virginia	Gauley Bridge Disaster	1934
U.S. Congress	Gauley Bridge Disaster Hearings	1936
Vermont	Granite Industry Set Dust Limits	1937
U.S. Congress	Mine Safety Hearings	1940
U.S. Congress	Mine Safety Hearings	1956
U.S. Congress	Occupational Safety and Health Act	1970
NIOSH	Recommended 50 $\mu g/m^3$	1974
IARC	Implication of silica as a carcinogen	1987

prevalence of silicosis reported earlier in different dusty exposure groups.[29] Understanding of the dose-response relationships has led to the formulation of exposure limits in occupational workplaces. From 1971 to the present, crystalline silica standards have been under continual re-evaluation, and decremental changes in permissible exposure limits at work sites were set by the Occupational Safety and Health Administration (OSHA). The current OSHA permissible exposure limit (PEL) for respirable crystalline silica is 100 $\mu g/m^3$ for an 8-hour work exposure. The National Institute for Occupational Safety and Health (NIOSH), charged with developing scientific information on the types and extent of exposures to occupational hazards, has recommended an exposure limit of 50 $\mu g/m^3$ for up to 10 h/d during a 40-hour work week.[41]

Despite the existence of remarkable engineering controls and protective devices, cases of silicosis continue to occur. In 1983 NIOSH estimated that approximately 3.2 million workers at 238,000 worksites were potentially exposed to crystalline silica and a significant number of workers in several industries had elevated rates of silicosis. The U.S. Department of Labor estimates that nearly 60,000 workers are at risk of developing some degree of silicosis. If these estimates are considered conservative and valid, the outlook for silicosis as a continuing threat is substantial and burdensome to health care management. NIOSH published several intelligence bulletins in recent years documenting the occurrence of acute silicosis in silica flour mills, sandblasting operations, surface coal mine drilling, and railway bed workers.[42–45] A 1992 NIOSH ALERT described 23 cases of silicosis from exposure to rock drilling.[46] In addition to this, the relationship between silica exposure, silicosis, and the development of lung cancer has received increased attention in recent years.[47,48]

In conclusion, silicosis as an occupational disease has long been recognized (Table 1). In spite of major advances in our understanding of its etiology and the importance of dust control, major pockets of overexposure and disease still exist.

REFERENCES

1. **Collis, E. L.,** Industrial pneumoconiosis with special reference to dust phthisis, *Public Health,* London, 28, 252–292, 1915.
2. **Ruffer,** 1921, Cited by George Rosen in *The History of Miner's Diseases. A Medical and Social Interpretation,* Schuman's Press, New York, 1943, 7.
3. **Zaidi, S. H.,** *Experimental Pneumoconiosis,* The Johns Hopkins Press, Baltimore, 1969, 11–25.
4. **Rosen, G.,** *The History of Miner's Diseases. A Medical and Social Interpretation,* Schuman's Press, New York, 1943.

5. **Agricola, G.,** *De Re Metallica,* Translation by Hoover, H.C. and Hoover, L., New York, 1950, 214.
6. **Van Diemerbroeck, I.,** Anatomie corporis humani, *Utrecht,* 2, 13, 1672, Cited by Hunter, D., 1984.
7. **Ramazzini, B.,** *Diseases of Worker,* Hefner Publishing, New York, 1964, 250.
8. **Hunter, D.,** *The Diseases of Occupations,* 5th ed., The English Universities Press, 1984, 915–1020.
9. **Thackrah, C. T.,** *The Effects of Arts, Trades and Professions on Health and Longevity,* 2nd ed., Longmans, U.K., 1832.
10. **Peacock, T. B.,** Millstone makers phthisis, siliceous matter found in lungs, *Trans. Path. Soc.,* London, 12, 36, 1861.
11. **Greenhow, E. H.,** *Trans. Path. Soc.,* London, 16, 59, 1865.
12. **Zenker, F. A.,** *Dtsch. Arch. Klin. Med.,* 116, 2, 1866.
13. **Visconti,** 1870, Cited by Rovinda, C.L. in Un case di silicosi del pulmone con analist chemica, *Ann. Chim.,* 1871.
14. **Allison and Miller, H.,** *My Schools and School Masters,* Edinburgh, 1869.
15. **Haldane, J. S., Martin, J. S., and Thomas, R. A.,** Report on the Health of Cornish Miners, Cmd. 2091, Her Majesty's Stationary Office, London, 1904.
16. **Haldane, J. S.,** *Seventh Rep. Explos. in Mines Comm.,* London, 1914a.
17. **Haldane, J. S.,** *Second Rep. of the Roy Comm. in Metal Mines and Quarries,* London, 1914b.
18. **Sutherland, C. L. and Bryson, S.,** Report on recurrence of silicosis among sandstone workers, Her Majesty's Stationary Office, London, 1929.
19. **Sutherland, C. L., Bryson, S., and Keating, N.,** Report on the occurrence of silicosis among granite workers, Her Majesty's Stationary Office, London, 1930.
20. **Peterson, F.,** Anthracosis pulmonum, *Med. Rec.,* 32, 113, 1887.
21. **Canedy, F. J.,** Grinder's consumption, *Med. Surg. J.,* 117, 198–200, 1887.
22. **Betts, W. W.,** Chalicosis pulmonum or chronic interstitial pneumonia induced by stone dust, *JAMA,* 34, 70–74, 1900.
23. **Rosener, D. and Markowitz, G.,** *Deadly Dust: Silicosis and the Politics of Occupational Disease in Twentieth-Century America,* Princeton University Press, NJ, 1991.
24. **Hoffman, F. L.,** Silicosis and allied disorders. History and industrial importance, *Med. Serv. Bull. No. 1,* Pittsburgh, Air Hygiene Foundation of America, pp 45–49, 68–69, 1937.
25. **Lanza, A. J. and Childs, S. B.,** 1. Miners' consumption: a study of 433 cases of the disease among zinc miners in southwestern Missouri. II. Roentgen-ray findings in miners' consumption, *Public Health Bull. No. 85,* U.S. Government Printing Office, Washington, D.C., 1917.
26. **Russell, A. E., Britton, R. H., Thompson, L. R., and Bloomfield, J. J.,** The health of workers in dusty trades. II. Exposures to silicosis dust (granite industry), *Public Health Bull. No. 187,* U.S. Government Printing Office, Washington, D.C., 1929.
27. **Smith, A. R.,** Silicosis among rock-drillers, blasters and excavators in New York City, *J. Ind. Hyg.,* 11, 37, 1929.
28. House Committee on Labor Sub-committee: An investigation relating to health conditions of workers employed in the construction and maintenance of public utilities, HJ Res. 449, 74th Congress, 2603, 1936.
29. **Hosey, A. D., Trasco, V. M., and Ashe, H. B.,** Silicosis in Vermont granite industry-A progress report, *Public Health Serv. Publ. No. 557,* U.S. Government Printing Office, Washington, D.C., 1957.
30. **Trasko, V. M.,** Silicosis, a continuing problem, *Public Health Rep.,* 73, 839, 1958.
31. **Sappington, C. O.,** Discussion: The role of the x-ray in industrial hygiene, Ed., P.G. Dick, *Ind. Med.,* 4, 160–161, 1935.
32. **Cherniack, M.,** *The Hawk's Nest Incident,* Yale University Press, New Haven, 1986.
33. Hearings and Report on Mine Safety (metallic and non-metallic mines), 84th Congress, 1940.
34. **Hamilton, A.,** A mid-American tragedy, *Survey Graphic,* 29, 434, 1940.
35. **Bloomfield, J. J.,** A preliminary survey of the industrial hygiene problem in the United States, *Public Health Bull. No. 259,* U.S. Government Printing Office, Washington, D.C., 1940.
36. **Cummings,** *Fourth Saranac Laboratory Symposium on Silicosis,* Ed., B.E. Kuechle, Wisconsin Employers Mutual Liability Insurance Company, Wausau, 316–319, 1939.
37. **Petrie, L. M.,** Silicosis control in Georgia granite industries, Division of Industrial Hygiene, Georgia Department of Health, Atlanta, 1948.
38. Hearings and Report on Mine Safety (metallic and non-metallic mines), 84th Congress, 1956.
39. **Hosey, A. D., Trasko, V. M., and Ashe, H. B.,** Silicosis in Vermont granite industry. A progress report, Public Health Service, Pub. No. 557, U.S. Government Printing Office, Washington, D.C., 1957.
40. **Ashe, H. B. and Bergstrom, D. E.,** Twenty six years' experience with dust control in the Vermont granite industry, *Ind. Med. Surg.,* 33, 973–78, 1964.
41. National Institute for Occupational Safety and Health, Criteria for a recommended standard: Occupational exposure to crystalline silica, U.S. Department of Health, Education, and Welfare, Public Health Service, Centers for Disease Control, DHEW Publication No. (NIOSH) 75–120, pp 54–55, 60–61, 1974.
42. **Banks, D. E., Bauer, M. A., Castellan, R. M., and Lapp, N. L.,** Silicosis in surface coalmine drillers, *Thorax,* 38, 275–278, 1983.

43. **Goodman, G. B., Kaplan, P. D., Stachura, I., Castranova, V., Pailes, W. H., and Lapp, N. L.,** Acute silicosis responding to corticosteroid therapy, *Chest,* 101, 366–370, 1992.
44. **Parker, J. E., Lapp, N. L., Banks, D. E.,** Surface coal mine drillers and silicosis: the ten year West Virginia experience, *Am. Rev. Respir. Dis.,* 139, A490, 1989.
45. **Maksimovic, S. D. and Page, S. J.,** Quartz dust sources during overburden drilling at surface coal mines, *Ann. Am. Conf. Gov. Ind. Hyg.,* 14, 361–366, 1986.
46. U.S. Department of Health and Human Services, National Institute for Occupational Safety and Health, Health Hazard Evaluation Report, HETA 82–302–1461, 1992.
47. International Agency for Research on Cancer Monograph on the Evaluation of the Carcinogenic Risk of Chemicals to Humans. Vol. 42, Silica and Some Silicates, 42, Lyon, France, World Health Organization, IARC, pp 49, 51, 73–111, 1987.
48. **Hnizdo, E. and Slouis-Cremer, G. K.,** Silica exposure, silicosis and lung cancer: a mortality study of South African gold miners, *Br. J. Ind. Med.,* 48, 53–60, 1991.

Section I
Chapter 3

GUIDELINES AND LIMITS FOR OCCUPATIONAL EXPOSURE TO CRYSTALLINE SILICA

Frank J. Hearl

CONTENTS

I. INTRODUCTION

Crystalline silica has long been recognized as a significant health hazard for workers engaged in mining, sandblasting, construction, and other occupations where significant dust exposures occur. The historical development of dust samplers and control of dust levels in the occupational environment was motivated by the recognition that exposure to dust containing crystalline silica (with three crystalline polymorphs: α-quartz, cristobalite, and tridymite) produced disabling lung diseases including silicosis (chronic, acute, and accelerated), silico-tuberculosis, and possibly lung cancer.[1] Consequently, the evolution of occupational dust exposure limits and the industrial hygiene sampling techniques designed to measure compliance with those limits concentrated on the control of silica. A variety of devices have been used over the years to quantify workers' exposure to airborne dust levels including impingers with particle-counting analysis and filters coupled with cyclone preseparators followed with gravimetric mass analysis.[2–4] The following sections will describe the evolution of dust sampling techniques and the work place exposure limits that have been applied to control occupational dust exposures, particularly when the dust contained crystalline silica.

II. DEVELOPMENT OF EXPOSURE GUIDELINES

The Greenburg-Smith impinger, developed in 1925 by the U.S. Bureau of Mines, the American Society of Heating and Ventilating Engineers, and the U.S. Public Health Service, was used for more than 30 years as the dust sampling method of choice in U.S. mines and factories. A modified, smaller version of the impinger, known as the "midget impinger," was also used for measuring the particle-count concentration of dust.[5] The midget impinger was designed to be equivalent to the Greenburg-Smith impinger, except that it was more convenient for field use.[6]

Dust particles collected in the impinger solution were counted using a counting cell technique adapted from a method used to count plankton in water.[7] The impinger sampler effectively collected dust particles that had an aerodynamic diameter larger than 0.75 µm. The particles were collected by accelerating a

0-8493-4709-2/96/$0.00+$.50

dust-laden air stream through a nozzle at sonic velocity into a solution of water, ethanol, or mixtures of both.[8,9] Concentrations reported from impinger samples were usually stated in million particles per cubic foot of air sampled (mppcf). Rules for counting were not universally standardized. Many industrial hygienists rejected counts of particles with observed diameters larger than 10 μm since these were "not respirable."[4] Consequently, impinger count data were perceived to be highly inaccurate and subject to training and experience bias among counters.[7] The American Conference of Governmental Industrial Hygienists (ACGIH) recognized that the health risk of exposure to dust was directly related to the total dust concentration and to the concentration of crystalline silica (also known as quartz or "free silica") in the dust. In 1962, after reviewing available data on dust exposed populations, the ACGIH adopted a Threshold Limit Value (TLV) for dust containing crystalline silica.[10] The TLVs adopted by the ACGIH are not legally enforceable standards. The ACGIH was careful to point out that TLVs were intended for use by practicing industrial hygienists as *guidelines.* The TLVs were *not developed for use as legal standards*[11] [emphasis added]. The adopted respirable dust TLV was stated in the form of a formula such that the airborne dust TLV would be reduced with increasing concentration of crystalline silica:

$$\text{TLV} = \frac{250}{\%\text{quartz} + 5}\,\text{mppcf} \tag{1}$$

To apply this exposure limit, the concentration of crystalline silica (%quartz) was found through chemical analysis of bulk airborne or settled dust samples.[12–14] The TLV for that work site was then calculated using the formula above. The total dust level would be measured using the impinger sampler, and the result obtained would be compared to the calculated TLV. For example, if the %quartz was analyzed at 20%, the TLV would be calculated from Equation 1 to be 10 mppcf. Any dust sample for which the measured concentration was more than 10 mppcf would exceed the prevailing TLV. When cristobalite or tridymite is present, the ACGIH recommends using one-half the value calculated from the count formula for α-quartz. In 1970, to make the TLV consistent with a nuisance dust limit of 30 mppcf, the formula was revised to:

$$\text{TLV} = \frac{300}{\%\text{quartz} + 10}\,\text{mppcf} \tag{2}$$

For both formulas, the prescribed measurement method was the impinger coupled with particle count analysis.[10]

Based on a growing body of literature in the U.S.[15] and the findings of the Johannesburg Pneumoconiosis Conference,[16] the ACGIH proposed a respirable dust TLV based on size-selective gravimetric sampling in 1968. Using findings from the U.S. Public Health Service, a gravimetric respirable crystalline silica TLV of 0.1 mg/m^3 was believed to provide equivalent protection to the existing 10 mppcf total dust concentrations applied to the Vermont Granite sheds, where the crystalline silica concentration had been measured at 25%.[17] Besides the crystalline silica TLV, the ACGIH decided to limit size-selected respirable dust to 5 mg/m^3. The ACGIH reasoned that the respirable dust TLV would limit the total dust concentration to 15 mg/m^3, based on an assumption that the respirable dust was approximately one-third of the total dust concentration. Using these limits for crystalline silica and respirable dust, the ACGIH proposed and adopted a respirable mass TLV formula analogous to the existing particle count formula (Equation 2) for control of respirable dust:

$$\text{TLV} = \frac{10}{\%\text{quartz} + 2}\,\text{mg}/\text{m}^3 \tag{3}$$

As with the particle count formula, the ACGIH recommended that the crystalline silica polymorphs, cristobalite and tridymite be limited to one-half of the value computed for the TLV for α-quartz. The %quartz value used in the formula was to be found from airborne samples except where it was decided that other methods were acceptable.[7]

In 1986, the ACGIH adopted a revised silica TLV that required the direct measurement of respirable crystalline silica with a TLV of 0.1 mg/m^3 for α-quartz and 0.05 mg/m^3 for cristobalite and tridymite. They also eliminated the "nuisance dust" TLV of 5 mg/m^3 respirable dust, replacing that with a "particles not otherwise classified" (PNOC) limit of 10 mg/m^3 taken as total dust.[10,11] There is no guidance currently provided by the ACGIH to apply the additive-mixture formula to silica and other pneumoconiosis-producing dusts. Recent studies by Morrow and co-workers have shown that overloading the lungs with an insoluble dust produced a retardation of clearance mechanisms, leading to impairment of normal lung function.[18] These data may provide justification for application of the additive-mixture formula when considering combined exposures of silica and other respirable dusts.

A recommended exposure limit (REL) was published by the National Institute for Occupational Safety and Health (NIOSH) covering crystalline silica. In 1976, NIOSH recommended that exposure to crystalline silica, including its polymorphs α-quartz, cristobalite, and tridymite, be limited to a combined 0.05 mg/m³ as a time-weighted average during a 40-hour work week.[19] This REL was intended to prevent silicosis; however, NIOSH is presently evaluating the findings which led the International Agency for Research on Cancer (IARC) to determine that crystalline silica is a potential human carcinogen.[20] Their assessment was based on findings of sufficient evidence for the carcinogenicity of crystalline silica in experimental animals and limited evidence for the carcinogenicity of crystalline silica to humans.[21]

III. DERIVATION OF THE SILICA TLV FORMULA

The intent of the ACGIH TLV committee was to control crystalline silica below 0.1 mg/m³, while maintaining concentrations of respirable dust below 5.0 mg/m³. However, the approach they selected to accomplish this also embodied the additive-mixture formula. In practice, the additive-mixture formula is infrequently applied by industrial hygienists. The additive-mixture formula, prescribed for mixtures which affect the same organ system with similar pathology is defined by Equation 4:

$$\frac{C_1}{TLV_1} + \frac{C_2}{TLV_2} + \ldots + \frac{C_i}{TLV_i} = 1 \quad \textbf{(4)}$$

where C_i is the concentration of species *i*, and TLV_i is the TLV for species *i*.[11] When the sum of the terms exceeds unity, then the TLV of the mixture is exceeded.

Let C_Q be the airborne concentration of crystalline silica in mg/m³, with a TLV of 0.1 mg/m³; and let C_D be the airborne concentration of respirable dust in mg/m³, with a TLV of 5.0 mg/m³. The additive-mixture formula, combined with the proposed limits for crystalline silica and respirable dust, describes the relationship between C_Q and C_D at their mixture TLV as:

$$\left(\frac{C_Q}{0.1}\right) + \left(\frac{C_D}{5.0}\right) = 1 \quad \textbf{(5)}$$

The defining equation for percent crystalline silica is:

$$\%\text{quartz} = \left(\frac{C_Q}{C_D}\right) \times 100 \quad \textbf{(6)}$$

Multiplying Equation 5 by $(10/C_D)$ gives:

$$\left\{\left(\frac{C_Q}{C_D}\right) \times 100\right\} + 2 = \left(\frac{10}{C_D}\right) \quad \textbf{(7)}$$

Substituting %quartz from Equation 6 into the term in braces in Equation 7 and rearranging gives:

$$C_D = \frac{10}{\%\text{quartz} + 2} \text{mg/m}^3 \quad \textbf{(8)}$$

Therefore, the respirable mass TLV adopted by the ACGIH in 1970 incorporated a crystalline silica TLV of 0.1 mg/m³ and a respirable dust TLV of 5.0 mg/m³, consistent with the use of the additive-mixture formula. The previously recommended particle-count formula used by the ACGIH, being of the same mathematical formulation, also embodied the mixture formula based on a silica TLV of 2.5 mppcf and a total dust TLV of 50 mppcf. The mixture formula provided for further reduction of the computed TLV when more toxic silicates, such as mica, soapstone, and talc, which had TLVs of 20 mppcf, were present.[22]

IV. THE DEFINITION OF RESPIRABLE DUST

Critical to the evaluation of silica exposures is the definition of respirable dust and the means of measuring respirable dust concentrations. The definition of respirable dust has been the focus of many symposia, journal articles, and technical committee deliberations. In 1968, the ACGIH established the first size-selective TLV for pneumoconiosis producing dusts. They proposed a specific definition for respirable dust after considering information on pulmonary deposition in humans. The definition specified several points on the collection efficiency curve, which gives the fraction of particles that pass through a size-selective preseparator and are collected on a filter for gravimetric analysis.[23] These defining points are presented in Table 1. In their most current edition, the ACGIH has proposed an intended change to the respirable dust definition by increasing the 50% collection efficiency point from 3.5 to 4 μm, harmonizing this definition with the definition adopted by the international community.[11]

Another approach to the definition of respirable dust was to define respirable dust as dust that is collected by a particular instrument. In the U.S., that instrument has been the 10-mm nylon cyclone. Since the 10-mm nylon cyclone's collection efficiency curve shifts with changes in the operating flow rate, there has been controversy about whether the flow rate should be 1.4 L/min, 1.7 L/min, or 2.0 L/min.[24–29] After examining the flow rate bias curves, which measure the difference between the ACGIH respirable dust collection efficiency curve and the sampler's observed performance, the ACGIH decided that 1.7 L/min should be used for sampling respirable dust. Although NIOSH has not adopted a particular definition of respirable dust, the NIOSH Manual of Analytical Methods, in Method 0600 ("Nuisance Dust, Respirable"), recommended using the 10-mm nylon cyclone at a sampling flow rate of 1.7 L/min.[30]

When respirable dust and silica are sampled in coal mines, the 10-mm nylon cyclone is prescribed with a sampling flow rate of 2.0 L/min and a 1.38 multiplication factor applied to the resulting concentrations. This factor converts the cyclone-measured dust concentration to an equivalent measurement that would have been made with a Medical Research Establishment (MRE) horizontal elutriator.[28] The 38% positive correction applied to the cyclone-collected respirable dust provides adjustment for dust in the size range from 3.5 to 7 μm, where the MRE instrument has a higher collection efficiency than the cyclone. The relation of the coal mine dust standard to the MRE instrument was necessary because the U.S. respirable coal mine dust standard was originally based on British epidemiological data, where the dust concentrations were measured using the MRE instrument. The collection efficiency of a 10-mm nylon cyclone shifts when operated at 2.0 L/min. It collects fewer large particles compared to operation at 1.7 L/min. Since the size-selection differs, and since the 1.38 correction factor is applied to the measured concentrations, silica sampling data from coal mine dust compliance sampling programs cannot be directly compared to results obtained in other industries or for non-coal mines where the 1.7 L/min sampling flow rate is routinely used.

V. FEDERAL REGULATION OF OCCUPATIONAL EXPOSURE TO CRYSTALLINE SILICA

The standards which regulate exposure to crystalline silica in the U.S. are dependent upon the industry classification of the site being evaluated. The separate development and evolution of labor laws regulating

TABLE 1
ACGIH Definition of Respirable Dust

Aerodynamic Diameter (Unit Density Sphere), μm	Percent Passing Selector
≤2	90%
2.5	75%
3.5	50%
5.0	25%
10.	0%

safety and health in general industry, construction, agriculture, maritime industries, and mining produced a confusing web of rules relevant to silica permissible exposure limits. The particular rules that were adopted generally evolved from the recommended ACGIH TLV discussed above.

The present Federal regulation concerning occupational exposure to silica in general industry is derived from the Walsh-Healy Public Contracts Act of 1936. The Walsh-Healy Act required employers with government contracts exceeding $10,000, to comply with prescribed health and safety standards.[31] Under this act, the 1968 ACGIH TLVs were incorporated by regulation (41 CFR 50.204).[19] The provisions of Section 6(a) of the Occupational Safety and Health Act of 1970, allowed the U.S. Department of Labor to "...by rule promulgate as an occupational safety and health standard... any established Federal standard...." Using this authority, and recognizing the Walsh-Healy regulations as "established Federal standards," the Occupational Safety and Health Administration (OSHA) adopted the 1968 TLVs as exposure limits for general industry in the U.S.[32] In 1968, the ACGIH TLV for silica was described by the formulas previously presented in Equations 1 and 3 and was adopted as a respirable dust permissible exposure limit (PEL) as:

$$PEL = \frac{250}{\%quartz + 5} mppcf$$

or

$$PEL = \frac{10}{\%quartz + 2} mg/m^3 \quad \textbf{(9)}$$

For the "respirable dust" PELs described above, the particle count formula describes a measurement made with an impinger sample for total dust. The formula based on particle mass describes a PEL based on sampling with a particle size selector having collection characteristics described in Table 1. In addition to these respirable dust limits, OSHA also adopted a total dust PEL based on mass sampling using the formula:

$$PEL = \frac{30}{\%quartz + 2} mg/m^3 \quad \textbf{(10)}$$

Modern chemical techniques, including x-ray diffraction and infrared analysis, are currently used to measure the silica concentration in the sampled dust.[33]

In 1989, the OSHA PEL for crystalline silica in non-mining industrial work places was changed to a PEL of 0.1 mg/m^3 for α-quartz and 0.05 mg/m^3 for cristobalite and tridymite measured directly as respirable dust.[34] However, in July 1992, the U.S. Court of Appeals for the Eleventh Circuit vacated the new OSHA rules on administrative procedural grounds. Consequently, OSHA has instructed its field offices to enforce the exposure limits which existed prior to promulgating the 1989 rule.[35]

The current OSHA limit for construction and maritime industries is a total dust limit expressed in mppcf based on the formula:[36]

$$PEL = \frac{250}{\%quartz + 5} mppcf \quad \textbf{(11)}$$

In these industries the particle mass formula, based on cyclone-collected respirable dust, does not apply. There are no current silica limits for agriculture.

Federal regulations providing for health and safety in mining were authorized by the Metal and Non-metallic Mine Safety Act of 1966, the Federal Coal Mine Health and Safety Act of 1969, and the Federal Mine Safety and Health Act of 1977. The mining industry was subdivided by these regulations into several categories: coal mining, metal and non-metal mining; and then subclassified further as surface or underground mining. Each segment has prescribed separate rules for regulating exposure to respirable dust and silica.

In coal mines, both surface and underground, when crystalline silica is present at a concentration greater than 5%, the 2.0 mg/m^3 respirable dust standard (RDS) is reduced according to the formula:[37,38]

$$RDS = \frac{10}{\%quartz} mg/m^3 \quad (12)$$

The enforcement procedure is to collect as few as one respirable crystalline silica sample on a working section to find the %quartz that will apply for that location. If the %quartz is greater than 5%, then the section must maintain an RDS below that computed using Equation 12. Note that the RDS samples are collected using a 10-mm nylon cyclone operating at 2.0 L/min, and the collected mass is multiplied by a 1.38 MRE correction factor as discussed in the preceding sections. These coal mine regulations do not include cristobalite and tridymite in the regulatory system.

For surface metal and non-metal mines, the Mine Safety and Health Administration (MSHA) adopted, by regulation, the air quality standards outlined in the ACGIH TLVs for 1973.[39] Underground metal and non-metal mines also adopted, by incorporation into regulation, the 1973 ACGIH TLVs.[40] These regulations included the 1970 particle count TLV change previously described, such that the regulations prescribe a total dust PEL for α-quartz in terms of mppcf and a respirable mass PEL in terms of mg/m^3 according to the following formulas:

$$PEL = \frac{300}{\%quartz + 10} mppcf$$

or

$$PEL = \frac{10}{\%quartz + 2} mg/m^3 \quad (13)$$

In addition, a total mass PEL was incorporated from the 1973 ACGIH TLVs according to the formula:

$$PEL = \frac{30}{\%quartz + 3} mg/m^3 \quad (14)$$

The 1973 ACGIH TLVs also prescribe that where cristobalite or tridymite are present the limit should be reduced to one-half the value obtained from the count or mass formula for α-quartz. By incorporation, this aspect of the silica TLV is also a part of the PEL computation.[41]

VI. SUMMARY

The control of occupational exposure to crystalline silica in the form of α-quartz, cristobalite, and tridymite has been the focus of attention for occupational health professionals over the past 75 years. Progress in measurement methodology along with improved understanding of the disease process and dose-response relationships lead to an evolving set of exposure limit guidelines. Coincident with these evolving limits was the sequential enactment of landmark occupational safety and health legislation covering mining, general industry, construction, agriculture, and maritime industries. As each law was enacted, a set of prevailing exposure limits was adopted, including limits for the various forms of crystalline silica in combination with other airborne dusts. These occurrences have left a complex weave of regulations relating to crystalline silica.

The current recommendations from NIOSH are to control exposures to all forms of crystalline silica below concentrations of 0.05 mg/m^3, while NIOSH is reviewing the data on carcinogenicity. The ACGIH recommends a TLV for α-quartz of 0.1 mg/m^3, and a TLV of 0.05 mg/m^3 for cristobalite and tridymite. Both recommendations prescribe respirable mass sampling rather than using impinger count methods. The 1989 proposed rules from the Department of Labor represented an attempt to consolidate U.S. federal regulations controlling silica at levels described by the present ACGIH TLVs. This attempt was rescinded by the courts on administrative procedural grounds. However, the technical basis for unifying these exposure limits to a fixed respirable crystalline silica PEL was fundamentally sound.

REFERENCES

1. **Peters, J. M.,** Silicosis, in *Occupational Respiratory Diseases*, Eds., Merchant, J.A., Boehlecke, B.A., Taylor, G., Pickett-Harner, M., DHHS(NIOSH) Publication No. 86–102, (1986).
2. **Glenn, R. E. and Kraft, B.,** Air Sampling for Particulates, in *Merchant, J.A., Boehlecke, B.A., Taylor, G., and Pickett-Harner, M., Occupational Respiratory Diseases*, DHHS (NIOSH) Publication No. 86–102, Superintendent of Documents, Washington D.C., 69–82, 1986.
3. **Lioy, P. J., Lippmann, M., and Phalen, R. F.,** Rationale for particle size-selective air sampling, *Annu. Am. Conf. Ind. Hyg.*, 11, 27–34, 1984.
4. **Lippmann, M.,** Size-Selective Health Hazard Sampling, in *Lioy, P.J., and Lioy, M.J.Y., Air Sampling Instruments*, 6th ed., ACGIH, Cincinnati, H1–H22, 1983.
5. **Mercer, T. T.,** *Aerosol Technology in Hazard Evaluation*, Academic Press, New York, 1973, 151–154.
6. **Drinker, P. and Hatch T.,** *Industrial Dust*, 2nd ed., McGraw-Hill, New York, 1954, 147–155.
7. **Ayer, H. E.,** The proposed ACGIH mass limits for quartz: review and evaluation, *Am. Ind. Hyg. Assoc. J.*, 30, 117–125, 1969.
8. **Hall, F. E., Kupel, R. E., and Harris, R. L.,** Particle settling times in ethyl alcohol-water mixtures as affected by variables in impinger sampling, *Am. Ind. Hyg. Assoc. J.*, 26, 537–543, 1965.
9. **Jacobson, M., Terry, S. L., and Ambrosia, D. A.,** Evaluation of some parameters affecting the collection and analysis of midget impinger samples, *Am. Ind. Hyg. Assoc. J.*, 31, 442–445, 1970.
10. American Conference of Governmental Industrial Hygienists, Documentation of the Threshold Limit Values and Biological Exposure Indices, Fifth ed., ACGIH, Cincinnati, 523–525, 1986.
11. American Conference of Governmental Industrial Hygienists 1992–1993, Threshold Limit Values for Chemical Substances and Physical Agents and Biological Exposure Indices, ACGIH, Cincinnati, pp. 29, 32–33, 41–44, 50–51, 1992.
12. **Talvitie, N. A.,** Determination of quartz in presence of silicates using phosphoric acid, *Anal. Chem.*, 23(4), 623–626, 1951.
13. **Talvitie, N. A. and Hyslop, F.,** Colorimetric determination of siliceous atmospheric contaminants, *Ind. Hyg. J.*, 19, 54–58, 1958.
14. **Talvitie, N. A.,** Determination of free silica: gravimetric and spectrophotometric procedures applicable to air-borne and settled dust, *Am. Ind. Hyg. Assoc. J.*, 25, 169–178, 1964.
15. **Morrow, P. E.,** Evaluation of inhalation hazards based upon the respirable dust concept and the philosophy and application of selective sampling, *Am. Ind. Hyg. Assoc. J.*, 25, 213–236, 1964.
16. **Orenstein, A. J.,** Proceedings of the Pneumoconiosis Conference, Johannesburg, 1959, Little, Brown & Co., Boston, 1960.
17. **Ayer, H. E., Sutton, G. W., and Davis, I. H.,** Size-selective gravimetric sampling in dusty industries, *Am. Ind. Hyg. Assoc. J.*, 29, 336–341, 1968.
18. **Morrow, P. E., Muhle, H., and Mermelstein, R.,** Chronic inhalation study findings as a basis for proposing a new occupational dust exposure limit, *J. Am. Coll. Tox.*, 10(2), 297–289, 1991.
19. National Institute for Occupational Safety and Health, Criteria for a Recommended Standard...Occupational Exposure to Crystalline Silica. DHEW(NIOSH) Publication No. 75–120, 1974.
20. National Institute for Occupational Safety and Health, Testimony of the National Institute for Occupational Safety and Health on the Occupational Safety and Health Administrations Notice of Proposed Rule on Air Contaminants, 29 CFR Part 1910, Docket No. H-020, Washington, D.C., August 1, 1988.
21. International Agency for Research on Cancer, IARC Monographs on the Evaluation of the Carcinogenic Risk of Chemicals to Humans — Silica and Some Silicates. Vol. 42, 39–143, Lyon, France, 1987.
22. American Conference of Governmental Industrial Hygienists, Threshold Limit Values of Air-borne Contaminants for 1968. (sic) ACGIH, Cincinnati, 1968.
23. Aerosol Technology Committee, Guide for respirable mass sampling, *Am. Ind. Hyg. Assoc. J.*, 31, 133–137, 1970.
24. **Bartley, D. L. and Breuer, G. M.,** Analysis and optimization of the performance of the 10-mm cyclone, *Am. Ind. Hyg. Assoc. J.*, 43, 520–528, 1982.
25. **Caplan, K. J., Doemeny, L. J., and Sorenson, S. D.,** Performance characteristics of the 10-mm cyclone respirable mass sampler: part I — monodisperse studies, *Am. Ind. Hyg. Assoc. J.*, 38, 83–95, 1977.
26. **Ettinger, H. J., Partridge, J. E., and Royer, G. W.,** Calibration of two-stage air samplers, *Am. Ind. Hyg. Assoc. J.*, 31, 537–545, 1970.
27. **Knuth, R. H.,** Recalibration of size-selective samplers, *Am. Ind. Hyg. Assoc. J.*, 30, 379–385, 1969.
28. **Tomb, T. F. and Raymond, L. D.,** Evaluation of the Penetration Characteristics of a Horizontal Plate Elutriator and of a 10-mm Nylon Cyclone Elutriator, U.S. Bureau of Mines Report of Investigations No. USBM-RI-7367, 1970.
29. **Tomb, T. F. and Treaftis, H. N.,** Review of Published Experimental Calibrations Performed on the 10 Millimeter Nylon Cyclone, Mining Enforcement and Safety Administration, Informational Report 1040, 1976.

30. National Institute for Occupational Safety and Health, Manual of Analytical Methods, Third ed., Method 0600-Nuisance Dust, Respirable, Revised February 15, 1984. DHHS(NIOSH) Publication No. 84–100, 1984.
31. **Ashford, N.,** *Crisis in the Workplace: Occupational Disease and Injury,* MIT Press, Cambridge, 1976, 51–52.
32. Code of Federal Regulations, *Labor,* Title 29: Part 1000, 1989.
33. National Institute for Occupational Safety and Health/Bureau of Mines, Collaborative Tests of Two Methods for Determining Free Silica in Airborne Dust, DHHS (NIOSH) Publication No. 83–124, 1983.
34. Department of Labor, 29 CFR Part 1910 – Air Contaminants; Final Rule, Federal Register, v. 54, no. 12, 2521–2523, January 19, 1989.
35. Occupational Safety and Health Reporter, OSHA Instructs Field Offices to Enforce Exposure Limits in Effect Before 1989 Rule, Bureau of National Affairs, Inc., Washington, D.C., 1754, March 24, 1993.
36. Department of Labor, 29 CFR Part 1910, et al. Air Contaminants; Proposed Rule, *Fed. Regist.,* v. 57, no. 114, book 2, 26214–26216, June 12, 1992.
37. Code of Federal Regulations, Mineral Resources, Title 30: Parts 70, 1992.
38. Code of Federal Regulations, Mineral Resources, Title 30: Parts 71, 1992.
39. Code of Federal Regulations, Mineral Resources, Title 30: Parts 56, 1992.
40. Code of Federal Regulations, Mineral Resources, Title 30: Parts 57, 1992.
41. American Conference of Governmental Industrial Hygenists, TLVs Threshold Limit Values for Chemical Substances in Workroom Air Adopted by ACGIH for 1973. ACGIH, Cincinnati, 1973.

Section I
Chapter 4

CLINICAL FEATURES OF SILICOSIS

Daniel E. Banks

CONTENTS

I. INTRODUCTION

Silicosis was first reported by the ancient Greeks and is as old as the history of man. The prevalence of this illness apparently peaked in the last half of the 19th century and the early part of this century. The aggressive industrialization of America, the development of powered tools which generated massive amounts of respirable size dust particles, the failure to recognize a latency period between exposure and development of disease, an inadequate (or perhaps careless) understanding of the relationship between dust exposure and disease, and respiratory protection proven to be inadequate has resulted in a series of epidemics of silicosis which have caused the premature death of many workers.[1–11]

Since the recognition of the dose-relatedness of this disease and the initiation of and compliance with effective dust control measures, the prevalence of silicosis has decreased dramatically.[12–14] The current U.S. Occupational Safety and Health Administration permissible exposure limit (PEL) for respirable free silica is 100 $\mu g/m^3$.[15] In some mines and quarries, compliance with this level has been achieved by instituting wetting techniques and improving ventilation; yet, in industries such as sandblasting, silica mining, and rock drilling, workers remain potentially exposed to many times the acceptable limit of respirable free silica (Table 1). In the U.S., particles much less toxic than silica are available for blasting, and since 1974, the National Institute for Occupational Safety and Health (NIOSH) has recommended substitution of non-silica containing particles in abrasive blasting.[16,17] Where silica sand is used in blasting, epidemics of very aggressive silicosis have recurred, even in developed countries where safe exposure limits are defined and respiratory protection is available[18] (Figure 1).

0-8493-4709-2/96/$0.00+$.50

TABLE 1
Major Industries with Silica Exposure

Occupation	Exposure
Mining	Silica contaminants in mined material.
Milling	Dry, finely ground silica (silica flour) is used for abrasives and filler.
Quarrying and stone work	Slate, granite, and sandstone exposures.
Foundry work	Silica is used as a mold; fettling and chipping produce fine particles but are necessary to make a better molded product.
Sandblasting	Ship building, oil rig maintenance, and preparing steel for painting are major sources of exposure.
Pottery making	Crushing flint and fettling are major sources of exposure.
Glassmaking	Sand is used to polish and as an abrasive.
Boiler work	Cleaning boilers may result in exposure to fine particulate quartz dust derived from coal and refractory brick dust.

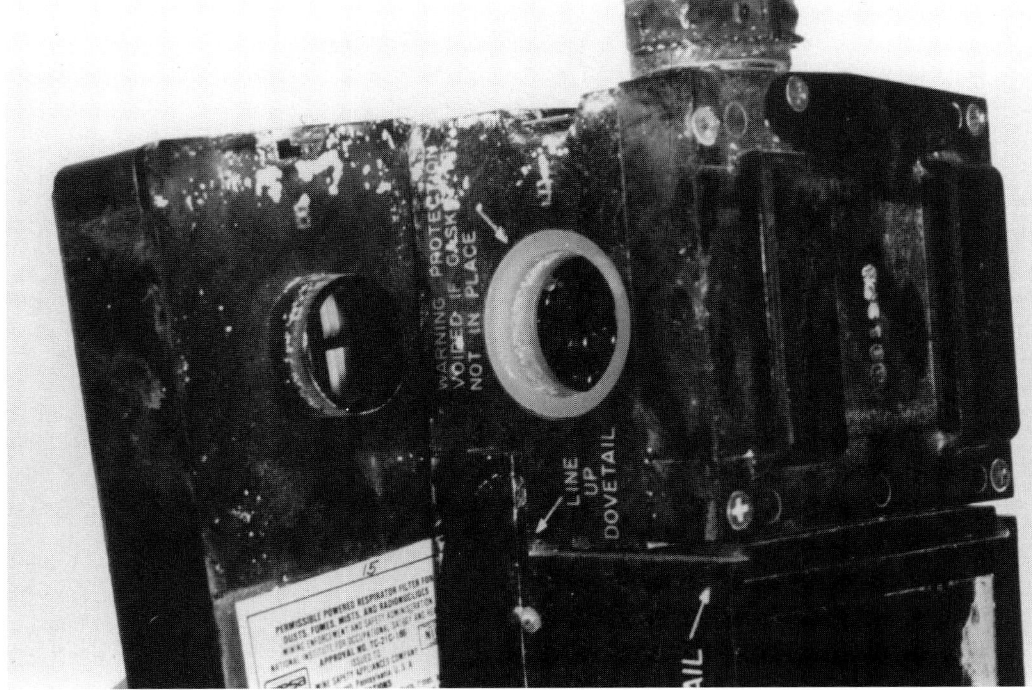

FIGURE 1 This respiratory protective device shows fine silica dust within the apparatus. Technologically sophisticated attempts such as this to protect the worker from excessive dust exposure are inadequate when faced with very fine particles.

II. DETERMINANTS OF SILICOSIS

Silicon dioxide, or silica, is the earth's most abundant mineral. Silicosis, the pulmonary disease caused by the inhalation of silica particles, occurs in workers consistently exposed to respirable size (0.5–10.0 microns in diameter) silica particles at levels exceeding those recognized to be safe. Although host factors such as genetics, smoking, and underlying disease may play roles in the development of silicosis, the primary determinants of whether a worker develops disease are the silica dose in ambient air (including the percentage of free crystalline silica in the dust particles), the duration of dust exposure, whether the silica is crystalline, and the particle size.

For example, hard-rock mining exposures appear to affect smokers and nonsmokers differently.[19,20] In never-smokers with dust exposure, a restrictive effect may occur, as reflected by decreasing total lung capacity and residual volume. Yet, in smokers with this same dust exposure, the mean effect was increasing total lung capacity and residual volume and a decreasing diffusion capacity when adjusted for alveolar volume. Furthermore, greater airflow limitation occurred in dust-exposed compared to nondust-exposed smokers.

There is little information concerning the effect of cigarette smoking on the lung function of workers with silicosis. Most studies have attempted to identify the effects of silicosis by radiographic category on lung function and have been unable to identify clear differences attributable to cigarette smoking.[21–24] Irwig and Rocks[25] compared lung function parameters in 110 pairs of silicotic and nonsilicotic miners matched for numerous parameters including smoking category. There was no significant difference in the spirometric values between the two groups, implying that dust exposure was the most important determinant of outcome in lung function.

In a more recent report, an additive effect of cigarette smoking and silica inhalation has been recognized. In a population of black South African gold miners with a very high percentage of silicosis (857/1197 miners) studied in a cross-sectional manner, 67% of the workers had bronchitis, including 45% of the nonsmokers.[26] When adjusted for smoking and other demographic parameters, there was a dose-dependent decline in FEV_1 (forced exploratory volume in 1 second), FVC (forced vital capacity), and DLCO (diffusing capacity of the lung for carbon monoxide). In this group, the effect of 25 years of dust exposure was associated with an additional decline of 8 ml per year in FEV_1, while the effect of 25 "pack years" (years smoking times packs smoked per day) of cigarette smoking resulted in an additional decline of 7 ml per year. In this report, the loss in lung function appeared dependent on silicosis category and not current dust exposure.

Only respirable size particles are deposited in the alveoli. Particles less than 1 μm in diameter are believed to be the most fibrogenic. Depending on particle size, up to 80% of the silica dust deposited in the alveoli is quickly cleared. It is the small fraction of retained particles which initiates the fibrogenic process. It is not surprising, therefore, that the duration of exposure, the amount of exposure, and the content of free crystalline silica in the dust are the most important determinants of progression of this disease.[27] Although there are numerous jobs where the risk for silicosis exists, exposures to finely milled silica in the production of silica flour (a material used as a filler or as an abrasive), sandblasting, drilling into siliceous rock (Figure 2), and grinding and chipping among foundry workers are examples of jobs where potentially life-threatening exposure to respirable size particles occurs, where the silica content of the particle is high, and where silicosis can develop unless action is taken to protect the worker.

In the Vermont granite workers' industry engineering controls have been implemented and the prevalence of silicosis nearly eradicated. The effect of silica dust (from granite grinding and chipping) exposure on this population serves as the backbone of the federal regulations for permissible silica exposure.[28–32] Investigators who have studied this industry have recorded a legacy of workers with premature death from silicosis and mycobacterial disease beginning in the early parts of this century. Earlier this century, two studies were performed on this population within a 20 year span. Each showed serious granite dust-induced lung disease with the premature death of workers employed in the granite industry.[4,5] However, beginning in the 1950s, there was evidence that institution of dust control measures had produced a safer workplace.[6,33,34] A recent landmark paper by Graham, et al., showed that the mandated current levels of permissible granite dust exposures in these workers are protective.[35] In the same year a report from England detailed aggressive silicosis in stone masons, showing how severe silicosis can be in the same industry when adequate respiratory protection is not used.[36]

III. THE EFFECT OF SILICA DUST ON LUNG FUNCTION

There are two primary respiratory risks to the worker who has silica exposure. The first is the development of simple silicosis — typically with no or little impairment — with the potential to progress to conglomerate silicosis (also known as progressive massive fibrosis) — a disease capable of inducing severe respiratory disability and a shortened life span.[37,38] In silicosis, depending on the overall dust burden and the rate of disease development, silicotic nodules, the histologic hallmark of this disease, may begin *de novo* or continue to enlarge even after exposure has ceased. For this reason, the physician's initial response to the diagnosis of silicosis should be to recommend that the worker cease silica exposure. Even if the worker ceases exposure, this does not guarantee that the disease will not progress. Attempting to lessen dyspnea is an important part of the treatment for this illness. This includes therapy with inhaled bronchodilators and theophylline preparations. There are no proven methods for halting the progression of this illness or reversing silica-induced impairment.

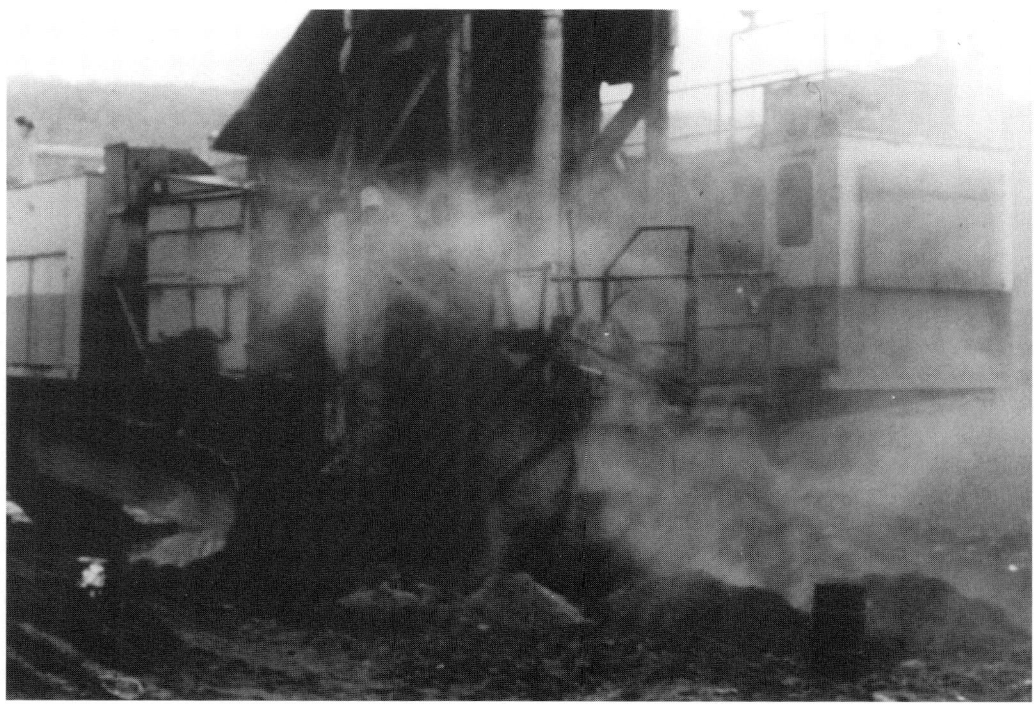

FIGURE 2 This is a photo of a surface coal mine drilling machine in action. After these holes are bored, explosive charges are inserted and detonated. In this way, the overburden is disturbed so that it may be removed and the underlying coal seam exposed. The risk of exposure in this occupation is not to coal but to siliceous rock overlying the coal seam. An operator is required to sit in the cab adjacent to the drilling apparatus in order to monitor drilling progress. Such work can be exceedingly dangerous because of the dust hazard. These machines generate overwhelming amounts of respirable size dust, typically with a high free crystalline silica content.

The second risk is the development of mycobacterial infection with ensuing respiratory impairment. It appears that silica exposure, even in the absence of silicosis, predisposes the worker to mycobacterial infection.[39] In some silica exposed workers, silicotic nodules are present but of an inadequate profusion to allow for a radiographic diagnosis of silicosis.[40] Yet, the mechanisms of fibrogenesis are underway and cellular and humoral features which alter immunologic mechanisms and which may also be a result of silica-induced immunologic impairment are present.[41–51] Mycobacterial infection in a silicotic worker has the very great potential to hasten the development of respiratory impairment and shorten the worker's life. Identifying changes in the chest radiograph of an individual with silicosis over a relatively short time period means superimposed mycobacterial infection until proven otherwise. A new infiltrate, coalescence of nodules in the upper lung fields, an acute chest illness, or cavitation of a pre-existing lesion are reasons for great concern and demand an aggressive search for mycobacterial organisms.

Although not studied in a systematic fashion, it is clinically reasonable to undertake yearly chest radiographs and application of a purified protein derivative (PPD) skin test in those with silicosis. If the PPD becomes positive without clinical evidence of active tuberculosis, at least a year of isoniazid therapy is indicated.[52–54] Many advocate longer, even life-long, antituberculous prophylactic therapy in this setting because of the very real possibility of extensive irreversible damage to the silicotic lung by this organism.[55]

Few reports have described the effect of silica dust inhalation on respiratory function among workers without silicosis. Among South African gold miners with silica dust exposure, Hnizdo[56] showed that cigarette smoke and dust exposure resulted in an additive loss of the FEV_1. For example, the expected 5 year loss in FEV_1 in a 50-year-old underground miner with a 60 pack year cigarette smoking history was 689 ml. In the same miner without a smoking history, the FEV_1 decline was 236 ml. In this population, the contribution of tobacco smoking was substantially greater than that of dust. Nonsmoking miners in the highest dust concentration had greater lung function than non-miners who smoked a package of cigarettes per day. Yet, the nonsmoking silicotics group had a significantly lower FEV_1 than nonsmokers without silicosis. Furthermore, in this same group of miners, workers exposed to silica dust who smoke were at a higher risk of dying from chronic obstructive lung disease than those not exposed to silica dust.[57]

In Cowie's previously cited work,[26] underground miners with silica exposure, but without silicosis, had supranormal values for FVC, FEV_1, and DLCO. In autopsied lungs from silica-exposed miners, emphysema was exceedingly rare unless concomitant cigarette smoking had been a part of the miner's lifestyle.[58] Overall, unless silicosis is recognized, the effects of silica exposure in the work place is thought unlikely to cause clinically important lung function declines.

IV. THE DIAGNOSIS OF SILICOSIS

There are three requisites for the diagnosis of silicosis. First, the worker must provide a history of silica exposure sufficient to cause this illness. Second, the chest radiograph must show opacities consistent with silicosis. Third, no underlying illnesses should be present which mimic silicosis. The most common diseases which might mimic silicosis include a miliary distribution of mycobacterial or fungal organisms, or in an unusual circumstance, sarcoidosis. Although respiratory symptoms and lung function impairment commonly are present, neither is necessary for the diagnosis of silicosis.

The first diagnostic criterion which must be addressed by the physician, determining whether the worker's occupational silica exposure is sufficient to cause silicosis, can be difficult. This requires knowledge about the work place environment and the worker's exposures. The most important information includes knowledge regarding the length of employment, exposure measurements (if available), and a recognition of whether the worker was provided effective respiratory protection. A reasonable starting point is the view that silicosis occurs in association with industrial processes where the silica particle is made respirable size. This is the common thread among occupations where silicosis is a clearly recognized risk (e.g., sandblasting, drilling into siliceous rock, or exposure to finely milled silica [silica flour]). Without manipulation of the silica particle so that it becomes respirable size, the particle is trapped in the upper airway defenses, and silicosis does not occur. Furthermore, the adequacy of respiratory protection devices are highly variable.[7] Silicosis can certainly occur in workers even though they use personal respiratory protection. To begin with, since each respirator has a limit beyond which the dust level exceeds the protective capacity, the worker may be using a respiratory protective device which is inadequate for the amount of dust present. Second, the worker may be using the wrong type of respirator. As an example, respiratory protective devices are designed to protect for the specific exposure. If a solvent mask were used for dust protection, the effectiveness would be compromised. Third, the respiratory protection may be ill-fitting. Finally, because these protective devices are associated with an increased work of breathing, which makes work more difficult, the worker may not use effective available protection. How some workers develop silicosis (or greater or lesser extents of this illness) while employed in the same general work area may be related to the adequacy of respiratory protection. Information regarding the silica dust levels in the work place can also provide important information. However, this approach cannot be guaranteed to represent the complete picture. Cases of acute silicosis in surface coal mine drillers have been reported where the measured dust levels were within normal limits.[9] In this report, the measurements were not representative of the overwhelming dust exposures which induced very aggressive silicosis, nor were there measurements of the percentage of free crystalline silica in the measured mine dust. Therefore, although dust measurements can be helpful, understanding the conditions under which the samples were collected and having confidence that these measurements accurately represent the work place environment is essential. Sometimes this information can only be understood by going to the work place and observing how the work is performed.

When the three clinical requirements for the diagnosis of silicosis are met, additional evaluation of the worker is not necessary to make the diagnosis. On occasion, the diagnosis cannot be made clinically. In these instances, histologic examination of lung tissue is necessary. Situations when this might be necessary occur when the exposure history is uncertain or when the differential diagnosis includes a malignant tumor (sometimes considered when the coalesced lesions of progressive massive fibrosis are recognized as unilateral or asymmetric). This consideration may arise more frequently because of the interest in silica as a potential carcinogen.[59–64] Other illnesses have radiographic features which mimic silicosis. These include rheumatoid nodules[65] (referred to as Caplan's syndrome when this occurs in the presence of pneumoconiosis), infectious processes, or sarcoidosis. Each may need to be ruled out by histologic assessment. When tissue for diagnostic analysis is required, the traditional view has been that an open lung biopsy is preferred in order to lessen the chance of complication of pneumothorax induced by a transbronchoscopic lung biopsy.[66] The increased risk for pneumothoraces may be explained by the knowledge that the upper zones are stiff while emphysematous changes are present in the lower zones. Although the small sample attained by transbronchial lung biopsy may sometimes be inadequate for diagnosis, bronchoalveolar lavage and transbronchial biopsy with energy dispersive x-ray analysis have been used together to aid in the diagnosis of silicosis. In one reported example, a worker employed as a sandblaster, the bronchoalveolar lavage fluid showed a neutrophilic alveolitis, silica was shown to be present in the macrophages by energy dispersive x-ray analysis (although no birefringent crystal particles were found), and the transbronchial biopsy showed fibrocellular nodules in the parenchyma consistent with silicosis.[67]

A. APPROACHES TO CATEGORIZING SILICOSIS

Silicosis can be categorized in two ways. Most commonly, the disease is categorized by findings on the chest radiograph.

B. CLASSIC SILICOSIS

Classic silicosis is separated into simple silicosis and progressive massive fibrosis. These two presentations are radiographically different, but are grouped together under the category of classic silicosis because they are a part of the radiographic spectrum of this illness. On the chest radiograph, simple silicosis is recognized as a profusion of small (less than 10 mm in diameter) rounded opacities (nodules) predominant in the upper lung zones (for an unknown reason, retention of silica particles are favored in the upper lung zones). In some, these small opacities gradually enlarge and coalesce to form larger, usually bilateral, upper zone opacities of similar sizes (more than 10 mm in diameter) recognized as conglomerate silicosis or progressive massive fibrosis.

In some workers with relatively low silica exposure, inhaled silica is more efficiently cleared from the alveolar spaces into the regional chest lymph nodes. In these instances, the chest radiograph reveals peripheral calcification of the hilar (and sometimes mediastinal) lymph nodes with only a minimal or no background of small rounded opacities (figures 3, 4). These are described as "eggshell calcifications" and appear to be a radiographic pattern seen consistently in silicosis. Workers with such radiographic findings are without symptoms attributable to these calcified nodes. An unusual case of such mediastinal nodes eroding through the airway wall and causing tracheobronchial obstruction has recently been reported.[68] In most workers with silica exposures who develop silicosis, however, the lung cannot effectively clear dust and nodules form in the pulmonary parenchyma, sometimes in association with "eggshell calcifications" in the lymph nodes.

In addition to the radiographic features of classic silicosis described above, the other radiographic presentation occurs rarely and is referred to as acute silicosis.[69–71] This is the result of an overwhelming exposure to free crystalline silica over several years. In addition, it may also be that excessive exposure to "freshly fractured silica," material shown to have considerably more free radical oxygen species than "stale" or "old" fractured silica, is more fibrogenic.[72] In some with acute silicosis, the chest radiograph appears as a basilar alveolar filling pattern (identical to that seen in pulmonary alveolar proteinosis) without rounded opacities or lymph node calcifications. This is termed silico-proteinosis. With time, these features progress from a pattern of lower zone alveolar filling to large masses of coalesced parenchymal tissue, typically bilateral but not always symmetrical, in the mid- and lower zones. In others with very excessive silica exposures, the radiographic features are those of simple silicosis which progresses to conglomerate silicosis in a very short time frame, which is consistent with acute silicosis. The explanation for the very different radiographic response of an alveolar filling pattern vs. a very aggressive nodular silicosis in the face of an overwhelming silica exposure is not known but might reflect an important difference in an individual's pulmonary lymphatic drainage.[73]

Silicosis can also be categorized by the duration from initial exposure to the recognition of the disease. The time frames are imprecise, but this approach is useful because of its relevance to prognosis. Classic silicosis develops slowly. Usually 10 to 30 years (a working lifetime) are required from the beginning of exposure to the recognition of radiographic manifestations. In a minority, the nodules of simple silicosis coalesce to become progressive massive fibrosis. Accelerated silicosis occurs infrequently and appears radiographically as simple silicosis which develops after less than 10 years of excessive silica exposure.

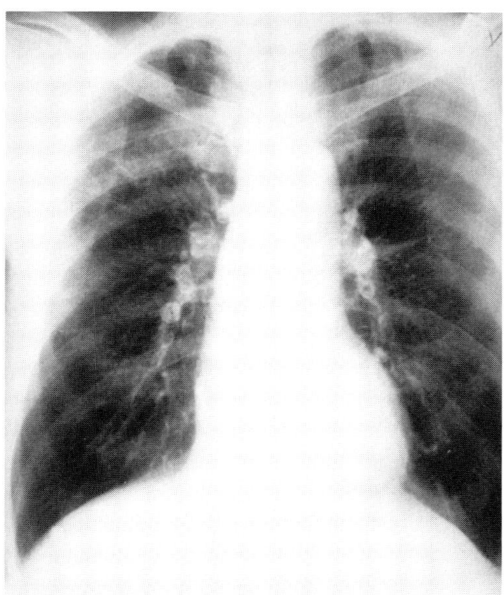
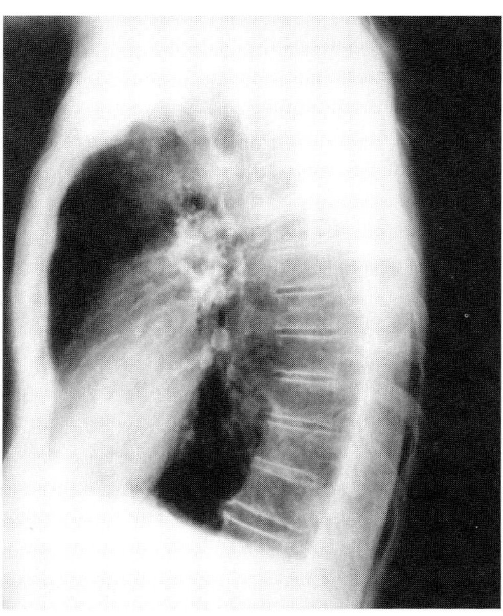

FIGURES 3 AND 4 These postero-anterior and lateral chest radiographs are of a 58-year-old man who worked on the railway for 23 years. His job was to load coal onto trains powered by steam and then to load the coal by shovel into the firebox of the steam engine. He had other duties which required him to spread sand on the tracks, a feature necessary to provide adequate traction for trains travelling the mountains of Eastern Pennsylvania.

These radiographs show a minimal amount of small rounded opacities consistent with pneumoconiosis. What is most remarkable about these films are the peripheral "eggshell" calcifications outlining the hilar and mediastinal nodes. (Radiographs courtesy of Edwin J. Morgan, M.D.).

The development of silicosis after such a short time signals that the worker is at great risk for the immunologic sequelae of silicosis[74–77] and for the development of progressive massive fibrosis. Finally, acute silicosis occurs over a fewer number of years and is associated with an inexorable progression towards a respiratory death.

1. Simple Silicosis

Workers with simple silicosis are usually without chest symptoms. Some, however, report a chronic productive cough, a feature likely due to dust-induced bronchitis. Physical examination of the chest is usually unremarkable. Coarse adventitious sounds which may be present are the result of co-existing bronchitis.

Roentgenographically, simple silicosis presents itself as an upper zone distribution of rounded opacities less than one centimeter in diameter. In miners, these opacities have the same distribution as the nodules described in simple coalworkers' pneumoconiosis but are generally larger and more dense.[78] Peripheral "eggshell" calcifications are sometimes present in the hilar and mediastinal lymph nodes.

Attempts have been made to identify workers with preclinical silicosis before changes are evident on chest radiographs. A high-resolution computerized tomographic (CT) scan of the chest, a technique which has increased the effectiveness of imaging in interstitial lung diseases, has been used to detect parenchymal nodulation before these features are evident on plain chest films. Compared to the usual CT scan of the chest, a high-resolution CT scan allows for high-definition, thin-section scans (1–2 mm compared to 8–10 mm "cuts" by the usual technique of CT scanning) (Figures 5,6). The result is much finer resolution of parenchymal detail, better recognition of the type and distribution of regular and irregular opacities[79–82] and thus, a better understanding of the most likely interstitial lung disease. Importantly, when compared to the chest radiograph, the use of high-resolution CT scan has not added to our ability to diagnose silicosis earlier in a worker's career,[83,84] however, the use of high-resolution CT scans has allowed for the recognition of early "coalescence" of nodules and an earlier diagnosis of progressive massive fibrosis.

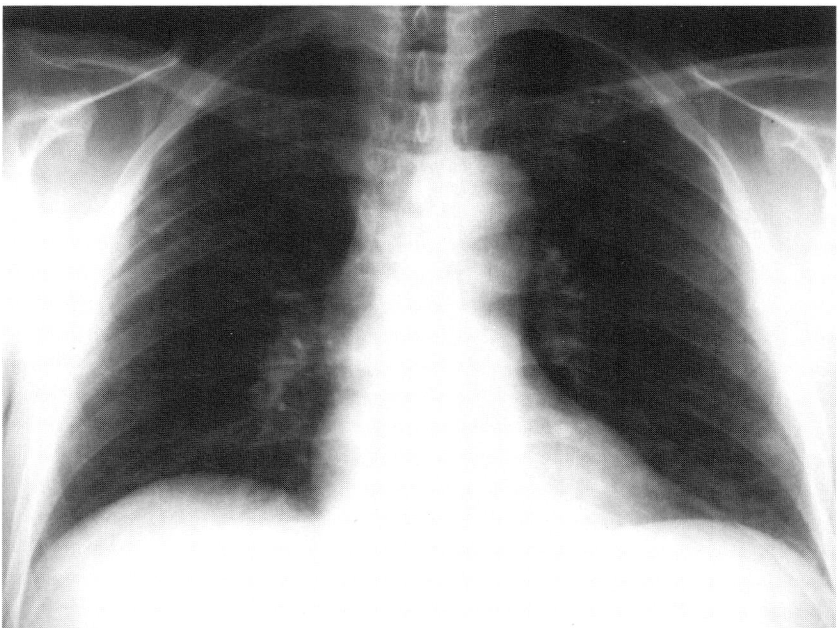

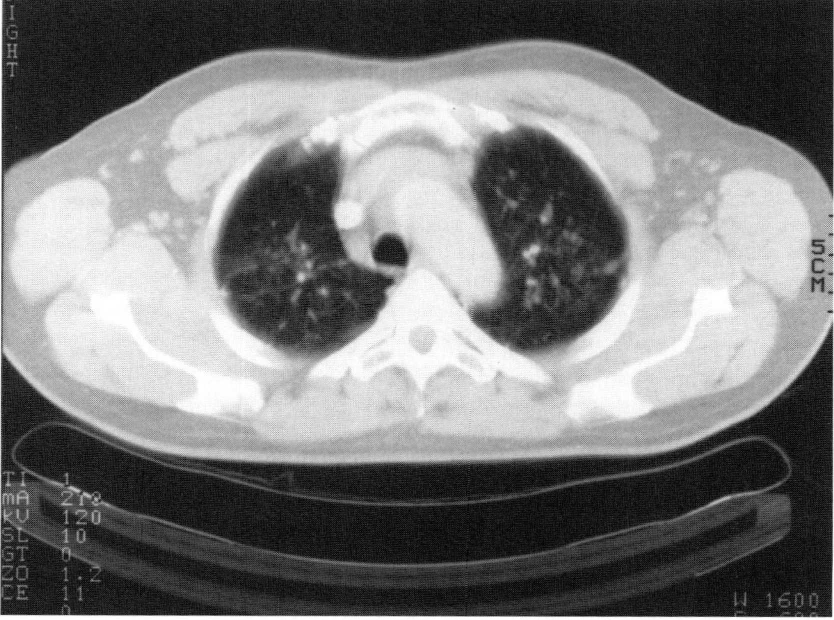

FIGURES 5 AND 6 The chest radiograph is from a 51-year-old, non-smoking underground miner who served as a roof bolter for approximately half of his 24 years of underground mining. The chest radiograph shows prominent parenchymal nodulations in the upper lung zones consistent with simple silicosis. The lung function tests were within normal limits. The CT scan shows these parenchymal nodules to be located in the posterior part of both upper zones. The nodules are discrete and without evidence of coalescence. A high-resolution CT scan was not available.

Pulmonary function studies in simple silicosis do not usually demonstrate functional impairment. Yet, there is a trend towards restriction in total lung capacity and compliance as the extent of profusion of small rounded opacities increases. This is most clearly manifested as overt restriction in some workers with progressive massive fibrosis. As the disease progresses, reduction in compliance usually precedes the

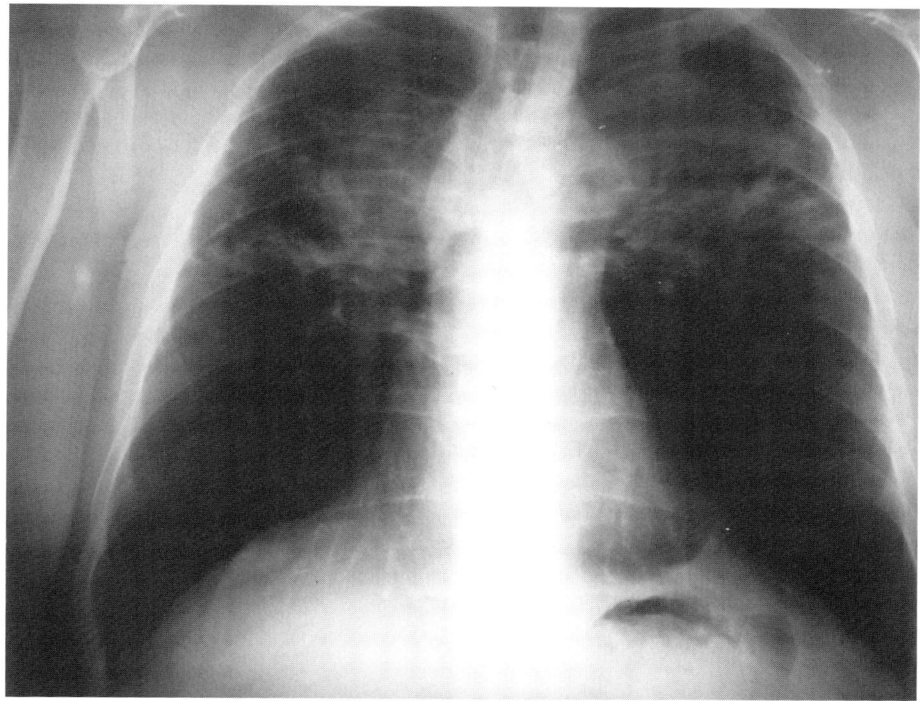

FIGURE 7 This chest radiograph is of a 38-year-old never-smoker employed as a surface coal mine driller from 1973 to 1986. The radiograph was taken one year after he stopped working at the mine. He has cough, morning sputum production, and dyspnea on exertion. Chest examination revealed a quiet chest without adventitious sounds. Lung function tests showed an FVC of 4.88 L (96% predicted), FEV_1 of 2.09 L (53% predicted), and a ratio of 43%. The diffusion capacity and the diffusion capacity adjusted for alveolar volume (KCO) were within normal limits. The chest radiograph shows large opacities in both upper zones of International Labor Office (ILO) category "B" and a background of minimal small rounded opacities. Although no earlier radiographs were available, the development of such severe disease in such a young man implies an accelerated progression of silicosis. In this case, the lung function tests show obstruction rather than the typical changes of restrictive impairment most commonly associated with progressive massive fibrosis.

reductions in vital capacity or forced expiratory flow rate. Few nonsmoking, dust-exposed workers with simple silicosis develop air flow abnormalities.[85,86] In a sophisticated study using high-resolution computed tomography (CT) scans of the chest to identify the presence of emphysema in workers with simple silicosis, Kinsella, et al., noted that simple silicosis did not cause significant emphysema and that it was the degree of emphysema, rather than the extent of simple silicosis, that determined the level of respiratory function. In those with progressive massive fibrosis, emphysema occurred frequently but was not different among smokers and nonsmokers.[87]

2. Progressive Massive Fibrosis

Progressive massive fibrosis is the result of the conglomeration of small rounded opacities. It has been traditionally recognized that progressive massive fibrosis develops on a background of advanced simple silicosis. Yet, not all coal miners who develop progressive massive fibrosis have an underlying advanced degree of simple coal workers' pneumoconiosis.[88] Whether this is also the case with silicosis has not been described (Figure 7).

The respiratory symptoms present in a worker with progressive massive fibrosis are again variable. They range from only a chronic productive cough to exertional dyspnea and, in some, ultimately to respiratory failure. With time, however, the progressive coalescence of silicotic nodules impairs the function of the underlying pulmonary parenchyma and results in progressive respiratory impairment.

Physical examination demonstrates decreased breath sounds on auscultation (explained by the emphysematous changes associated with progressive massive fibrosis) and, if the illness is extensive, signs of cor pulmonale and impending respiratory failure. Crackles do not occur as a result of the fibrotic changes, and finger clubbing, if present, is attributable to another etiology.

The chest roentgenogram reveals confluent nodules greater than one centimeter in diameter which occur on a background of small rounded opacities, which is recognizable as simple silicosis. The confluence of these nodules begins posteriorly and peripherally and migrates centrally. As with simple silicosis, progressive massive fibrosis develops most prominently in the upper lobes. As these upper lobe fibrous masses progressively enlarge, the hila are retracted upward and the lower zones become hyperinflated and appear as bullous emphysema. The presence of these upper zone opacities is often discussed in the context of possible neoplastic processes in the lung, particularly if they are not symmetrical. Importantly, progressive massive fibrotic lesions are relatively thin and plate-like and are located in the peripheral and posterior aspects of the upper lung zones. These radiographic features are sometimes helpful in separating the lesions of progressive massive fibrosis from a malignant etiology for these pulmonary masses.

Pulmonary function studies initially demonstrate a decrease in compliance followed by decreases in lung volume and diffusing capacity. If bronchial distortion and lower zone hyperinflation are present, the forced expiratory time is likely to be prolonged and airflow obstruction is measurable. Deterioration in lung function commonly occurs despite discontinuing silica exposure. The likelihood of progression directly correlates with the duration and concentration of silica exposure, as well as the presence or absence of mycobacterial infection.

C. ACCELERATED SILICOSIS

Accelerated silicosis is radiographically identical to classic silicosis except that the time from initial exposure to silica to the development of a radiographic diagnosis of silicosis, and the pulmonary function changes attributable to silicosis, occur over a shorter time and are often exaggerated. Accelerated silicosis is associated with a relatively rapid progression from the radiographic changes of simple silicosis to progressive massive fibrosis with ensuing severe respiratory impairment and a shortened life span (Figures 8, 9).

Silicotics have an increased prevalence of autoimmune serology, elevated gamma globulin levels, and an increased frequency of connective tissue disease, particularly scleroderma. Alternatively, concomitant connective tissue disease may also influence the course of pneumoconiosis. In 1953, Caplan noted that the course of coal workers' pneumoconiosis in workers with dust exposure could be influenced by co-existing rheumatoid arthritis. Upper zone large opacities appeared more frequently in the lungs of workers with underlying rheumatoid arthritis.

The role of the generally stimulated immune system is not well understood in this disease. Antinuclear antibodies and elevated immunoglobulin levels have not correlated with the baseline profusion category of the chest radiograph, the rate of chest radiographic progression, or the rate of lung function decline in sandblasters with silicosis.

D. ACUTE SILICOSIS

Acute silicosis, the most aggressive form of silicosis, occurs over a short duration of exposure to overwhelmingly high concentrations of respirable free silica. The worker progresses to disabling chest symptoms and severe respiratory impairment, which invariably leads to death due to respiratory failure. Although patients with this form of silicosis may have some features of classic silicosis, there are distinct clinical, radiographic, and histologic differences.

In 1969, Buechner reported four sandblasters with acute silicosis and coined the term silico-proteinosis.[18] At autopsy, these sandblasters had periodic acid Schiff (PAS), positive-staining proteinaceous material filling the alveolar spaces, silica particles in the lung, and histologic changes of alveolar proteinosis. However, a review of the literature prior to Buechner's description suggests that many of the earlier patients had similar histologic features. Suratt reported the same presentation in tombstone sandblasters.[3] Chapman reported the histology to show localized areas of basilar "bronchopneumonia" in which the alveoli were filled with a pink staining edema fluid with a high protein content.[71] Gardner confirmed the uniqueness of this presentation by showing the most common lesion to be an alveolar exudate in which few, if any, cells could be identified.[90] Silico-proteinosis is a descriptive term of the histologic findings of the lungs in those who develop silicosis over a very short period of time (acute silicosis) and not a separate entity.

Workers with acute silicosis have been reported to have an irritative, sometimes productive, cough, weight loss, fatigue, and occasionally, pleuritic pain. Symptoms begin usually one to three years after the initial exposure; however, in very rare examples, symptoms occurring less than a year after beginning

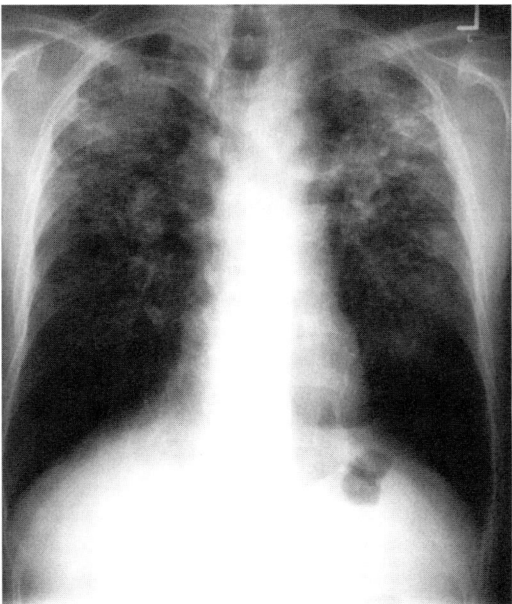

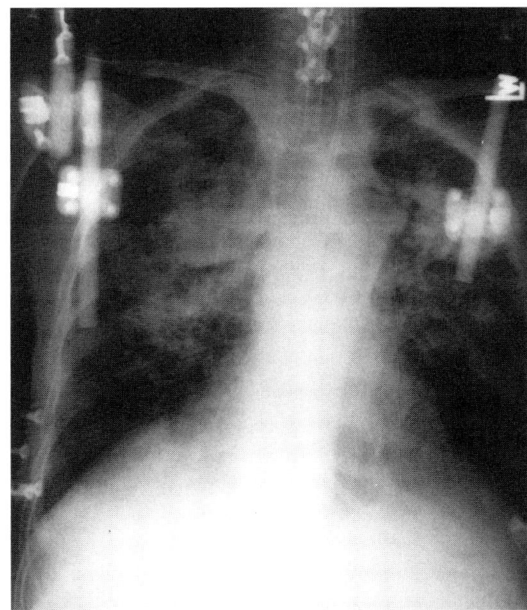

FIGURES 8 AND 9 These radiographs are from a 55-year-old man who was first seen in 1988 and later in 1992. He provided a 75 pack year smoking history and had worked as a rock driller for approximately 20 years. Mycobacterial infection was searched for but not found. A PPD was non-reactive. The dramatic worsening of the radiograph over just four years reflects an accelerated course associated with a shortened life span. The chest radiographs show the way the coalescence of opacities in the upper zones occur and form progressive massive fibrotic lesions. The neck brace in the second radiograph was a part of therapy for a traumatic neck injury.

sandblasting have been reported. Unlike the quiet chest examination of classical silicosis, crackles are usually present and likely reflect alveolar and airway fluid. Patients rapidly develop cyanosis, symptoms of cor pulmonale, and respiratory failure. Survival after the onset of symptoms is typically less than four years. Mycobacterial and fungal infections frequently complicate the clinical course.

The chest radiograph typically reveals bilateral basilar alveolar filling with air bronchograms.[70,91] The diffuse alveolar filling is best described as a ground-glass appearance. Histologically small rounded opacities can sometimes be identified, but they are not easily recognized on the chest radiograph. Progression of the chest radiograph occurs over a relatively short time. Areas of alveolar filling progress to large masses which are similar to those seen in progressive massive fibrosis but somewhat larger and often located in the mid, compared to upper, zones. Tracheal distortion is common and a result of the parenchymal distortion with stress placed on the trachea. The process of radiographic progression is accelerated in these workers by a superimposed mycobacterial infection.

Acute silicosis can usually be diagnosed on the basis of a history of employment in an occupation where the opportunity for overwhelming silica exposure exists and where the clinical features and chest radiograph are consistent with this illness. If a review of the lung tissue becomes necessary for an accurate diagnosis, an open lung biopsy is recommended. Despite appropriate therapy for any underlying chest infection, the worker's lung function continues to deteriorate. Perhaps the best differential diagnosis of these very unusual chest radiographs includes alveolar proteinosis, bronchiolitis obliterans with organizing pneumonia, desquamative interstitial pneumonitis, and lipoid pneumonia. These entities can usually be excluded on a clinical basis.

V. CONCLUSION

The prevention of silicosis has not yet been achieved. If the past leads the way to the future, then it is by no means guaranteed that this disease can ever be totally abolished. Cases continue despite aggressive enforcement policies by regulatory agencies, attempts at dissemination of very readable materials aimed at workers and management,[92,93] and respiratory dust exposure standards which appear protective and are in place. It is more than frustrating for all parties to see reports of aggressive silicosis in young workers. Perhaps, like the crusade against drunk driving, a determined effort through the contemporary methods of communication might enlighten American society and its workers about the very destructive health effects of silica exposure. Furthermore, both the physician and the affected worker are helpless when a diagnosis of silicosis has been made, and there is no way to affect the natural history of the processes that are underway. What must be developed is a type of "salvage therapy" that has the potential to reverse, or at least dramatically lessen, the aggressive natural history of silicosis that develops over relatively short time periods. Perhaps, if the illness cannot be prevented, an approach to lessen the effect of the fibrosis induced by this dust can be developed.

ACKNOWLEDGMENT

Supported in part by National Institute for Occupational Safety and Health grant #U60/CCU306149–01.

REFERENCES

1. **Betts, W. W.,** Chalicosis pulmonum or chronic interstitial pneumonia induced by stone dust, *JAMA,* 34, 70–74, 1900.
2. **Banks, D. E., Morring, K., Boehlecke, B. A., Althouse, R., and Merchant, J. A.,** Silicosis in silica flour workers, *Am. Rev. Respir. Dis.,* 124, 445–450, 1981.
3. **Suratt, P. M., Winn, W. C., Brody, A. R., Bolton, W. K., and Giles, R. D.,** Acute silicosis in tombstone sandblasters, *Am. Rev. Respir. Dis.,* 115, 521–529, 1977.
4. **Russell, A. E., Britten, E. H., Thompson, L. R., and Bloomfield, J. J.,** The health of workers in dusty trades — II. Exposure to siliceous dust (granite industry), Public Health Bull. No. 187, U.S. Treasury Department, Public Health Service, 1929.
5. **Russell, A. E.,** The health of workers in dusty trades — VII. Restudy of a group of granite workers, Public Health Bull. No. 269, Federal Security Agency, U.S. Public Health Service, Washington, D.C., 1941.
6. **Hosey, A. D., Trasko, V. M., and Ashe, H. B.,** Control of silicosis in the Vermont granite industry: progress report, Publication 557, U.S. Department of Health, Education and Welfare, Washington, D.C., 1957.
7. **Glindmeyer, H. W. and Hammad, Y.,** Contributing factors to sandblaster's silicosis: inadequate respiratory protection equipment and standards, *J. Occup. Med.,* 30, 917–921, 1988.
8. **Davies, C. N.,** Inhalation risk and particle size in dust and mist, *Br. J. Ind. Med.,* 6, 245–253, 1949.
9. **Banks, D. E., Bauer, M. A., Castellan, R. M., and Lapp, N. L.,** Silicosis in surface coalmine drillers, *Thorax,* 38, 275–278, 1983.
10. **Fleming, D., Maynard, D., McKinney, B., Perrotta, D. M., Schulze, L., and Pichette, J.,** Silicosis: Clusters in sandblasters-Texas, and occupational surveillance for silicosis, *Morbidity and Mortality Weekly Report,* 39, 433–437, 1990.
11. **Amandus, H. E. and Piacitelli, G.,** Dust exposures at U.S. surface coal mines in 1982–1983, *Arch. Environ. Health,* 42, 374–381, 1987.
12. National Institute for Occupational Safety and Health, Criteria for a recommended standard. Occupational exposures to crystalline silica, Washington, D.C., U.S. Department of Health, Education and Welfare, Public Health Service, Centers for Disease Control, 1974, 54–55.
13. Work related lung disease surveillance report, U.S. Department of Health and Human Resources, Public Health Service, Centers for Disease Control, National Institute for Occupational Safety and Health, 1991, 27.
14. **Graham, W. G. B., Ashikaga, T., Hemenway, D., Weaver, S., and O'Grady, R. V.,** Radiographic abnormalities in Vermont granite workers exposed to low levels of granite dust, *Chest,* 100, 1507–1515, 1991.
15. Office of Federal Register, Code of federal regulations: occupational safety and health standards. Subpart Z: Air contaminants-permissible exposure limits. Table-1-A, Washington D.C., Office of the Federal Register, National Archives and Records Administration, 1989 (29 CFR 1910.1000).
16. **MacKay, G. R., Stettler, L. E., Kommineni, C., and Donaldson, H. M.,** Fibrogenic potential of slags used as substitutes for sand in abrasive blasting operations, *Am. Ind. Hyg. Assoc. J.,* 41, 836–842, 1980.
17. **Stettler, L. E., Procter, J. E., Platek, S. F., Carolan, R. J., Smith, R. J., and Donaldson, H. M.,** Fibrogenicity and carcinogenic potential of smelter slags used as abrasive blasting substitutes, *J. Toxicol. Environ. Health,* 25, 35–36, 1988.
18. **Buechner, H. A. and Ansari, A.,** Acute silico-proteinosis, *Dis. Chest,* 55, 274–284, 1969.

19. **Manfreda, J., Sidwall, G., Maini, K., West, P., and Cherniack, R. M.,** Respiratory abnormalities in employees of the hard rock mining industry, *Am. Rev. Respir. Dis.*, 126, 629–634, 1982.
20. **Kreiss, K., Greenberg, L. M., Kogut, S. J. H., Lezotte, D. C., Irvin, C. G., and Cherniak, R. M.,** Hard rock mining exposures affect smokers and nonsmokers differently, *Am. Rev. Respir. Dis.*, 139, 1487–1493, 1988.
21. **Teculescu, D. B., Stanescu, D. C., and Pilat, L.,** Pulmonary mechanics in silicosis, *Arch. Environ. Health*, 14, 461–468, 1967.
22. **Becklake, M. R., DuPreez, L., and Lutz, W.,** Lung function in silicosis of the Witswatersrand gold miner, *Am. Rev. Tuberc.*, 77, 400–412, 1958.
23. **Ehrlich, R. I., Rees, D., and Zwi, A. B.,** Silicosis in the non-mining industry on the Witswatersrand, *S. Afr. Med. J.*, 73, 704–708, 1988.
24. **Jones, R. N., Weill, H., and Ziskind, M.,** Pulmonary function in sandblasters silicosis, *Bull. Physiopath. Respir.*, 11, 589–595, 1975.
25. **Irwig, L. M. and Rocks, P.,** Lung function and respiratory symptoms in silicotic and nonsilicotic gold miners, *Am. Rev. Respir. Dis.*, 117, 429–435, 1978.
26. **Cowie, R. L. and Mabena, S. K.,** Silicosis, chronic airflow obstruction, and chronic bronchitis in South African gold miners, *Am. Rev. Respir. Dis.*, 143, 80–84, 1991.
27. **Hughes, J. M., Jones, R. N., Gilson, J. C., Hammad, Y. Y., Samimi, B., Hendrick, D. J., Turner-Warwick, M., Doll, N. J., and Weill, H.,** Determinants of progression in sandblasters' silicosis, *Ann. Occup. Hyg.*, 26, 701–712, 1982.
28. Criteria for a recommended standard...Occupational exposure to crystalline silica, U.S. Department of Health, Education and Welfare, Public Health Service, Centers for Disease Control, National Institute for Occupational Safety and Health, HEW publication No. (NIOSH) 75–120, 1974.
29. **Theriault, G. P., Burgess, W. A., DiBernardinis, L. J., and Peters, J. M.,** Dust exposure in the Vermont granite sheds, *Arch. Environ. Health*, 28, 12–17, 1974.
30. **Theriault, G. P., Peters, J. M., and Fine, L. J.,** Pulmonary function in Vermont granite shed workers, *Arch. Environ. Health*, 28, 18–22, 1974.
31. **Theriault, G. P., Peters, J. M., and Johnson, W. M.,** Pulmonary function and roentgenographic changes in granite shed exposure, *Arch. Environ. Health*, 28, 23–27, 1974.
32. **Graham, W. G. B., O'Grady, R. V., and Dubuc, B.,** Pulmonary function loss in Vermont granite workers, *Am. Rev. Respir. Dis.*, 123, 25–28, 1981.
33. **Ashe, H. B.,** Silicosis and dust control, *Public Health Rep.*, 70, 983–985, 1955.
34. **Ashe, H. B. and Bergstrom, D. E.,** Twenty six years experience with dust controls in the Vermont granite industry, *Ind. Med. Surg.*, 33, 73–78, 1964.
35. **Graham, W. G. B., Ashikaga, T., Hemenway, D., Weaver, S., and O'Grady, R. V.,** Radiographic abnormalities in Vermont granite workers exposed to low levels of granite dust, *Chest*, 100, 1507–1514, 1991.
36. **Seaton, A., Legge, J. S., Henderson, J., and Kerr, K. M.,** Accelerated silicosis in Scottish stonemasons, *Lancet*, 337, 341–344, 1991.
37. **Westerholm, P.,** Silicosis: Observations on a case register, *Scand. J. Work Environ. Health*, 1–86 (suppl 6), 1980.
38. **Finkelstein, M., Kusiak, R., and Suranyi, G.,** Mortality among miners receiving compensation for silicosis in Ontario: 1940–1975, *J. Occup. Med.*, 24, 663–667, 1982.
39. **Sherson, D. and Lander, F.,** Morbidity of pulmonary tuberculosis among silicotic and nonsilicotic foundry workers, *J. Occup. Med.*, 32, 110–113, 1990.
40. **Craighead, J. E. and Vallyathan, N. V.,** Cryptic pulmonary lesions in workers occupationally exposed to dust containing silica, *JAMA*, 244, 1939–1941, 1980.
41. **Craighead, J. E., Kleinerman, J., Abraham, J. L., Gibbs, A. R., Green, F. H. Y., Harley, R. A., Ruettner, J. R., Vallayathan, N. V., and Juliano, E. B.,** Diseases associated with exposure to silica and nonfibrous silicate minerals, *Arch. Pathol. Lab. Med.*, 112, 673–720, 1988.
42. **Bowden, D. H. and Adamson, I. Y. R.,** The role of cell injury in the continuing inflammatory response in the generation of silicotic pulmonary fibrosis, *J. Pathol.*, 144, 149–161, 1984.
43. **Adamson, I. Y. R. and Bowden, D. H.,** Role of polymorphonuclear leukocytes in silica-induced pulmonary fibrosis, *Am. J. Pathol.*, 117, 37–43, 1984.
44. **Lugano, E. M., Dauber, J. H., and Daniele, R. P.,** Acute experimental silicosis, *Am. J. Pathol.*, 109, 27–36, 1982.
45. **Callis, A. H., Sohnle, P. G., Mandel, G. S., and Mandel, N. S.,** The role of complement in experimental silicosis, *Environ. Res.*, 40, 301–312, 1986.
46. **Christman, J. W., Emerson, R. J., Graham, W. G. B., and Davis, G. S.,** Mineral dust and cell recovery from the bronchoalveolar lavage of healthy Vermont granite workers, *Am. Rev. Respir. Dis.*, 132, 393–399, 1985.
47. **Lowrie, D. B.,** What goes wrong with the macrophage in silicosis? *Eur. J. Respir. Dis.*, 63, 180–182, 1982.
48. **Schmidt, J. A., Oliver, C. N., Lepe-Zunige, J. L., Green, I., and Gery, I.,** Silica-stimulated monocytes release fibroblast proliferation factors identical to interleukin 1, *J. Clin. Invest.*, 73, 1462–1472, 1984.
49. **Martin, T. R., Altman, L. C., Albert, R. K., and Henderson, W. R.,** Leukotriene B_4 production by the human alveolar macrophage: a potential mechanism for amplifying inflammation in the lung, *Am. Rev. Respir. Dis.*, 129, 106–111, 1984.

50. **Bitterman, P. B., Wewers, M. D., Rennard, S. I., Adelberg, S., and Crystal, R. G.,** Modulation of alveolar macrophage driven fibroblast proliferation by alternative macrophage mediators, *J. Clin. Invest.,* 77, 700–708, 1986.
51. **Davis, G. S.,** Pathogenesis of silicosis: current concepts and hypotheses, *Lung,* 164, 139–154, 1986.
52. **Snider, D. E.,** The relationship between tuberculosis and silicosis, *Am. Rev. Respir. Dis.,* 118, 455–460, 1978.
53. **Baras, G.,** Silico-tuberculose en Suisse, *Schweiz. Med. Wochenschr.,* 100, 1802–1805, 1970.
54. **Cowie, R. L., Langton, M. E., and Becklake, M. R.,** Pulmonary tuberculosis in South African gold miners, *Am. Rev. Respir. Dis.,* 139, 1086–1089, 1989.
55. **Morgan, E. J.,** Silicosis and tuberculosis, *Chest,* 75, 202–203, 1979.
56. **Hnizdo, E.,** Loss of lung function associated with exposure to silica dust and with smoking and its relation to disability and mortality in South African gold miners, *BJIM,* 49, 472–479, 1992.
57. **Hnizdo, E.,** Combined effect of silica dust and tobacco smoking on mortality from chronic obstructive lung disease in gold miners, *Br. J. Ind. Med.,* 47, 656–664, 1990.
58. **Hnizdo, E., Sluis-Cremer, G. K., and Abramowitz, J. A.,** Emphysema type in relation to silica dust exposure in South African gold miners, *Am. Rev. Respir. Dis.,* 143, 1241–1247, 1991.
59. **Hessel, P. A., Sluis-Cremer, G. K., and Hnizdo, E.,** Silica exposure, silicosis, and lung cancer: a necropsy study, *Br. J. Ind. Med.,* 47, 4–9, 1990.
60. **Wu, K.-G., Fu, H., Mo, C.-Z., and Yu, L.-Z.,** Smelting, underground mining, smoking, and lung cancer: a case-control study in a tin mine area, *Biomed. Environ. Sci.,* 2, 1–8, 1989.
61. **Heppleston, A. G.,** Silica, pneumoconiosis, and carcinoma of the lung, *Am. J. Ind. Med.,* 7, 285–294, 1985.
62. **Lynge, E., Kurppa, K., Kristoferson, L., Malker, H., and Sauli, H.,** Silica dust and lung cancer: results from the Nordic occupational mortality and cancer incidence registers, *J. Nat. Cancer Inst.,* 77, 883–889, 1986.
63. **Goldsmith, D. F., Guidotti, T. L., and Johnston, D. R.,** Does occupational exposure to silica cause cancer?, *Am. J. Ind. Med.,* 3, 423–440, 1982.
64. **McDonald, J. C.,** Silica, silicosis, and lung cancer, *Br. J. Ind. Med.,* 46, 289–291, 1989.
65. **Caplan, A.,** Certain unusual radiologic appearances in the chest of coalminers suffering from rheumatoid arthritis, *Thorax,* 8, 29–30, 1953.
66. **Ziskind, M., Jones, R. N., and Weill, H.,** Silicosis, *Am. Rev. Respir. Dis.,* 113, 643–665, 1976.
67. **Nugent, K. M., Dodson, R. F., Idell, S., and DeVillier, J. R.,** The utility of bronchoalveolar lavage and transbronchial lung biopsy combined with energy-dispersive x-ray analysis in the diagnosis of silicosis, *Am. Rev. Respir. Dis.,* 140, 1438–1441, 1989.
68. **Cahill, B. C., Harmon, K. R., Shumway, S. J., Mickman, J. K., and Hertz, M. I.,** Tracheobronchial obstruction due to silicosis, *Am. Rev. Respir. Dis.,* 145, 719–721, 1992.
69. **Dee, P., Suratt, P., and Winn, W.,** The radiographic findings in acute silicosis, *Radiology,* 126, 359–363, 1978.
70. **Sampson, H. L.,** The Roentgenogram in so-called "acute" silicosis, *Am. J. Pub. Health,* 23, 1237–1239, 1933.
71. **Chapman, E. M.,** Acute Silicosis, *JAMA,* 98, 1439–1441, 1932.
72. **Vallyathan, V., Shi, X., Dalal, N. S., Irr, W., and Castranova, V.,** Generation of free radicals from freshly fractured silica dust: potential role in acute silica-induced lung injury, *Am. Rev. Respir. Dis.,* 138, 1213–1219, 1988.
73. **Eden, K. G. and von Seebach, H. B.,** Atypical quartz dust induced pneumoconiosis in SPF rats. Aspects of the role of the lymphatic system in the pathogenesis of silicosis, *Virchows Arch. A.* 372, 1–9, 1976.
74. **Lippman, M., Eckert, H. L., Hahon, N., and Morgan, W. K. C.,** Circulating antinuclear and rheumatoid factors in coal miners. A prevalence study in Pennsylvania and West Virginia, *Ann. Intern. Med.,* 79, 807–811, 1973.
75. **Jones, R. N., Turner-Warwick, M., Ziskind, M., and Weill, H.,** High prevalence of antinuclear antibodies in sandblasters silicosis, *Am. Rev. Respir. Dis.,* 113, 393–395, 1976.
76. **Rodnan, G. P., Bendek, T. G., Medsger, T. A., and Cammarata, R. J.,** The association of progressive systemic sclerosis with coal miners' pneumoconiosis and other forms of silicosis, *Ann. Intern. Med.,* 66, 323–329, 1967.
77. **Haustein, U. F., Zeigler, V., Hermann, K., Melhorn, J., and Schmidt, C.,** Silica-induced scleroderma, *J. Am. Acad. Dermatol.,* 22, 444–448, 1990.
78. **Anderson, W. H., Hamilton, G. L., and Dorsett, B. E., Jr.,** A comparison of coal miners exposed to coal dust and those exposed to silica dust, *Arch. Environ. Health,* 1, 540–547, 1960.
79. **Muller, N. L. and Miller, R. R.,** Computed tomography of chronic infiltrative lung disease. Part 1, *Am. Rev. Respir. Dis.,* 142, 1206–1215, 1990.
80. **Muller, N. L. and Miller, R. R.,** Computed tomography of chronic infiltrative lung disease. Part 2, *Am. Rev. Respir. Dis.,* 142, 1440–1448, 1990.
81. **Mathieson, J. R., Mayo, J. R., Staples, C. A., and Muller, N. L.,** Chronic diffuse lung disease: comparison of diagnostic accuracy of CT and chest radiography, *Radiology,* 171, 111–116, 1989.
82. **Bergin, C. J., Coblentz, C. L., Chiles, C., Bell, D. Y., and Castellino, R. A.,** Chronic lung disease: specific diagnosis by using CT, *Am. J. Roentgenol.,* 152, 1183–1188, 1989.
83. **Begin, R., Bergeron, D., Samson, L., Boctor, M., and Cantin, A.,** CT assessment of silicosis in exposed workers, *Am. J. Roentgenol.,* 148, 509–514, 1987.
84. **Bergin, C. J., Muller, N. L., Vedal, S., and Chan-Yeung, M.,** CT in silicosis: correlation with plain films and pulmonary function tests, *Am. J. Roentgenol.,* 147, 477–483, 1986.

85. **Teculescu, D. B., Stanescu, D. C., and Pilat, L.,** Pulmonary mechanics in silicosis, *Arch. Environ. Health,* 14, 461–468, 1967.
86. **Jones, R. N., Weill, H., and Ziskind, M.,** Pulmonary function in sandblasters silicosis, *Bull. Physiopath. Resp.,* 11, 589–595, 1975.
87. **Kinsella, M., Muller, N., Vedal, S., Staples, C., Abboud, R. T., and Chan-Yeung, M.,** Emphysema in silicosis. A comparison of smokers with non-smokers using pulmonary function testing and computed tomography, *Am. Rev. Respir. Dis.,* 141, 1497–1500, 1990.
88. **Hodous, T. K. and Attfield, M. D.,** Progressive massive fibrosis developing on a background of minimal simple coal workers' pneumoconiosis. Proc. VIIth International Pneumoconiosis Conference. National Institute for Occupational Safety and Health, Department of Health and Human Services, (NIOSH) Publ. No. 90–108, Part 1, 123–126.
89. **Middleton, E. L.,** The present position of silicosis in industry in Britain, *Br. Med. J.,* 2, 485–489, 1929.
90. **Gardner, L. U.,** Pathology of so-called silicosis, *Am. J. Public Health,* 23, 1240–1249, 1933.
91. **Sampson, H. L.,** The Roentgenogram in so-called "acute" silicosis, *Am. J. Public Health,* 23, 1237–1239, 1933.
92. Centers for Disease Control Alert: Request for assistance in preventing silicosis and deaths from sandblasting, U.S. Department of Health and Human Services, Public Health Service, CDC, National Institute for Occupational Safety and Health, Department of Health and Human Services (NIOSH) Publ. No. 92–102.
93. Centers for Disease Control Alert: Request for assistance in preventing silicosis and deaths in Rock drillers, U.S. Department of Health and Human Services, Public Health Service, CDC, National Institute for Occupational Safety and Health, Department of Health and Human Services, (NIOSH) Publ. No. 92–107.

Section I
Chapter 5

PATHOLOGIC RESPONSES TO INHALED SILICA

Francis H. Y. Green and Val Vallyathan

CONTENTS

I. INTRODUCTION

Silicosis is defined as pulmonary disease resulting from the inhalation of crystalline silica. In the human, silicosis manifests as four pathologically distinct entities: acute silicosis (silicolipoproteinosis), accelerated silicosis, chronic simple silicosis, and complicated silicosis. Complicated silicosis develops to progressive massive fibrosis by the conglomeration of nodular lesions. Rheumatoid pneumoconiosis, silicotuberculosis, and scleroderma are also associated with silica exposure.

The components of the silicotic response have strong temporal and exposure associations. Acute silicosis and accelerated silicosis have short latency periods (several months to several years) and are associated with intense, brief exposures. Chronic simple silicosis and complicated silicosis, by contrast, are more likely to occur a decade or more after first exposure and are associated with lower levels of

0-8493-4709-2/96/$0.00+$.50

exposure over long periods of time. However, overall cumulative exposure (exposure level × duration) may be similar in patients presenting with different types of disease.

Although this classification and the general principles enumerated concerning latency and exposure apply to most cases of silicosis, certain qualifications apply. First, this disease classification describes a spectrum of changes that may exist in transitional forms (e.g., accelerated silicosis has features in common with both acute silicosis and chronic simple silicosis). Second, the various distinctive lesions may co-exist in the same lung (e.g., pulmonary alveolar proteinosis may be seen in patients with silicotic massive fibrosis).[1] Third, the features of silicosis may be modified by the presence of other minerals in the dust (see Chapter 4, Section II).

The number of workers at risk for developing silicosis remains high. The National Institute for Occupational Safety and Health (NIOSH) estimated in 1986 that 2.3 million workers were exposed to quartz dust.[2] Every year, approximately, 1,500 cases of silicosis are diagnosed in the U.S.[3] It is likely that many more cases remain undiagnosed.

However, silicosis is now rare in populations of workers exposed to quartz levels averaging less than the current permissible limit of 100 $\mu g/m^3$.[3] Most cases today occur in poorly regulated or unregulated industrial settings or in situations where the exposure was not recognized. Unusual sources of exposure resulting in silicosis include inhalation of crack cocaine,[4] scouring powder,[5] exposure in the electronics industry,[6] grinding maize,[7] farming,[8] living in desert-like terrain,[9,10] and the cutting of gemstones.[11,12] Exposure to silica-containing dust can also result in cryptic pulmonary disease that is not detected radiologically. Craighead and Vallyathan described small fibrotic lesions associated with deposits of crystalline silica in post mortem specimens of 15 granite workers who lacked radiological evidence of pneumoconiosis.[13]

It is important to bear in mind that silica is not a single entity. Free silica (silicon dioxide) occurs in crystalline and amorphous forms. The major crystalline phases are quartz, cristobalite, tridymite, stishovite, and coesite. In general, the toxicity of the crystalline forms of silica is directly related to the temperature and pressure at which the minerals have formed. Thus, tridymite is more toxic than quartz, and cristobalite is more toxic than tridymite.[14,15] Free silica may also exist in cryptocrystalline forms in which minute grains of quartz are cemented together with amorphous silica. Flint, chert, and chalcedony are examples of cryptocrystalline forms of silica. Diatomite and vitreous silica are examples of amorphous silica. In and of itself, amorphous silica is relatively nontoxic; however, in the industrial setting, heating and processing may convert the amorphous silicon dioxide into microcrystalline particles of tridymite and cristobalite. In a critical review, Parkes concluded that studies showing a toxic effect of amorphous silica can largely be accounted for by the presence of contaminating crystalline forms (see Chapter 1, Section II).

Amorphous silica can also exist in biogenic form and may have a fibrous morphology. It occurs in many food crops and in dry plant matter. SiO_2 concentrations have been measured at up to 12% by weight in rice, 3.4 to 5% in wheat and up to 16.4% in corn.[16] A major source of release of this biogenic silica is the burning of wheat, stubble, grass, and sugarcane leaf. Airborne amorphous fibers generated during sugarcane leaf burning were found to measure between 3.5 and 65 microns in length with a mean length of 12 microns and an average diameter of 0.6 microns. The biologic significance of these fibers is uncertain; however, epidemiologic studies have associated biogenic silica with increased risk for cancers of the upper digestive tract and of the lungs and pleural cavities.[16]

II. PATHOGENESIS AND MORPHOGENESIS

Crystalline silica is one of the most toxic minerals known. It is ubiquitous in the environment, and exposure to fine particulates of crystalline silica are common in the industrial and environmental setting. The pathogenesis of silicosis has been extensively researched (see Chapter 1, Section III). Crystalline silica is toxic to a wide range of animal species, including man. Individual susceptibility does not appear to be an important factor in the development of silicosis. Cumulative exposure, intensity of exposure, and latency are the most important factors in determining the type and progression of silicosis in humans.[17]

Examination of human lungs and lungs from experimental animals at various stages and severity of disease indicates that the classic silicotic nodule evolves through a series of immature forms. The evolution of these lesions can be interpreted as an attempt by the body to sequester the silica particles from sensitive tissues and cells. The earliest lesions consist of aggregates of macrophages and histiocytes, which assume a granulomatous arrangement. Lymphocytes are seen within the lesion at this stage. With further maturation, the histiocytic cells assume the characteristics of fibroblasts and the amount of collagen increases. Gradually over a period of several months to several years, the connective tissue fibers become circularly orientated to the center of the lesion. At this stage, the lesion can be confidently diagnosed as a silicotic nodule. Over a period of several years to decades the nodules become more acellular, histiocytic cells and lymphocytes disappear from the body of the lesion, and the collagen fibers become more hyalinized. Finally, central necrosis, calcification, or secondary infection with mycobacteria may occur.

Radiographic studies have shown that silicosis tends to progress even in the absence of continuing exposure.[11,17] It is not possible to determine from autopsy material whether this growth occurs as a result of a chronic stimulus for collagen deposition from silica dust already present within the nodule, or results from the accretion of newly deposited or redistributed dust to its surface.

The mechanism(s) of silica toxicity has remained elusive. Investigations into the pathogenesis of silicosis have focused on four broad areas of research:

A. PHYSICAL AND CHEMICAL PROPERTIES OF PARTICULATE SILICA

On an equivalent weight or surface area basis, the toxicity of silica is much greater than other nonfibrous mineral dusts found in the occupational setting. Theories based on the reaction of silanol (hydroxyl) groups on the particle surface, or hydrogen donation by polymeric silicic acid to form complexes with phospholipids in cell membranes, do not adequately explain the toxicity of silica.[18,19] The formation of silica free radicals on the particle surface may be a factor in the cytotoxicity of the silica.[20–22] The greatest production of free radicals occurs when the mineral is freshly fractured.[21] As the dust ages, free radical formation is reduced. This factor may account for differences in toxicity seen in animal and epidemiologic studies. Other surface properties such as charge, shape (edge effects), and surface area may also play a role in the toxicity of silica but have not been extensively investigated. The toxicity of silica can be markedly reduced by coating of the particle surface or chemical modification. Surface modification experiments include such compounds as organosilane,[23] surfactant,[24,25] polyvinylpyridine-N-oxide (PNO),[26] and aluminum compounds.[27]

B. DEPOSITION, CLEARANCE, AND RETENTION OF SILICA PARTICLES

Several observations indicate that lymphatic injury and obstruction to the lymphatic clearance pathways may be important factors in the pathogenesis of silicosis. Morphologic studies indicate that silica is more likely to be retained in the lung than an "inert" dust or amorphous silica[28–30] and that silica particles become concentrated at convergence points for clearance pathways.[31] At low exposure concentrations, when alveolar clearance mechanisms are presumably intact, the lung parenchyma of silica dust-exposed workers are usually free of disease, and silicotic nodules are only seen in the tracheo-bronchial and intrapulmonary lymph nodes.[32] Once a certain exposure threshold has been breached, it is likely that silica injures lymphatic vessels, impeding clearance of the particles.[33] This would explain the characteristic distribution of parenchymal silicotic nodules along the lymphatic routes in the pleura, interlobular septa and bronchopulmonary rays. At even greater exposure levels, lesions are seen throughout the pulmonary interstitium, and the alveoli become flooded with lipoproteinaceous material (silicolipoproteinosis). These features would indicate that lung liquid clearance is inhibited. Thus lymphatic obstruction could also be a factor in the progressive accumulation of lipoproteinosis material in acute and accelerated silicosis.

C. INTERACTION OF SILICA PARTICLES WITH CELL MEMBRANES, CELLS, TISSUES, AND ORGANS

Regardless of the mechanism, there is extensive evidence that quartz particles are membranolytic and cytotoxic to macrophages and other cells. For further discussion of the many interactions between silica particles and cellular components, see Chapter 1, Section III.

D. CELLULAR AND HUMORAL RESPONSES ASSOCIATED WITH DISEASE AND DISEASE PROGRESSION

Exposure to quartz results in the release of inflammatory cytokines, such as tumor necrosis factor (TNF-α), interleukin-1 (IL-1), interleukin-6 (IL-6), and platelet-derived growth factor (PDGF) from macrophages and possibly from other cells. These cytokines modulate the inflammatory and fibroblastic

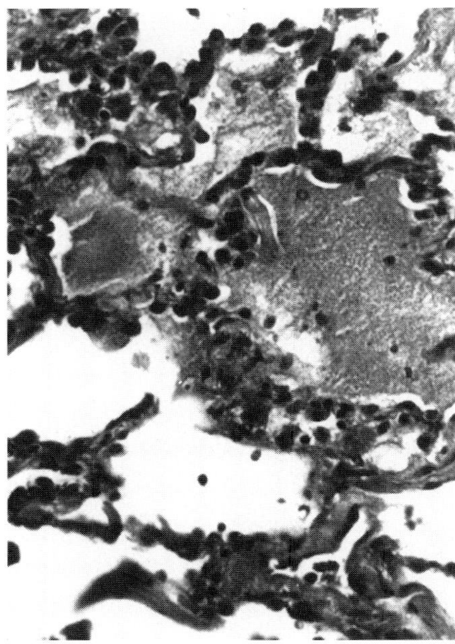

FIGURE 1 Acute silicolipoproteinosis in a 33 year surface coal miner (rock driller). Open lung biopsy section showing granular material within the alveoli.

response and interact, in ways that are currently not understood, to produce the classic nodular and other pathologic features of silicosis. In addition, release of proteolytic enzymes following membrane damage may also play a role in promoting leakage of fluid from blood vessels and lymphatics and in the development of emphysema (see section M.). Activation of T-lymphocytes by inflammatory cytokines may also play an important role in disease progression and systemic effects.[34] A detailed discussion of these factors is beyond the scope of this chapter (see Section III).

III. PATHOLOGICAL FEATURES

A. SILICOLIPOPROTEINOSIS (ACUTE SILICOSIS)

Acute silicolipoproteinosis is a rapidly progressive form of silicosis with a high mortality rate. It follows intense exposure to crystalline silicon dioxide, usually in the form of quartz, but also to the more fibrogenic polymorphs, cristobalite and tridymite. It may develop after only six months of such exposure. It has been described in workers involved in tunneling,[35] sandblasting,[36] silica flour mill operations,[37] rock drilling, and in the ceramic industry.[38,39] These activities produce fine particles of quartz (<1 μm) with cleaved or sheared surfaces rich in relatively short-lived free radicals of Si and SiO.[20,21] Small particle size and "freshness" of the particle surface are important factors in silica particle toxicity.

The lungs from fatal cases at autopsy are heavy and firm, and their cut surfaces exude glistening fluid. The lungs may have a slightly nodular texture. The gross appearances of the lungs are similar to those observed in other forms of alveolar lipoproteinosis.[40] The gross appearances should be distinguished from acute pulmonary edema. In this condition, the lungs are softer and exude frothy blood-tinged fluid, which is maximal in the dependent zones.

Microscopically, the fluid within the alveoli in alveolar lipoproteinosis bears a superficial resemblance to classic alveolar edema. However, it is a deeper pink on hematoxylin and eosin (H&E) stained sections and at high magnification it has a finely granular appearance (Figure 1) and may contain cholesterol clefts. The material stains magenta with periodic acid-Schiff method (PAS) and is resistant to diastase digestion. It is nonreactive with traditional mucin stains.[39,40] It contains abundant lipid which is best seen on frozen sections stained by Oil Red O or Sudan Black. There is usually an associated chronic interstitial pneumonitis. Granulomatous inflammation and early silicotic nodules may also be seen. These inflammatory and fibrotic changes, when present, help to differentiate silicolipoproteinosis from other forms of alveolar lipoproteinosis which do not have an interstitial or inflammatory component. Birefringent particles may be seen within the alveoli on polarizing microscopy; however, in most cases the particles are below the limits of resolution of the light microscope (<0.5 μm). The alveoli are lined by prominent type II cells which have been shown to be both hypertrophic and hyperplastic.[41] Surfactant apoprotein has been demonstrated immunohistochemically in human lungs showing alveolar lipoproteinosis.[42] This is associated with increases in surfactant phospholipids and surfactant proteins.[41] Electron microscopy of the alveolar material shows that it largely consists of multilaminated structures, membranous vesicles, granules, and other electron opaque materials. Abnormal tubular myelin-like multilaminated structures account for 30 to 60% of the total particulate volume.[43]

Silica is one of many agents that can increase phospholipid levels in the lung. These include oxidant gases, particulates, soluble agents, and therapeutic agents with amphiphilic cationic properties (see Chapter 8, Section III). A history of exposure to dust or fumes has been elicited in about half the reported cases of alveolar lipoproteinosis,[40] including exposure to wood dust, kaolin, aluminium, cement, welding fumes, and cadmium, in addition to silica. Backscatter electron microscopy in combination with X-ray microanalysis of the alveolar material has been used to demonstrate particulates in 78% of cases of lipoproteinosis.[44] These particles are usually very small and below the resolution of the light microscope.

Experimental studies have shown that silica induces hyperplasia and hypertrophy of alveolar type II cells associated with massive accumulation of intracellular and extracellular phospholipids in the lung. The number of lamellar bodies is also greatly increased in the hypertrophic cells, indicating increased biosynthesis of phospholipid and surfactant protein-A.[45–47] Enhanced secretion alone cannot account for the progressive accumulation of the surfactant materials. Recent experimental evidence indicates that imbalances between biosynthesis, secretion, and clearance are also important.[48] Because of the many morphological and biochemical similarities between human and experimental silicosis, it is likely that similar mechanisms are involved in the pathogenesis of human disease. Silica may be a particularly potent inducer of alveolar-lipoproteinosis in view of its cytotoxic effects on the alveolar capillary membrane,[49] leading to alveolar flooding. Analysis of fluid from patients with alveolar lipoproteinosis reveals large amounts of protein in addition to phospholipid.[41] Serum proteins and, in particular, fibrinogen are potent inhibitors of surfactant activity,[50,51] and they may, in part, account for the loss of normal surface active properties of material extracted from lung specimens.[52]

B. ACCELERATED SILICOSIS

This form of the disease is associated with high to moderately intense exposure and has a latency of 1 to 14 years. It has been described in men exposed to dust in silica flour mill operations,[37] during the manufacture of slate pencils, and in shipyard sandblasters[53] and stonemasons.[36]

In this condition, the exudative alveolar response of acute silicosis[54] may progress to a predominantly interstitial process characterized by chronic inflammation and the formation of cellular fibrotic nodules. The latter contain histiocytic cells enmeshed in a variable amount of mature and immature collagen and reticulin. Some of the lesions have the appearance of granulomas (Figure 2); others show a greater number of fibroblasts with circular orientation of the collagen fibers. The latter are the immature form of the hyalinized classic nodule of chronic simple silicosis described below. From the description it can be seen that accelerated silicosis occupies an intermediate position, showing some of the features of acute silicosis at one extreme and of chronic nodular silicosis at the other.

C. CHRONIC SIMPLE SILICOSIS

This is the most common form of lung disease associated with the inhalation of crystalline silica. The disease may take several decades of low intensity exposure to become apparent on the chest radiograph. Thereafter the disease may progress slowly over many years. Epidemiologic studies based on chest radiography have shown that the overall density and size of the silicotic nodules are primarily determined by cumulative exposure and latency.

The characteristic pathologic lesion is the silicotic nodule. Macroscopically, the nodules appear as rounded, firm to hard regions of fibrosis that are sharply demarcated from the surrounding lung parenchyma (Figure 3). They range in size from a few millimeters to several centimeters in diameter. The nodules are more common in the upper and posterior regions of the lung and frequently involve the visceral pleura. They are seen in greatest density in regions of the lung rich in lymphatic channels. These sites include pleura, interlobular septa, and peribronchial connective tissues. They are not confined to

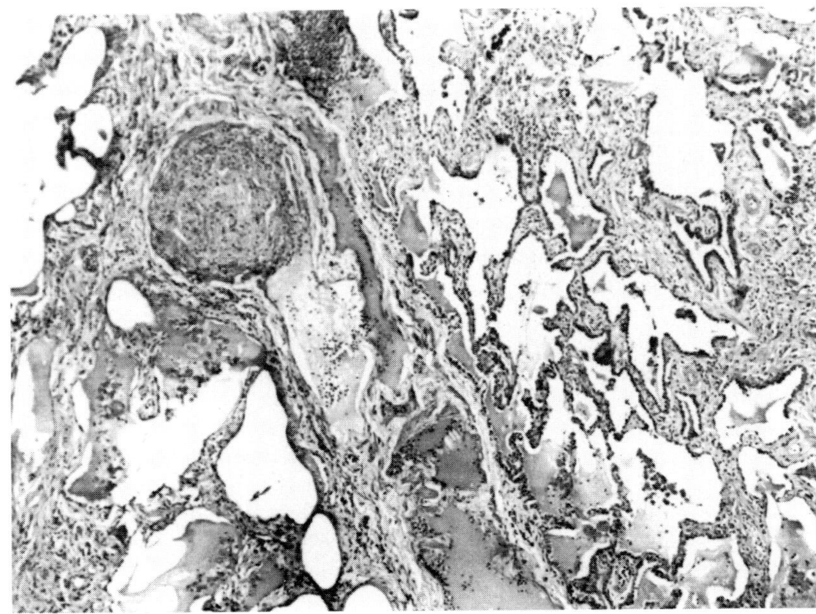

FIGURE 2 Accelerated silicosis. Low magnification view showing thickened alveolar septa lined by hyperplastic type II cells and enclosing lipoproteinacous material. An evolving silicotic nodule is seen at bottom left.

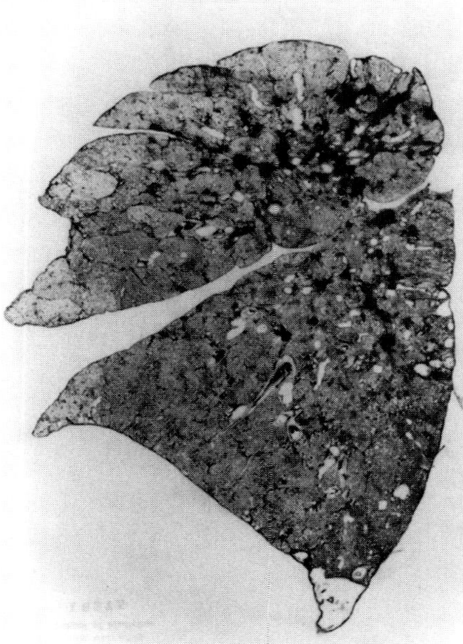

FIGURE 3 Chronic simple silicosis in a coal miner. Whole lung section showing round silicotic nodules predominantly in the upper zone of the lung. Many of the nodules have pale centers, and there is a tendency of the nodules to coalesce.

these sites, however, and may originate in any part of the lung parenchyma, including the peripheral interstitium and even within the alveoli.[55] The center of the cut surface of the classic lesion is pale but may become pigmented due to concomitant exposure to carbonaceous dust. They frequently show calcification.

The microscopic appearance of the simple silicotic nodule is characteristic and unlikely to be confused with other pathologies. In its mature form, the nodule is composed of concentrically arranged, whorled bundles of hyalinized collagen showing variable calcification within the center (Figure 4). The nodule itself may be relatively free of pigmentation but is usually surrounded by a more cellular periphery consisting of dust-containing macrophages, fibroblasts, reticulin, and occasional lymphocytes. Polarizing microscopy reveals dull, birefringent particles, consistent with quartz, primarily within the center of the hyalinized nodule. Brightly birefringent particles with acicular and needle-shaped profiles, indicative of silicates, are also commonly present and tend to be concentrated at the periphery of a lesion. Identification of the chemical nature of the particles can be performed *in situ* on 5 μm paraffin sections using backscatter electron imaging and X-ray microanalysis (Figure 5).[56]

Parenchymal silicosis is almost invariably associated with the development of silicotic nodules within the lymph nodes. However, the reverse is not true, and many individuals develop nodules in the lymph nodes without having parenchymal silicosis.[32,33] It is therefore important not to make the diagnosis of silicosis based on examination of lymph nodes alone.

D. SILICA CONTENT OF HUMAN LUNGS

The mean number of exogenous mineral particles in the lungs of urban dwellers without specific occupational exposures has been shown to be approximately 508 (±417 SD) × 10^6 per gram of dry lung.[57] Approximately 18% of these mineral dust particles had a chemistry consistent with silica. The other major mineral species were aluminum silicates (38%), rutile (10%), iron oxide (6%), and magnesium (3%). This burden of mineral dust was not associated with the development of disease. By contrast, the lungs of patients with silicosis may contain up to 16,000 × 10^6 exogenous mineral particles per gram of dry lung of which up to 50% may be silica.[57] Gravimetric analyses of silica content of normal lungs have shown that approximately 0.1 to 0.2% of dry tissue is comprised of silica dust and pulmonary lymph nodes may contain from 0.23 to 0.6% silica.[14] The silica content of silicotic lungs may be as high as 20% of the dry weight[35] but more commonly is in the range of 2 to 5%.[58,59]

E. PROGRESSIVE MASSIVE FIBROSIS

Silicotic progressive massive fibrosis (PMF) is a large fibrotic lesion that is somewhat arbitrarily distinguished from the classic nodule on the basis of size. The Silicosis and Silicate Disease Committee of NIOSH recommended that PMF be defined as a lesion greater than 2 cm in diameter.[39] However, the radiologic definition of PMF, established by the International Labor Office (ILO), defines PMF as an opacity on the chest X-ray that is 1 cm in diameter or greater.[60] The situation is further complicated by the fact that radiologic size, assessed on the chest film, may not be identical to pathologic size due to the divergence of the X-ray beam from its source to the film. A radio-dense nodule with an actual size of 1 cm situated in the anterior thorax will appear approximately the same size on a standard postero-anterior film; whereas the same nodule in the posterior thorax would appear approximately 15% larger.[133] For this reason, and because there are important legal implications in making a diagnosis of PMF, we recommend that pathologists document the exact size of the larger nodular lesions in the lungs of a patient with silicosis.

PMF is formed by the coalescence and agglomeration of smaller nodules. It is usually symmetrically bilateral and may undergo cavitation. It is associated with destruction of the lung parenchyma and broncho-vascular structures. Marked distortion of the adjacent lung is seen due to contraction of the fibrosis (Plate 1*). Mycobacterial infection should be suspected in cases showing cavitation and appropriate attempts made to isolate and identify the organisms.

Histologically, PMF shows discrete and coalescing silicotic nodules enclosing areas of cavitation and necrosis (Figure 6). Silicotic alveolar proteinosis may be present adjacent to the areas of fibrosis.[1] Elastic stains are useful in these advanced lesions to demonstrate widespread destruction of blood vessels and airways.

F. PLEURAL AND LYMPH NODE LESIONS

Subpleural silicotic nodules are a common feature of silicosis. They appear as pale elevated domes above the pleural surface surrounded by a zone of black pigmentation. They have been termed candle wax

* Plate 1 follows page 50.

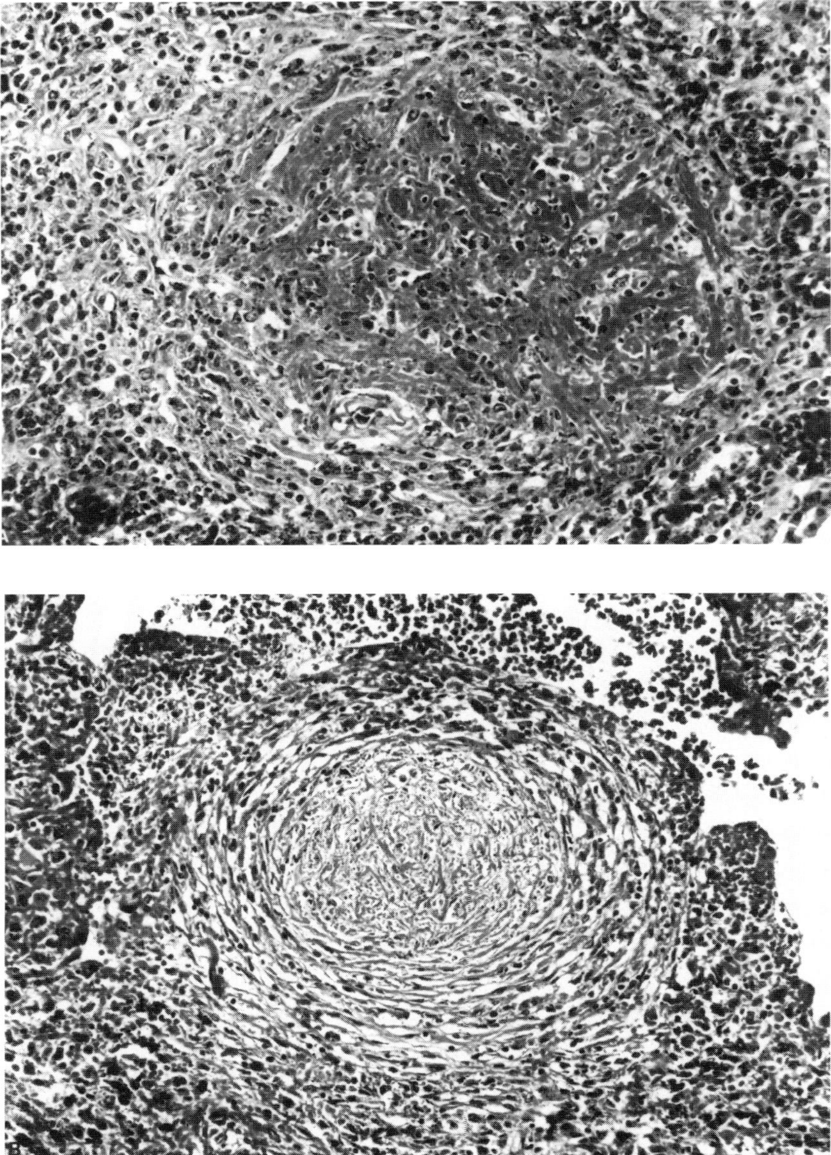

FIGURE 4 Chronic simple silicosis. The four photomicrographs show the classic silicotic nodule at varying stages of evolution. A. Silicotic nodule in granulomatous phase. The lesion is composed predominantly of histiocytic cells, collagen fibers, and lymphocytes. The orientation of the collagen fibers is not apparent at this stage. B. Cellular fibrotic nodule containing irregularly arranged collagen at center with circularly arranged collagen at the periphery. Histiocytes and lymphocytes are prominent in this lesion. C. More mature nodule: the center of the lesion is acellular and avascular. Small amounts of dust are trapped within the circularly orientated collagen fibers. A cellular mantle of macrophages and pigment is seen at the periphery. D. Mature nodule in late stages. The outline of the nodual is circular, apart from a small mantle of dust and macrophages. The nodual is composed entirely of dust and collagen, and the center has become calcified.

lesions because of these characteristic features.[39] Histologically, the nodules have a hyalinized core with the concentric arrangement of collagen fibers seen in the classic silicotic nodule (Figure 7A). The overlying pleura is fibrotic. Adjacent lesions may coalesce to form a network of lesions. Pleural pearls have been described in association with these lesions and may represent sequestration of subpleural nodules into the pleural cavity[134] (Figure 7B). Silicotic pleural lesions should not be confused with asbestos pleural plaques which form on the parietal aspect of the pleural surface.

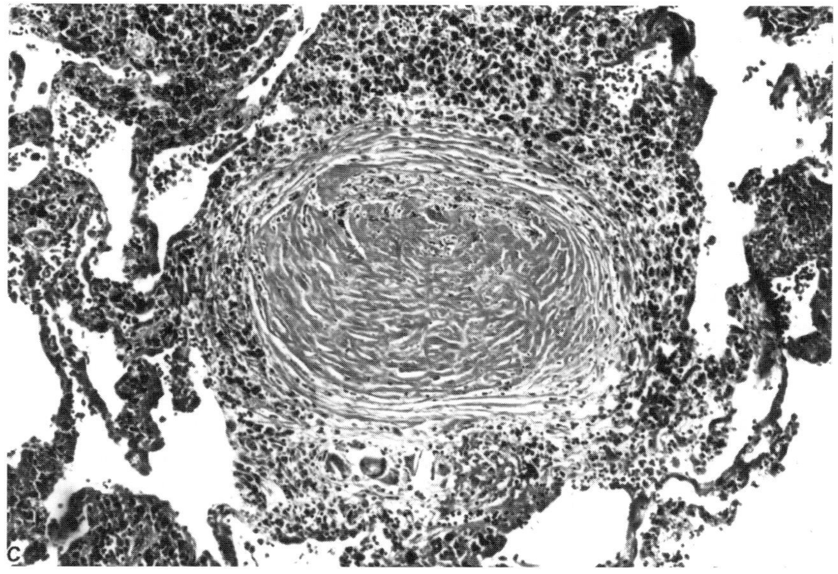

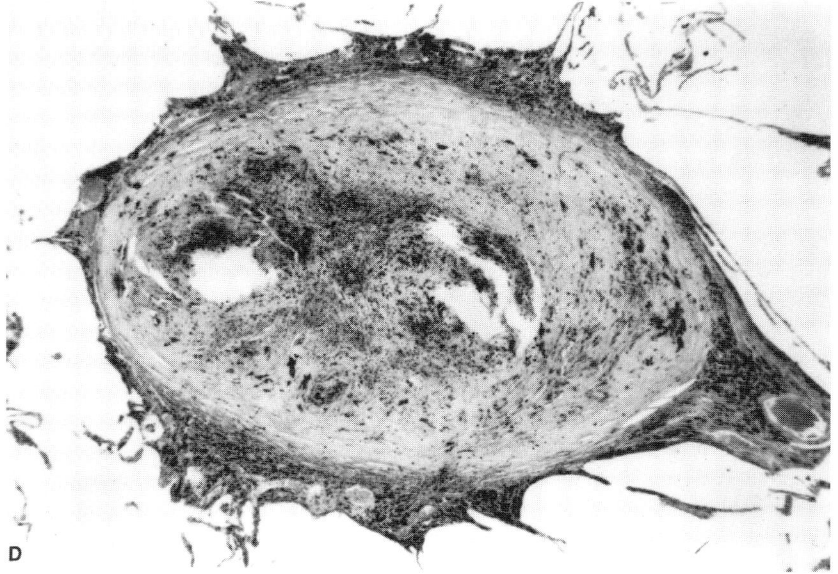

FIGURE 4 (continued)

Exposure to silica is also associated with the development of fibrotic nodules in the hilar lymph nodes (Figure 8),[32,33] and at distant sites (see section P.). It has been suggested that the development of fibrotic nodules in the lymph nodes may predispose to the subsequent development of parenchymal silicosis[33] due to the obstruction of the lymphatic drainage of the lung with resultant increase in lung dust burden.

G. MIXED DUST PNEUMOCONIOSIS

This term was originally applied by Uehlinger in 1946 to a form of nodular fibrosis caused by free silica in combination with less fibrogenic dusts such as iron oxide, silicates and coal.[61] The term is only applied to those situations where the silica is inhaled at the same time as the other dusts.[14] Mixed dust fibrosis has been described in workers in the following industries: hematite mining (free silica and iron oxide), slate quarrying (quartz, muscovite),[62] iron and steel foundries (quartz, tridymite, or cristobalite

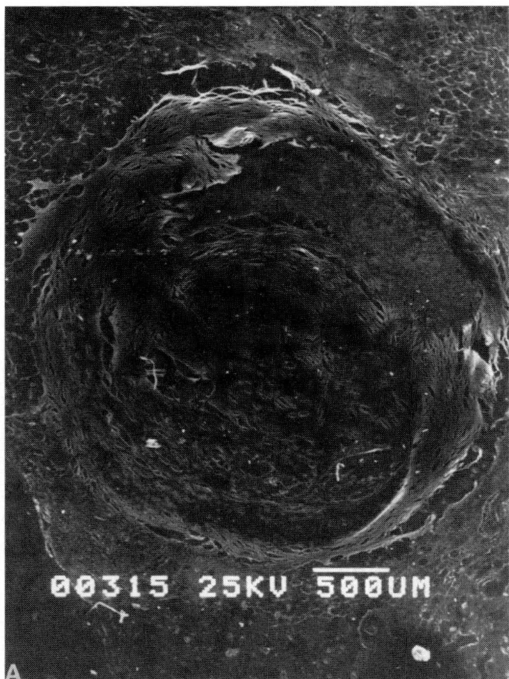

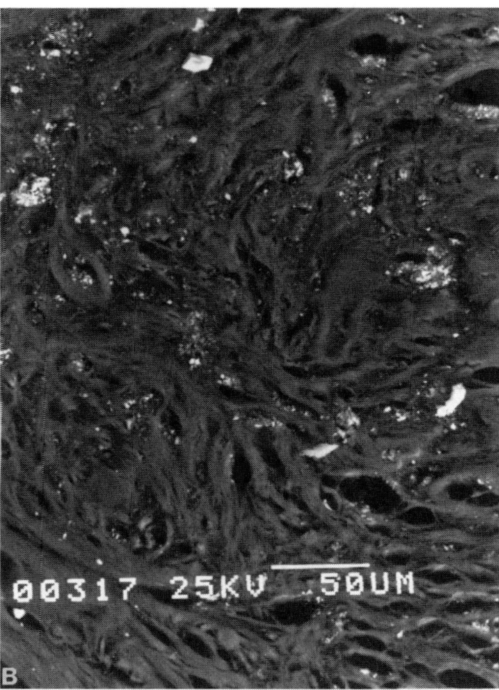

FIGURE 5 Scanning electron micrographs of a 5 micron, deparaffinized section of silicotic nodule mounted on a carbon stub. A. The orientation of the collagen fibers is apparent when viewed in secondary electron mode. B. Backscattered electron image from center of lesion showing large numbers of high atomic number particles embedded in the collagenous stroma. X-ray microprobe analysis of these particles (data not shown) revealed that the majority had a chemistry consistent with silicon dioxide.

and iron oxide), welding (quartz and iron oxide fumes), oil shale mining (quartz, mica, and kaolin), ceramic and china clay industry (quartz, kaolinite, and mica), coal mining (quartz, aluminosilicates, carbonates, and feldspars), and manufacture of silicon carbide abrasives[63,64] and other dusts.[14,65]

The amount of quartz in the dust varies but is usually less than 20%; above this level, the pathology more closely resembles classic nodular silicosis.[15] A variety of experimental and human evidence indicates that quartz is less fibrogenic in the presence of these other minerals. The ability of coal dust to reduce quartz fibrogenesis is considerable. In one experiment, Rhesus monkeys exposed to coal dust containing 40% quartz failed to produce classic silicotic lesions.[66] This mitigating effect has also been studied in rats where it was thought that it resulted from non-quartz silicates and other minerals in the coal.[67] Iron oxide is potent at mitigating fibrogenesis in experimental situations.[68] Studies of deceased miners also indicate that iron hydroxide may be effective in preventing quartz fibrogenesis.[69] Metallic aluminum dust and aluminum lactate have also been used to inhibit silicosis in experimental animals.[27,70,71] Based on the results of the early studies, aluminum inhalation was employed in an attempt to prevent the development of silicosis in gold miners during the early 1940s to the mid 1950s.[14] The results of these trials were not successful.[14,72]

The distribution of the nodules of mixed dust fibrosis is similar to that seen for silicosis and coal workers' pneumoconiosis (CWP).[39,73] The nodules range in size from 2 mm to 1 cm or more and may show varying degrees of pigmentation depending on the composition of the dust. The mixed dust nodule has a more irregular border than the classic silicotic nodule, and the fibrosis tends to extend out into the surrounding lung parenchyma.

Microscopically, the nodules show irregularly arranged, interlacing bundles of collagen and reticulin fibers interspersed with dust. The concentric arrangement of fibers typical of the classic silicotic nodule is not seen. The dust is uniformly distributed throughout the nodule, and polarizing microscopy commonly reveals brightly birefringent silicates in addition to occasional particles of the less birefringent quartz. A distinctive feature of the mixed dust nodule is an irregular or serpiginous border, with

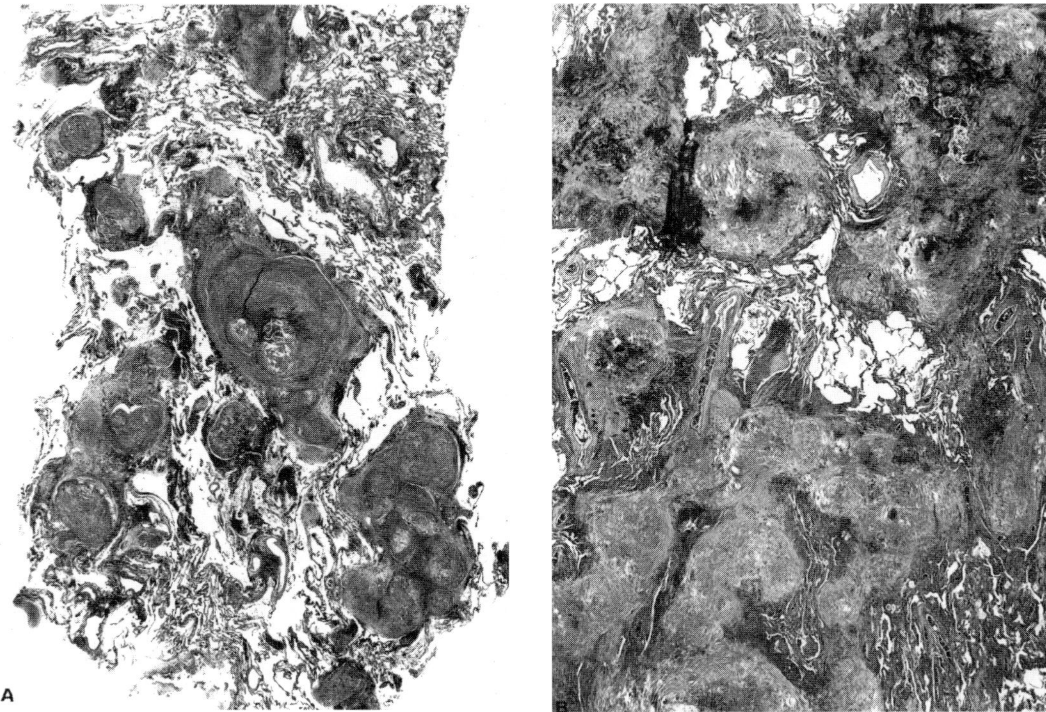

FIGURE 6 Silicotic progressive massive fibrosis. A. Section of lung from miner with advanced simple silicosis showing fusion of discrete silicotic nodules to form massive lesions. B. More advanced stage of silicotic progressive massive fibrosis showing fusion of multiple nodules to form large conglomerate areas of fibrosis in which the outlines of individual nodules can still be discerned. Several areas within the fibrosis show cavitation, a feature characteristic of massive fibrosis.

finger-like extensions into the adjacent interstitium (Figure 9). Although calcification and necrosis can occur, these features are uncommon. Massive fibrosis and tuberculous pneumoconiosis may arise in association with mixed dust fibrosis. Macules, interstitial fibrosis, and ferruginous bodies may also be associated with mixed dust pneumoconiosis.[39]

H. SILICOSIS IN COAL WORKERS

Exposure to quartz at underground and surface coal mines depends on a number of factors including the thickness of the seam, the composition of the adjacent rock strata, faults and undulations, method of mining, and specific job of the miner. Miners employed in transportation, roof bolting, and tunnel drilling are at much greater risk of developing silicosis than miners employed in other job categories.[32,75–77] Marked regional differences in the prevalence of silicosis have been found. In an autopsy study of U.S. underground coal miners, a very high prevalence of silicosis (35%) was noted in miners previously employed in the eastern anthracite coal fields of Pennsylvania. This finding is in keeping with epidemiologic studies documenting a high prevalence of pneumoconiosis in anthracite miners.[78] By state, Pennsylvania had the highest overall prevalence of silicosis (15%) followed by Wyoming and Utah (14.2%), West Virginia (13.7%), Colorado (9.5%), Virginia (6.5%), Illinois (5.2%), Kentucky (4.5%), and Ohio (4.1%).[32]

Although the majority of nodular lesions in coal workers can be considered to be of the mixed dust variety, classic silicotic nodules are also seen in the lungs of coal workers. Many of these contain a central hyalinized and concentrically arranged core of collagen surrounded by a heavily pigmented border of irregularly arranged collagen and reticulin (Figure 10). A study of autopsy specimens from U.S. underground coal workers submitted to the National Coal Workers Autopsy program revealed that 12.5% of the population showed classic silicotic nodules in the lung parenchyma. A much larger proportion (53%) showed silicotic nodules in the tracheobronchial lymph nodes (Table 1).[32] Furthermore, an exposure-response relationship was noted for both extent and severity of silicotic lesions in the lung parenchyma.

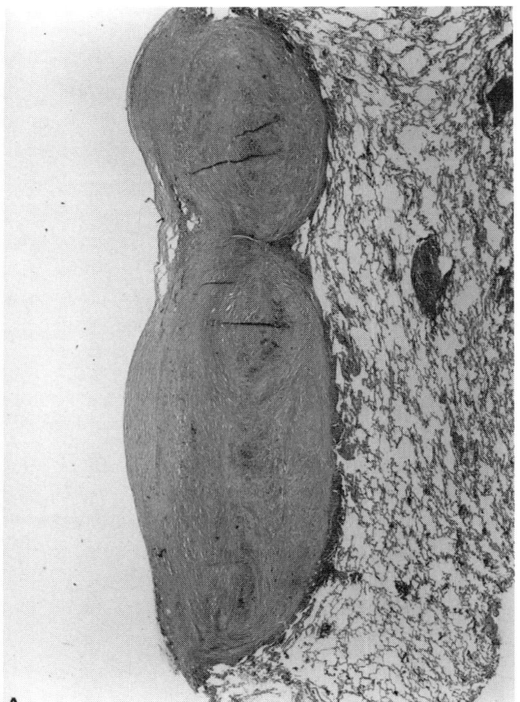

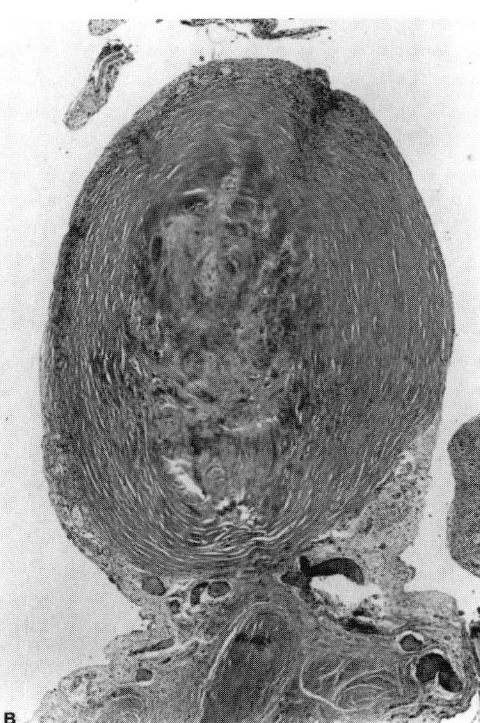

FIGURE 7 Pleural lesions: A. Subpleural silicotic nodule:[23] This section shows two fused nodules with characteristic concentric arrangement of the collagen fibers. The surface of the nodule projects from the pleural surface and compresses the adjacent underlying lung. B. Pleural Pearl: the silicotic nodule projects from the pleural surface. Other lesions were detached from the pleural surface.

A reliable diagnosis of silicosis in coal workers can only be made at autopsy or lung biopsy,[39,73] as it is impossible on routine chest radiography to distinguish the nodules of CWP from those of silicosis.[60] It is also possible by pathologic examination to distinguish silicotic nodules from those associated with infections (for example, tuberculosis and histoplasmosis) and from nonspecific scars in the lung. A radiographic feature that does appear to correlate with the presence of silicosis pathologically is the presence of r-type opacities.[79,80] However, this is a statistical association and is of limited usefulness in the diagnosis of an individual case. A radiographic sign that is thought to be indicative of silicosis is egg-shell calcification of the tracheo-bronchial and hilar lymph nodes.[14] Calcification is a nonspecific response to injury and may be seen in inflammatory and infectious conditions as well as chronic fibrosing conditions such as silicosis. Moreover, the high prevalence of silicotic nodules in tracheo-bronchial lymph nodes in U.S. coal miners in the absence of parenchymal lesions would indicate that the sign has little diagnostic usefulness for predicting the presence of parenchymal silicosis.[32]

I. RHEUMATOID PNEUMOCONIOSIS

Rheumatoid pneumoconiosis is a rare condition characterized by rapidly evolving large radiologic opacities, particularly in the peripheral areas of the lung in patients with rheumatoid disease or with sera positive for rheumatoid factor.[14] Macroscopically, the lesions exhibit alternate laminations of light and dark areas due to zones of dust deposited within areas of necrosis. They range in size from 0.5 to 5 cm, tend to be located in the periphery of the lung, and, unlike PMF, occur against a background of mild pneumoconiosis. They have a similar appearance to those seen in coal workers.[39,55] Microscopically they consist of a central zone of fibrinoid necrosis surrounded by pallisaded histiocytes and variable numbers of polymorphous neutrophils, lymphocytes, and fibroblasts. They can only be reliably distinguished from mycotic and mycobacterial infectious nodules through culture and appropriate histologic stains.

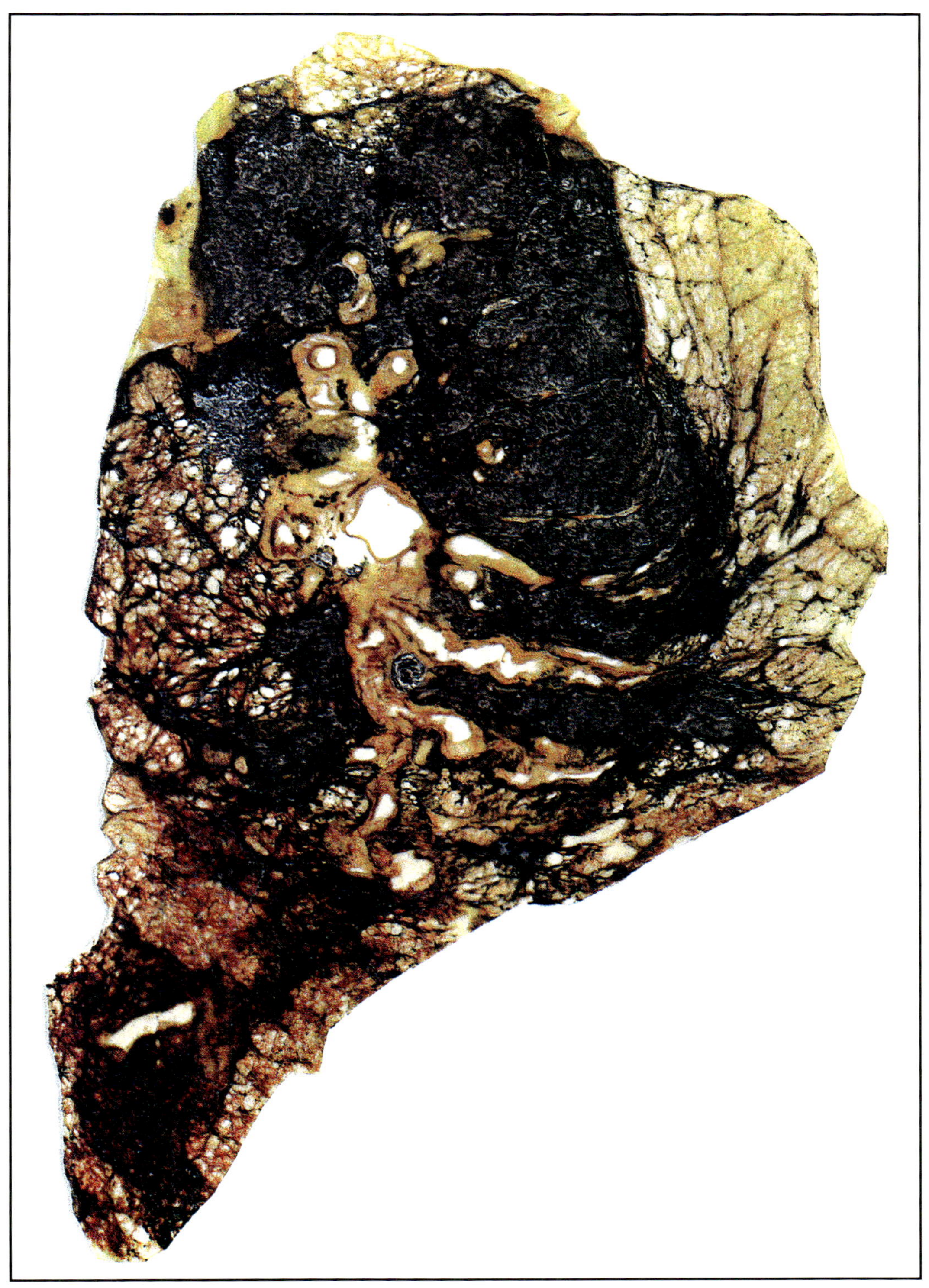

SECTION I, CHAPTER 5, PLATE 1

Whole lung section of silicotic progressive massive fibrosis.

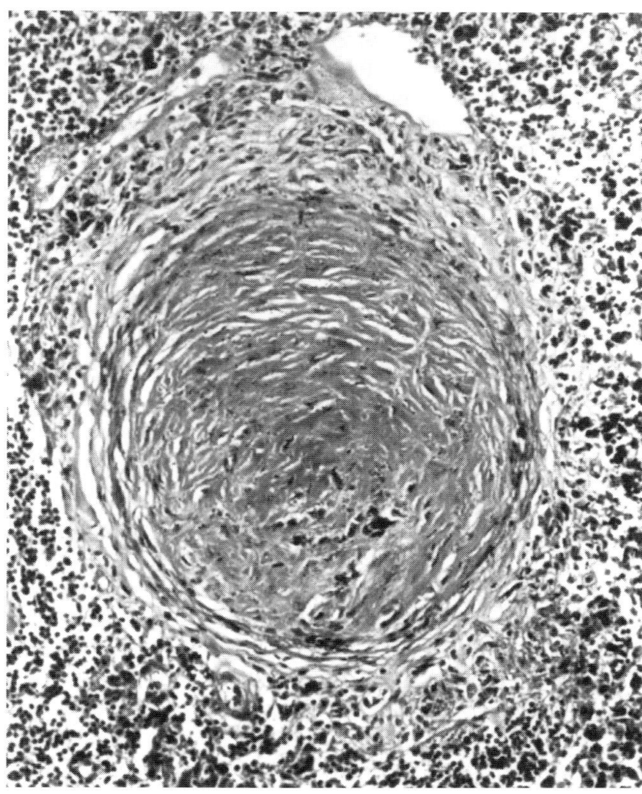

FIGURE 8 Silicotic nodule in a lymph node. The nodule is morphologically identical to those found in the pulmonary parenchyma. The periphery consists of lymphoid tissue.

J. SILICO-TUBERCULOSIS

Tuberculosis is a common complication of silicosis that may occur at any stage in the evolution of the disease but is more likely to occur in older workers with severe grades of silicosis.[14,81] Historically, death from tuberculosis among miners has been of epidemic proportions.[82,83] In the early 20th century, the average working life of a black South African gold miner was 5 years,[84] and pulmonary tuberculosis was a major contributor to death in virtually every instance.[85] Indeed, the association of mining with tuberculosis has been so strong that a clear distinction between silicosis alone and silicosis with tuberculosis was not made until 1935.[86] Since that time the incidence of tuberculosis has progressively decreased with the initial enforcement of dust control measures in 1912, the development of drug regimens that could cure tuberculosis in 1950, and the institution of short-course chemotherapy in 1977.[82] Despite these advances the incidence of tuberculosis remains high in black South African gold miners. A group of 1,153 gold miners without evidence of tuberculosis at entry in 1984 was followed for 7 years by a routine mine surveillance program for detection of tuberculosis.[81] The incidence of tuberculosis increased from 1% per annum for 335 men without silicosis to 2.2% in miners with Category I silicosis, to 2.9% for those with Category 2, and to 6.3% for those with Category 3. An increased risk for pulmonary tuberculosis with higher grades of silicosis has also been reported in a recent study of Danish foundry workers.[87]

The clinical features vary, but rapid radiologic progression, cavitation (unilateral), and hemoptysis are all highly suspicious of tuberculous infection in a person with pre-existing silicosis. Tuberculosis in a person exposed to silica dust may be difficult to distinguish from PMF and rheumatoid pneumoconiosis, both clinically and pathologically; hence, a high degree of suspicion combined with appropriate bacteriologic study is required to establish the diagnosis.

The predilection of mycobacteria to colonize and proliferate in silicotic lung tissue is not confined to *M. tuberculosis*. Other pathogenic mycobacteria: *M. avium-intracellulare*, *M. scrofulaceum*, and *M.*

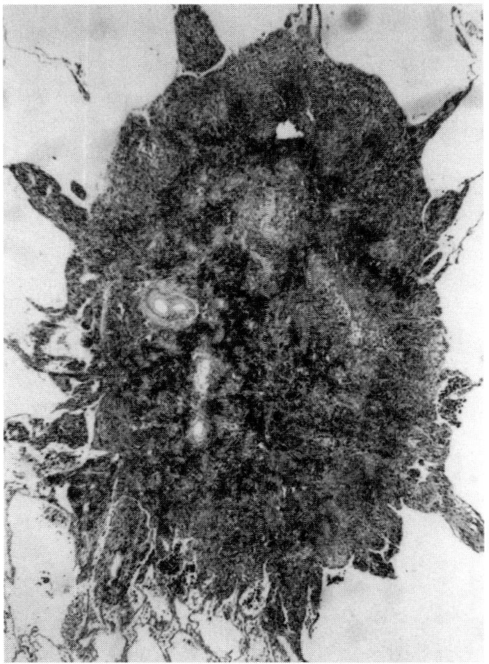

FIGURE 9 Characteristic mixed dust nodule in a coal worker. Note that the nodule is composed of interlacing bundles of collagen mixed with pigment and that there is no central orientation of the collagen fibers. The irregular serpiginous borders are characteristic of the mixed dust nodule.

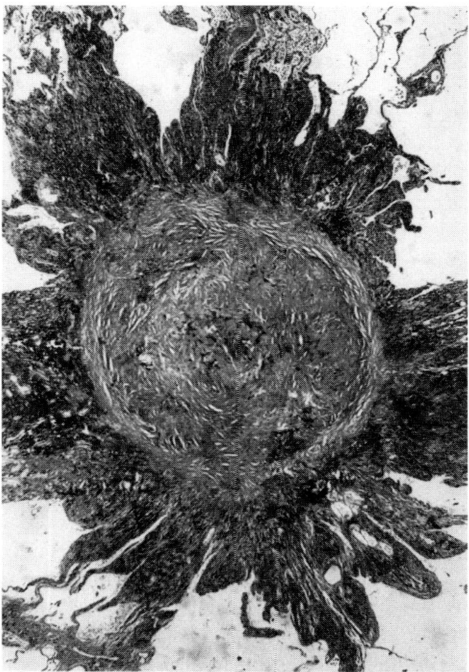

FIGURE 10 Silicotic nodule in a coal miner. The lesion is composed of a central silicotic nodule with characteristic circular arrangement of the collagen fibers surmounted by an irregular mantle of pigment, collagen, and reticulin extending out into the adjacent interstitum. These lesions have the appearance of classic silicotic nodules at the center and mixed dust nodules at the periphery, sometimes referred to as *anthracosilicosis* in the literature. (From Churg, A. and Green, F.H.Y., *Pathology of Occupational Lung Diseases*, Igaku-Shoin Medical Publishers, New York, 1988, 138.)

TABLE 1
Silicotic Nodules, Coal Dust Nodules, and Coal Macules in U.S. Coal Miners at Autopsy

Pathologic Type	Percent Positive
Silicotic nodule (parenchyma)	12.6
Silicotic nodule (lymph node)	52.9
Mixed dust nodules (parenchyma)	18.9
Coal dust macules	45.6

Data from U.S. National Coal Workers Autopsy Study.

kansasii have also been implicated, and nonpathogenic mycobacteria such as photochromogenic and nonphotochromogenic mycobacteria may colonize the lung and be isolated in the sputum.[88] The potentiating effect of silica dust on tuberculosis infection has been confirmed in other species[89] for both pathogenic and nonpathogenic strains of mycobacteria.[90] The mechanism that accounts for the enhancement of mycobacterial infection is not known with certainty. Most theories implicate the pulmonary macrophage. *In vitro* experimental studies have shown that macrophages dusted with silica are unable to kill mycobacterium tuberculosis[91,92] or even usually nonpathogenic mycobacteria.[93] However, the relevance of these studies to human disease is uncertain, as macrophages obtained from men with silicosis have been shown to have normal viability and function.[94]

It is of interest that tuberculosis and silicosis both favor the apices of the lung. It has been proposed that this is not fortuitous but results from impaired clearance mechanisms in this region.[95] Although this concept would provide a unifying hypothesis for the synergism between the two diseases, it would not account for the finding of increased extrapulmonary tuberculosis in men with silicosis.[81] The latter would implicate a systemic abnormality of immune function.

K. INTERSTITIAL FIBROSIS

Diffuse or focal interstitial fibrosis may be seen in association with the nodular lesions of chronic silicosis (Figure 2). This form of pulmonary fibrosis is more common in workers exposed to a combination of silica and silicates[96] and workers exposed to diatomaceous earth which contains a high concentration of cristobalite.[97,98] The interstitial fibrosis is usually of mild severity but may be sufficiently severe to result in honeycombing and respiratory failure.

L. VASCULAR LESIONS AND COR PULMONALE

Chronic cor pulmonale is defined as right ventricular hypertrophy due to structural or functional abnormalities of the lungs.[99] Advanced silicosis is associated with the development of pulmonary hypertension and cor pulmonale.[100,101] A recent case-control study of 732 South African gold miners showed that the risk for cor pulmonale increased with severity of silicosis.[102] Both chronic hypoxia and vascular obliterative changes probably contribute to the development of the cor pulmonale. The latter are common in silicosis due to the encroachment of silicotic nodules and lesions of massive fibrosis on the pulmonary vessels. Elastin stains are useful for the demonstration of obliterated and partially obliterated blood vessels in, and adjacent to, the lesions of silicosis.

M. EMPHYSEMA AND CHRONIC AIRFLOW OBSTRUCTION

Mortality studies of white South African gold miners have shown an association between cumulative dust exposure and death from chronic respiratory diseases (bronchitis, emphysema, and pneumoconiosis).[103–106] In these studies, both smoking and silica dust exposure were demonstrated to be major risk factors. Post-mortem examination of 1,553 lungs from autopsied white South African gold miners showed a positive association between cumulative dust exposure and both centriacinar and panacinar emphysema.[107] Centriacinar, but not panacinar emphysema, was also associated with the presence of silicosis in the lung. Animal experimental studies have also linked silica dust exposure with the subsequent development of small airway lesions and emphysema.[108] The emerging findings, with respect to the association between emphysema and silica dust exposure, are similar to those found for coal miners.[55]

N. AIRWAY LESIONS

Direct extension of silicotic lesions into the airway walls is a rare complication of silicosis[6] and is the only noninfectious cause of broncholithiasis.[109] Patients present with cough, hemoptysis, lithoptysis, pneumonia, fistula formation, and varying degrees of airway obstruction. Biopsy of the lesion may reveal florid granulation tissue and/or secondary infection overlying the calcified silicotic nodule.[6]

O. SILICOSIS AND LUNG CANCER

The relationship between silica exposure, silicosis, and lung cancer is controversial and has yet to be adequately resolved. Human epidemiologic and case registry studies have on balance shown that workers in industries exposed to silica, or individuals with silicosis, have a higher mortality from lung cancer than control populations[110–112] (see Chapter 2, Section V). Unfortunately most of these studies have not been adequately controlled for possible effects of confounding factors such as exposure to cigarette smoke, asbestos, polycyclic hydrocarbons, and radon gas. Furthermore, no clear dose-response relationship has been demonstrated in the positive studies. Animal studies have in general shown increased lung tumors in animal inhalation studies,[113] and, based on these data, the International Agency for Research on Cancer (IARC) classified silica as probable human carcinogen in 1987.[114] The relevance of the animal studies can be questioned as the studies show species and gender differences and little evidence for a dose-response relationship.[111] Moreover, recent evidence implicates particle loading rather than a specific agent as the trigger for development of lung tumors in rodents[115] (see also Chapter 1, Section V).

Unfortunately, very few pathologic studies have been conducted on appropriate populations. Well controlled pathologic studies could be used to determine whether silica influences the distribution of cell types (histogenesis), and microanalytical procedures could be used to determine the amount of silica and the presence of other mineral types, such as asbestos, and metals, such as arsenic. An autopsy study of South African gold miners found an increased prevalence of lung cancer in miners with silicotic nodules in the lymph node but not of the lung parenchyma.[116] The author speculated that reduced lymphatic clearance as a result of silica exposure may impede clearance of inhaled carcinogens.

P. SYSTEMIC EFFECTS OF SILICA EXPOSURE

Silica exposure is associated with local and systemic alterations in immune function.[3,38,103,117] These latter effects may account for the association of silicosis with scleroderma,[93,118] renal abnormalities,[119,120] hepatic abnormalities,[121] rheumatoid pneumoconiosis,[14,122] and susceptibility to infection with mycobacterium *tuberculosis* and *mycobacterium* avium *intracellulare*.

Scleroderma in association with silica exposure may be atypical in that the skin disease is often localized[123] and that other features of scleroderma, such as Raynaud's phenomena, microstoma, and systemic involvement, may be absent.[14] A recent survey of male patients with scleroderma in East Germany revealed that 93 of 120 (78%) had evidence of long term exposure to silica dust.[118] Antinuclear antibodies, antibodies against double stranded DNA, and anticentromere antibodies together with abnormalities of collagen metabolism were found in some, but not all, patients. The investigators proposed that crystalline particles of silica activate macrophages to release lymphokines and monokines, which in turn activate fibroblasts to synthesize collagen and glycosaminoglycans. They also proposed that silica may act as an adjuvant to increase immuno-reactivity. A more direct local effect of silica particles on the skin cannot be ruled out in view of a recent finding of silica particles within the skin of patients with systemic sclerosis.[124]

The renal lesions associated with silica exposure are varied. They include: segmental necrotizing glomerulonephritis and arteriolitis,[120] focal mesangial proliferation,[119] degenerative changes of the proximal tubular cells,[119] and acute glomerulonephritis associated with the deposition of IgM and C3 component of complement.[125] Increased silicon content in the kidney has been demonstrated in some cases.[14]

Q. SILICOSIS IN ANIMALS

Animals exposed to free silica in the natural environment show pathologic lesions remarkably similar to those seen in humans. Environmental silicosis has been described in birds,[126] horses,[127] New Zealand kiwis,[128] and camels.[129] Animals exposed to silica dust under controlled experimental conditions also show many of the same features of human silicosis including acute silicosis (silicotic lipoproteinosis) and the formation of granulomatous and collagenous nodules. Species demonstrating these effects include rats, hamsters, guinea pigs, monkeys, and mice.[49,130–132] Features of acute silicosis and granulomatous reactions are the most frequently described histopathologic lesions. Classic silicotic nodules and massive fibrotic reactions occur but are less common. These differences probably reflect the time scales involved rather than intrinsic differences in species response to silica.

REFERENCES

1. **Honma, K. and Chiyotani, K.,** Pulmonary alveolar proteinosis as a component of massive fibrosis in cases of chronic pneumoconiosis, *Zentralbl. Pathol.,* 137, 414–417, 1991.
2. **Sanderson, W. T.,** The U.S. population at risk to occupational respiratory diseases, in Occupational Respiratory Disease, Merchant, J.A., Ed., DHHS (NIOSH), Publ. No. 86–102, 739–759, 1986.
3. **Graham, W. G.,** Silicosis, *Clin. Chest Med.,* 13, 253–267, 1992.
4. **O'Donnell, A. E., Mappin, F. G., Sebo, T. J., and Tazelaar, H.,** Interstitial pneumonitis associated with "crack" cocaine abuse, *Chest,* 100, 1155–1157, 1991.
5. **Dumontet, C., Biron, F., and Vitrey, D.,** Acute silicosis due to inhalation of a domestic product, *Am. Rev. Respir. Dis.* 143, 880–882, 1991.
6. **Cahill, B. C., Harmon, K. R., Shumway, S. J., Mickman, J. K., and Hertz, M. I.,** Tracheobronchial obstruction due to silicosis, *Am. Rev. Respir. Dis.,* 145, 719–721, 1992.
7. **Grobbelaar, J. P. and Bateman, E. D.,** Hut lung: a domestically acquired pneumoconiosis of mixed aetiology in rural women, *Thorax,* 46, 334–340, 1991.
8. **Sherwin, R. P., Bauerman, M. L., and Abraham, J. L.,** Silicate pneumoconiosis in farmworkers, *Lab. Invest.,* 40, 576–582, 1979.
9. **Bar-Ziv, J. and Goldberg, G. M.,** Simple siliceous pneumoconiosis in Negev bedouins, *Arch. Environ. Health,* 29, 121–126, 1974.
10. **Norboo, T., Angchuk, P. T., Yahya, M., Kamat, S. R., Pooley, F. D., Corrin, B., Kerr, I. H., Bruce, N., and Ball, K. P.,** Silicosis in a Himalayan village population: role of environmental dust, *Thorax,* 46, 341–343, 1991.
11. **Ng, T. P., Tsin, T. W., O'Kelley, F. J., et al.,** A survey of the respiratory health and silica exposed gemstone workers in Hong Kong, *Am. Rev. Respir. Dis.,* 135, 1249–1254, 1987.
12. **White, N. W., Chetty, R., and Bateman, E. D.,** Silicosis among gemstone workers in South Africa: tigers-eye pneumoconiosis, *Am. J. Ind. Med.,* 19, 205–213, 1991.
13. **Craighead, J. E. and Vallyathan, N. V.,** Cryptic pulmonary lesions in workers occupationally exposed to dust containing silica, *JAMA,* 244, 1939–1941, 1980.
14. **Parkes, W. R.,** Diseases due to free silica, in *Occupational Lung Disorders,* Butterworth and Co., London, 1982, pp. 134–174, 175–232.
15. **Goldstein, B. and Rendall, R. E. G.,** The relative toxicities of the main classes of minerals, in *Pneumoconiosis,* Proceedings of the International Conference, Johannsberg, Shapiro, H. A., Ed., Oxford University Press, Capetown, 429–434, 1969.
16. **Boeniger, M., Hawkins, M., Marsin, P., and Neuman, R.,** Occupational exposure to silicate fibers and PAH's during sugarcane harvesting, *Ann. Occup. Hyg.,* 32, 153–169, 1988.
17. **Hughes, J. M., Jones, R. N., Gilson, J. C., Haymad, Y. Y., Semeene, B., Hendrick, D. J., Turner-Warwick, M., Doll, J., and Weill, H.,** Determinants of progression in sandblasters' silicosis, *Ann. Occup. Hyg.,* 26, 701–711, 1973.
18. **Heppleston, A. G.,** Environmental lung disease, in *Pathology of the Lung,* Thurlberg, J. R., Ed., Thieme Medical Publishers, New York, 1988, 591–686.
19. **Bagchi, N.,** What makes silica toxic?, *Br. J. Ind. Med.,* 49, 163–166, 1992.
20. **Vallyathan, V., Shi, X., Delal, N. S., Irr, W., and Castranova, V.,** Generation of free radicals from freshly fractured silica dust. Potential role in acute silica induced lung injury, *Am. Rev. Respir. Dis.,* 138, 1213–1219, 1988.
21. **Shi, X., Dalal, N. S., and Vallyathan, V.,** ESR evidence for the hydroxyl radical formation in aqueous suspension of quartz particles and its possible significance to lipid peroxidation in silicosis, *J. Toxicol. Environ. Health,* 25, 237–245, 1988.
22. **Ghio, A. J., Kennedy, T. P., Schapira, R. M., Crumblis, A. L., and Hoidal, J. R.,** Hypothesis: is lung disease after silicate inhalation caused by oxygen generation? *Lancet,* 336, 967–969, 1990.
23. **Vallyathan, V., Kang, J. H., Van Dyke, K., Dalal, N. S., and Castranova, V.,** Response of alveolar macrophages to *in vitro* exposure to freshly fractured versus aged silica dust: the ability of Prosil 28, an organosilane material, to coat silica and reduce its biological reactivity, *J. Toxicol. Environ. Health,* 33, 303–315, 1991.
24. **Wallace, W. E., Keane, M. J., Mike, P. S., Hill, C. A., Vallyathan, V., and Regad, E. D.,** Contrasting respirable quartz and kaolin retention of lecithin surfactant and expression of membranolytic activity following phospholipase A2 digestion, *J. Toxicol. Environ. Health,* 37, 391–409, 1992.

25. **Emerson, R. J. and Davis, G. S.,** Effect of alveolar lining material-coated silica on rat alveolar macrophages, *Environ. Health Perspect.,* 51, 81–84, 1983.
26. **Nash, T., Allison, A. C., and Harrington, J. S.,** Physico-chemical properties of silica in relation to its toxicity, *Nature,* 210, 259–261, 1966.
27. **Begin, R., Cantin, A., Mesa, S., Dufresne, A., Perreault, G., and Sebastien, P.,** Aluminum inhalation in sheep silicosis, *Int. J. Exp. Pathol.,* 74, 299–307, 1993.
28. **Klosterkötter, W. and Einbrodt, H. J.,** Quantitative tiexperimentelle Untersuchungen über den Abtransport von Staub aus den Lugen in die regionalen Lymphknoten, *Arch. Hyg.,* 149, 367–384, 1965.
29. **Driscoll, K. E., Maurer, J. K., Lidenschmidt, R. C., Romberger, D., Rennard, S. I., and Crosby, L.,** Respiratory tract responses to dust, *Toxicol. Appl. Physiol.,* 106, 88–101, 1990.
30. **Warheit, D. B., Hansen, J. F., and Hartsky, M. A.,** Physiological and pathophysiological pulmonary responses to inhaled nuisance-like or fibrogenic dusts, *Anat. Res.,* 231, 107–118, 1991.
31. **Brody, A. R., Roe, N. W., Evans, J. N., and Davis, G. S.,** Deposition and translocation of inhaled silica in rats, *Lab. Invest.,* 47, 533–542, 1982.
32. **Green, F. H. Y., Althouse, R., and Webber, K. C.,** Prevalence of silicosis at death and underground coal miners, *Am. J. Ind. Med.,* 16, 605–615, 1989.
33. **Murray, J., Webster, I., Reid, G., and Kielkowski, D.,** The relation between fibrosis of hilar lymph glands and the development of parenchymal silicosis, *Br. J. Ind. Med.,* 48, 267–269, 1991.
34. **Hubbard, A. K.,** Role for T-lymphocytes in silica-induced pulmonary inflammation, *Lab. Invest.,* 61, 46–52, 1989.
35. **Smith, C. S. and Wikoff, H. L.,** The silica content of the lungs of a group of tunnel workers, *Am. J. Public Health,* 23, 1250–1254, 1933.
36. **Seaton, A., Legge, J. S., Henderson, J., and Kerr, K. M.,** Accelerated silicosis in Scottish stonemasons, *Lancet,* 337, 341–344, 1991.
37. **Banks, D. E., Morring, K. L., Boehlecke, B. A., et al.,** Silicosis in silica flour workers, *Am. Rev. Respir. Dis.,* 124, 445, 1981.
38. **Davis, G. S.,** The pathogenesis of silicosis, *Chest,* 89, 166S–169S, 1986.
39. **Craighead, J. E., Kleinerman, J., Abraham, J. L., Gibbs, A. R., Green, F. H. Y., Harley, R. A., Rüttner, J. R., Vallyathan, V., and Juliano, E. B.,** Diseases associated with exposure to silica and non-fibrous silicate minerals, *Arch. Pathol. Lab. Med.,* 112, 673–720, 1988.
40. **Dail, D. H.,** Metabolic and other diseases, Chapter 22 in *Pulmonary Pathology,* 2nd ed., Dail, D.H., and Hammer, S.P., Ed., Springer-Verlag Inc., 1993, 745–751.
41. **Hook, G. E. R.,** Alveolar proteinosis and phospholipidoses of the lungs, *Toxic Pathol.,* 19, 482–513, 1991.
42. **Singh, G., Katyal, S. L., Bedrossian, C. W. M., and Rogers, R. M.,** Pulmonary alveolar proteinosis. Staining for surfactant apoprotein in alveolar proteinosis and in conditions stimulating it, *Chest,* 83, 82–86, 1983.
43. **Gilmore, L. B., Tally, F. A., and Hook, D. E.,** Classification and morphometric quantitation of insoluble materials from the lungs of patients with alveolar proteinosis, *Am. J. Pathol.,* 133, 252–264, 1988.
44. **McEuen, D. D. and Abraham, J. L.,** Particulate concentrations in pulmonary alveolar proteinosis, *Environ. Res.* 17, 334–339, 1978.
45. **Miller, B. E., Dethloff, L. A., and Hook, G. E. R.,** Silica-induced hypertrophy of type II cells in the lungs of rats, *Lab. Invest.,* 55, 153–163, 1986.
46. **Miller, B. E., Chapin, R. E., Pinkerton, K. E., Gilmore, L. B., Merinport, R. R., and Hook, G. E.,** Quantitation of silica-induced type II cell hyperplasia by using alkaline phosphatase histochemistry in glycol methacrylate embedded lung, *Exp. Lung Res.,* 12, 135–148, 1987.
47. **Miller, B. E., Bakewell, W. E., Catal, S. L., Singh, G., and Hook, G. E.,** Induction of surfactant protein (SP-A) biosynthesis and SP-A mRNA in activated type II cells during acute silicosis in rats, *Am. J. Respir. Cell. Mol. Biol.,* 3, 217–226, 1990.
48. **Dethloff, L. A., Gladden, B. C., Gilmore, L. B., and Hook, G. E.,** Kinetics of pulmonary surfactant phosphatidylcholine metabolism in the lungs of silica treated rats, *Toxicol. Appl. Pharmacol.,* 98, 1–11, 1989.
49. **Bowden, D. H. and Adamson, I. Y. R.,** The role of cell injury in the continuing inflammatory response in the generation of silicotic pulmonary fibrosis, *J. Pathol.,* 144, 149–161, 1984.
50. **Seeger, W., Stöhr, G., Wolf, H. R. D., and Neuhof, H.,** Alteration of alveolar surfactant function due to protein leakage: special interaction with fibrin monomer, *J. Appl. Physiol.,* 58, 326–338, 1985.
51. **Green, F. H. Y., Schurch, S., De Sanctis, G. T., Wallace, J. A., Cheng, S., and Prior, M.,** Effects of hydrogen sulphide exposure on surface properties of lung surfactant, *J. Appl. Physiol.,* 70, 943–949, 1991.
52. **Kuhn, C., III, Gyorkey, F., Levine, B. E., and Rimirez-Rivera, J.,** Pulmonary alveolar proteinosis: a study using enzyme histochemistry, electron microscopy and surface tension measurements, *Lab. Invest.,* 15, 492–509, 1966.
53. **Ziskind, M., Weill, H., Anderson, A. E., Sammi, B., Neilson, A., and Waggenspack, C.,** Silicosis in shipyard sandblasters, *Environ. Res.,* 11, 237–243, 1976.
54. **Begin, R. O., Cantin, A. M., Boileau, R. D., and Bisson, G. Y.,** Spectrum of alveolitis in quartz exposed human subjects, *Chest,* 92, 1061–1067, 1987.
55. **Green, F. H. Y.,** Coal workers' pneumoconiosis and pneumoconiosis due to other carbonaceous dust, in *Pathology of Occupational Lung Disease,* Churg, A., and Green, F.H.Y., Eds., Igaku-Shoin, New York, 1988, 89–154.

56. **Craighead, J. E. and Vallyathan, N. V.,** Cryptic pulmonary lesions in workers occupationally exposed to dust containing silica, *JAMA,* 244, 1939–1941, 1980.
57. **Stettler, L. E., Platek, S. F., Groth, D. H., Green, F. H. Y., and Vallyathan, V.,** Particle contents of human lungs, in *Electron Microscopy and Forensic Occupational and Environmental Health Sciences,* Basu, S., Millot, J.R., Eds., Plenum Press, New York, 1986, 217–226.
58. **Sweany, H. C., Porsche, J. D., and Douglass, J. R.,** Chemical and pathologic study of pneumoconiosis with special emphasis on silicosis and silico-tuberculosis, *Arch. Pathol.,* 22, 593–633, 1936.
59. **Foweather, F. S.,** Silicosis and the analyst, *Analyst,* 64, 779–787, 1939.
60. International Labor Office, Guidelines for the use of the International classification of radiographs of the pneumoconiosis, Revised Ed., ILO, Occupational Safety and Health, Series No. 22 (Ref. Revision 80), Geneva, ILO, 1980.
61. **Uehlinger, E., Übermischstaubpneumo-Koniosen,** *Schweiz. Z. Pathol. Bakt.,* 9, 692–700, 1946.
62. **Craighead, J. E., Emerson, R. J., and Stanley, D. E.,** Slate workers pneumoconiosis, *Hum. Pathol.,* 23, 1098–1205, 1992.
63. **Masse, S., Begin, R., and Cantin, A.,** Pathology of silicon carbide pneumoconiosis, *Mod. Pathol.,* 1, 104–108, 1988.
64. **Hayashi, H. and Kajita, A.,** Silicon carbide in lung tissue of a worker in the abrasive industry, *Am. J. Ind. Med.,* 14, 145–155, 1988.
65. **Gibbs, A. R. and Wagner, J. C.,** Diseases due to silica, in *Pathology of Occupational Lung Disease,* Churg, A., and Green, F.H.Y., Eds., Igaku-Shoin, New York, 1988, 155–176.
66. **Weller, W. and Ulmer, W. T.,** Inhalation studies of cold-quartz dust mixture, *Ann. N.Y. Acad. Sci.,* 200, 142, 1972.
67. **Martin, J. C., Daniel-Moussard, H., Le Bouffant, L., and Policard, A.,** The role of quartz in the development of coal workers' pneumoconiosis, *Ann. N.Y. Acad. Sci.,* 200, 127–142, 1972.
68. **Gross, P., Westrick, M. L., and McNerney, J. M.,** Experimental silicosis: the inhibitory effect of iron, *Dis. Chest,* 37, 35–41, 1960.
69. **Reichel, G., Bauer, H.-D., and Bruckmann, E.,** The action of quartz in the presence of iron hydroxides in the human lung, in *Inhaled Particles and Vapors IV,* Walton, W.H., Ed., Pergamon Press, Oxford, 1977, 403–410.
70. **Denny, J. J., Robson, W. D., and Irwin, D. A.,** Prevention of silicosis by metallic aluminum, *Can. Med. Assoc. J.,* 40, 213–228, 1939.
71. **Webster, I.,** Prevention of silicosis, *S. Afr. Pneumoconiosis Rev.,* 4, 11–12, 1968.
72. **Kennedy, M. C. S.,** Aluminum powder inhalations in the treatment of silicosis of pottery workers and pneumoconiosis of coal miners, *Br. J. Ind. Med.,* 13, 85–99, 1956.
73. **Kleinerman, J., Green, F. H. Y., Laqueur, W., Taylor, G., Harley, R., Pratt, P., Wyatt, S., and Naeye, R.,** Pathology standards for coal workers' pneumonoconiosis, *Arch. Pathol. Lab. Med.,* 103, 375–431, 1979.
74. **Craighead, J. E., Emerson, R. J., and Stanley, D. E.,** Slate workers' pneumoconiosis, *Hum. Pathol.,* 23, 1098–1205, 1992.
75. **Banks, D. E., Bauer, M. A., Castolin, R. M., and Lapp, N. L.,** Silicosis in surface coal mine drillers, *Thorax,* 38, 275–278, 1983.
76. **Seaton, A., Dick, H. A., Dodgson, J., and Jacobsen, M.,** Quartz and pneumoconiosis in coal miners, *Lancet,* 2(8258), 1272–1275, 1981.
77. **Walton, W. H., Dodgson, J., Paddern, G. G., and Jacobsen, M.,** The effect of quartz and other non-coal dusts of coal workers pneumoconiosis, in *Inhaled Particles IV,* Vol. II, Walton, W.H., Ed., Pegamon Press, Oxford, 1977, 669–690.
78. **Morgan, W. K. C., Burgess, D. B., Jacobsen, G., O'Brien, R. L., Pendergrass, E. P., Reger, R. B., and Shoub, E. P.,** The prevalence of coal workers' pneumoconiosis in US coal miners, *Arch. Environ. Health,* 27, 221–226, 1973.
79. **Ruckley, V. A., Furney, J. M., and Chapman, J. S.,** Comparison of radiographic appearances with associated pathology and lung dust content in a group of coal workers, *Br. J. Ind. Med.,* 41, 459–467, 1984.
80. **Davis, J. M. G., Chapman, J., Collings, P., Douglas, A. N., Ferney, J., Lamb, D., and Ruckley, V. A.,** Variations in the histological patterns of the lesions of coal workers in Britain and their relationship to lung dust content, *Am. Rev. Respir. Dis.,* 128, 118–124, 1983.
81. **Cowie, R. L.,** The epidemiology of tuberculosis in gold miners with silicosis, *Am. J. Respir. Crit. Care Med.,* 150, 1460–1462, 1994.
82. **Cowie, R. L.,** The five ages of pulmonary tuberculosis and the South African goldminer, *S. Af. Med. J.,* 76, 566–567, 1989.
83. **Agricola, G.,** *De Re Metallica,* 1556, translated by Hoover, H.C., and Hoover, L., in *The Mining Magazine,* London, 1912.
84. **Gordon, D.,** Dust and history, *Med. J. Aust.,* 2, 161–166, 1954.
85. **Watkins-Pitchford, W.,** The silicosis of the South African gold mines and the changes produced in it by legislative and administrative effort, *J. Ind. Hyg.,* 9, 109–139, 1927.
86. **Simson, F. W. and Strachan, A. S.,** Silicosis and tuberculosis: Observations on the origin and character of silicotic lesions, Publ. XXXVI of the South African Institute of Mining and Research, 6, 367–406, 1935.
87. **Sherson, D. and Lander, F.,** Morbidity of pulmonary tuberculosis among silicotic and nonsilicotic foundry workers in Denmark, *J. Occup. Med.,* 32, 110–113, 1990.

88. **Schepers, G. W. H., Smart, R. H., Smith, C. R., Dworski, M., and Delahant, A. B.,** Fatal silicosis with complicating infection by an atypical acid-fast photochromic bacillus, *Ind. Med. Surg.*, 27, 27–36, 1958.
89. **Policard, A., Gernez-Rieux, C., Tacquet, A., Martin, J. C., Devulder, B., and LeBouffant, L.,** Influence of pulmonary dust load on the development of experimental infection by mycobacteria Kansasii, *Nature (London)*, 216, 177–178, 1967.
90. **Gardner, L. U.,** Silicosis and its relationship to tuberculosis, *Am. Rev. Tuburc.*, 29, 1–7, 1934.
91. **Allison, A. C. and Hart, D. A. P.,** Potentiation by silica of the growth of mycobacterium tuberculosis in macrophage cultures, *Br. J. Exp. Pathol.*, 49, 465–476, 1968.
92. **Ebina, T., Takahashi, Y., and Hasuike, T.,** Effects of quartz powder on tubercle bacilli and phagocytes, *Am. Rev. Respir. Dis.*, 82, 516–527, 1960.
93. **Ziskind, M., Jones, R. N., and Weill, H.,** Silicosis. The state of the art, *Am. Rev. Respir. Dis.*, 113, 643–665, 1986.
94. **Christman, J. W., Emerson, R. J., Graham, G. B., and Davis, G. S.,** Mineral dust and cell recovery from the bronchoalveolar lavage of healthy Vermont granite workers, *Am. Rev. Respir. Dis.*, 132, 393–399, 1985.
95. **Goodwin, R. A. and Des Prez, R. M.,** Apical localization of pulmonary tuberculosis, chronic pulmonary histoplasmosis and progressive massive fibrosis of the lung, *Chest*, 83, 801–805, 1983.
96. **Honma, K. and Chiyotani, K.,** Diffuse interstitial fibrosis in non-asbestos pneumoconiosis: a pathological study, *Respiration*, 60, 120–126, 1993.
97. **Vigliani, E. C. and Mottura, G.,** Diatomaceous earth silicosis, *Br. J. Ind. Med.*, 4, 148–160, 1948.
98. **Pintar, K., Funahashi, A., and Siegesmund, A.,** A diffuse form of pulmonary silicosis in foundry workers, *Arch. Pathol. Lab. Med.*, 100, 535–538, 1976.
99. World Health Organization, Chronic cor pulmonale, Report of an expert committee, 27, 594–615, Circulation 1963.
100. **Rüttner, J. R. and Gassmann, R.,** Lungengefäßveränderungen bei Silikose und ihre Beziehungen zum Cor pulmonale chronicum, Staub., 3, 459–470, 1957.
101. **Gough, J.,** Pathological changes in the lungs associated with cor pulmonale, *Bull. N.Y. Acad. Med.*, 13, 24, 1965.
102. **Murray, J., Reid, G., Kielkowski, D., and deBeer, M.,** Cor pulmonale and silicosis: a necropsy based case-control study, *Br. J. Ind. Med.*, 50, 544–548, 1993.
103. **Wyndham, C. H., Bezuidenhout, B. N., Greenacre, M. J., and Sluis-Cremer, G. K.,** Mortality of middle aged white South African gold miners, *Br. J. Ind. Med.*, 43, 677–684, 1986.
104. **Becklake, M. R., Irwig, L., Kielowski, D., Webster, I., deBeer, M., and Landau, S.,** The predictors of emphysema in South African gold miners, *Am. Rev. Respir. Dis.*, 135, 1234–1241, 1987.
105. **Cowie, R. L. and Mabena, S. K.,** Silicosis, chronic airflow limitation, and chronic bronchitis in South African gold miners, *Am. Rev. Respir. Dis.*, 144, 1423–1424, 1991.
106. **Hnizdo, E.,** Loss of lung function associated with exposure to silica dust and with smoking and its relation to disability and mortality in South African gold miners, *Br. J. Ind. Med.*, 49, 472–479, 1992.
107. **Hnizdo, E., Sluis-Cremer, G. K., and Abramowitz, J. A.,** Emphysema type in relation to silica dust exposure in South African gold miners, *Am. Rev. Respir. Dis.*, 143, 1241–1247, 1991.
108. **Wright, J. L., Harrison, N., Wiggs, B., and Churg, A.,** Quartz but not iron oxide causes air-flow obstruction, emphysema, and small airways lesions in the rat, *Am. Rev. Respir. Dis.*, 138, 129–135, 1988.
109. **Dickson, G. F., Donnerberg, R. L., Schonfeld, S. A., and Whitcomb, M. E.,** Advances in the diagnosis and treatment of broncholithiasis, *Am. Rev. Respir. Dis.*, 129, 1028–1030, 1984.
110. **Amandus, H. E., Castellan, R. M., Shy, C., Heineman, E. F., and Blair, A.,** Reevaluation of silicosis and lung cancer in North Carolina dusty trades workers, *Am. J. Ind. Med.*, 22, 147–153, 1992.
111. **Pairon, J. C., Brochard, P., Jaurand, M. C., and Bignon, J.,** Silica and lung cancer: a controversial issue, *Eur. Respir. J.*, 4, 730–744, 1991.
112. **Ng, T. P., Chang, S. L., and Lee, J.,** Mortality of a cohort of men in a silicosis register: further evidence of an association with lung cancer, *Am. J. Ind. Med.*, 17, 163–171, 1990.
113. **Holland, L. M.,** Crystalline silica and lung cancer: a review of recent experimental evidence, *Regulatory Toxicol. Pharmacol.*, 12, 224–237, 1990.
114. International Agency for Research on Cancer, Monographs on the evaluation of the carcinogenic risk of chemicals to humans, Vol. 42, IARC, Lyon, 1987, 111.
115. **Mauderly, J. L.,** Contribution of inhalation bioassays to the assessment of human health risks from solid airborne particles. Proceeding from the 4th International Symposium, Toxic and Carcinogenic Solid Particles in the Respiratory Tract, 1993, ILSI Press, Washington, D.C., in press.
116. **Hnizdo, E. and Slouis-Cremer, G. K.,** Silica exposure, silicosis, and lung cancer: a mortality study of South African gold miners, *Br. J. Ind. Med.*, 48, 53–60, 1991.
117. **Schuyler, M. R., Ziskind, M., and Salvaggio, J.,** Cell-mediated immunity in silicosis, *Am. Rev. Respir. Dis.*, 116, 147–151, 1977.
118. **Haustein, U. F., Ziegler, V., Herrmann, K., Mehlhorn, J., and Schmidt, C.,** Silica-induced scleroderma, *J. Am. Acad. Dermatol.*, 22, 444–448, 1990.
119. **Pouthier, D., Duhoux, P., and Van-Damme, B.,** Pulmonary silicosis and glomerular nephropathy. Apropos of one case, *Nephrologie*, 12, 8–11, 1991.

120. **Arnalich, F., Lahoz, C., Picazo, M. L., Monereo, A., Arribas, J. R., Martinez-Ara, A. J., and Vazquez, J. J.,** Polyarteritis nodosa and necrotizing glomerulonephritis associated with long-standing silicosis, *Nephron,* 51, 544–547, 1989.
121. **Liu, Y. C., Tomashefski, J., McMahon, J. T., and Petrelli, M.,** Mineral associated hepatic injury. A report of seven cases with X-ray microanalysis, *Hum. Pathol.,* 22, 1120–1127, 1991.
122. **Klockars, M., Koskela, R. S., Jarvinen, E., Kolari, P. J., and Rossi, A.,** Silica exposure and rheumatoid arthritis: a follow up study of granite workers 1940–81, *Br. Med. J.,* 294, 997–1000, 1987.
123. **Jablonska, E.,** *Scleroderma and pseudoscleroderma,* Dowden, Hutchinson & Ross, Stroudsburg, PA, 1975.
124. **Mehlhorn, J., Ziegler, V., Keyn, J., and Vetter, J.,** Quartz crystals in the skin as a cause of progressive systemic scleroderma, *Z. Gesamte Inn. Med. Ihre Grenzgeb.,* 45, 149–154, 1990.
125. **Giles, R. D., Stergill, B. C., Suratt, P. M., and Boltin, W. K.,** Massive proteinuria and acute renal failure in a patient with acute silicoproteinosis, *Am. J. Med.,* 64, 336–342, 1978.
126. **Evans, M. G., Slocombe, R. F., and Schwartz, L. D.,** Pulmonary silicosis in captive ring necked pheasants: definitive diagnosis by electron probe X-ray microanalysis, *Vet. Pathol.,* 25, 239–241, 1988.
127. **Schwartz, L. W., Knight, H. D., Whittig, L. D., Mulloy, R. L., Abraham, J. L., and Tyler, N. K.,** Silicate pneumoconiosis and pulmonary fibrosis in horses from the Monterey-Carmel peninsula, *Chest,* 80, 82S–85S, 1981.
128. **Smith, B. L., Poole, W. S. H., and Martinvitch, D.,** Pneumoconiosis in the captive New Zealand kiwi, *Vet. Pathol.,* 10, 94–101, 1973.
129. **Hansen, H. J., Jama, F. M., Nilsson, C., Norrgren, L., and Abdurahman, O. S.,** Silicate pneumoconiosis in camels. *Zentralbl. Veterinaermed. Reihe A.,* 36, 789–796, 1989.
130. **Hannothiaux, M. H., Scharfman, A., Wastiaux, A., Cornu, L., Van Brussel, E., Lafitte, J. J., Sebastien, P., and Roussel, P.,** An attempt to evaluate lung aggression in monkey silicosis: hydrolases, peroxidase and antiproteases activities in serial bronchoalveolar lavages, *Eur. Respir. J.,* 4, 191–204, 1991.
131. **Seki, J., Kawanami, O., Yoneyama, H., and Hara, F.,** Analysis of cells in bronchoalveolar lavage and ultrastructure of lung tissues in experimental silicosis, *Nipon-Kiobo-Shikkan-Gakkai-Zasshi,* 31, 686–693, 1993.
132. **Gross, P. and deTreville, R. T. P.,** Experimental "acute" silicosis, *Arch. Environ. Health,* 17, 720–725, 1968.
133. **MacGregor, J. H.,** unpublished observations.
134. **Rashid, A.-M. H. and Green, F. H. Y.,** Pleural Pearls following silicosis: a histological and electron microscopic case study, *Histopathology,* 26, 84–87, 1995.

Section II
Current Concepts Concerning Physiochemical Properties of Silica

Section II
Chapter 1

THE STRUCTURE OF CRYSTALLINE SiO_2

Gretchen Mandel and Neil Mandel

CONTENTS

I. INTRODUCTION

Silicon makes up almost 28% of the Earth's crust. Due to this abundance, the silica minerals are very important to many aspects of modern mining, industry, and construction; however, they are a major health risk. Silica is a term referring to the family of SiO_2 crystal structures, the most common of which is quartz.[1] The bonding geometry of silicon is highly variable, and five different SiO_2 crystal structures have been characterized — quartz, cristobalite, coesite, tridymite, and stishovite.[2] The different crystalline structures based on the SiO_2 repeat are termed dimorphs of SiO_2. Three of these dimorphs — quartz, cristobalite, and tridymite — have two closely related, temperature-dependent, crystallographic structures which are denoted as α (high) or as β (low) temperature structures.

On the Periodic Chart, silicon is in the same column as carbon. Under normal conditions, silicon, like carbon, forms four bonds in a tetrahedral array using the four unpaired electrons in its 2s and 2p electron shells. Each oxygen atom is shared by two silicon tetrahedra, and each silicon atom is surrounded by four nearest neighbor oxygen atoms, thus forming the SiO_2 stoichiometry. The tetrahedral SiO_2 structures are coesite, cristobalite, quartz, and tridymite. However, under extreme pressure and heat, the silicon atoms can be forced into a more dense octahedral bonding array. The intense pressure causes one pair of electrons from the lower energy 1s shell to split apart and form two additional bonds making a total of six bonds in an octahedral configuration. The octahedral SiO_2 mineral is stishovite.

This chapter describes the basic crystallographic structure of the five dimorphs of SiO_2, as well as the most probable molecular structures on representative crystal faces. Since the emphasis of this monograph is the disease conditions associated with these structures, we have included discussion on possible correlations between crystal structure, crystal surface structure, and biologic reactivity for the various dimorphs.

TABLE 1
The Crystallographic Data for the Crystal Structures of the SiO_2 Minerals Described in this Chapter

Name	a(Å)	b(Å)	c(Å)	α(°)	β(°)	γ(°)	Space Group	References
Coesite	7.173	12.328	7.175	90	120	90	C2/c	3,4
α-Cristobalite	4.978	4.978	6.948	90	90	90	$P4_12_12$	5,6
α-Quartz	4.913	4.913	5.404	90	90	120	$P3_12$	7
Stishovite	4.179	4.179	2.665	90	90	90	P4/mnm	2,8
β-Tridymite	5.03	5.03	8.22	90	90	120	P6/mmc	2,14

II. CRYSTALLOGRAPHIC AND INTERATOMIC BONDING CONSIDERATIONS

Every crystal is a three-dimensional lattice containing repeating blocks of unit structure (defined as the unit cell), which are in perfect orientation necessary to create an overall large single block (crystal). Unit cells are defined with three axial lengths and three interaxial angles: *a*(Å), *b*(Å), *c*(Å), α(°), β(°), and γ(°). Atoms and molecules in the unit cell, and therefore in the overall structure, are positioned in very symmetrical patterns, which can be defined with symmetry transformations such as 60°, 120°, or 180° rotations or as mirrored pairs of atoms or molecules. Crystallographically, there are only 230 combinations of symmetry operations which allow atoms and molecules to pack into three-dimensional lattices in a thermodynamically stable pattern that will fill all the space in a crystal. Table 1 lists the lattice constants, space groups, and references for the structures described in this chapter.

In order to describe the molecular structure on growth or fracture faces of a crystal, it is necessary to define the faces in crystallographic terms which represent planes that are passed through the basic unit cell. This process is based on a set of three integers called Miller indices that indicate which of the unit cell axes the plane bisects. For example, the (100) plane intercepts the *a* axis one unit cell from the origin and does not intercept either the *b* or *c* axes, i.e., this plane is parallel to the plane containing the *b* and *c* axes.

The indexing of crystal morphology and crystal growth or fracture faces is usually done by a combination of X-ray crystallographic and optical or polarizing microscopic techniques. Most of the SiO_2 particulate load seen in the pneumoconioses is dust that is primarily composed of ground crystals. When quartz is ground, the cleaved crystal surfaces are not smooth, but rather they contain conchoidal depressions which are composed of a series of wide steps with a spectrum of Miller index planes neighboring and intermixing with defined crystal growth faces.[1] This chapter describes the molecular structures on the primary crystal growth faces as a representation of the surface structure on the most common fracture faces.

Table 2 details the average bonding atomic geometry around the silicon atoms in each of the SiO_2 dimorphs. This table highlights the structural differences between the various crystals. The silicon-oxygen distance is nearly constant for all the tetrahedral structures, but when the silicon atom is forced into octahedral coordination, this distance is stretched by as much as 0.4 Å. As expected, the O–Si–O angle most clearly reflects the tetrahedral vs. octahedral coordination geometry. These differences in

TABLE 2
The Average Atomic Geometry of the SiO_4 Coordination Sphere for the Various Structures. Values are the Mean Followed by the Standard Deviation

Name	Si–O–Si Angle(°)	Si–O Distance(Å)	O–Si–O Angle(°)	%Occupied Vol.
Coesite	129.94 ± 11.98	1.61 ± 0.02	109.47 ± 0.93	67.8
α-Cristobalite	146.71 ± 0.09	1.60 ± 0.01	109.47 ± 1.26	54.4
α-Quartz	143.90 ± 0.00	1.61 ± 0.00	109.47 ± 0.67	61.8
Stishovite	114.58 ± 23.03	1.78 ± 0.02	180 or 90	100.1
β-Tridymite	180	1.55 ± 0.02	109.47 ± 0.77	53.6

crystallographic bonding geometry translate into differences in surface atomic structures for all the SiO_2 dimorphs.

The structure of each of the SiO_2 minerals is presented in a series of four figures. Oxygen atoms are denoted by the larger, light grey spheres, and the silicon atoms are denoted by the smaller dark grey spheres. The first figure in each series, Figures 1, 5, 9, 13, and 17, shows the molecular packing and bonding connectivity in the unit cell with a ball and stick representation. The set of second figures, Figures 2, 6, 10, 14, and 18, also shows the unit cell contents in the same orientation, but the atoms now have van der Waals radii,[10] presenting a more realistic molecular space filling view of the structures. The space-filling figures contain a better perspective of the overlapping of the atoms in the various structures. The basic differences in the molecular bond parameters in the various structures lead to differences in molecular packing, with some structures appearing more densely packed than others. In Table 2 we have attempted to quantitate these differences in packing with a parameter we call the % occupied volume. The % occupied volume is defined as the percentage ratio of the difference between the volume of the unit cell based on the lattice constants (Vol.) and the sum of the volume occupied by all the atoms in the structure against the volume of the unit cell.[11] The spherical volume of the atoms is calculated using van der Waals radii (r).

$$\%\ \text{occupied vol.} = \frac{\text{Vol.} - \Sigma\, 4/3\, \pi r^3}{\text{Vol.}} \tag{11}$$

Figures 3, 7, 11, 15, and 19 present a view of a representative crystal face using a ball and stick drawing of the structures. Each of these figures is followed by a space-filling view in the same orientation, Figures 4, 8, 12, 16, and 20. For each structure, the face view shown only includes atoms from the top layer of the structure. The thickness of these layers varies between 4.6Å (stishovite) and 5.03Å (tridymite), except for that of coesite which is 7.2Å thick. Since a single SiO_4 tetrahedra is about 5.4Å thick, the face views shown for cristobalite, quartz, stishovite, and tridymite are all approximately the thickness of a single tetrahedra. The ball and stick view of the coesite face, Figure 3, shows that three silicon atoms and three oxygen atoms bond together forming six-membered rings. The coesite face is a sheet of parallel chains of six-membered rings. The coesite face shown is thicker than those of the other SiO_2 structures in order to accommodate the thickness of these rings.

The atoms in the pseudo six-membered rings in all of the structures have been denoted with small black dots. The average distance between the oxygen atoms that make up the pseudo hexagonal arrays of the crystal faces have been determined and are listed in Table 3 as the O– –O distance (Å). The differences in the O– –O distances can be visualized in the surface structures in Figures 4, 8, 12, 16, and 20 by noting that the white area between the atoms represents the openness of the structure. The amount of unoccupied space, or degree of openness in the tetrahedral structures, is greater than that observed for the more densely packed octahedral mineral. The surfaces of the various dimorphs have different surface oxygen atom structures. As can be seen in the space-filling figures, the surface oxygen atom structures have varying degrees of depth between the highest and the lowest oxygen atoms. In Table 3, we have attempted to quantitate this observation by defining the vertical offset distance between the highest and

TABLE 3
The Bonding Parameters of the Hexagonal Packing Arrays on the Crystal Surfaces for the Various Structures

Structure	Face	O– –O Distance(Å)	Vertical Offset(Å)
α-Quartz	100	5.16	1.0
α-Cristobalite	100	4.59	1.03
β-Tridymite	100	5.18	1.15
Coesite	001	4.70	0.60
Stishovite	100	2.84	0.50

Note: The hexagons are neither regular nor planar, so geometries given here are averages of representative values. The vertical offset is that distance between the highest and lowest surface available oxygen atoms on the crystal planes shown in the van der Waals space-filling figures.

the lowest oxygen atoms on the various surfaces described in this chapter. The program Chem3D® allows for real time rotation and viewing of the structure along a defined plane. The program also allows for distance and angle calculations. These two capabilities were used to first identify selected atoms on the surface structure and then to obtain the distances needed for the vertical offset calculations.

All drawings presented in this chapter were prepared using the program Chem3D® from the Molecular Modeling System, (Cambridge Scientific Computing, Inc.) running on a Macintosh IIci® computer. The Chem3D® algorithm requires that all atoms have a set of x, y, and z coordinates and that all molecular contacts be noted by atom sequence numbers. Crystallographic programs for generating coordinates and finding bonding pairs were part of our crystallographic single crystal program package, CRYSP.[12]

III. THE STRUCTURES

A. COESITE

The structure of coesite is presented in Figures 1 through 4. Figure 1 shows the unit cell. Figure 2, which uses van der Waals atomic radii for space filling representation, shows that there is some unoccupied volume and some degree of atomic roughness on the coesite crystal surfaces. The ball and stick view of the 001 face, Figure 3, emphasizes the symmetrical nature of the coesite structure. Since the *a* and *c* axial lengths are almost equal and the β angle is 120°, coesite has a pseudo-hexagonal structure. This figure shows that three silicon atoms and three oxygen atoms bond together forming six-membered rings. This figure also shows the rather open nature of the coesite structure. All of the open spaces visible in Figure 3 are sealed at the bottom by the atomic matter in the next layer below in the three-dimensional structure. The SiO_2 structures with large O––O and small offset distances (Table 3) have wide, shallow surface pockets at the atomic level. Coesite is an example of this kind of surface packing structure.

B. α-CRISTOBALITE

The structure of α-cristobalite is presented in Figures 5 through 8. The structure of β-cristobalite evidences very small distortions from that of α-cristobalite. The unit cell representation of α-cristobalite is shown in Figure 5. The two oxygen atoms at the top center of the unit cell are bonded to two different silicon atoms in the unit cell above that pictured, i.e., the unit cell translated up by one in the z direction. On the 100 face, Figure 7, the cristobalite bonding pattern evidences a trigonal array of surface oxygen atoms approximately 4.59 Å on a side. Six trigonal arrays form one hexagonal ring which, by default, is also 4.59 Å on a side. The surface array is composed of lines of elevated oxygen atoms which are separated from each other by the *c* axis (6.948 Å) and lines of lower oxygen atoms which are similarly separated by the same distance. This molecular packing appears to be trigonal or hexagonal because the two lines are offset by one half of the *c* axis (3.474 Å) creating a staggered pattern. The lines of elevated oxygen atoms are 1.03 Å above the lower lines, the offset distance. The molecular pockets on this surface of α-cristobalite are wide, but the offset distance is intermediate compared to the other structures.

C. α-QUARTZ

The two dimorphs of quartz have closely related structures. If α-quartz is heated above 575° under proper conditions, it transforms into β-quartz. The three-dimensional structure of α-quartz is shown in Figures 9 through 12. As shown in the unit cell representation of α-quartz, Figure 9, the structure is composed of three-dimensional networks of SiO_4 tetrahedra connected at vertices. The silicon atoms lie on three interpenetrating hexagonal lattices which have a spiral arrangement with respect to each other in the vertical direction. Because this view is down the *a* axis, the unit cell above the one shown is offset to the left by one half the *a* axis (2.46 Å). This offset allows each silicon tetrahedron to nestle into the depression made by the four tetrahedra in the layer below when they pack together.

As can be seen in Figure 11, the 100 face, the surface oxygen atoms are spaced in a rectangular array with dimensions 4.91 by 5.40 Å which are the lengths of the *b* and *c* axes. The diagonal distance across the rectangle is 7.30 Å. There are two lower oxygen atoms in the middle of the rectangle with a vertical offset of 1.00 Å.

D. STISHOVITE

The structure of stishovite is shown in Figures 13 through 16. As shown in the unit cell representation of stishovite, Figure 13, the structure contains a compact crystal packing pattern. Rutile, as well as many

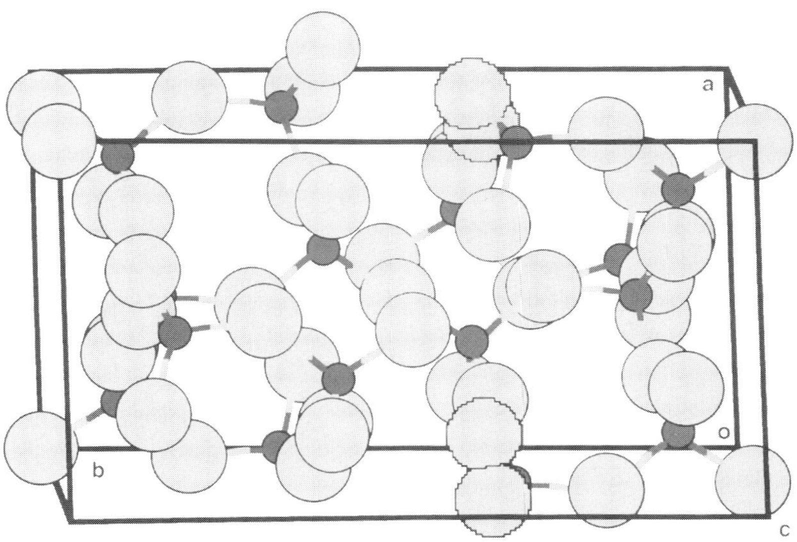

FIGURE 1 The ball and stick representation of the unit cell structure of coesite.

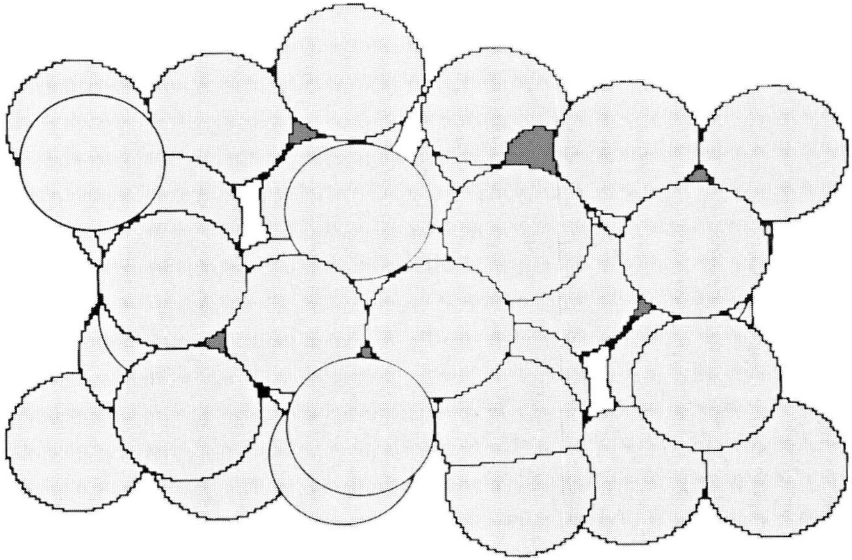

FIGURE 2 The space-filling view of the coesite unit cell.

other quadrivalent metal dioxides, share this compact crystal packing structure pattern.[9] Of all the SiO_2 structures, stishovite has the smallest O– –O distance, which combined with the smallest vertical offset, translates into a smooth layer of negative charges. The stishovite structure has a very box-like molecular appearance. This is especially clear in the space-filling representation of the stishovite unit cell, Figure 14. The hexagonal array on the 100 surface of stishovite is composed of rows of elevated oxygen atoms interspersed by rows of lower oxygen atoms. This hexagonal array has four 2.778 Å and two 2.958 Å sides. The 2.958 Å bonds and two of the 2.778 Å bonds involve atoms from both the elevated and lower rows of oxygen atoms. The vertical offset is 0.50 Å. These combined parameters translate into an efficiently packed octahedral lattice.

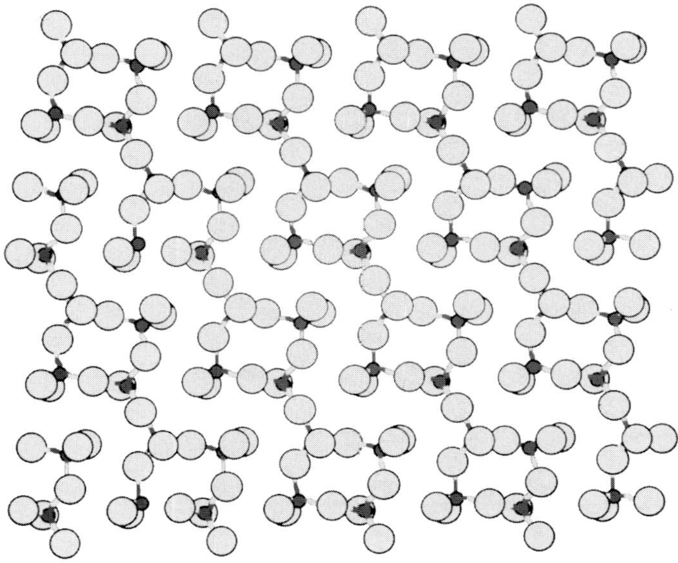

FIGURE 3 The ball and stick representation of the 001 face of coesite. This view shows an area of 17.6 × 16.5 Å. The depth of view is 7.2 Å.

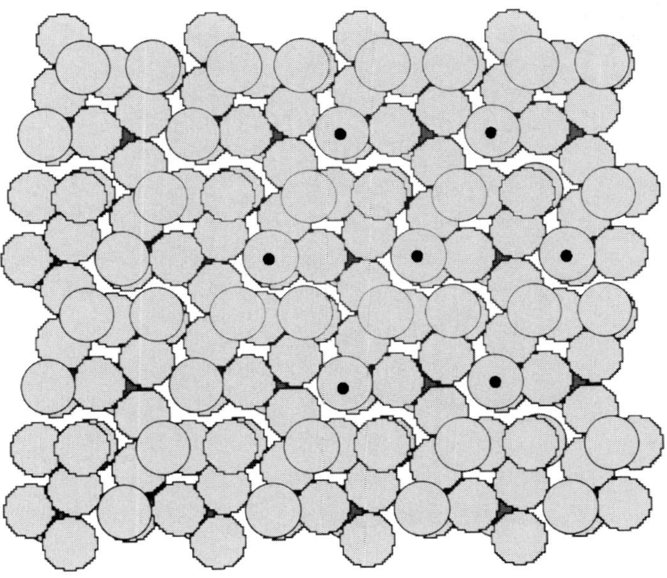

FIGURE 4 The space-filling view of the 001 face of coesite.

Stishovite is a very rare form of SiO_2 and is only found in a few geologic locations. Research groups have been forced to use rutile, a TiO_2 isostructural substitute for stishovite, in many of their biologically related studies. Although rutile is a TiO_2 structure, the two structures are identical crystallographically (isostructural), and it is a reasonable assumption that crystal growth and fracture plane structure will be identical in the two structures.

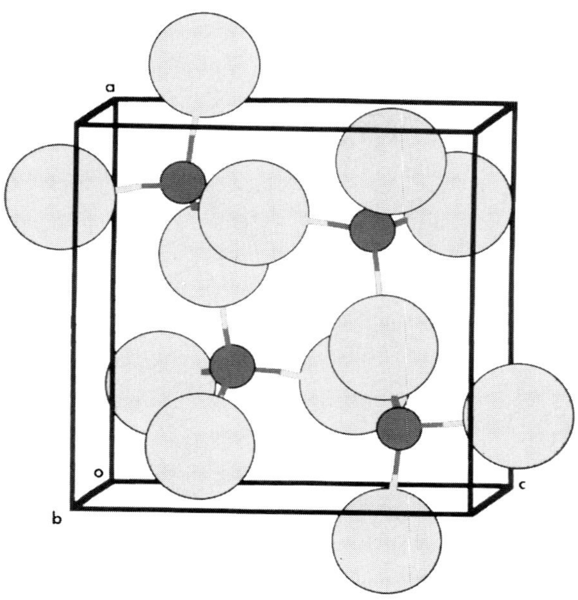

FIGURE 5 The ball and stick representation of the unit cell structure of α-cristobalite.

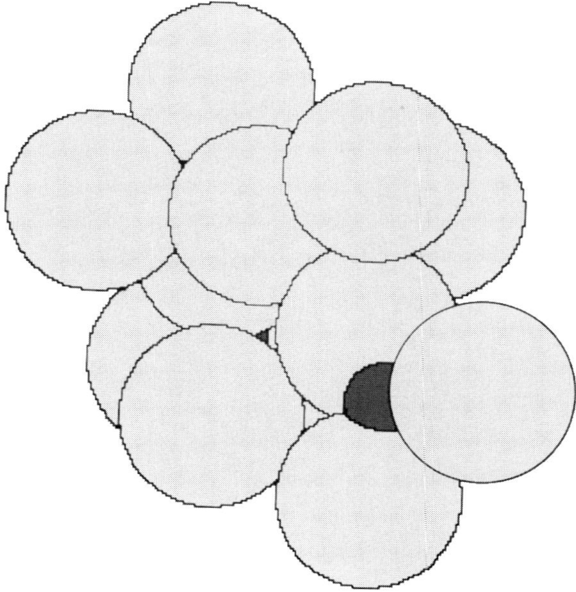

FIGURE 6 The space-filling view of the α-cristobalite unit cell.

E. β-TRIDYMITE

The structure of β-tridymite is shown in Figures 17 through 20. Tridymite has two other dimorphs stable below 200°C. One structure is an intermediate form while the other is low (α) tridymite. Both dimorphs are related to β-tridymite. As shown in Figure 17 and detailed in Table 2, the Si–O–Si angle in tridymite is 180°. Of all the structures, β-tridymite has the shortest Si–O bond distance while

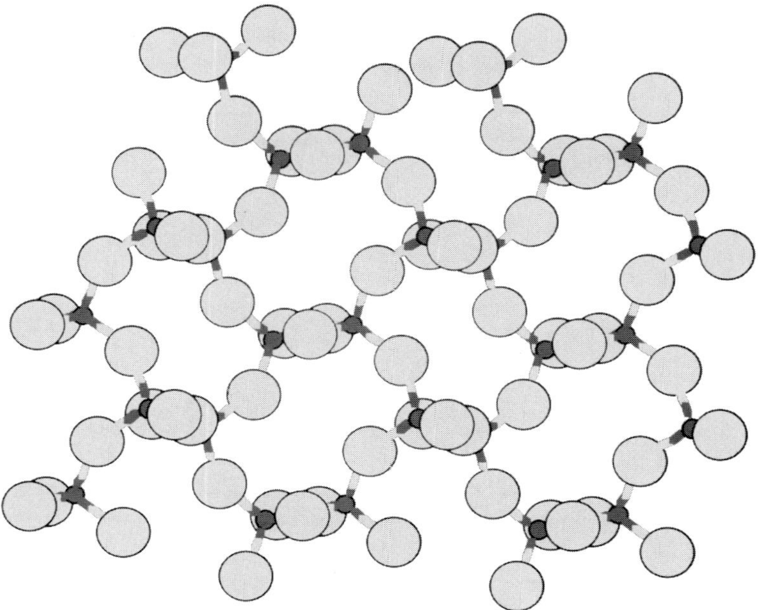

FIGURE 7 The ball and stick representation of the 100 face of α-cristobalite. This view shows an area of 14.9 × 17.3 Å. The depth of view is 5.0 Å.

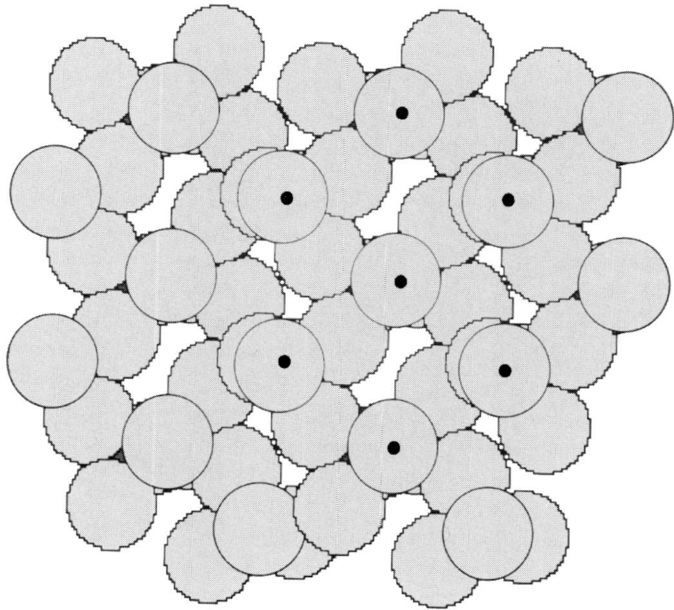

FIGURE 8 The space-filling view of the 100 face of α-cristobalite.

maintaining the ideal O–Si–O tetrahedral angle of 109.47°. The energy gained from the formation of these tight interatomic bonds with ideal bonding geometry offsets the energy lost in forming the Si–O–Si angle of 180°. As shown in the ball and stick representation of the 100 face, Figure 19, the silica tetrahedra form rings. Unlike the other tetrahedral surface structures for the other dimorphs, there are six silicon atoms

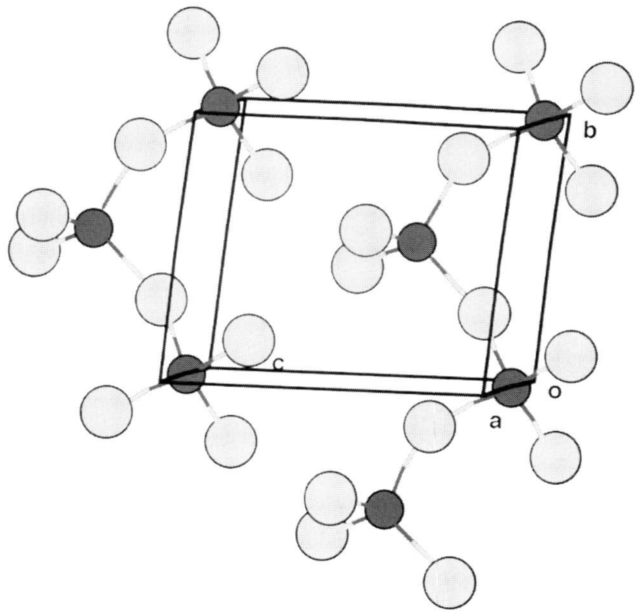

FIGURE 9 The ball and stick representation of the unit cell structure of α-quartz.

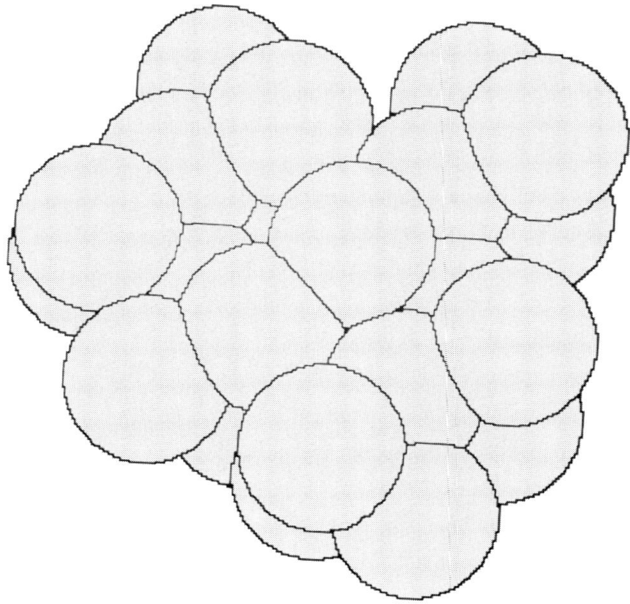

FIGURE 10 The space-filling view of the α-quartz unit cell.

and six oxygen atoms bonded together in β-tridymite forming twelve-membered rings. This arrangement presents a trigonal or hexagonal array of surface available oxygen atoms. Like the surface topography of cristobalite, the pockets on this surface of β-tridymite are wide and intermediate in vertical offset distances compared to the other structures.

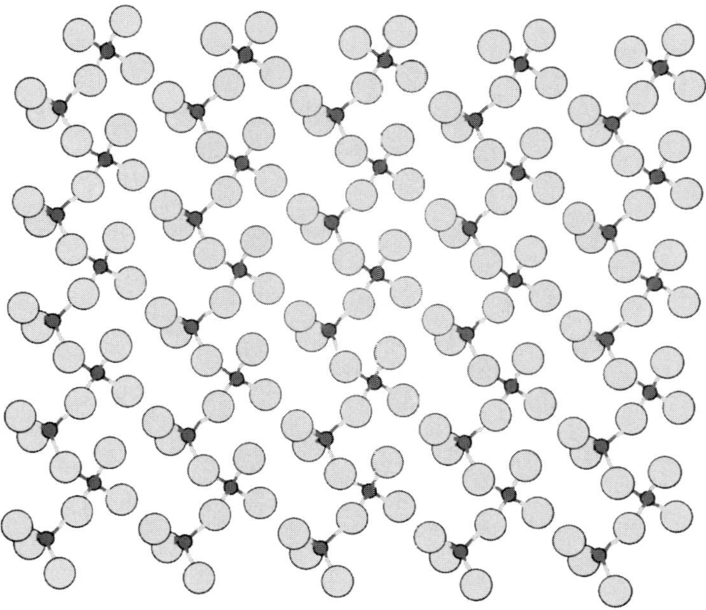

FIGURE 11 The ball and stick representation of the 100 face of α-quartz. This view shows an area of 24.6 × 27.0 Å. The depth of view is 4.9 Å.

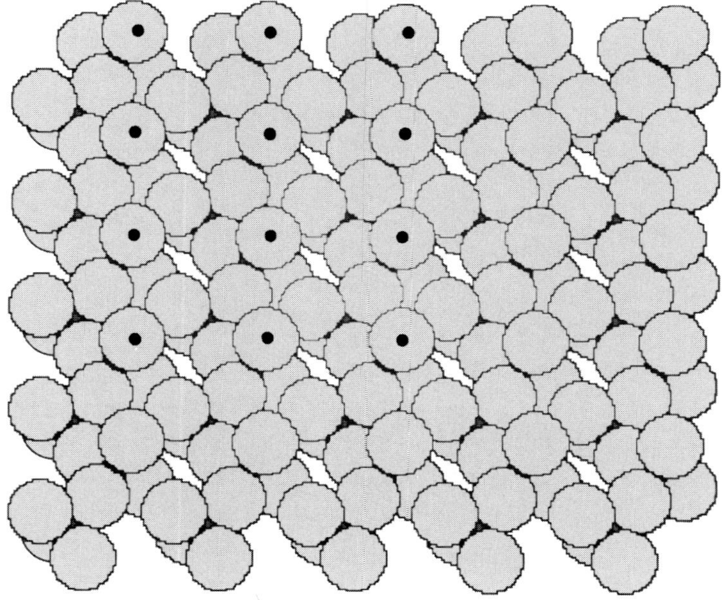

FIGURE 12 The space-filling view of the 100 face of α-quartz.

IV. SUMMARY

Comparing the various SiO_2 structures described in this chapter highlights the fact that differences in the molecular bonding within a crystal structure result in differences in molecular packing on the crystal surface. The bonding parameters presented in Table 2 show the broad spectrum of Si–O–Si and O–Si–O

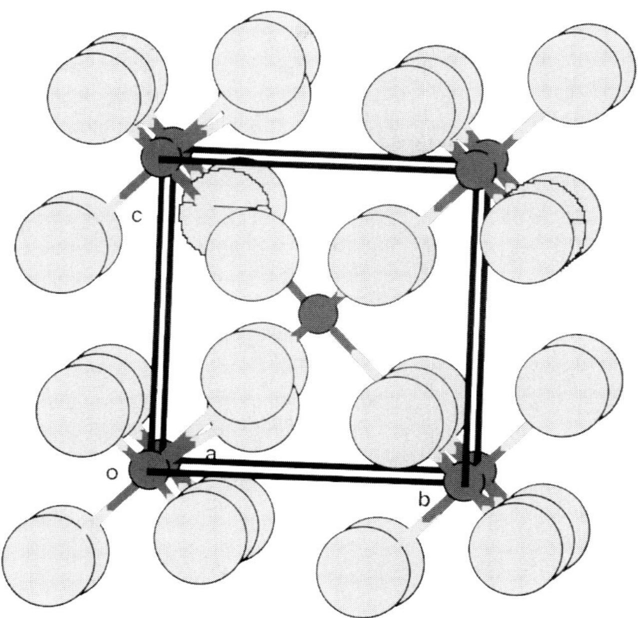

FIGURE 13 The ball and stick representation of the unit cell structure of stishovite.

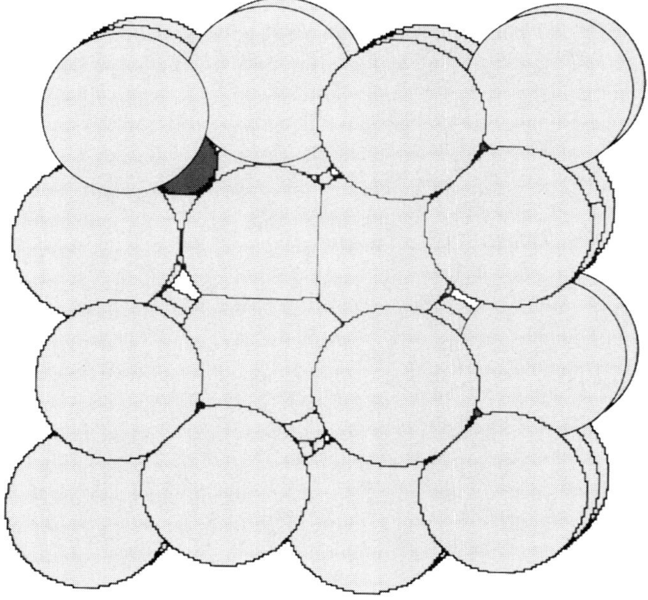

FIGURE 14 The space-filling view of the stishovite unit cell.

angles observed in the SiO_2 structures. The bond angle differences about the Si atom are related to the tetrahedral or octahedral coordination geometries. The differences in the molecular arrays on the crystal faces have potential significance in determining a crystal's effective biologic activity since any interaction between a crystal and a biologic structure such as a membrane will be based on a molecular contact between the atoms on crystal surfaces and the biologic molecular structure. As shown in the van der Waals space-filling views of the SiO_2 crystal surfaces, oxygen atoms will be the reactive molecular

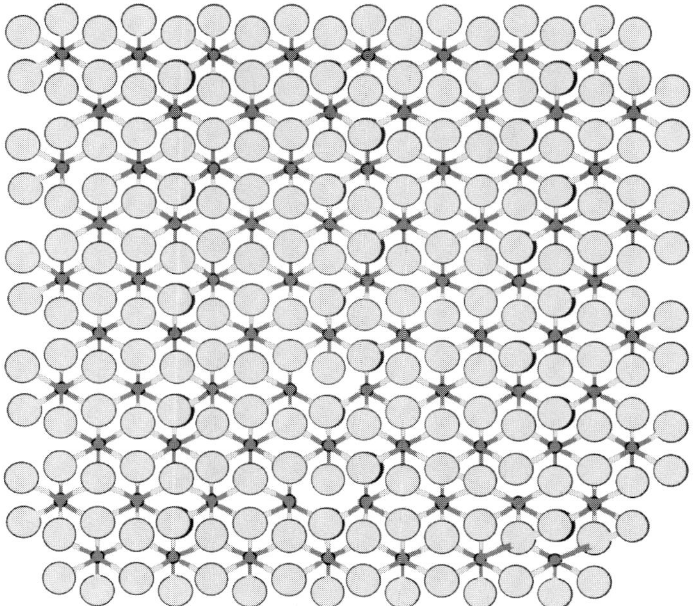

FIGURE 15 The ball and stick representation of the 100 face of stishovite. This view shows an area of 23.0 × 21.0 Å. The depth of view is 4.6 Å.

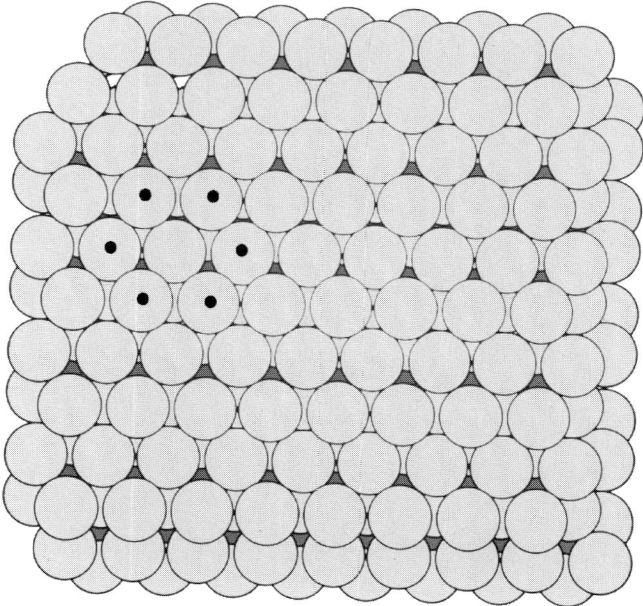

FIGURE 16 The space-filling view of the 100 face of stishovite.

interaction atoms. The molecular description of the structure of these surface oxygen atoms as described by the O– –O distances, the vertical offset distance from the highest to the lowest oxygen atom array, and the % occupied volume indicates that the various SiO_2 structures are quantitatively different at their surface structure level. We suggest that these surface structural differences can be correlated with a crystal's effective biologic activity.

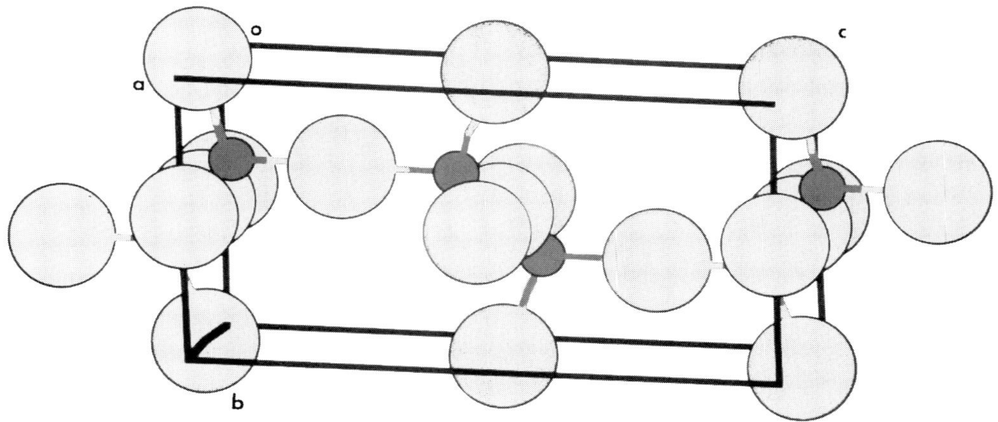

FIGURE 17 The ball and stick representation of the unit cell structure of β-tridymite.

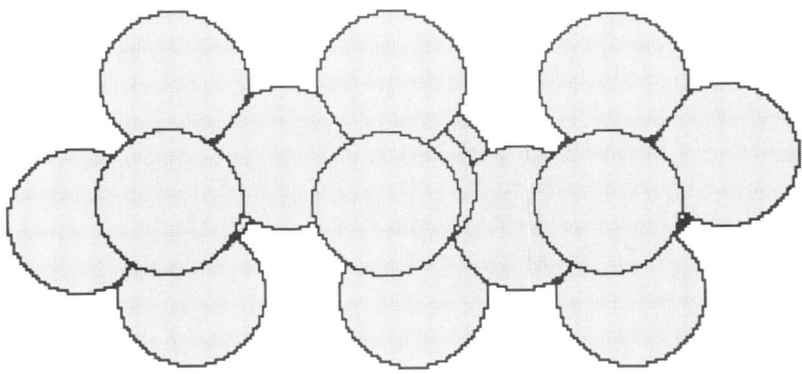

FIGURE 18 The space-filling view of the β-tridymite unit cell.

We have attempted to correlate these structural differences with biologic markers of crystal toxicity. When crystals are incubated with RBCs, toxic crystals induce a rupture of the cell membrane, termed membranolysis. When crystals are instilled intratracheally into the lungs of mice, toxic crystals induce the synthesis of hydroxyproline due to localized inflammation and as part of the development of fibrosis. Figure 21 shows the correlation of three structural parameters, the percent occupied volume normalized to quartz, the O––O distance, and the vertical offset distance with two biologic markers of crystal reactivity — the level of hydroxyproline synthesis in mice exposed to the SiO_2 dimorphs[11] and the % hemolysis of RBCs.[13]

The normalized % occupied volume is a function which describes the basic crystal structure. The O––O distance and the vertical offset distance are parameters which describe specific surface structural characteristics. As shown in Figure 21, as the occupied volume decreases indicating a more open structure, the biologic reactivity as measured by the hydroxyproline levels and the % hemolysis increases. This correlation is not linear since the occupied volume is virtually identical in stishovite and coesite, but it is reduced in cristobalite and further reduced in tridymite. Similarly, the hydroxyproline levels and % hemolysis levels are similar in stishovite and coesite, and then increase in cristobalite and tridymite.

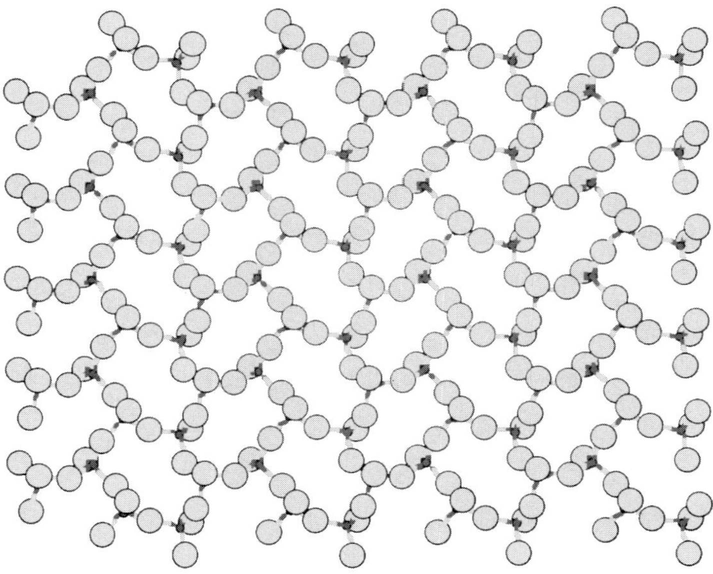

FIGURE 19 The ball and stick representation of the 100 face of β-tridymite. This view shows an area of 25.1 × 32.9 Å. The depth of view is 5.0 Å.

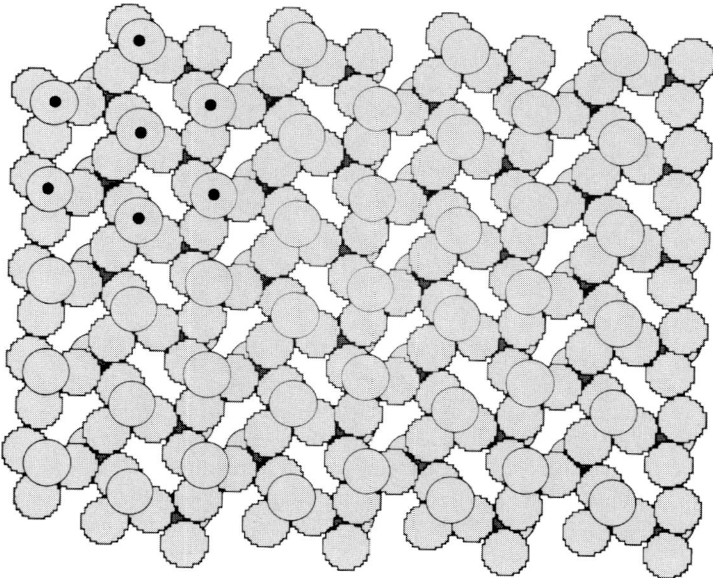

FIGURE 20 The space-filling view of the 100 face of β-tridymite.

The vertical offset distance appears to be an important mediator of biologic reactivity. In stishovite and coesite, the offset distance is comparable as is the hydroxyproline levels. In cristobalite, tridymite, and quartz the offset distance increases as does the hydroxyproline level. This suggests that the vertical offset distance is the primary structural element which can be correlated with the synthesis of hydroxyproline and that the depth of the molecular pockets on a crystal surface are important in mediating crystal-cell

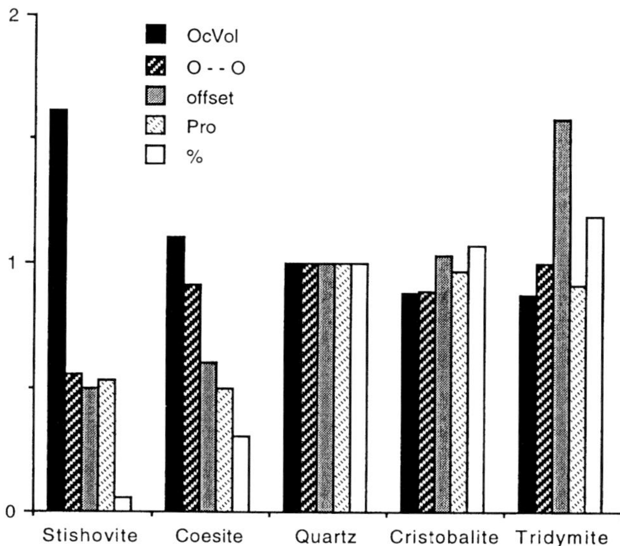

FIGURE 21 Biological reactivity and atomic geometries of the surface oxygen atoms on the crystal faces described in this chapter. All values have been normalized by dividing by the quartz value, thereby setting the quartz values to one. The O– –O and the vertical offset (offset) distances are taken from Table 3. The biological data are Pro for hydroxyproline as a measure of fibrosis,[11] and % for % hemolysis as a measure of crystal-induced RBC membrane lysis.[12]

interactions. This relationship is dependent on an oxygen atom array structure on the crystal surfaces which can be matched with a supportive molecular array on the cell surface. In tridymite, even though the molecular pockets are significantly deeper compared to stishovite, coesite, and cristobalite, the O– –O distance is apparently beyond an acceptable level to induce an increased biologic response that would be predicted based solely on the vertical offset distance. Therefore, biologic reactivity of the SiO_2 structures is dependent on both the molecular surface topography and the O– –O molecular lattice on crystal surfaces.

The structural dependence of crystal-induced membranolysis in RBCs appears to be primarily dependent on the O– –O distance. As the O– –O distance increases from stishovite to coesite, so does the % lysis. Similarly, as the O– –O distance increases from cristobalite to tridymite, so does the % lysis. It is not clear why the trend from stishovite to tridymite is not more linear, except as discussed above: the vertical offset distance appears to be a major structural variable that probably also influences crystal-cell interaction in crystal-induced membranolysis.

This data suggest that the vertical offset distance and the O– –O distance must both be considered when analyzing the structural dependence for a crystal's effective biologic reactivity. It must be recognized that in quartz these structural variables are ideal for a significant biologic response and that the predicted biologic reactivity would be quartz > tridymite > cristobalite > coesite > stishovite.

REFERENCES

1. **Cornelius, S. H., Ed.,** *Dana's Manual of Mineralogy,* 16th ed., John Wiley & Sons, New York, 1952.
2. **Wycoff, R. W. G.,** *Crystal Structures,* 2nd ed., Vol. 1, Interscience Publishers, New York, 312–322, 1963.
3. **Araki, T. and Zoltai, T.,** Refinement of a coesite structure, *Z. Kristallogr.,* 129, 381, 1969.
4. **Zoltai, T. and Buerger, M. J.,** The crystal structure of coesite, the dense high-pressure form of silica, *Z. Kristallogr.,* 111, 129, 1959.
5. **O'Keeffe, M. and Hyde, B. G.,** Cristobalites and topologically-related structures, *Acta Crystallogr.,* B32, 2923, 1976.

6. **Dollase, W. A.,** Reinvestigation of the structure of low cristobalite, *Z. Kristallogr.*, 121, 369, 1965.
7. **Young, R. A. and Post, B.,** Electron density and thermal effects in alpha quartz, *Acta Crystallogr.*, 15, 337, 1962.
8. **Chao, E. C. T., Fahey, J. J., Little, J., and Milton, D. J.,** Stishovite, SiO_2, a very high pressure new mineral from Meteor Crater, Arizona, *J. Geophys. Res.*, 67, 419, 1962.
9. **Cromer, D. T. and Herrington, K.,** The structures of anatase and rutile, *J. Am. Chem. Soc.*, 77, 4708, 1954.
10. **Pauling, L.,** *The Nature of the Chemical Bond and the Structure of Molecules and Crystals: An Introduction to Modern Structural Chemistry,* Cornell University Press, Ithaca, 1960, 256–260.
11. **Wiessner, J. H., Henderson, J. D., Sohnle, P. G., Mandel, N. S., and Mandel, G. S.,** The effect of crystal structure on mouse lung inflammation and fibrosis, *Am. Rev. Respir. Dis.*, 138, 445, 1988.
12. **Mandel, G. S. and Mandel, N. S.,** A crystallographic structure package for a minicomputer-CRYSP78, *Am. Cryst. Assoc. Abstracts 2,* 6, 77, 1979.
13. **Kozin, F., Millstein, B., Mandel, G., and Mandel, N.,** Silica-induced membranolysis: a study of different structural forms of crystalline and amorphous silica and the effect of protein adsorption, *J. Colloid Interface Sci.*, 88, 326, 1982.
14. JCPDS Powder Diffraction Files, International Centre for Diffraction Data, Swarthmore, PA, File No. 14–260, 1992.

Section II
Chapter 2

THE STRUCTURE OF SILICA SURFACES IN RELATION TO CYTOTOXICITY

Peter P. Bolsaitis and William E. Wallace

CONTENTS

I. INTRODUCTION

Many or most chemical processes and physical interactions involving solid materials occur at their surface. A reduction of particle size, and the resulting increase in surface area per unit weight of material, generally increases the reactivity of solid materials. Hence the structure and composition of any material at its surface, more than its bulk composition, determine many of its chemical and physical properties. Unfortunately most analytical techniques used for the chemical characterization of materials tend to sample the bulk of the material, or a layer much deeper than the surface layer active in interactions with the environment. For ultrapure materials the issue may be of little consequence, but most materials found in nature are not pure, and impurities contained in the bulk tend to segregate to the surface by virtue of thermodynamic equilibrium effects. Also, by interaction with its environment, any solid material will tend to adsorb impurity atoms or molecules at its surface.

Consequently, surface characteristics play a dominant part in defining properties of ultrafine particles (respirable dusts and aerosols). This review focuses in particular on those properties that define the biological activity and toxicity of respirable-size, silica-based particles.

Since silica and its derivatives can be produced in a greater variety of forms and structures than most other chemical materials, numerous applications of silica exist, especially for the high-specific surface area, amorphous variety, where surface chemistry plays a dominant role. Silica-based materials include adsorbants and dessicants, catalysts, fillers, lubricants, thickening agents, paints, and other widely used materials. In Chapter 6 of his treatise on the chemical properties of silica, Iler presents a comprehensive review (with more than 500 references) of the wealth of data available on the structure and properties of silica and silica surfaces (Iler, 1979).

0-8493-4709-2/96/$0.00+$.50

Earlier reviews on the effect of surface characteristics of respirable particles on their pathogenic activity can be found in articles by Heffernan and Green (1928), Scheel, et al., (1954), and Monterra and Low (1973). Nolan, et al., (1981) review subsequent research with emphasis on those aspects of surface chemistry of respirable particles that may affect biological processes.

Although silica and several other minerals comminuted to the size of respirable particles can produce disease in man when inhaled, knowledge about the mechanisms of interaction of particle surfaces with biochemical materials leading to pathogenic reactions is still, at this time, on the level of hypothesis undergoing laboratory tests. Furthermore, little of the knowledge about the surface structure characteristics of silica particles has been integrated into the numerous biological investigations dealing with the potential toxicity of these materials.

In reviewing research results on the surface characteristics of respirable silica-based materials, one must distinguish between those dealing with "pure" materials, which emphasize the structure of the surfaces (including effects of trace impurities) of the various polymorphs of silica, and those dealing with "naturally formed" particles, in which impurities abound and several phases may co-exist within a single particle. Evidence exists, for example, suggesting that the cytotoxicity of "pure" or freshly formed quartz surfaces, as can be produced in the laboratory or during the drilling of high quartz-content rocks, differs in intensity and nature from that of quartz particles whose surfaces have been exposed to contamination and weathering processes.

II. STRUCTURE OF SILICA AND OF SILICA SURFACES

Silica occurs in nature in several crystalline structures and amorphous forms. The more common crystalline forms of silica are α- and β-quartz, α- and β-tridymite (each with several substructural variations), and α- and β-cristobalite. Structures stable at high temperatures and high pressures, such as keatite, coesite, and stishovite may also be found under ordinary conditions as metastable phases (Frondel, 1962; Sosman, 1965).

Table 1 summarizes the basic crystallographic data for the more common phases of silica. Of these crystalline materials, α-quartz is by far the most commonly found in nature and the most extensively studied for its structure and properties.

Common amorphous forms of silica include silica quenched from the molten state (glass), silica condensed and agglomerated from the vapor phase ("aerogels," commonly known by trade names like Aero-Sil, and Cab-O-Sil), and silica gels obtained by precipitation from liquid solutions. Silica particles formed from aerosols or colloidal solutions are typically aggregates of extremely fine (0.01 to 0.1 μm) primary particles and have large specific surface area (from about three to several hundred square meters per gram).

Surface structures developed on fine, pure silica particles are derived from the structure and properties of the bulk material. Pulverized dusts of crystalline silica result from comminution processes by two principal mechanisms: *fracture,* which results from the propagation, under stress, of pre-existing defects in the crystalline structure; and *cleavage,* occurring as an explosive rupture along atomic planes with lowest surface energy (greatest planar atomic density). Since the preferential planes of fracture differ among crystalline structures, comminuted particles of each of the crystalline silica polymorphs will have, on average, different atomic structures on their surface planes. α-quartz belong to the relatively complex trigonal trapezohedral class of the hexagonal system, and many different facets configure the basic crystal unit (Ford, 1957).

Many researchers have studied the cleavage and fracture planes in quartz resulting from different comminution processes and found (1010), (1011), (0111), and (0001) to be the most abundant. The assessment of the occurrence of such planes is only semiquantitative, but the source material and the comminution process appear to affect, to some extent, the facets preferentially developed (Bloss, 1957; Bloss and Gibbs, 1963; Christie, et al., 1964; Hammond, et al., 1973).

Interaction with water, either in aqueous suspensions or in normal atmospheres, critically affects the nature of silica surfaces. Terminal siloxane (–O–Si–O–) bonds define the surface of calcined, dry silica. Such surfaces are chemically and biologically quite inert (Razzaboni, et al., 1988). However, silica has a pronounced affinity for water. It hydrolyzes and adsorbs water readily, and the hydrolyzed silica surface terminates in silanol (–Si–OH) groups. The acidic (hydrogen-bond forming) character of the hydroxyl groups is generally associated with adsorption to cell membranes and the initiation of the cytotoxic or fibrogenic processes.

TABLE 1
Stability Ranges of Crystalline Phases of Silica

Modification	Symmetry system	Symmetry class	Temp. range (°C)	Stability
Quartz				
low (α-)	Hexagonal; rhombo hedral subd.	$D_3(32)$	–273 → 573	stable
high (β-)	Hexagonal; hexagonal subd.	$D_2(622)$	573 → 867	stable
Tridymite				
S-I	Orthorhombic		–273 → 64	metastable
S-II			64 → 117	metastable
S-III	Hexagonal	hemihedral(?)	117 → 163	metastable
S-IV	Hexagonal	holohedral(?)	163 → 210	metastable
S-V			210 → 475	metastable
S-VI	Hexagonal	C_6(mmc)	475 → 867	metastable
			867 → 1470	stable
M-I			–273 → 117	metastable
M-II			117 → 163	metastable
M-III			>163	metastable
Cristobalite				
low (α-)	Tetragonal	$D_4(422)$	–273 → 272	metastable
high (β-)	Isometric	O_h(m3m)	272 → 1470	metastable
			1470 → 1723	stable
Coesite	Monoclinic	C2/c	~300 → 1700 (~15 to 40 kbars)	stable
Keatite	Tetragonal	$D_4(422)$	400–500 (0.8–1.3 kbars)	stable
Stishovite			1200 → 1400 (~160 kbars)	stable

Adapted from Frondel, C., *Dana's System of Mineralogy*, 1962, pp. 1–8.
Adapted from Sosman, R. B., *The Phases of Silica*, 1964, p. 22.

The behavior of silica, particularly quartz, particles in aqueous media is also complex because of the capability of silica surfaces to adsorb one or more layers of silicic acid (H_2SiO_3) forming a Beilby layer of amorphous or partly polymerized silica (Holt and King, 1955; Baumann, 1966). For example, this effect results in "passivation" of quartz particles after boiling in water inside glass containers (Wallace, et al., 1988). Thus, the possible presence of a Beilby layer on crystalline quartz particles and a resulting alteration of biological activity must also be accounted for when characterizing their cytotoxicity. A complete characterization of silica surfaces and their properties must deal with water as a complementary constituent.

Contaminants constitute another important factor defining surface properties of particles. Even high purity quartz contains trace amounts of impurities that will concentrate along particular crystallographic planes or defects within the solid and affect the relative ease of cleavage or fracture along particular planes. This may result in an *ab initio* contamination of the surface facets developed during comminution.

III. SILICA SURFACES AND CYTOTOXICITY

The relative frequency of occurrence of various surface planes on silica particles of different crystal structures, especially in relation to their toxicity or activity in biological systems, may be the reason why such activity has been reported to vary between respirable size particles of different crystalline structure. Several investigations have been conducted on this topic; however, the results are not fully consistent. Early experiments conducted *in vitro* and with different animal models suggested that, for the silica polymorphs most frequently tested, the intensity of response follows the order tridymite > cristobalite > quartz > fused silica (glass), (Langer, 1978).

However, Stalder and Stöber (1965) tested the hemolytic activity of dusts of different crystalline modifications and found the following response sequence: tridymite ≅ quartz > cristobalite ≅ vitreous silica > coesite >> stishovite; and Kessel, Monaco, and Marchisio (1963) investigated the cytotoxic activity of the same materials in contact with guinea pig peritoneal macrophages and found tridymite, quartz, and cristobalite to be of similar activity while fused silica was essentially inert.

Subsequently, Kozin and co-workers (1982) have tested the hemolytic activity of different forms of silica in contact with human erythrocytes and found that on a per-unit-area basis quartz is twice as active as tridymite and cristobalite and more hemolytic than stishovite and fused silica, by factors of 8 and 100, respectively. And, more recently, Wiessner and co-workers (1988) have reported results on hemolytic activity and on inflammation and fibrosis in mouse lungs induced by particles of quartz, cristoballite, trydimite, and coesite, using a narrow size fraction of particles (~2 μm) with nearly equal specific surface areas. Their results on hemolysis show the activities of tridymite, cristobalite, quartz, and coesite in ratios of 1.14:1.05:1.00:0.26. The activity differences of tridymite, cristobalite, and quartz are within the range of experimental error. The lung fibrosis tested showed tridymite, cristobalite, and quartz to cause essentially the same response, while coesite proved inert.

A critical analysis, taking into account particle sizes, specific surface areas, experimental uncertainties, and experimental errors, indicates only small differences between the reported cytotoxicities of the three most common crystalline forms of silica (quartz, cristobalite, and tridymite), when compared on an equal particle number and surface area basis (Pandurangi and Seehra, 1991).

The reported correlations of cytotoxicity or biological activity with the crystalline structure of dust particles generally ignore, however, the possible presence of trace impurities on particle surfaces. Robok and Klosterkötter (1973) and, more recently, Tourmann and Kaufmann (1989) have found that even relatively pure, respirable mine dusts derived from quartz sands from different sources exhibit large differences in cytotoxicity measured by TTC (2,3,5-triphenyl-tetrazole chloride) reduction activity. Strübel and Rinn (1987) have shown that exposure of quartz particles to solutions that contain ions dissolved from different clay minerals can change the acidity of the quartz surface (affecting the dissociation ability of surface silanol groups) and with it the *in vitro* cytotoxicity (as measured by an LDH test with alveolar macrophages of guinea pigs). Similarly Kuhn (1992) has observed marked differences in the cytotoxicity of pure quartz (Min-U-Sil) and amorphous silica (Cab-O-Sil) particles when washed with deionized and nondeionized distilled water.

IV. INSTRUMENTAL METHODS FOR CHARACTERIZING SILICA SURFACES

Several physical methods have been used in recent years to identify, quantify, and correlate measurable physical properties of silica particles with their cytotoxicity. They include electrophoretic mobilities ("zeta-potentials"), thermally stimulated luminescence (TSL), electron spin resonance (ESR), infrared spectroscopy, laser microprobe mass analysis (LAMMA), and composition profiling with energy dispersive X-ray analysis (EDXA).

A. ELECTROPHORETIC MOBILITY

Bergman and Langrish (1972) studied the electrophoretic mobilities of silica powders of different crystalline structures in an attempt to relate this property, dependent largely on the surface charge characteristics of the particles, to their biological activity. Although a marked difference between the electrophoretic mobilities of the various material was found (quartz > tridymite > cristobalite ≅ vitreous silica), no obvious correlation could be established with their cytotoxicity.

B. THERMALLY STIMULATED LUMINESCENCE

The high sensitivity of TSL of silica on surface treatment (Robok and Klosterköter, 1973) has lead to further investigations on the possibility of relating this physical property of silica dust surfaces to their cytotoxicity. Kriegseis, et al. (1975), conducted an extensive study of TSL from quartz and other silica-based particles with variously treated surfaces and possible correlations between TSL and cytotoxicity. They found no correlation between absolute intensities of TSL peaks and either cytotoxicity or quartz content of the different dust samples. However, upon adsorption of water, alcohol, or acetone on a silanol (–Si–OH) bonded surface of quartz-containing materials, a very marked increase in the 171 K TSL peak was observed. The authors concluded that this increase in observed luminescence intensity resulted from hydrogen bonding of oxygen or hydroxyl groups onto the silanol surface. In many mechanisms proposed for cytotoxicity and fibrogenicity, this type of bonding between particles and cell membranes represents the first step in the particle-cell membrane interaction leading to cytotoxicity. A correlation of the cytotoxicity of the dust with the relative increase in 171 K luminescence was found but not with the quartz content of the materials.

More recently Kriegseis and Scharmann (1987) have developed improved luminescence methods for the determination of free quartz surfaces in mine dusts. An improvement in the accuracy of thermoluminescence measurements results from composition-dependent correcting for absorption of the emitted lights. The improved method utilizes the fact that SiO_2 materials exhibit a very intense radioluminescence during irradiation at 77 K, which decreases sharply at higher temperatures (~170 K). This characteristic step allows the quartz-specific proportion of the signal to be distinguished from the radioluminescence of other materials present in a mine dust and thus to establish the quartz fraction present in the material. Contrary to thermoluminescence, which is primarily a surface phenomenon, radioluminescence of quartz is a bulk effect. The calculation of extinction coefficients from radioluminescence data simplifies the calculation of the unmasked quartz surface from thermoluminescence measurements. Using this method, the authors have determined that mine dusts from sources located in two different areas (Ruhr and Saar), although of similar bulk quartz content, contain markedly different amounts of free or "clean" quartz surfaces (Kriegseis, Ruediger, and Scharmann, 1987).

C. ELECTRON SPIN RESONANCE

Hochstrasser and Antonini (1972) have measured and described in detail the ESR spectrum of freshly formed silica and quartz surfaces and the nature of the "dangling bonds" formed in fracture. They also showed these dangling bonds to be the preferential sites of adsorption for CO_2 molecules. They further noted the transient nature of these dangling bonds or surface free radicals and identified the diffusion of trace impurities to the surface as one of the main mechanisms for elimination of these surface radicals (passivation).

A high concentration of free radicals on freshly formed quartz particle surfaces may be the root cause of acute silicosis, as has been observed in instances where pure quartz rock has been drilled (e.g., the infamous New River Hawks Nest tunnel incident), causing particularly high cytotoxicity of the resulting dusts. Formation of fresh quartz surfaces could be associated with any rock drilling process, and thus a particular interest for free radicals on quartz surfaces has emerged.

In recent years ESR has been successfully employed by several groups of investigators to characterize and quantify the surface concentration of free radicals in freshly formed quartz dusts and to relate it to cytotoxic effects [Bolis, et al. (1983); Fubini, et al. (1987); Shi, et al. (1988); Vallyathan, et al. (1988)].

Bolis, et al. (1983), measured energies of adsorption for water molecules to identify highly reactive sites on freshly formed quartz surfaces which could also be related to unsaturated valencies ($-Si^{\cdot}$, $-SiO^{\cdot}$) on the freshly formed surface. Subsequently, Fubini, et al., have used these results to postulate mechanisms for the formation of several partially reduced oxygen species on the silica surface that could help explain the proposed, lipid-peroxidation mechanism for the membranolytic action of silica.

Shi, et al. (1988), have demonstrated that freshly ground quartz particles can induce the formation of $OH^{\cdot}$ radicals in aqueous suspensions, a likely active species in the peroxidation reactions leading to silicosis. Vallyathan, et al. (1988), have further quantified the formation and decay of free radicals on quartz particle surfaces and related the enhanced activity of the "freshly formed" surfaces to increased biological activity measured by several different protocols. According to these findings the grinding of quartz results in approximately 10^{18} $Si^{\cdot}$ and $Si\text{-}O^{\cdot}$ radicals per gram of dust. The concentration of these radicals decreases with aging in air with a half-life of approximately 30 hours, while its ability to generate $OH^{\cdot}$ radicals in aqueous suspension decreases with a half-life of approximately 20 hours. Compared to aged-quartz dust, the freshly ground dust showed a 1.5-fold increase in cytosolic LDH from alveolar macrophages, a more than thirty-fold increase in hemolytic activity, and a three-fold increase in the ability to induce lipid peroxidation.

D. LASER MICROPROBE MASS ANALYSIS

This technique consists of vaporizing and partly ionizing with a laser beam a small volume of material near the surface of a particle. The ions generated are identified with a time-of-flight, mass spectrometer. LAMMA has proven useful for probing the chemical composition of single, respirable-size particles at shallow penetrations, near the particle surface.

Tourmann and Kaufmann (1989) employed this technique successfully to distinguish between particles with clean, uncontaminated, quartz surfaces and those containing some level of impurities. They studied quartz sand samples from eight different deposits by this method and were able to correlate the cytotoxicity of the materials with the relative number of "clean" quartz particles in the sample. A similar correlation could not be established with the total quartz content of the materials.

E. EDXA DEPTH PROFILING

A technique similar to LAMMA, but nondestructive of the volume sampled, has been demonstrated by Wallace, et al. (1990, 1992), using low-voltage, scanning-electron microscopy-X-ray analysis. Respirable-sized particles of high-quartz content from a clay mine, several coal mines, and a tunneling site were examined for aluminum and silicon content by a scanning electron microscopy, energy-dispersive, X-ray analysis at incident energies of 5 to 20 keV. The results, combined with a model for calculating the silicon fraction of the signal as a function of the incident electron energy and beam penetration, show that a significant fraction of "quartz" particles collected from some mixed-dust atmospheres have heterogeneous structure with an aluminosilicate coating occluding a silica core. The method is described at greater length in Section II, Chapter 4.

F. INFRARED SPECTROSCOPY

The identification and quantification of surface bond structure, as well as of species adsorbed onto silica surfaces, has become possible with the development of special infrared spectroscopy techniques.

Although IR absorption spectrometry has been used for more than two decades for the analysis of adsorption complexes on high surface area materials (Little, 1966; Bell and Hair, 1980), the recent advent of fast-scanning IR Michelson interferometers with Fourier-transform analysis of signals has greatly enhanced the surface analysis capabilities of the instrument (Griffith and de Haseth, 1986). With this new generation of Fourier transform IR (FTIR) instruments, the sensitivity of detection by surface-specific techniques such as photoacoustic and diffuse reflectance spectroscopies has increased sufficiently to register signals associated with surface vibrational modes. Hoffmann and Knözinger (1987) have used FTIR techniques to characterize the far IR spectrum associated with the torsional and stretching modes of OH groups on silica surfaces. They used time-resolved IR spectroscopy to characterize the physical and chemical sorption of water on silica surfaces in the 25 to 1100°C temperature range. Hoffmann's and Knözinger's research, as well as most other IR studies of silica surfaces, has been conducted on amorphous, fumed silica materials of large, specific surface areas. The most outstanding feature of the surface-related FTIR spectrum of this amorphous silica is a sharp band at 3748 cm^{-1} which decreases in intensity and shifts to higher frequencies after treating the material at increasingly higher temperatures. This shift results from the change of the bonding characteristics of the surface silanol groups from hydrogen-bonded vicinal groups on the fully hydrated surface (absorption band at ~3745 cm^{-1}) to free, single silanol groups (absorption band at 3749 cm^{-1}) for the nearly dehydroxylated surface.

Kriegseis, et al. (1975), have previously reported IR spectra for several quartz dusts of different origins which did not exhibit the 3749 cm^{-1} band characteristic of the amorphous silicas. They observed, however, different surface-related bands on the different dusts and identified two bands, one at 3610 cm^{-1} and the other at 3685 cm^{-1}, whose intensities correlate in inverse proportion with the cytotoxicity of the dust.

Pandurangi, et al. (1990), have conducted a comparative study of the FTIR spectra and hemolytic activities of amorphous, high-surface area silica and high purity quartz dusts. In this study the 3749 cm^{-1} band, as well as bands at 3619 cm^{-1} and 3695 cm^{-1}, were detected for the quartz sample, although the former is much weaker than the latter. The concentration of surface silanol groups was varied with different thermal treatment and shown to correlate with hemolytic activity for both amorphous silica and quartz.

V. RESPIRABLE QUARTZ PARTICLES IN MINE DUSTS

As has been alluded above, the purity level of quartz particles surfaces is a primary variable affecting its cytotoxic behavior. Impurities inside the siliceous material play a role in the formation of cleavage facets of essentially pure material, and the adsorption of impurities from the environment further affect the properties of particle surfaces. For quartz and other siliceous material particles present in dusts formed from coal or other mines, the surface characteristics and their effect on properties may be expected to be much more complex. Although inhaled mine dusts are known to be a dominant cause of pneumoconioses, fibrosis, and silicosis in humans, and acute silicosis resulting from inhalation of pure, or nearly pure quartz dusts is well documented, it has not been possible to establish a quantitative relationship between the pathogenicity of mine dusts (particularly coal mine dusts) and their quartz content.

Extensive studies conducted over the past 25 years of the characteristics of coal mine dust from different mines and different stratigraphic horizons from across the countries of the European community and the incidence of silicosis among workers engaged in these mines has shown no correlation between the quartz content of the dusts and their level of pathogenicity (Hurley, et al., 1982; Le Bouffant, 1988; Robok and Bauer, 1988). Similar results have been reported for mineral dusts from different mines in the U.S. (Walton, et al., 1977; Razzaboni, et al., 1991; Wallace, et al., 1992).

Within particular coal mining regions [Germany (Saar and Ruhr), Great Britain, and France (Lorraine and Pas de Calais)], it has been found that stratigraphic horizons of higher-ranking seams are associated with a higher incidence of silicosis than those with lower-ranking seams (Hejny, Robok, and Armbruster, 1989). The fact that the weight fraction of silica is not a sufficient criterion for estimating the risk of silicosis has also been demonstrated by dusts from iron ore mines of the Salzgitter region of Germany (Bauer, 1986). In spite of high quartz contents detected in these dusts by X-ray diffraction methods, no incidence of silicosis has been found among the workers of these mines.

These observations show that the mass fraction of quartz alone does not define its cytotoxicity; rather, factors, directly or indirectly related to the stratigraphic horizon of the dust source, which affect the structure, composition, and chemical nature of the quartz particle surfaces, may define their cytotoxicity. A number of studies have been conducted recently to obtain more detailed information on the surface structure of respirable-size quartz particles encountered in mining environments that may relate to their cytotoxic and fibrogenic potential.

Smith, et al. (1991), have studied the morphology of respirable quartz particles in relation to the mineralogical characteristics of the source rock. They examined a large number of respirable-size quartz particles in the airborne dust and in the source rocks of three coal mines and compared the morphologies of these particles to those of similar size particles formed by mechanical crushing of quartz samples. The mechanically-broken grains typically have the form of slivers or shards and terminate at high atomic-density cleavage planes. Such surfaces were not observed in similar-size particles collected in the mine dust or obtained by grinding the corresponding source rocks. These latter particles were generally found to be rounded with no apparent cleavage faces or sharp edges.

The source rocks in question were shales and mudstones. This suggests that the shape of the quartz particles found in the source rock and released to the atmosphere during mining operations has been determined, in this case, by the mineralogical history of the rock and not by mechanical fracturing during the process. The sedimentary nature of the rocks implies that their constituent particles have been in transport and in contact with aqueous media for hundreds of millions of years. The rounding of the particles could have occurred by two principal mechanisms: abrasion during the sedimentation process or preferential reaction (e.g., hydrolysis) of the material located at the edges and corners of the grains. Quartz particles smaller than 0.2 μm are rarely, if ever, found in sedimentary rock samples, suggesting that the increased reactivity of these particles leads to hydrolysis and the formation of clay. The increased reactivity derives from the smaller radius of curvature (increased energy of the atoms located at the particle surface) and the higher chemical activity of atoms located at the edges and corners of crystalline particles.

The hydrolysis and formation of aluminosilicates at the surface of micron-sized particles may also be the cause of the occlusion of quartz particle surfaces by clay, as has been determined by Wallace, et al. (1990), in a study of the composition profile of high silica content, respirable particles from clay mines. In a similar study, Tourmann and Kaufmann (1989) used laser microprobe mass analysis to study the depth composition profiles of surface layers of quartz particles in different quartz reference materials and in three mineral-rich dust filter samples. They found that the toxicological data for the dusts studied correlated with the fraction of unoccluded or unmasked quartz particles in each sample rather than with the total mass fraction of quartz.

The reduction of the toxicity of quartz by adsorbed foreign material may be visualized as a mechanical masking or blocking effect by adsorbed particles; however, the presence of surface impurities also may affect the chemical activity of quartz. Strübel and Rinn (1987) have studied the changes in surface acidity of quartz particles resulting from their reaction in aqueous media with illitic and kaolinitic clay minerals and the effect of surface acidity on cytotoxicity. The basic phenomenon under scrutiny was the dissociation behavior of the surface silanol groups at different pH and electrolyte concentration. The results show a reduction in surface acidity of quartz after reaction with clay minerals and a concurrent reduction in the cytotoxicity to alveolar macrophages of guinea pigs.

The possible cytotoxicity or fibrogenicity of particles of different composition adhering to quartz particles complicates the effect of occlusion on the cytotoxicity of quartz surfaces. Several studies indicate that some silicates (kaolinite, muscovite, montmorrilonite, illite, feldspars, etc.) induce some pathogenic effects of their own. Le Bouffant, et al. (1977), report that intratracheal injections of kaolinite, illite, and muscovite into lungs of rats caused fibrogenicity, although lower than that resulting from similar doses of quartz dust. More recently, Rosmanith, et al. (1989), have reviewed the experimental work on cytotoxicity and fibrogenicity of various silicates and report experimental results on kaolinite, muscovite, and feldspar. These results, obtained from intratracheal tests conducted on rats, show that all three silicates tested elicit fibrogenicity. Muscovite, the most potent of the three, exhibits an activity equal to about 10% of that obtained with quartz (50 mg of muscovite generated an effect comparable to that obtained with 5 mg of quartz).

Shape analysis also permits the evaluation of the history of formation of respirable-size particles. Dumm and Hogg (1991), for example, have developed a scheme of shape analysis with the specific aim of distinguishing between angular and more rounded particles. Their two-parameter ("angular variability" and "elongation index") is shown to be consistent with visual observations and capable of distinguishing quartz dust particles produced by different grinding procedures. This method, combined with the observation of Smith, et al. (1991), on the shape of quartz particles in mine dusts, suggests a method for quantifying the relative amount of "freshly formed," or relatively clean quartz surfaces in any given dust sample.

VI. SILICA SURFACE ADSORPTION OF BIOMOLECULES

The adsorption of lipids or proteins on the surface of silica and other minerals has been studied extensively as the first step of the complex mechanisms that lead to mineral-surface induced membranolysis, *in vitro* cytotoxicity and pulmonary fibrosis. Iler (1979) has reviewed much of this literature, and a continuing review of current research has been provided by the North Atlantic Treaty Organization Advanced Science Institutes Series on the Effects of Mineral Dusts on Cells.

Hydrogen bond formation between quartz surface silanol groups and phosphate groups was an early suggestion for the mechanism of membranolysis. Its role in silicosis was postulated by Allison and colleagues to be damage to the lysosomal membrane following particle phagocytosis by pulmonary macrophages, resulting in cell death or damage.

It has been suggested that hemolysis by mineral surface of asbestos fiber and of quartz may be due to an adsorption of cell membrane phospholipid constituents onto the mineral surface. In studies by Jaurand, et al. (1980 a,b), of the adsorption of phospholipid liposomes and red blood cell membrane on native and treated chrysotile asbestos and DQ12 silica, a linear relationship was found between the concentration of dust needed to give 100% hemolysis in an *in vitro* system and the reciprocal of the specific adsorption capacity of the dust for dipalmitoyl phosphatidylcholine (DPPC). That is, there was a correlated hyperbolic relationship between hemolytic activity and adsorption capacity for DPPC.

A suggested mechanism for such membranolysis by membrane lipid adsorption on mineral surface is electrostatic interaction between silica surface silanol sites and the positively charged trimethylammonium group of any particular diacyl phosphatidylcholine.

The DPPC molecule consists of two hydrophobic palmitic acid residues esterified to a glycerol; onto the third glycerol carbon a choline group is esterified through a phosphate. The phosphate is acidic; the choline at the end of the molecule contains a fixed positive charge trimethylammonium nitrogen. Thus an electrostatic interaction is posited between the positive charge of the choline and the acidic silanol groups of the mineral surface. This interaction is suggested to lead to adsorption of membrane phospholipids with consequent distortion and rupture of the membrane.

This model predicts differing membranolytic activity as a function of the ratio between the areas of silica surface and of the membrane. Predictions are consistent with data from a test system of *in vitro* hemolysis induced by varying concentrations of spherical particles of amorphous silica of 15 nm particle diameter. Percent hemolysis after a given time versus silica concentration was non-linear with a maximum at the concentration for which the total surface area of applied silica was the same order of magnitude as the total surface area of exposed membrane. These results are interpreted in terms of the potential for maximum distortion of the membrane at such relative silica concentration. In that study, hemolysis was found to be inhibited by the addition of the soluble tetramethylammonium bromide. The inhibition was shown not to be related to coagulation of the silica particles and was suggested to be due to adsorption of the tetramethylammonium ion, essentially competing with lipid choline for the surface silanol sites.

These mechanisms for cytotoxicity induction as a result of the primary interaction of silica surface silanol adsorption of plasma or lysosomal membrane do not provide an immediate basis for distinguishing the pathogenic potential between various silica structures and silicates. Iler (1979) notes that the significant cytotoxicities of amorphous silica are not necessarily contradictory to the apparent lower fibrogenic potential of amorphous silica in comparison with crystalline polymorphs. This may be due to the lack of definition of amorphous silica pathogenic potential separate from the drastic difference in size of particles between typical crystalline and amorphous silica exposures. A similar seeming contradiction, that silicate clay and crystalline silica express comparable *in vitro* cytotoxicities for comparable size and surface area dusts but appear to have differing potentials for *in vivo* induction of fibrosis in animal models, has been suggested to reside in additional biochemical reactions with other functional groups on the aluminoisilicate surface. This is discussed in Section IV, Chapter 1.

A number of surface structural features and associated mechanisms may be involved in the cause or the modification of silica cytotoxicity, from physisorption by surface silanols to peroxidation or other energetic reactions by excited surface states. The exposure situations under which various surface functions and mechanisms may be prominent, as between mature and freshly fractured silica surface; the possible role for surface order of the active sites, as between amorphous and crystalline silica; and the surface properties which distinguish the fibrogenic potential from the cytotoxic potential, as between quartz and clay, still are subject to investigation.

REFERENCES

Antonini, J. F. and Hochstrasser, G., Surface states of pristine silica surfaces II. UHV studies of the CO_2- adsorption-desorption phenomena, *Surf. Sci.*, 32, 644–664, 1972.

Bauer, H. D., Staubbewertung und Staubbekampfung Schwerpunkte der Silikoseforschung, *Kompass*, 96, 456–461, 1986.

Baumann, H., Adsorption von Kieselsaure an Quartz, *Naturwissenschaften*, 53, 177–178, 1966.

Bell, A. T. and Hair, M. L., Vibrational Spectroscopies for Adsorbed Species, ACS Symposium 137, American Chemical Society, Washington, D.C., 1980.

Bergman, I. and Langrish, B., Silica powders of respirable size: The effect of methods of comminution and pretreatment on electrophoretic mobility, *Electroanal. Chem. Interfacial Electrochem.*, 34, 203–210, 1972.

Bloss, F. D., Anisotropy of fracture in quartz, *Am. J. Sci.*, 255, 214–225, 1957.

Bloss, F. D. and Gibbs, G. V., Cleavage in quartz, *Am. Mineral.*, 48, 821–838, 1963.

Bolis, V., Fubini, B., and Venturello, C., Surface characterization of various silicas. A tentative correlation between the energies of adsorption sites and the different biological activities, *Therm. Anal.*, 28(2), 249–258, 1983.

Christie, J. M., Griggs, D. T., and Carter, N. L., Experimental evidence of basal slip in quartz, *J. Geol.*, 72, 734–756, 1964.

Depasse, J. and Warlus, J., Relation of the toxicity of silica and its affinity for trimethylammonium groups, *J. Colloid Interface Sci.*, 56(3), 618, 1976.

Depasse, J., Mechanism of the Haemolysis by Colloidal Silica, in *In Vitro Effects of Mineral Dusts*, Brown, R.C., Ed., Academic Press, London, 125–130, 1980.

Dumm, T. F. and Hogg, R., Characterization of Particle Shape, Proc. of the 3rd Symposium on Respirable Dust in the Mineral Industries, Frantz, R.L. and Raman, R.V. Eds., Society for Mining, Metallurgy, and Exploration, Inc., Littleton, CO, 283–288, 1991.

Ford, W. E., *A Textbook of Mineralogy*, J. Wiley, New York, 1957.

Frondel, C., *Systems of Mineralogy (Vol. III): Silica Minerals*, John Wiley, New York, 1962.

Fubini, B., Bolis, V., and Giamello, E., The surface chemistry of crushed quartz dust in relation to its pathogenicity, *Inorg. Chim. Acta*, 138, 193–197, 1987.

Griffiths, P. R. and de Haseth, J. A., *Fourier Transform Infrared Spectrometry,* J. Wiley, New York, 1986.

Hammond, C., Moon, C. F., and Smalley, I. J., High voltage electron microscopy of quartz particles from post-glacial clay soils, *J. Mater. Sci.,* 8, 509–513, 1973.

Harington, J. S. and Alison, A. C., Tissue and cellular reaction to particles, fibers, and aerosols retained after inhalation, in *Handbook of Physiology-Reaction to Environmental Agents,* Lee, D.H.K., Ed., American Physiological Society, Washington, D.C., 263–283, 1977.

Heffernan, P. and Green, A. T., The method of action of silica dust in the lungs, *J. Ind. Hyg.,* 10, 272–278, 1928.

Hejny, H., Robok, K., and Armbruster, L., On the question of quartz evaluation in mine dusts from coalmining and its specific harmfulness, Silicosis Report/North-Rhine Westphalia, 17, 139–158, 1989.

Hochstrasser, G. and Antonini, J. F., Surface states of pristine silica surfaces I. ESR studies of Es' dangling bonds and of CO_2- adsorbed radicals, *Surf. Sci.,* 32, 644–664, 1972a.

Hoffmann, P. and Knözinger, E., Novel aspects of mid and far IR Fourier spectroscopy applied to surface and adsorption studies on SiO_2, *Surf. Sci.,* 188, 181–198, 1987.

Holt, P. F. and King, D. T., Solubility of silica, *Nature,* 175, 514–515, 1955.

Hurley, J., Burns, T., Copland, T., Dodgson, J., and Jacobson, M., Coalworkers simple pneumoconiosis and exposure to dust at 10 British coal mines, *Br. J. Ind. Med.,* 39, 120–127, 1982.

Iler, R. K., *The Chemistry of Silica,* John Wiley and Sons, New York, 1979.

Jaurand, M. C., Chemical and photoelectron spectroscopy analysis of the adsorption of phospholipid model membrane and red blood cell membrane onto chrysotile fibers, *Br. J. Ind. Med.,* 37, 169, 1980.

Jaurand, M. C., Reiner, A., and Bignon, J., The adsorption of phospholipids and red blood cell membranes on chrysotile fibers, in *in Vitro Effects of Mineral Dusts,* Brown, R.C., Ed., Academic Press, London, 1980, 125–130.

Kessel, R. W. I., Monaco, L., and Marchisio, M. A., The specificity of the cytotoxic action of silica — a study *in vitro, Br. J. Exp. Pathol.,* 44, 351–364, 1963.

Kozin, F., Millstein, B., Mandel, G., and Mandel, N., Silica-induced membranolysis: a study of different structural forms of crystalline and amorphous silica and the effects of protein adsorption, *J. Colloid Interface Sci.,* 88, 326–337, 1982.

Kriegseis, W., Biederbrick, R., Boese, J., Robok, K., and Scharmann, A., Investigation into the determination of the cytotoxicity of quartz dust by physical methods, in *Inhaled Particles and Vapours,* Vol. IV, Walton, W.A., Ed., British Office of Health and Safety, Edinburgh, Pergamon Press, London, 1975, 345–359.

Kriegseis, W., Ruediger, R., and Scharmann, A., Determination of free quartz surfaces in coal mine dust using an improved luminescence measurement, Silicosis Report/North-Rhine Westphalia, 16, 97–102, 1987.

Kriegseis, W. and Scharmann, A., An improved method for determining the free quartz surface in coal mine dust using luminescence measurements, Silicosis Report/North-Rhine Westphalia, 16, 91–96, 1987.

Kuhn, D., Hershey Medical Center, PA, Private Communication, 1992.

Langer, A. M., Crystal faces and cleavage planes in quartz as templates in biological processes, *Q. Rev. Biophys.,* 11, 543–575, 1978.

Le Bouffant, L., Daniel, H., and Martin, J. C., Die Rolle des Quarzes bei der Bildung pneumokoniotischer lasionen beim Steinkohlen-Bergarbeiter, EGKS Series Arbeitshygiene und Arbeitsmedizin v. 19, Luxemburg, 1977.

Le Bouffant, L., Gemeinschaftsforschung: Untersuchungen der Beziehungen zwischen den epidemiologischen Ergebnissen und der Schadlichkeit der Feinstaube im Kohlenbergbau, CEC Report EUR 10872, Health Protection in Mining, 1988.

Little, L. H., *Infrared Spectra of Adsorbed Species,* Academic Press, New York, 1966.

Monterra, C. and Low, M. J. D., Reactive silica: Novel aspects of the chemistry of silica surfaces, *Ann. N.Y. Acad. Sci.,* 220, 133–244, 1973.

Nash, T., Allison, A. C., and Harrington, J. S., Physicochemical properties of silica in relation to its toxicity, *Nature,* 210, 259, 1966.

Nolan, R. P., Langer, A. M., Harington, J. S., Oster, G., and Selikoff, I. J., Quartz hemolysis as related to its surface functionalities, *Environ. Res.,* 26, 503–520, 1981.

Pandurangi, R. S., Seehra, M. S., Razzaboni, B. L., and Bolsaitis, P., Surface and bulk infrared modes of crystalline and amorphous silica particles: a study of the relation of surface structure to cytotoxicity of respirable silica, *Environ. Health Perspect.,* 86, 327–336, 1990.

Pandurangi, R. S. and Seehra, M. S., Hemolytic Ability of Different Forms of Silica and Role of the Surface Silanol Species, Proc. of 3rd Symposium on Respirable Dusts in the Mineral Industries, Frantz, R.L. and Ramani, R.V., Eds., SMME, Littleton, CO, 121–125, 1991.

Razzaboni, B. L., Rainey, L., Wallace, W. E., Vallyathan, V., and Bolsaitis, P., A Micro-hemolysis Assay for Monitoring Mineral Dusts, Proc. of 3rd Symposium on Respirable Dusts in the Mineral Industries, Frantz, R.L. and Ramani, R.V., Eds., Society of Mining and Metallurgical Engineers, Littleton, CO, 111–115, 1991.

Razzaboni, B. L., Bolsaitis, P., Wallace, W. E., and Keane, M. J., Effect of thermal treatment on the surface characteristics and hemolytic activity of respirable size silica particles, Proc. of the VIIth International Pneumoconioses Conference, Pittsburgh, PA, NIOSH-ILO, 215–230, 1988.

Robok, K. and Klosterkötter, W., Investigations into the specific toxicity of different SiO_2 and silicate dusts, *Staub Reinhart. Luft* (in English), 33, 60–63, 1973.

Robok, K. and Bauer, H. D., Investigations into the specific fibrogenicity of mine dusts in hardcoal mines of countries in the European Community, Proceedings of the VIIth International Pneumoconioses Conference, Pittsburgh, PA, NIOSH-ILO, 280–283, 1988.

Rosmanith, J., Hilscher, W., Hessling, B., Schyma, S. B., and Ehm, W., The fibrogenic action of kaolinite, muscovite, and feldspar, Silicosis Report/North-Rhine Westphalia, 17, 305–322, 1989.

Scheel, L. D., Smith, B., VanRiper, J., and Fleischer, E., Toxicity of silica. II. Characteristics of protein films adsorbed by quartz, *Arch. Ind. Hyg.*, 9, 29–36, 1954.

Shi, X., Dalal, N. S., and Vallyathan, V., ESR evidence for the hydroxyl radical formation in aqueous suspension of quartz particles and its possible significance to lipid peroxidation, *J. Toxicol. Environ. Health,* 25, 237–245, 1988.

Smith, D. K., Mutmansky, J. M., Klimkiewicz, M., and Marks, J. A., Quartz Particulate Behavior During the Mechanical Mining of Coal Seams, Proc. of the 3rd Symposium on Respirable Dust in the Mineral Industries, Frantz, R.L. and Raman, R.V., Eds., Society for Mining, Metallurgy, and Exploration, Inc., Littleton, CO, 239–251, 1991.

Sosman, R. B., *The Phases of Silica,* Rutgers University Press, New Brunswick, NJ, 1964.

Stalder, K. and Stober, W., Haemolitic activity of suspensions of different silica modifications and inert dusts, *Nature,* 207, 874–875, 1965.

Strübel, G. and Rinn, G., Empirical investigations into the acidity of quartz surfaces and the effectiveness of surface masking, Silicosis Report/North-Rhine Westphalia, 16, 103–109, 1987.

Tourmann, J. L. and Kaufmann, R., LAMMA investigations of SiO_2-dusts and mineral-rich coalmine dusts in relation to their toxicity, Silicosis Report/North-Rhine Westphalia, 17, 111–118, 1989.

Vallyathan, V., Shi, X., Dalal, N. S., Irr, W., and Castranova, V., Generation of free radicals from freshly fractured silica dust: potential role in acute silica-induced lung injury, *Am. Rev. Respir. Dis.,* 138, 1213–1219, 1988.

Wallace, W. E., Harrison, J., Keane, M. J., Bolsaitis, P., Eppelsheimer, D., Poston, J., and Page, S. J., Clay occlusion of respirable quartz particles detected by low voltage scanning electron microscopy-X-ray analysis, *Ann. Occup. Hyg.,* 34, 195–204, 1990.

Wallace, W. E., Harrison, J. C., Grayson, R. L., Keane, M. J., Bolsaitis, P., Kennedy, R. D., Wearden, A. Q., and Attfield, M. D., Aluminosilicate surface contamination of respirable quartz particles from coal mine dusts and from clay works dusts, *Ann. Occup. Hyg.,* 38, suppl. 1, pp. 439–445, 1994.

Wallace, W. E., Hill, C. A., Keane, M. J., Page, S. J., Bolsaitis, P., Razzaboni, B. L., Vallyathan, V., and Mike, P., Alteration of Respirable Quartz Cytotoxicity by Thermal Treatment in Aqueous Media, Proceedings of the VIIth International Pneumoconioses Conference, Pittsburgh, PA, NIOSH-ILO, 215–230, 1988.

Walton, W. E., Dodgson, J., Hadden, G. G., and Jacobsen, M., The effect of quartz and other non-coal dusts on coal workers pneumoconiosis, in *Inhaled Particles IV,* Pergamon Press, Oxford, 1977, 669–689.

Wiessner, J. H., Henderson, J. D., Sohnle, P. G., Mandel, N. S., and Mandel, G. S., The effect of crystal structure on mouse lung inflammation and fibrosis, *Am. Rev. Respir. Dis.,* 138, 445–450, 1988.

Section II
Chapter 3

ROLE OF SURFACE FREE RADICALS IN THE PATHOGENICITY OF SILICA

Vincent Castranova, Nar S. Dalal, and Val Vallyathan

CONTENTS

I. INTRODUCTION

Silica can exist in either a crystalline or amorphous form. Evidence suggests that crystalline silica is more inflammatory and cytotoxic than amorphous silica.[1,2] Quartz is the most common form of crystalline silica. Silica is used in glass manufacturing, pottery making, and sandblasting. Quartz dust is also generated in foundries, mining, tunnelling, quarrying, and granite carving.

Silicosis is a fibrotic lung disease produced by inhalation of crystalline silica. Chronic silicosis may occur 20 to 40 years after initial exposure and is characterized by the development of concentric hyalinized nodular lesions in the upper lobes of the lungs. As the disease progresses from a simple to complicated form, these fibrotic lesions become larger and more numerous, and pulmonary function decreases.[3]

Acute silicosis is associated with the generation of freshly fractured silica dust in occupations such as sandblasting, rock drilling, tunnelling, and silica milling. Acute silicosis is characterized by the rapid onset (1 to 3 years after initial exposure) of dyspnea, fatigue, cough, and weight loss. Acute silicosis is associated with alveolar proteinosis and the development of diffuse, rather than nodular, fibrosis.[4]

Since acute silicosis is associated with grinding, milling, or fracturing of the crystalline structure of silica, it is possible that freshly generated cleavage planes have surface properties which make them more reactive to lung tissue and, thus, result in the rapid development of pulmonary disease. This chapter presents evidence to support the hypothesis that radicals are generated on cleavage planes of silica, which result in greater cytotoxicity and pathogenicity of this silica dust.

II. GENERATION OF RADICALS ON THE SURFACE OF SILICA

Figure 1 is a representation of crystalline quartz. The molecular structure of quartz is silicon dioxide (SiO_2), arranged as a three-dimensional crystal. When quartz is cut, ground, or milled, the crystal is

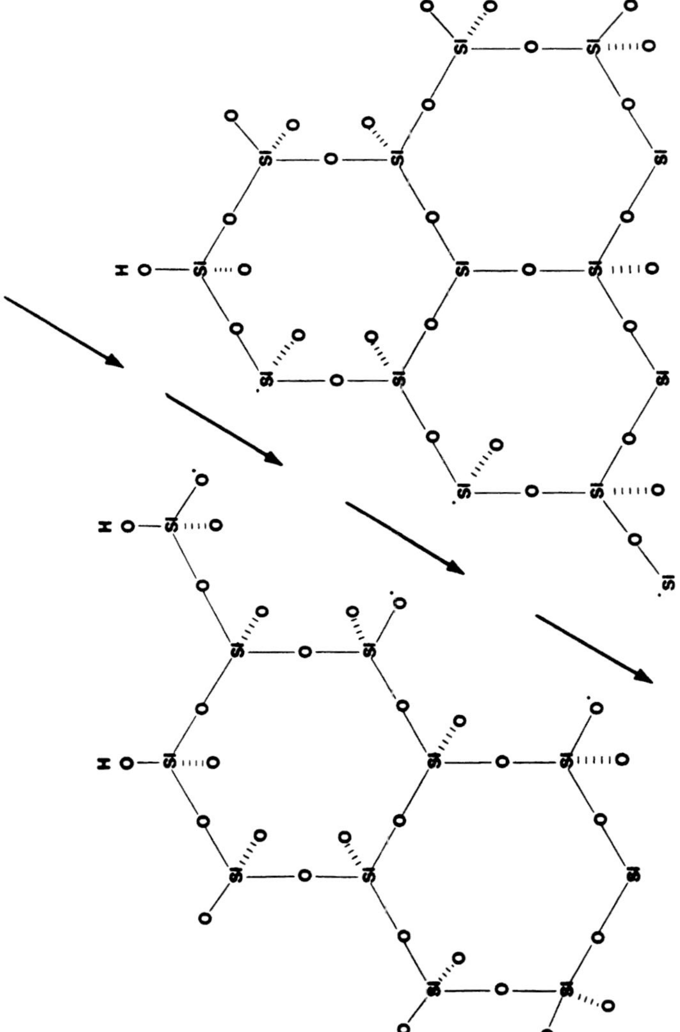

FIGURE 1 Crystalline lattice of quartz. Splitting Si–O bonds during fracturing generates $\dot{\text{Si}}$ and Si–$\dot{\text{O}}$ on the fracture surfaces.

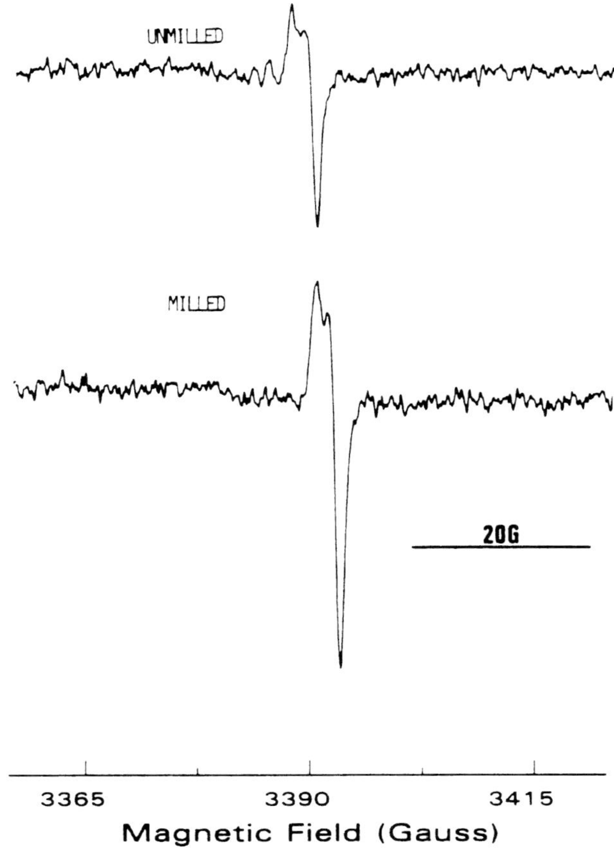

FIGURE 2 ESR spectra of unmilled and air jet milled silica. ESR spectra were obtained at X-band (~9.49 GHz) using a Varian E109 ESR spectrometer. All measurements were conducted at room temperature. The following settings were used: receiver gain = 4×10^4; modulation amplitude = 2 G; scan time = 240 sec; and field = 3380 ± 200 G.

fractured and $\dot{Si}$ and Si–$\dot{O}$ radicals theoretically should be generated on the cleavage surfaces. If surface free radicals exist on freshly fractured silica, their presence should be detectable using electron spin resonance (ESR) spectroscopy.[5]

Figure 2 presents typical ESR signals for native and milled silica. Native silica particles exhibit a small ESR signal. However, fracturing silica in a jet mill results in a significant increase in ESR signal intensity. This augmented signal is centered around g = 2.0015 which is characteristic of silicon-based radicals ($\dot{Si}$ and Si–$\dot{O}$), i.e., the so-called E-center.[6,7]

The relative intensity of the ESR signal, measured as signal height peak-to-peak, increases with the extent of fracturing. Figure 3 demonstrates that silica ground for 8 min with a ball mill exhibits a 7-fold greater ESR signal than silica ground for 1 min. This enhanced activity reflects a greater number of broken bonds and more silicon radicals on the fracture surfaces. These surface radicals decay with time after grinding, i.e., as ground silica is stored or aged. Approximately 80% of the ESR signal intensity decreases following first order kinetics with a $T_{1/2}$ of 30 h in air (Figure 4). The $T_{1/2}$ accelerates to a few minutes when fractured silica is stored in aqueous medium. Note that in air, 20% of the ESR signal remains detectable even after 4 weeks of storage.

The decay of silicon-based surface radicals in air can be increased by elevating the temperature. However, such an effect is not significant until relatively high temperatures (>200°C) have been reached (Figure 5).

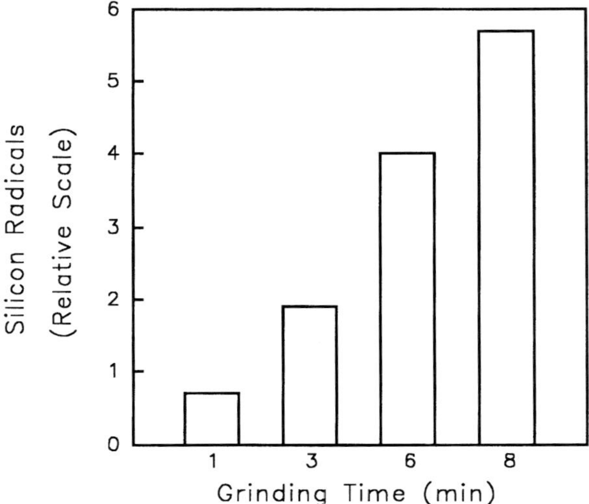

FIGURE 3 Relationship between generation of silicon-based radicals and grinding time. Silica was ground with an agate ball mill for various times before measurement of surface radicals with an ESR spectrometer. Data modified from Shi, Dissertation, West Virginia University, 1988.

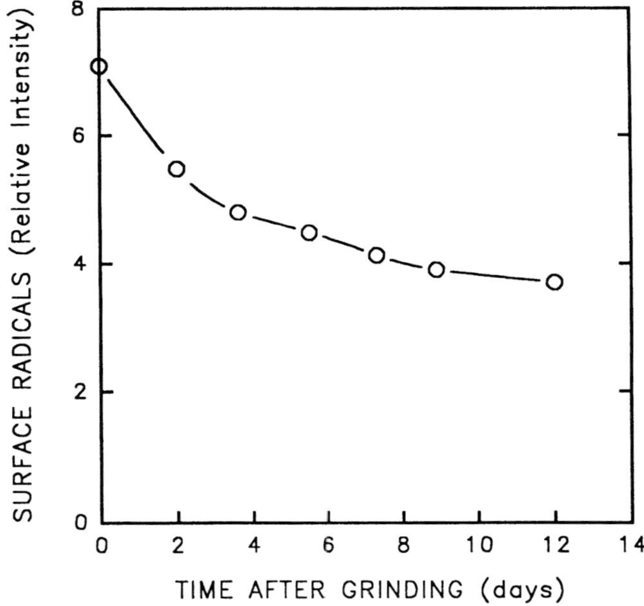

FIGURE 4 Decay of silicon-based surface radicals with time after grinding. Silica was ground with an agate ball mill. ESR intensity was determined immediately following grinding and after this ground sample was stored at 22°C in the dark, in air. (Data modified from Vallyathan et al., *Am. Rev. Respir. Dis.*, 138, 1213, 1988.)

Activation of particle surfaces after fracturing can also be determined by comparing the light emitted from freshly ground silica vs. ground silica which has been aged (stored) in air. Freshly fractured silica generates 4.4-fold more light than silica aged for 3 h after grinding (Figure 6). The $T_{1/2}$ for the decay in light emission is approximately 37 min, i.e., much shorter than the decay time for silicon-based surface radicals. This suggests that immediately after grinding, surface radicals are in an excited state. Rapidly, these radicals are converted to ground state radicals, emitting energy in the form of light. After reaching a ground state, this fractured silica can decay to the nonradical form.

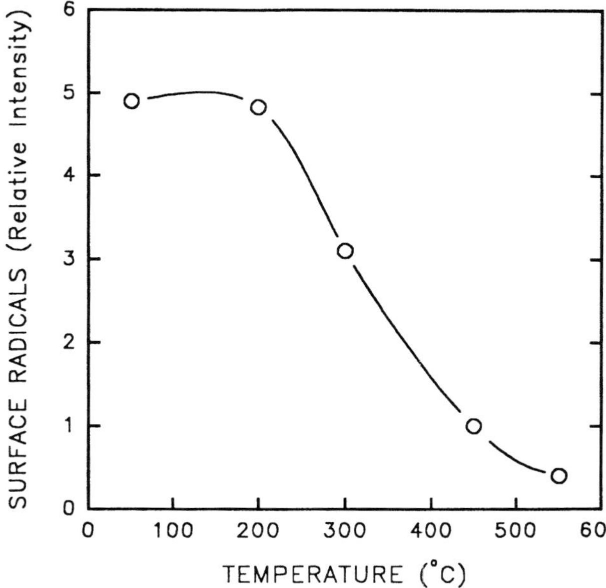

FIGURE 5 Decay of silicon-based surface radicals at elevated temperatures. Silica was ground with an agate ball mill then heated at various temperatures for 30 min prior to measurement of the ESR signal. (Data modified from Dalal et al., Proc. of the 7th International Pneumoconiosis Conf., 1424, 1990.)

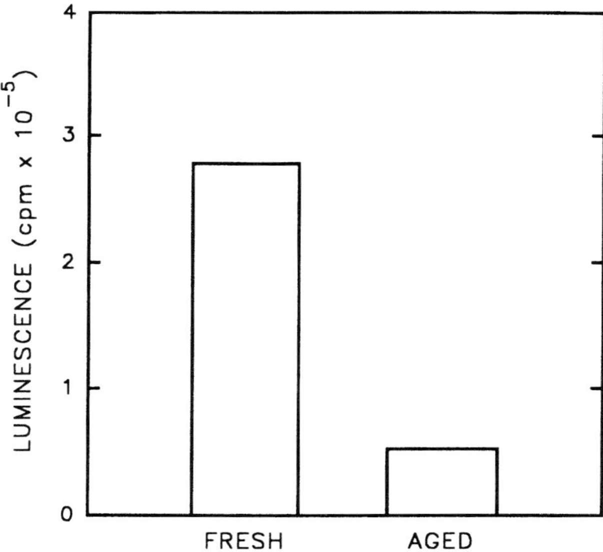

FIGURE 6 Surface activity of silica measured as luminescence. Light emission was measured immediately after grinding for 30 min with an agate ball mill (fresh) or 3 h after grinding (aged). (Data modified from Castranova et al., *Effects of Mineral Dusts on Cells,* Springer-Verlag, Berlin, 1989, 181, and Dalal et al., Proc. of the 7th International Pneumoconiosis Conf., 943, 1990.)

III. GENERATION OF HYDROXYL RADICALS BY FRESHLY GROUND SILICA

In aqueous media, these $\dot{S}i$ and Si–$\dot{O}$ radicals on the fracture planes of quartz can generate highly reactive hydroxyl radicals ($^{\cdot}OH$), which can be detected by ESR spectroscopy using an hydroxyl radical

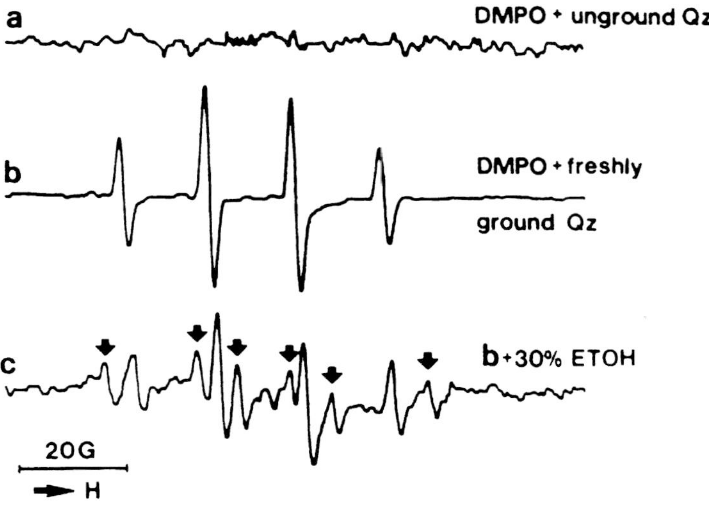

FIGURE 7 ESR spectra of silica in aqueous media containing 100 m*M* DMPO. Spectrum is with: (a) unground silica, (b) silica ground with an agate ball mill, and (c) ground silica plus 30% ethanol. Spectrometer settings were: receiver gain = 5 $\times 10^5$, modulation amplitude = 2 G, scan time = 100 sec, and field = 3460 ± 75 G. (Modified from Dalal et al., *Effects of Mineral Dusts on Cells,* Springer-Verlag, Berlin, 1989, 273.)

spin trap, DMPO (5,5-dimethyl-1-pyrroline-N-oxide).[13] As shown in Figure 7, freshly ground silica in aqueous medium containing 100 m*M* DMPO generates a substantial ESR signal compared to unground silica. This ESR signal is centered around g = 2.0059 and exhibits a 1:2:2:1 quartet pattern with a splitting of 14.9 G, which is characteristic of a DMPO-˙OH adduct.[14] The generation of ˙OH in aqueous medium can be verified further by quenching with ethanol, an ˙OH scavenger. Indeed, ethanol reacts with ˙OH to produce ethanolyl radicals, depresses the 1:2:2:1 ESR signal typical of a DMPO-˙OH adduct, and forms a DMPO-$\dot{C}HOCH_3$ adduct, indicated by arrows in Figure 7c.[14]

As with $\dot{S}i$ and Si–$\dot{O}$ generation, ˙OH production increased as fracturing became more extensive (Figure 8). For example, the potential for silica to generate ˙OH is 4-fold greater after 10 min of grinding than following 1 min of milling. The capacity of fractured silica to generate ˙OH decreases with aging in air, exhibiting a $T_{1/2}$ of approximately 1 d for the first order component of this decay curve. As with the presence of $\dot{S}i$ and Si–$\dot{O}$ surface radicals, fractured silica maintains some potential to generate ˙OH, even after 4 d of storage in air (Figure 9).

The magnitude of the DMPO-˙OH signal generated by freshly cleaved silica in aqueous medium is substantially decreased in the presence of the hydrogen peroxide (H_2O_2) scavenger, catalase, or the iron chelator, desferal (Figure 10). These data imply that the Fenton reaction plays a role in the generation of ˙OH.[17] Under this scheme, quartz contains trace amounts of ferrous iron as an impurity and, upon fracturing, generates H_2O_2 in aqueous medium to initiate the production of ˙OH as follows:[18]

1. $Si–\dot{O} + H_2O \rightarrow SiOH + {}^{\cdot}OH$
2. $Si–\dot{O} + {}^{\cdot}OH \rightarrow SiOOH$
3. $SiOOH + H_2O \rightarrow SiOH + H_2O_2$
4. $Fe^{2+} + H_2O_2 \rightarrow Fe^{3+} + {}^{\cdot}OH + OH^-$

IV. *IN VITRO* CYTOTOXICITY OF FRESHLY GROUND VS. AGED SILICA

Previously presented data indicate that grinding or milling silica cleaves bonds in the crystal lattice of quartz and generates silicon-based radicals on the fracture planes. These surface radicals react with water to generate the highly reactive species, ˙OH. As fractured silica ages, the ability to generate radicals declines.

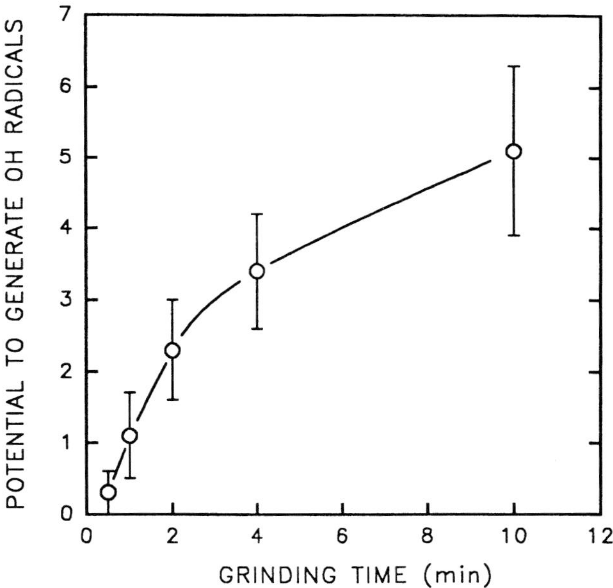

FIGURE 8 Potential of silica to generate hydroxyl radicals in aqueous medium vs. grinding time. Silica was ground with an agate ball mill. ESR spectra were measured in media containing 100 m*M* DMPO. (Modified from Dalal et al., Proc. of the 7th International Pneumoconiosis Conf., 250, 1990.)

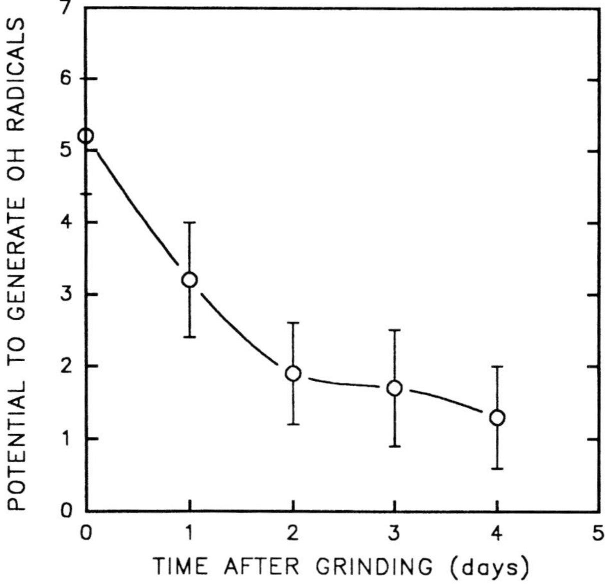

FIGURE 9 Relationship between hydroxyl radical generation and time after grinding. Silica was ground in an agate ball mill. ESR spectra were measured in media containing 100 m*M* DMPO at various times after storage of the milled dust in air, at 22°C, in the dark. (Modified from Dalal et al., Proc. of the 7th International Pneumoconiosis Conf., 250, 1990.)

Radicals, such as ·OH, are highly reactive with biological tissue and have been implicated in various disease processes.[19] The question is whether the radicals associated with freshly fractured silica cause it to be more toxic and inflammatory than aged silica.

Data presented in Figure 11 indicate that freshly fractured silica causes lipid peroxidation *in vitro*. This reactivity decays rapidly as the ground dust ages, decreasing by approximately 80% after storage for 4 d.

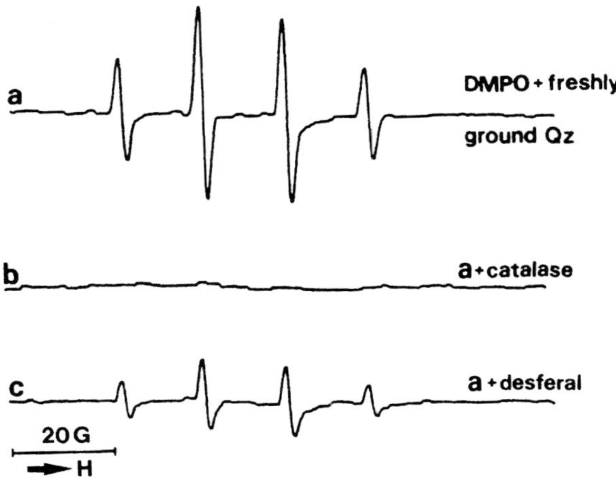

FIGURE 10 ESR spectra of freshly ground silica in media containing 100 m*M* DMPO. Spectrum is that for: (a) untreated ground silica, (b) ground silica in the presence of 5000 units/ml catalase, and (c) ground silica in the presence of 1 m*M* desferal. (Modified from Dalal et al., *Effects of Mineral Dusts on Cells,* Springer-Verlag, Berlin, 1989, 273.)

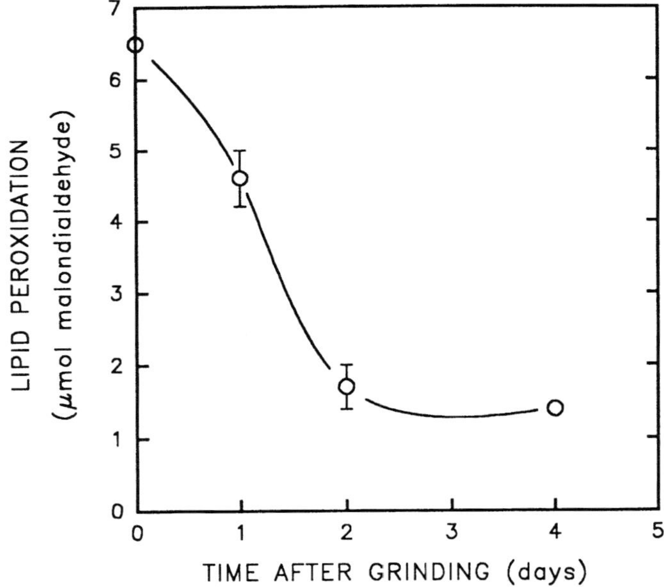

FIGURE 11 Decay in the ability of ground silica to peroxidize lipids with increasing storage time in air. Silica was ground with an agate ball mill. Lipid peroxidation was determined as malondialdehyde production following the treatment of linoleic acid (a polyunsaturated lipid) with 2.5 mg/ml silica for 1 h at 37°C. Malondialdehyde production was measured fluorometrically at an excitation wavelength of 515 nm and an emission of 555 nm. (Modified from Vallyathan et al., *Am. Rev. Respir. Dis.,* 138, 1213, 1988.)

Dalal, et al.,[20] have shown that the ability of silica to oxidize lipids strongly correlates with its ability to generate ˙OH in aqueous media.

Fresh silica is a potent lytic agent for red blood cells. The lytic potential of ground silica decreases by 97% after 4 d of storage in air (Figure 12). Freshly fractured silica is also more cytotoxic to alveolar macrophages than aged dust *in vitro.* As shown in Figure 13, fresh silica causes 47% more LDH (lactate dehydrogenase) release than dust stored in air for 2 d after grinding. The release of these cytosolic enzymes reflects loss of membrane integrity in these phagocytes. Silica-induced membrane damage in

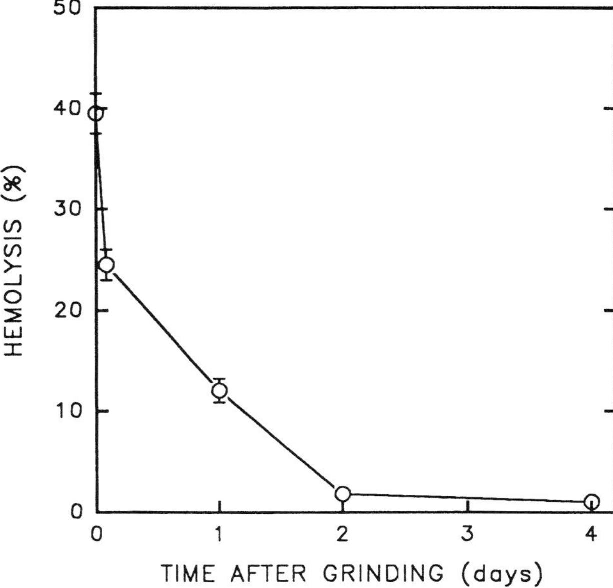

FIGURE 12 Hemolytic potential of ground silica vs. aging. Silica was ground with an agate ball mill. Silica was stored at room temperature in the dark, in air to age. Red blood cells (2% suspension) were treated with 10 mg/ml silica for 1 h at 37°C, and hemolysis was measured as the absorbance of the suspension supernate determined at 540 nm. (Modified from Dalal et al., *Effects of Mineral Dusts on Cells,* Springer-Verlag, Berlin, 1989, 265.)

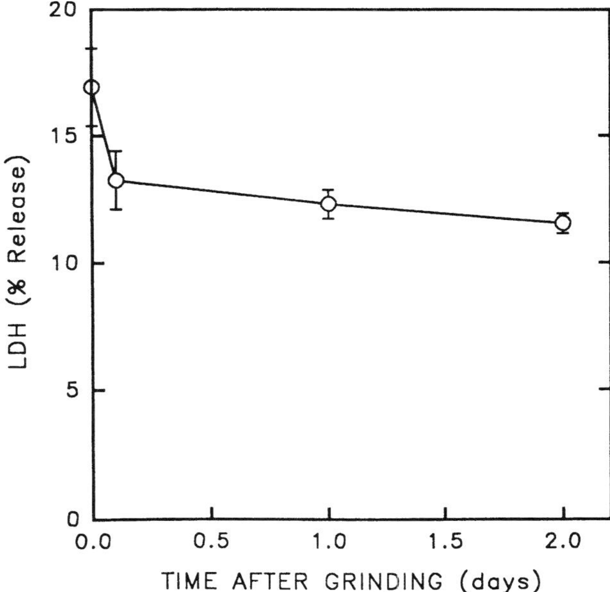

FIGURE 13 Effect of storage on the ability of ground silica to cause lactate dehydrogenase release from alveolar macrophages. Silica was ground with an agate ball mill and stored at room temperature in the dark, in air to age. LDH release from macrophages was measured spectrophotometrically at 340 nm following a 1 h treatment with 1 mg/ml silica. (Modified from Vallyathan et al. *Am. Rev. Respir. Dis.,* 138, 1213, 1988.)

alveolar macrophages can be verified by monitoring trypan-blue exclusion (Figure 14). Freshly cleaved silica is nearly 4-fold more potent in inducing membrane leakiness than fractured silica which has been stored in air for 2 weeks to age.

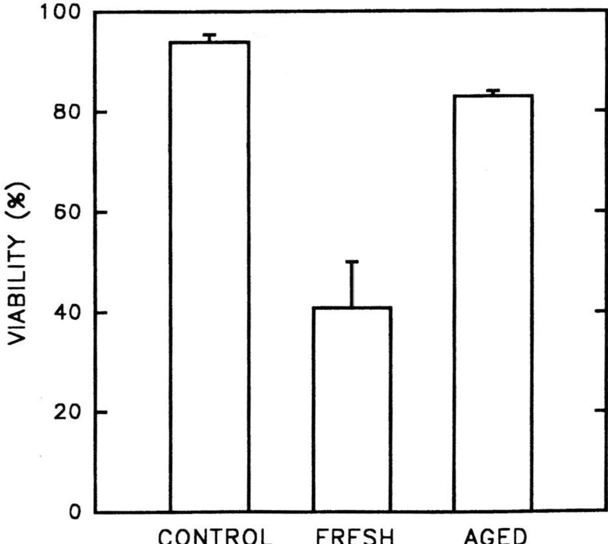

FIGURE 14 The effect of fresh or aged silica on the viability of alveolar macrophages. Silica was ground with an agate ball mill and used immediately (fresh) or 2 weeks (aged) after grinding. Viability of alveolar macrophages was measured as trypan-blue exclusion following a 30 min incubation of phagocytes at 37°C in the absence (control) or presence of 15 mg/ml silica. (Modified from Vallyathan et al., *J. Toxicol. Environ. Health,* 33, 303, 1991.)

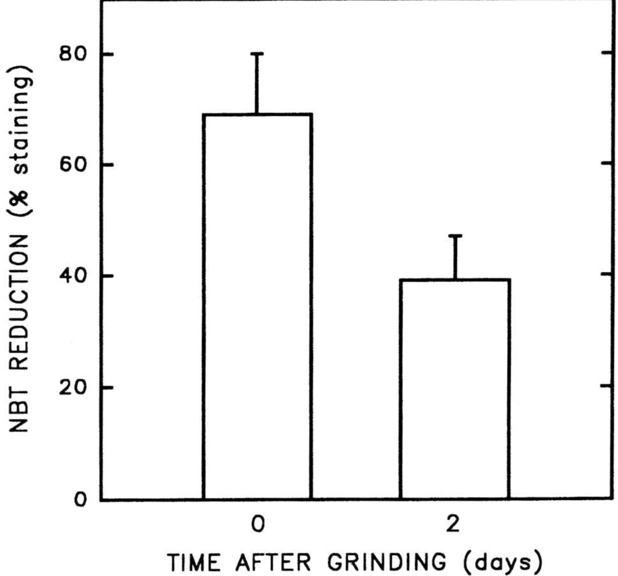

FIGURE 15 Effect of fresh vs. aged silica on superoxide anion release from alveolar macrophages. Superoxide anion production was measured histochemically as the reduction of nitro blue tetrazolium to formazan. (Modified from Vallyathan et al., *Am. Rev. Respir. Dis.,* 138, 1213, 1988.)

V. INFLAMMATORY POTENTIAL OF FRESHLY GROUND VS. AGED SILICA *IN VITRO*

The previous data indicate that fresh silica is more toxic to cells *in vitro* than aged silica. Further results indicate that fresh silica is also more inflammatory than aged silica; i.e., fresh silica is a more potent activator of oxidant generation by alveolar macrophages. Figure 15 shows that superoxide anion production

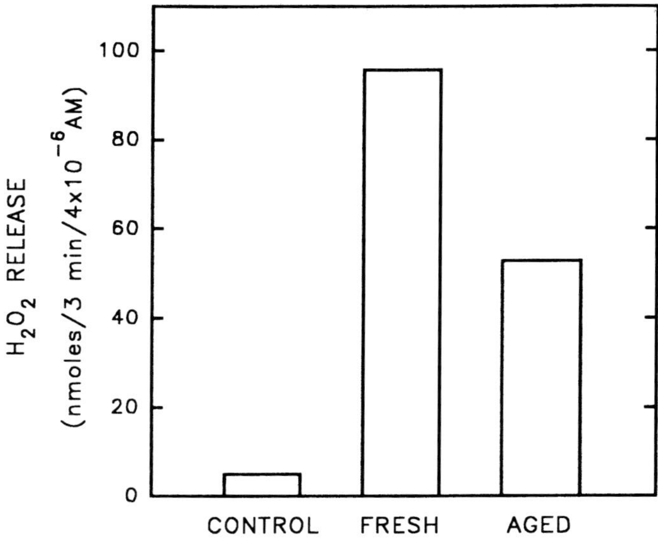

FIGURE 16 Ability of fresh or aged silica to stimulate hydrogen peroxide release from alveolar macrophages. Cells were exposed to 1 mg/ml fresh or aged (2 weeks) silica. H_2O_2 production was determined by monitoring the decrease in fluorescence of scopoletin at an excitation wavelength of 350 nm and an emission of 460 nm. (Modified from Kang, Dissertation, West Virginia University, 1990.)

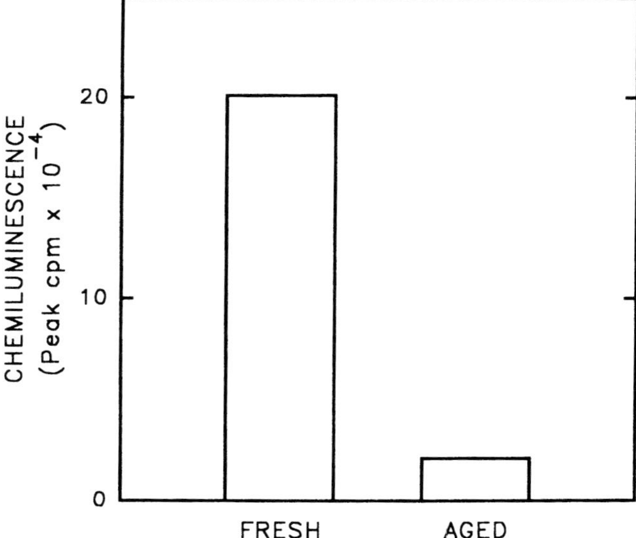

FIGURE 17 Silica-stimulated chemiluminescence from alveolar macrophages. Phagocytes (1×10^6 AM) were stimulated with 20 μg/ml freshly milled or aged (stored in air for 2 d after grinding) silica. Peak CL was measured 9 min after the addition of silica in the presence of lucigenin (2.5×10^{-8}M). CL data are silica-stimulated minus resting counts per minute (cpm). (Modified from Castranova et al., *Effects of Mineral Dusts on Cells,* Springer-Verlag, 1989, 181.)

by macrophages is 77% higher after exposure to freshly milled silica compared to fractured dust aged in air for 2 d. Similarly, silica-induced hydrogen peroxide release is 82% greater with fresh compared to aged dust (Figure 16). The enhanced potency of freshly fractured silica to stimulate alveolar macrophages is most evident using a chemiluminescence assay. As shown in Figure 17, silica-induced generation of light from alveolar macrophages is 9-fold greater using fresh, rather than aged, quartz.

TABLE 1
Cell Yield from Bronchoalveolar Lavage

Group	Total Cells	Alveolar Macrophages	RBC	Leukocytes
Control	5.70 ± 0.57	5.35 ± 0.59	0.10 ± 0.03	0.10 ± 0.01
Aged Silica	12.16 ± 1.55[a]	5.46 ± 0.80	1.48 ± 0.14[a]	4.75 ± 0.66[a]
Fresh Silica	23.73 ± 2.36[b]	6.73 ± 1.05[b]	5.83 ± 0.74[b]	10.70 ± 1.33[b]

Note: Values are means ± standard errors of 4 determinations (10^6 cells/rat). Rats were lavaged via a tracheal cannula with ten 8 ml aliquots of Ca^{2+}, Mg^{2+}-free phosphate buffered medium (145 m*M* NaCl, 5 m*M* KCl, 1.9 m*M* NaH_2PO_4, 9.35 m*M* Na_2HPO_4, and 5.5 m*M* dextrose; pH = 7.4). Total and differential cell counts were obtained using an electronic cell counter (Coulter Z_{BI}) equipped with a cell sizing attachment (Channelizer 256). Cell types were distinguished by their characteristic volume distributions. Leukocytes designate lymphocytes and granulocytes.

[a] Significantly greater than control ($p < 0.05$).
[b] Significantly greater than aged silica ($p < 0.05$).
Modified from Castronova, V., et al., 2nd International Symp. on Silica, Silicosis, and Cancer, 264–272 1993.

The data presented thus far indicate that fracturing silica generates silicon-based radicals and hydroxyl radicals which are associated with the direct toxicity of quartz. Furthermore, fresh silica is also a more potent stimulant of oxidant release from alveolar macrophages than aged quartz. The combination of particle-associated radicals and reactive species generated from silica-stimulated alveolar macrophages may overwhelm the antioxidant defense systems of the lung and result in the development of damage and disease.

VI. *IN VIVO* PULMONARY RESPONSE TO FRESHLY GROUND VS. AGED SILICA

In vitro data support the hypothesis that freshly ground silica is more cytotoxic and inflammatory than aged dust. Therefore, the next step was to verify this theory *in vivo.* For these *in vivo* exposures, fresh silica was generated in an air jet mill fitted with a polyurethane liner. Freshly milled silica was passed through a cyclone and either instilled into an inhalation chamber or collected in a bag and stored in air at room temperature for 2 months prior to aerosolization into the exposure chamber. Rats were divided into three groups: i.e., filtered air, freshly milled silica, and aged silica. Dust exposure was 20 mg silica/m^3 air, 5 h/d, 5 d/week, for 2 weeks. Measurement of exposures indicated that particle size (mass medium aerodynamic diameter ≈1.9 μm and count median circular area equivalent diameter ≈0.5 μm) and dust concentration (≈20 mg/m^3) did not differ significantly between the fresh and aged silica exposures. However, fresh silica exhibited an ESR signal for silicon-based radicals that was 54% greater than aged dust.[24]

After a two week exposure to 20 mg/m^3 silica, there is a substantial pulmonary reaction, as judged from cell differentials of bronchoalveolar lavage samples (Table 1). Total cells, red blood cells, and leukocytes (lymphocytes and granulocytes) are significantly elevated by 113%, 1380%, and 4650%, respectively, after exposure to aged silica. However, inhalation of freshly cleaved silica results in a substantially greater cellular reaction than aged silica: i.e., increasing total cells by 95%, red blood cells by 294%, and leukocytes by 125% above aged quartz. This inflammatory response is accompanied by lung damage measured as lung lipid peroxidation (Figure 18). Although aged silica exposure increases lung lipid peroxidation by 125% over control, inhalation of freshly milled silica causes 33% more damage than aged quartz.

Oxidants produced by alveolar macrophages may be responsible, in part, for this silica-induced lung damage. As shown in Table 2, inhalation of aged silica potentiates zymosan-stimulated chemiluminescence of alveolar macrophages by 847% above control. However, priming of alveolar macrophages is far greater after inhalation of fresh silica, yielding 176% more chemiluminescence than phagocytes from the

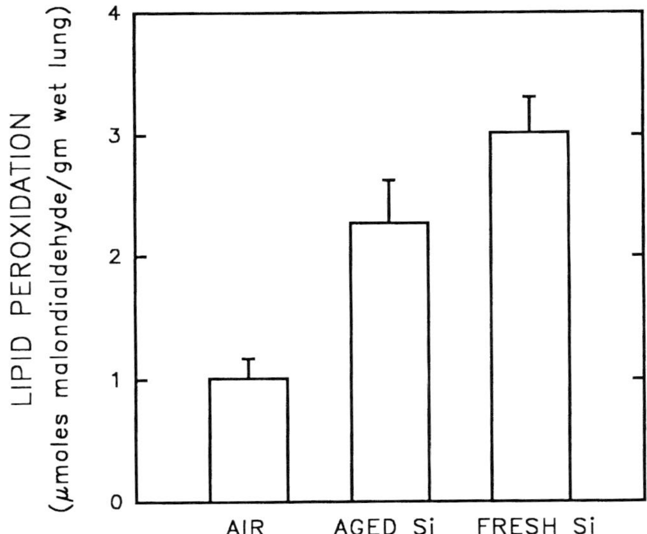

FIGURE 18 Lung lipid peroxidation in response to inhalation of fresh or aged silica. Lungs were exposed to freshly jet milled or aged (stored for 2 months) silica at 20 mg/m^3, 5 h/d, 5 d/week, for 2 weeks. Lipid peroxidation was measured spectrophotometrically as malondialdehyde formation. (Modified from Vallyathan et al., 2nd International Symp. on Silica, Silicosis, and Cancer, 263, 1993.)

TABLE 2
Chemiluminescence Generated from Alveolar Macrophages

Group	Zymosan-stimulated CL[a]	NO Synthase-dependent CL[b]
Control	29.34 ± 2.41	4.68 ± 1.04
Aged Silica	277.82 ± 13.08[c]	88.43 ± 9.84[c]
Fresh Silica	767.54 ± 79.85[d]	302.38 ± 45.27[d]

Note: Values are means ± standard errors of 4 experiments (cpm/0.75 × 10^6 AM). Chemiluminescence was measured at 37°C in the presence of 8 μg % luminol using a Berthold LB953 Luminometer. Cells were suspended in HEPES-buffered solution (145 m*M* NaCl, 5 m*M* KCl, 10 m*M* HEPES, 1 m*M* $CaCl_2$, and 5.5 m*M* dextrose; pH = 7.4).

[a] Zymosan-stimulated chemiluminescence was measured in the presence of 2 mg/ml unopsonized zymosan. Note that granulocytes do not respond to unopsonized zymosan.

[b] Nitric oxide synthase-dependent chemiluminescence was determined as the amount of zymosan-stimulated CL which was inhibitable by L-NAME (Nω-nitro-L-arginine methylester). Cells were preincubated for 10 min at 37°C with 1 m*M* L-NAME prior to the addition of zymosan and measurement of CL.

[c] Significantly greater than control ($p < 0.05$).

[d] Significantly greater than aged silica ($p < 0.05$).

Modified from Castranova, V., et al., 2nd International Symp. on Silica, Silicosis, and Cancer, 264–272, 1993.

aged silica-exposed animals. Evidence indicates that at least part of this increased chemiluminescence (CL) involves the generation of nitric oxide, since the NO synthase inhibitor, L-NAME (Nω-nitro-L-arginine methylester), significantly decreases this activity. Inhalation of aged silica increases NO synthase-dependent CL by 1790% above control. Again, fresh silica is a more potent inducer of NO synthase activity than aged silica, causing 242% more L-NAME-inhibitable CL.

VII. SUMMARY

Data presented in this chapter indicate that grinding or fracturing crystalline silica breaks Si–O bonds and generates $\dot{S}i$ and Si–$\dot{O}$ radicals on the cleavage planes. These surface radicals can react with water to generate ˙OH. This process seems to involve a Fenton type reaction. These surface and/or hydroxyl radicals are toxic to pulmonary cells both *in vitro* and *in vivo* causing increased lipid peroxidation and membrane leakiness. In addition, fresh silica is a more potent stimulator of reactive product generation by alveolar macrophages than aged silica. These reactive species include superoxide anion, hydrogen peroxide, nitric oxide, and peroxynitrite. In addition, cytokine production may also be elevated after inhalation of freshly fractured silica, since bronchoalveolar lavage yields high numbers of inflammatory cells following inhalation of freshly milled dust. Sandblasters, rock drillers, and silica flour millers are exposed to freshly fractured silica. Therefore, they may be at unique risk of suffering pulmonary damage and developing disease.

REFERENCES

1. **Warheit, D. B., Carakostas, M. C., Hartsky, M. A., and Hanson, J. F.,** Development of a short-term inhalation bioassay to assess pulmonary responses to carbonyl iron and silica, *Toxicol. Appl. Pharmacol.,* 107, 350–368, 1991.
2. **Warheit, D. B., Carakostas, M. C., Kelly, D. P., and Hartsky, M. A.,** Four-week inhalation toxicity study with ludox colloidal silica in rats: pulmonary cellular responses, *Fundam. Appl. Toxicol.,* 16, 590–601, 1991.
3. **Peters, J. M.,***Silicosis. Occupational Respiratory Diseases,* Merchant, J.A., Boehlecke, B.A., Taylor, G. and Pickett-Harner, M., Eds., DHHS (NIOSH) Publ. No. 86–102, 1986, 219–237.
4. **Banks, D. E.,** *Acute Silicosis. Occupational Respiratory Diseases,* Merchant, J.A., Boehlecke, B.A., Taylor, G. and Pickett-Harner, M., Eds., DHHS (NIOSH) Publ. No. 86–102, 1986, 239–241.
5. **Dalal, N. S., Suryan, M. N., Jafari, B., Shi, X., Vallyathan, V., and Green, F. H. Y.,** Electron spin resonance detection of reactive free radicals in fresh coal dust and quartz dust and its implication to pneumoconiosis and silicosis, in *Respirable Dust in the Mineral Industries: Health Effects, Characterization and Control,* Frantz, R.L. and Ramani, R.V., Eds., ACGIH Publ., 1988, 25–29.
6. **Hochstrasser, G., and Antonini, J. R.,** Surface states of pristine silica surfaces, *J. Surface Sci.,* 32, 644–664, 1972.
7. **Bolis, V., Fubini, B., and Venturello, G.,** Surface characterization of various silica, *J. Thermal Anal.,* 28, 249–257, 1983.
8. **Shi, X.,** ESR spin trapping applications to biochemical problems, Dissertation, West Virginia University, 1988.
9. **Vallyathan, V., Shi, X., Dalal, N. S., Irr, W., and Castranova, V.,** Generation of free radicals from freshly fractured silica dust: potential role in acute silica-induced lung injury, *Am. Rev. Respir. Dis.,* 138, 1213–1219, 1988.
10. **Dalal, N. S., Shi, X., and Vallyathan, V.,** Do silicon-oxygen radicals play a role in the quartz-induced hemolysis and fibrogenicity? Proc. of the 7th International Pneumoconiosis Conf., DHHS (NIOSH) Publ. No. 90–108, Part II, 1424–1428, 1990.
11. **Castranova, V., Vallyathan, V., Van Dyke, K., and Dalal, N. S.,** Use of chemiluminescence assays to monitor the surface characteristics and biological reactivity of freshly fractured vs aged silica, in *Effects of Mineral Dusts on Cells,* Mossman, B.T., and Begin, R.O., Eds., Springer-Verlag, Berlin, NATO ASI Series, Vol. H30, 1989, 181–188.
12. **Dalal, N. S., Vallyathan, V., Leelarasamee, N., Castranova, V., and Van Dyke, K.,** Chemiluminescence and biologic activity of freshly fractured silica, Proc. of the 7th International Pneumoconiosis Conf., DHHS (NIOSH) Publ. No. 90–108, Part II, 943–945, 1990.
13. **Finkelstein, E., Rosen, G. M., and Rauchman, E. J.,** Spin trapping of superoxide and hydroxyl radicals: practical aspects, *Arch. Biochem. Biophys.,* 200, 1–6, 1980.
14. **Buettner, G. R.,** The spin trapping of superoxide and hydroxyl radicals. *Superoxide Dismutase,* Oberly, L.W., Ed., CRC Press, Boca Raton, Vol. 2, 1984, 63–81.
15. **Dalal, N. S., Shi, X., and Vallyathan, V.,** Oxygenated radical formation by fresh quartz dust in a cell-free aqueous medium and its inhibition by scavengers, in *Effects of Mineral Dusts on Cells.,* Mossman, B.T. and Begin, R.O., Eds., Springer-Verlag, Berlin, NATO ASI Series, Vol. H30, 1989, 273–280.
16. **Dalal, N. S., Shi, X., and Vallyathan, V.,** Detection of hydroxyl radicals in aqueous suspension of fresh silica dust and its implication to lipid peroxidation in silicosis, Proc. of the 7th International Pneumoconiosis Conf., DHHS (NIOSH) Publ. No. 90–108, Part I, 250–253, 1990.
17. **Morehouse, K. M., and Mason, R. P.,** The transition metal-mediated formation of the hydroxyl free radical during the reduction of molecular oxygen by ferredoxin-ferredoxin: $NADP^+$ oxidoreductase, *J. Biol. Chem.,* 263, 1204–1211, 1988.

18. **Shi, X., Dalal, N. S., Hu, X. N., and Vallyathan, V.,** The chemical properties of silica particle surface in relation to silica-cell interactions, *J. Toxicol. Environ. Health,* 27, 435–454, 1989.
19. **Halliwell, B.,** Oxidants and human disease: some new concepts, *FASEB J.* 1, 358–364, 1987.
20. **Dalal, N. S., Shi, X., and Vallyathan, V.,** Role of free radicals in the mechanisms of hemolysis and lipid peroxidation by silica: comparative ESR and cytotoxicity studies, *J. Toxicol Environ. Health,* 29, 307–316, 1990.
21. **Dalal, N. S., Shi, X., and Vallyathan, V.,** Potential role of silicon-oxygen radicals in acute lung injury, in *Effects of Mineral Dusts on Cells,* Mossman, B.T., and Begin, R.O., Eds., Springer-Verlag, Berlin, NATO ASI Series Vol. H30, 1989, 265–272.
22. **Vallyathan, V., Kang, J. H., Van Dyke, K., Dalal, N. S., and Castranova, V.,** Response of alveolar macrophages to *in vitro* exposure to freshly fractured vs aged silica dust: the ability of Prosil 28, an organosilane material, to coat silica and reduce its biological reactivity, *J. Toxicol Environ. Health,* 33, 303–315, 1991.
23. **Kang, J. H.,** Possible mechanism and prevention strategies for silicosis, Dissertation, West Virginia University, 1990.
24. **Castranova, V., Pailes, W. H., Dalal, N. S., et al.,** Enhanced pulmonary response to the inhalation of freshly fractured silica as compared to aged dust exposure, 2nd International Symp. on Silica, Silicosis, and Cancer, Goldsmith, D.F., Ed., Western Consortium for Public Health, Berkeley, 264–272, 1993.
25. **Vallyathan, V., Pack, D., Hubbs, A., et al.,** Acute silicosis: etiology? 2nd International Symp. on Silica, Silicosis, and Cancer, Goldsmith, D.F., Ed., Western Consortium for Public Health, Berkeley, 263, 1993.

Section II
Chapter 4

SURFACE PROPERTIES OF SILICA IN MIXED DUSTS

William E. Wallace, Michael J. Keane, Joel C. Harrison, James W. Stephens, Patricia S. Brower, R. Larry Grayson, and Michael D. Attfield

CONTENTS

I. INTRODUCTION

Attempts to distinguish the contribution of quartz to the pathogenic potential of mixed-composition work place dusts are not without ambiguity. While exposure to pure respirable quartz is known to induce pulmonary fibrosis, epidemiological studies of workers exposed to mixed dusts have not always shown a clear role for quartz in disease induction. This anomaly has been extensively detailed in British and European epidemiological studies of coal workers' pneumoconiosis (CWP) and progressive massive fibrosis (PMF). Those studies generally have shown a correlation of disease prevalence with cumulative exposure to total respirable dust and coal rank, but not with the explicit quartz component of the cumulative dust exposure. A general hypothesis to explain the seeming failure of quartz, a strongly pathogenic agent for fibrosis, to contribute to CWP or PMF, especially when the other components of the dust are not so strong in isolation, is that the mass percent silica component of a dust, as conventionally measured, is not necessarily a measure of biologically available of toxic silica surface. Several methods are being used to characterize the degree of availability or purity of the surface of silica particles in mixed-composition dusts.

We review here a fraction of the literature of studies of silica exposure and CWP, and of experimental silicosis in lab animals exposed to mixed-composition dusts. One method used to detect surface "occlusion," or sub-micrometer coating, of aluminosilicate clay on respirable-sized silica particle is outlined. Application of the method to a set of Pennsylvania coal mine dusts is reviewed, demonstrating the occurrence of such clay occlusion of silica particles and showing that the fraction of such silica particles can significantly vary between exposure situations.

II. SILICA AND MIXED DUST PNEUMOCONIOSES

Epidemiological studies that have not correlated CWP or PMF prevalence with exposure to the quartz component of coal mine dust typically measure quartz content of respirable dust samples by X-ray diffraction or infrared spectroscopy, each of which essentially measures the mass-percent quartz in a bulk sample. The failure of correlation of such quartz exposure measurements and disease prevalence could be due either to an exacerbated activity of the quartz content in some dusts or to a diminution of pathogenic activity of the quartz in others. The latter possibility has led to a hypothesis that bulk analyses of the silica content of a coal mine dust may not be predictive of biological activity of the silica particle surface. For instance, heteroatomic surface contamination or surface occlusion by other minerals would not be evident.

British Institute of Occupational Medicine studies highlight a general experience that CWP and PMF prevalence do not necessarily correlate with exposure to the quartz content of coal mine dust. Epidemiological analyses, using chest radiographs of miners and infrared analyses of the quartz content of coal mine respirable dusts, found exposure-effect relationships with cumulative dust exposure but a lack of evidence of an overall effect of quartz in two studies of CWP and exposure to dust in British coalmines.[1,2] The latter study estimated cumulative exposures from 20 years of observation and compared them with three rounds of chest radiographs for 2600 of the miners involved throughout the study. On average, the percentage of men with CWP category 2/1 or more increased with cumulative dust exposure from near zero percent at 100 g.h/m^3 to near 10% at 400 g.h/m^3. The estimated probability of developing category 2/1 or more CWP vs. mean dust concentration over 35 years of exposure showed two extreme colliery specific differences, above and below the mean probabilities for the other eight collieries. These differences were not attributable to quartz. Their main results showed little evidence of an overall quartz effect and showed extreme colliery-related differences, the reason for which was not understood. Colliery differences were associated with various coal rank indices.

In Germany, investigations into the specific fibrogenicity of mine dusts in hardcoal mines of countries in the European community[3] have found correlations of disease with mine dust exposure and coal rank but not explicitly with quartz content. A review of 30 years of investigations into the specific fibrogenicity of mine dusts in hardcoal mines concluded that European and American hardcoal mine dusts have significantly different fibrogenicities between high- and low-rank coal collieries. There is a clear relationship between mass concentration of respirable dust and the occurrence of ILO category 2 radiological measure of lung change for any colliery. But the differences in occurrence at the same exposure levels between collieries could not be explained by reference to dust composition, including the quartz content as determined by X-ray diffraction or infrared spectroscopy measurements. Indeed, German experience was parallel to the British observations that the prevalence of disease was 10 times higher in high-rank vs. low-rank coal workers with the same cumulative dust exposure, while a lower cumulative quartz dust dose was seen in the high-rank coal mines. They also refer to studies of aluminum contamination of quartz being associated with a reduction in fibrogenicity during *in vivo* experiments on animals. This contamination is proposed to be aluminum substitution for silicon in the lattice of the mineral structure, perhaps distinct from a simple contaminant coating of quartz surface.

The correlation of CWP and PMF prevalence with rank is also seen in the U.S. In an investigation into the relationship between CWP and dust exposure in U.S. coal mines,[4] the various grades of CWP as determined by chest radiographs in the U.S. National Study of Coal Workers Pneumoconiosis showed a positive response with cumulative respirable-dust exposure, which depended significantly upon the regional location or rank of the coal mine. High-rank anthracite mining resulted in greater disease prevalence for a given cumulative exposure than did bituminous coal mining. The pattern was also seen within bituminous mining, with decreasing specific prevalence as rank decreased from central Pennsylvania-Johnstown area coal mines to western Pennsylvania-Pittsburgh area mines to mines in the midwestern U.S.

Animal exposure studies also have been used to examine the role of silica as conventionally measured in inducing disease, with results suggesting the need to determine the nature of the surface of silica particles and the role of that surface in pathogenic exposures.

Kriegseis[5] has studied surface composition of silica particles from German mine dusts using Auger spectroscopy and using a thermoluminescence method which gives an estimation of reactive quartz surfaces in an indirect manner. Five samples of respirable dusts from the Ruhr and Saar coal fields analyzed by scanning Auger spectroscopy revealed no clean surfaced quartz particles, i.e., particles whose surfaces were free of aluminum as determined by Auger elemental analysis. One sample, which induced fibrotic reactions in rats after intratracheal application, did not present a clean quartz surface even after argon sputtering to remove about 15 nm of the surface. Thus, the aluminum composition of the surface penetrated to a depth of at least several atomic layers. It was concluded that the surfaces of the quartz particles were essentially covered by inorganic material. Several possible explanations for fibrotic activity expression in the face of contaminated silica particles were advanced: silica is not the etiologic agent in the dusts; small sub-microscopic points of clean silica surface exist on the particles which could not be detected by Auger with a lateral resolution of 0.2 μm; such contaminants on quartz particle surfaces are removed in the lungs; and larger clean quartz surface areas exist on particles and are active agents but occur too infrequently to have been seen during the investigation.

In a set of studies of the effect of impurities and associated minerals on quartz toxicity, LeBouffant, et al.,[6] compared in the rat the *in vivo* toxicity of quartz which naturally occurred in coal mine dust, pure quartz, and quartz sands, using lung weight, lipids, collagen, and histological determination of nodular fibrosis. The study demonstrated that quartz inherent in coal dust does not express the toxic activity of equal challenges with pure quartz dust synthetically mixed in coal dust of low inherent quartz content. Extraction of the inherent quartz from coal and removal of contaminants from that quartz produced a material of toxicity comparable to that of pure quartz. Additionally, comparison of pure quartz and a set of sands found a six-month delay in the onset of manifest toxicity induced by the sands. And this delay was eliminated by removal of contaminants from the sands. It was concluded that all types of quartz have high intrinsic toxicity and that the apparent low toxicities of quartz in some naturally occuring dusts, e.g., some coal mine dusts, may be due to surface impurities or associated minerals. It was suggested that aluminum released from illite or kaolinite might combine with the surface of quartz and modify its toxicity.

III. DETECTING SILICA PARTICLE SURFACE ELEMENTAL HETEROGENEITY

The respirable-particle, surface-analysis method discussed below which analyzes X-ray spectra induced by electrons of different energies, was designed to address the silica anomaly from a hypothesis that pathogenic activity of respired quartz particles is associated with properties of and interactions with the particle surfaces. Individual particle surface features, invisible by bulk sample mass analysis, may occur and alter the biological availability of a fraction of quartz particles in a dust. Specifically, mineral coating or "occlusion" of the silica surface might affect the biological availability of the quartz component of the dust in exposures. In coal mining, clay aluminosilicate minerals are frequently seen in the infrared spectra or X-ray diffraction analyses of respirable dust samples, so possible association of clays was postulated. Therefore, a method was developed to distinguish a heterogeneously-structured particle, such as a stable clay coating on a silica particle, from a mixture or agglomeration of separable clay particles with a silica particle. A stably coated, non-agglomerate, single particle would present a biologically available clay, rather than silica, surface. Its contribution to a mass-analysis of silica dust exposure could thus confound epidemiological analyses of the role of quartz in CWP, PMF, or other occupationally induced diseases which use mass-analysis measures of exposure.

A technique was developed to detect substantial but sub-micrometer thick surface occlusions on respirable-sized mineral particles[7,8] by using scanning electron microscopy-energy dispersive X-ray analysis (SEM-EDX) on individual particles, modified by the use of multiple electron beam accelerating voltages. At high accelerating voltages, the electron beam samples deeper into the particle than at low voltages. Performing electron-beam excited X-ray analyses at two or more electron beam accelerating voltages permits elemental composition near the surface of a particle to be distinguished from underlying bulk elemental composition. The method can be applied using conventional SEM-EDX if the system can be operated at two or more electron beam accelerating voltages between 20 and 5 keV. At voltages down to 5 kilo-electron volts (keV), the K-alpha X-ray spectra can be used for elements up to calcium. Heavier elements are analyzed by using L-line and higher series, rather than K-line, X-ray spectra. This permits one to distinguish surface elemental composition inhomogeneity in the range from about 0.1 μm to about 1 μm thickness, in a non destructive fashion.

Auger spectrometry and X-ray photoelectron spectrometry can be used to analyze the elemental composition of material surfaces, for surface layer thicknesses from one atomic layer to about 0.001 to 0.01 μm deep. To distinguish the surface from the underlying material composition by Auger analysis, the surface must be analyzed, then destructively ion-etched to permit analysis of the underlying material. Incidental contamination, e.g., carbon from handling or solvents, can mask the surface of interest, requiring pre-treatment to bare the mineral surface for analysis. These problems are exacerbated if one is attempting to study specific components of mixed materials, e.g., quartz particles in mixed dusts. In that case, it may be impossible to pre-identify particles of a selected type for detailed surface analysis.

SEM-EDX nondestructively analyzes the overall composition first, permitting selection of particles or areas which are then subjected to near-surface analysis by use of lower electron beam voltages.

A particle is subjected first to electron beam-induced X-ray spectroscopic analysis with the electron beam accelerated to a kinetic energy of about 20 keV. The energy is chosen to be high enough to analyze to a selected depth and low enough to avoid surface damage. The ratios of the elemental X-ray signals are measured. Then, the electron beam energy is reduced in one or several steps. As the beam voltage is reduced the electrons excite X-rays to lesser depths. The limitation is that the electron energy must be greater than the photon energy of the elemental line to be excited. The effect of proximity of the excitation energy and X-ray energy can be accounted for to first order in the analysis, but it is recommended to use electron energies of at least twice the energy of the X-ray to be excited. For K-shell X-ray lines this means electrons with energies as low as 4 to 5 keV can be used to analyze silicon and lower atomic number elements. For elements above calcium, L-line or higher line spectra permit use of electron energy down to 3 to 5 keV for near surface analysis. Using two excitation voltages sequentially, such as 20 and 5 keV, the ratios of elemental line strengths are measured at each voltage, and then the ratios are compared to determine if there is heterogeneity of elemental composition with depth into the material. By using several voltages, composition with depth can be profiled; the depths are functions of the density of the material being analyzed and the differences between the excitation energies and the energies of the X-ray lines being excited.

Spectral line intensities versus applied electron beam accelerating voltage are interpreted in terms of a heterogeneous composition model of pure silica core particles occluded by a uniform aluminosilicate coating of equiatomic Si and Al and a homogeneous composition model of the particles as homogeneously distributed aluminum substitution in a silica matrix. The average lateral dimension of the particle is used as an estimate of the thickness; this is an approximation for silica but can fail for clays, which can tend to form plate-like particles.

A simple one-dimensional mathematical model with analytic solutions predicts the ratio of silicon to silicon plus aluminum fraction of signal $[I_{Si}/(I_{Si} + I_{Al})]$ vs. electron accelerating voltage. The heterogeneous structure of an aluminosilicate-occluded silica core is modeled as an aluminosilicate layer of equimolar Si and Al and thickness T on the front and back faces of a one-dimensional silica slab of total thickness D.

In SEM-EDX analysis, part of the incident electron kinetic energy generates characteristic elemental X-ray emissions by inelastic electron scattering within the particle. Ionization of an electron from a specific shell of a specific element can result in emission of a specific X-ray photon as the inner shell vacancy is filled by an outer shell electron. Within a differential thickness of material at a given depth in the particle, the intensity of a so-stimulated X-ray line is proportional to four parameters: the concentration of target atoms, the intensity of the electron beam in the thickness with adequate energy to stimulate the X-ray line, the cross-section for ionization of the target atom shell by those electrons, and the fluorescence yield, which is the probability that the ionization will result in that X-ray emission. As a simplified model, diminution of the electron beam intensity (I_e) with depth into the sample (z) can be modeled as a Beer's law process: $dI_e = -k_e I_e dz$.[9] One expression for the depth or "range" (R_i) to which an incident electron beam of electron kinetic energy V_o (keV) can excite an X-ray photon of characteristic energy V_i (keV), developed by C.A. Anderson and M.F. Hasler, is: $mR_i = 0.064 (V_o^{1.68} - V_i^{1.68})$, where R_i is in micrometers, and m is the density of the sample in gm/cc.[10] The extinction coefficient for Beer's law attenuation of the electron beam intensity with depth is taken as $k_{ei} = 3/R_i$. The cross section for ionization is a function of the logarithm of the ratio of electron energy at the site of excitation and the energy of the line to be excited. The model presented here approximates this simply as a function of incident electron and characteristic line energies: $k_{gi} = P_i (V_o - V_i)^{1.65}$, where P_i is the mole fraction of element i in the differential thickness of sample.[11] The fluorescence yield (w_i) is independent of the specifics of the ionization process, and tabulated values are available for the lines of interest here.[12] Attenuation of the intensity of emerging characteristic X-rays by a differential thickness of sample is also modeled by a Beer's law diminution with exponential coefficient k_{xi}; this coefficient is calculated as the mass percent composition-weighted summation of the X-ray mass attenuation coefficients for each element in the sample for the measured K-alpha line.[12]

The heterogeneous structure model predicts the measured fractional silicon signal $(I_{Si}/(I_{Si} + I_{Al}))$ as a function of incident electron energy with I_i, the intensity of the silicon (i = Si) or aluminum (i = Al) elemental X-ray, given by:

$$
\begin{aligned}
I_i = {} & \frac{g_{Ci} w_i}{k_{xCi} + k_{eCi}} \left[1 - e^{-(k_{xCi} + k_{eCi})T} \right] \\
& + \frac{g_{Bi} w_i}{k_{xBi} + k_{eBi}} e^{(-k_{eBi}(D-T) - k_{xCi}T)} \left[e^{k_{eBi}(D-2T)} - e^{-k_{xBi}(D-2T)} \right] \\
& + \frac{g_{Ci} w_i}{k_{xCi} + k_{eCi}} e^{(-k_{eCi}D - k_{xBi}(D-2T) - k_{xCi}T)} \left[e^{k_{eCi}T} - e^{k_{xCi}T} \right]
\end{aligned}
$$

where k_{Bi} and k_{Ci} are the extinction coefficients for electron beam intensity in the silica core (B) or clay coating (C), given by $3m_{B\text{ or }C}\,[0.064\,(V_o^{1.68} - V_i^{1.68})]^{-1}$, where: $m_{B\text{ or }C}$ is the density of the silica core or clay coating; V_o is the incident electron beam energy; V_i is the energy of the silicon (i = Si) or aluminium (i = Al) X-ray line; k_{xBi} and k_{xCi} are the extinction coefficients for silicon (i = Si) or aluminium (i = Al) X-rays in the core or coating; w_i is the probability of excitation of an X-ray rather than an Auger electron; g_{Bi} and g_{Ci} are the excitation coefficients for electron ionization of silicon (i = Si) or aluminum (i = Al) inner shell electrons by the incident electrons; D is the particle thickness; and T is the thickness of the aluminosilicate coating on the particle surface, calculated from a model of equi-atomic silicon and aluminum in a top and bottom coating on a pure silica core giving the overall particle composition measured at high voltage. The extinction coefficients and generation coefficients (values in reciprocal micrometers) for aluminosilicate coating (subscript 1) on a silica core (subscript 2) are given by:

$$k_{g1Si} = 0.5k_{g2Si} = 0.5\left(V_o - 1.740\right)^{1.65},$$

$$k_{g1Al} = 0.5\left(V_o - 1.487\right)^{1.65}, \quad k_{g2Al} = 0,$$

$$k_{e1Si} = k_{e2Si} = 3/R_{Si} = 117.2/\left(V_o^{1.68} - 1.740^{1.68}\right),$$

$$k_{e1Al} = k_{e2Al} = 3/R_{Al} = 117.2/\left(V_o^{1.68} - 1.487^{1.68}\right),$$

$$k_{r1Si} = 0.3643, \quad k_{r2Si} = 0.1820,$$

$$k_{r1Al} = 0.2653, \quad k_{r2Al} = 0.2818,$$

$$w_{Si} = w_{Al} = 0.038 \quad \text{for the K shell.}$$

For a homogeneous aluminosilicate particle of thickness D with actual molar ratio, Si/(Si + Al) = P, and composition, $Si_PO_{2P}Al_{(1-P)}O_{1.5(1-P)}$, this model gives a predicted signal $I_{Si}/(I_{Si} + I_{Al})$ vs. incident electron beam energy (V_o) with I_{Si} or I_{Al} given by the first term in Equation 1, with:

$$k_{gSi} = P\left(V_o - 1.74\right)^{1.65}, \quad k_{gAl} = (1-P)\left(V_o - 1.487\right)^{1.65},$$

$$k_{eSi} = 117.2/\left(V_o^{1.68} - 1.74^{1.68}\right),$$

$$k_{eAl} = 117.2/\left(V_o^{1.68} - 1.487^{1.68}\right),$$

$$k_{rSi} = 2.5(11.808 - 7.44P)/(51 + 9P) \quad \text{for the K - alpha silicon line}$$

and

$$k_{rAl} = 2.5(5.0109 + 1.7507P)/(51 + 9P) \quad \text{for the K - alpha aluminum line}$$

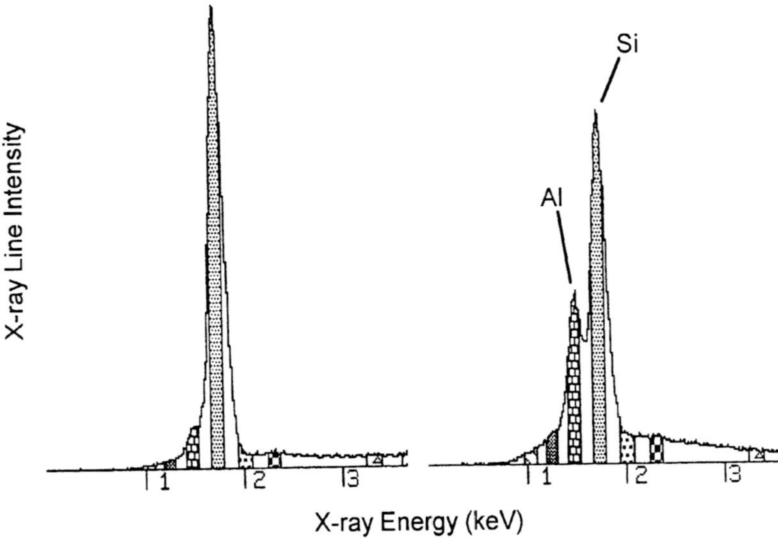

FIGURE 1 Silicon and aluminum X-ray line relative intensities induced by 20 keV (left spectra) and by 5 keV (right spectra) electron beams by SEM-EDX of a western-Pennsylvania coal mine dust particle of 2 μm size and silicon fraction of signal $I_{Si}/(I_{Si} + I_{Al}) = 0.955$ measured at 20 keV.

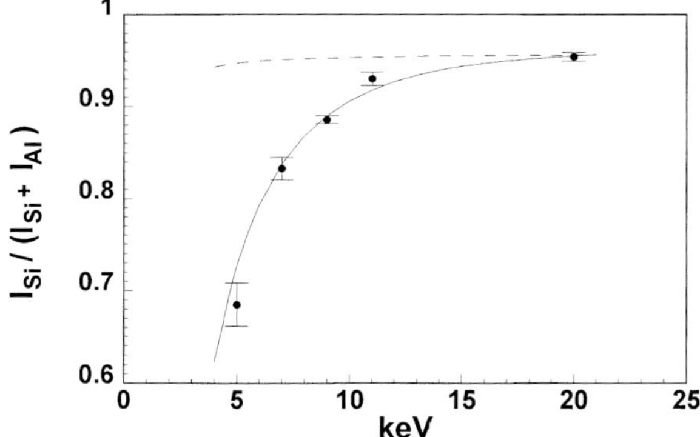

FIGURE 2 Theoretical and observed change in silicon fraction of signal, $I_{Si}/(I_{Si} + I_{Al})$, vs. electron beam accelerating voltage, for the particle of Figure 1. The dashed line is a homogeneous composition model prediction; the solid line is a clay-occluded silica particle model prediction. The data are the means and standard deviations of 5 measurements made at 20, 11, 9, 7, and 5 keV.

The homogeneous structure model also displays a decrease in fractional silica signal with applied voltage at lower incident electron energies, albeit significantly smaller than the decrease displayed by the heterogeneous model. The homogeneous particle behavior is due to the depth of excitation (R_i) and X-ray generation cross-section (k_{gi}) being functions of the difference between the applied electron kinetic energy and the characteristic X-ray energy excited. The ratios of these values for silicon and aluminum increase as the applied electron voltage is decreased, leading to a small drop in the silicon fractional signal at the lowest voltages. The decrease is much greater in the heterogeneous model, reflecting the actual compositional heterogeneity with depth.

Figures 1 and 2 demonstrate multiple voltage SEM-EDX analysis for a western-Pennsylvania, bituminous coal mine dust particle of lateral dimension between 1.5 and 2.5 μm and silicon fraction of signal of 0.955 measured at 20 keV. Figure 1 displays the SEM-EDX spectra of the particle taken at 20 keV and at 5 keV electron beam voltage, showing the change in the relative intensities of the silicon and aluminum

X-ray lines with beam voltage. Figure 2 shows the measured and predicted silicon fraction of signal, $I_{Si}/(I_{Si} + I_{Al})$, vs. electron beam accelerating voltage. The predicted values are calculated for a particle of 2 μm thickness and 95.5% silica fraction as measured at 20 keV. The clay-occluded silica model prediction is shown as a solid line, and the homogeneous particle model is shown as a dashed line. The data points show the means and standard deviations of five measurements each made at 20, 11, 9, 7, and 5 keV on the particle.

IV. SILICA OCCLUSION IN COAL MINE DUSTS

This method of multiple voltage SEM-EDX was applied to respirable particles collected at a set of coal mines across the state of Pennsylvania. Coal rank decreases across the state from anthracite in the east to bituminous in the central and western part of the state. Bituminous coal mined in the central-Johnstown area is higher in rank (carbon-to-hydrogen ratio) than bituminous mined in the western-Pittsburgh region of the state. The National Study of Coal Workers Pneumoconiosis (NSCWP) of the National Institute for Occupational Safety and Health, has found that the prevalence of the various degrees of CWP, including PMF, increases with coal rank for a given level of cumulative dust exposure.[4] Analyses were performed on two eastern Pennsylvania anthracite coal mine dust samples (A1-A2) three central Pennsylvania bituminous coal mine dust low-temperature-ashed (LTA) samples and one nonashed sample (C1-C4), and two western Pennsylvania bituminous coal mine LTA samples and a nonashed sample (W1-W3). The moisture- and ash-free carbon content of coals from those seams were 84% for A1-A2, 69% for C1-C4, and 64% for W1-W3. In a randomly selected field, all particles which did not image as overlaid or agglomerated particles were analyzed at 20 keV. Particles for which silicon (Si) accounted for 75% or more of the 20 keV-excited spectra line intensities for elements of atomic number equal to or greater than that of sodium were subjected to five measurements at both 20 and 5 keV. Some 20 particles were analyzed for each dust sample.

Particles in the 1 to 3 μm size range of a powdered aluminosilicate glass of 95% $I_{Si}/(I_{Si} + I_{Al})$ was used to represent the behavior of particles with homogeneous aluminum contamination throughout the particle. The value of 0.029 for change in silicon fraction measured at 20 and 5 keV represents the 90th percentile of the change in silicon fraction for this homogeneous control group (glass).

The change in silicon fraction was averaged over the 5 repeated measurements for each particle in each dust sample, and box plots, shown in Figure 3, were generated from the resulting data. In the box plots, the central 50% of the observations (interquartile range) is contained within the boxes, with the mean represented by a plus sign. The vertical 'whiskers' represent the 95th and 5th percentiles, and the circles (o) represent data points that fall outside those percentiles. The horizontal line at 0.029 represents the 90th percentile of the change in silicon fraction for the homogeneous control group (glass).

To test the hypothesis that each distribution of change in silicon fraction was identical to that of the control, the number of particles in each dust group with changes greater than the 90th percentile for the control group was determined, shown in Table 1. The probability of this number (or greater) occurring by chance was then computed using the binomial distribution with parameter ($p = 0.10$) and sample size equal to the number of particles. Comparisons of each dust sample distribution, with the cut-off limit, revealed that 80% of the particles from western-Pennsylvania dust samples and 54% of the particles from central-Pennsylvania dust samples were above the limit (p-value < 0.0001 in each case); only anthracite samples (20%) were compatible with the control group.

Change in silicon fraction with reduction in voltage were categorized into four ranges (<0.01, $0.01–<0.05$, $0.05–<0.10$, ≥ 0.10). Table 2 shows the differences in the distributions between the three mining regions and between samples within each region assessed using likelihood-ratio chi-squared statistics or Wilks's statistics. Across all nine Pennsylvania coal mine dust samples, the chi-square test showed lack of homogeneity (p-value < 0.0001), indicating a systematic difference between each coal mine sample. Significant lack of homogeneity existed between the three regional areas (p-value < 0.0001 in each case). The majority of the variation between the coal mine samples was associated with these differences between the regions. However, within each region the likelihood-ratio chi-squared statistic was not statistically significant (p-value > 0.05 for each case), indicating homogeneous groups. Anthracite mine dusts were similar to the control powdered aluminosilicate glass and so did not manifest significant fractions of aluminosilicate coated silica particles. Bituminous coal mine dusts were different from the control glass dust, indicating occlusion of significant fractions of the high-percentage silica mine dust particles.

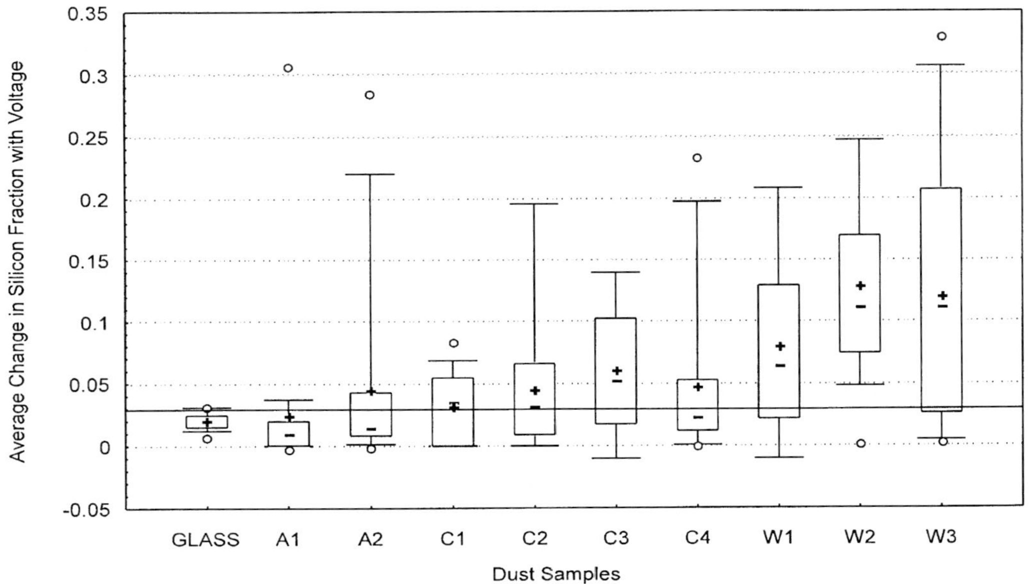

FIGURE 3 Distribution of the change in measured silicon fraction, $I_{Si}/(I_{Si} + I_{Al})$, with reduction in electron beam voltage from 20 to 5 keV, of the average repeated measurement per particle for some 20 particles in each of nine coal mine dust samples. In the box plots: the central 50% of the observations are contained within the boxes; a plus sign represents the mean; vertical 'whiskers' represent the 95th and 5th percentiles; and the circles (○) represent data points that fall outside those percentiles. The horizontal line at 0.029 represents the 90th percentile of the change in silicon fraction for the homogeneous control group of glass particles.

TABLE 1
The Distribution of the Number of Particles in Each Dust Group with Changes in Silicon Fraction Greater Than the 90th Percentile for the Control Group (Glass)

Coal Mine Dust Samples	Number of Particles >0.029	P-value[a]
Control (Glass)	2/21 = 0.10	0.635
Anthracite:		
A1	2/21 = 0.10	0.635
A2	6/20 = 0.30	0.011
Central Pennsylvania:		
C1	11/21 = 0.52	0.000
C2	9/17 = 0.53	0.000
C3	13/18 = 0.72	0.000
C4	8/20 = 0.40	0.000
Western Pennsylvania:		
W1	14/19 = 0.74	0.000
W2	21/22 = 0.95	0.000
W3	14/20 = 0.70	0.000

[a] P-value based on the binomial distribution with parameter p = 0.10 and sample sizes n = 17 through 22.

TABLE 2
The Likelihood-ratio Chi-squared Statistics for Testing Homogeneity of Change in Silicon Fraction with Reduction in Voltage for Dust Sample Groups.

Comparison Group	Df	Likelihood-Ratio[2]	P-value[a]
Overall Test Between 9 Samples	24	80.7	**
Between Anthracites (A1 and A2)	3	6.2	
Between Central Pennsylvania (C1, C2, C3, and C4)	9	16.5	*
Between Western Pennsylvania (W1, W2, and W3)	6	10.1	
Between Anthracite and All Bituminous	3	23.3	**
Between Central and Western Pennsylvania	3	24.6	**

[a] P-values represent the probability of homogeneity by chance alone, where blank = $p > 0.10$, ** = $p < 0.0001$, and * = $p < 0.10$.

Ongoing research is extending these analyses to other coal mines and to metal and non metal mines. The suggestion in the data that coal rank may be a predictor of frequency of particle occlusion cannot be validly inferred from these limited data; not all mines show this relationship, and limited current data distinguishes anthracite from all bituminous coal but does not distinguish far-west bituminous from central-Pennsylvania bituminous coals. The results do indicate that respirable-sized high-percentage silica particles found in some mines can exhibit surface aluminosilicate contamination or occlusion. It should be noted that all mine samples from all coal ranks contained particles with apparently non occluded quartz surface; under no circumstances should quartz particles from any mine be considered biologically harmless.

V. HYPOTHESES

Both epidemiological studies of human exposure to silica in mixed dusts and animal exposure experiments have indicated that induction of pneumoconioses does not necessarily correlate with the silica fraction of cumulative mixed-dust exposure. This has been subject to considerable study in the case of CWP and PMF. A general hypothesis is that the conventionally measured silica fraction of dust exposures is not necessarily a valid measure of exposure to silica surface, and that pathology stems from toxic interactions on true silica surface. Research has suggested that contaminants on the surface may diminish the biological availability of toxic surface sites by gross occlusion of the silica surface by mineralogically distinct material, e.g., clay. Research also has shown that homogeneous contamination of species other than silicon sometimes occurs in the silica matrix itself. It has been postulated that some such impurities within the silica may alter the surface toxicity substantially from that of pure quartz surface; the limiting suggestion, from the general paucity of pure quartz particles seen in coal mine dusts, has been that quartz is not involved in the etiology of CWP and PMF. There is insufficient data to determine immediately the conditions under which occluded quartz or homogeneously contaminated quartz is a contributor to pneumoconioses, or to determine if the non-occluded or non-contaminated fraction of silica in mixed dusts can be shown to correlate with disease prevalence. In part this is due to the difficulty in attempting to use *in vitro* cytotoxicity as an indicator of dust pathogenic potential for correlation with silica purity or occlusion. This difficulty arises from the comparable *in vitro* cytotoxicities of quartz and clay; a sample of clay, and thus of clay-occluded silica particles, will manifest prompt *in vitro* cytotoxicity comparable to that of the same amount (with comparable size and surface area) of pure quartz.[13] Thus, comparisons of pathogenic potential and silica exposure must be made on the basis of worker population epidemiological data, for which the surface properties of dust exposures typically were not investigated, or on the basis of *in vivo* animal model studies.

Multiple voltage SEM-EDX analyses of a set of American coal mine dusts indicate that a fraction of coal mine dust quartz particles can be surface occluded by aluminosilicate clay. The data reviewed here show that the fraction of silica particles evidencing such occlusion can vary between samples. The very limited number of samples reported is not sufficient to determine that coal rank is a factor in that frequency. Frequency of occlusion may be presumed, *a priori,* to depend on the specifics of dust generation at any particular time: the rank of the coal, the material being cut including mine floor or roof, the sedimentary or metamorphic nature of the rock, the nature and energetics of the cutting process which might include disaggregation of sedimentary strata or cleavage of new surface, or other mining activities such as the use of sand for friction on railway transport underground.

An additional factor in deconvolving the role of particle contamination in disease induction is the question of the persistance of the contaminating material under conditions of particle deposition and residence in the lung. Upon deposition in a pulmonary alveolus, a particle would first contact the hypophase which is rich in pulmonary surfactants. Limited tests have been performed on the durability of occluded silica particles upon a few hours incubation in surrogate pulmonary surfactant.[7] An aqueous dispersion of surfactant is made by ultrasonically mixing dipalmitoyl phosphatidyl choline (lecithin) and/or other components of pulmonary surfactant into physiological concentration saline at 37°C. Into this dispersion was mixed a dust previously found to contain silica particles with a high frequency of clay occlusion. The sample was mixed by briefly vortexing and then incubated in a rotary incubator at 37°C for 3 h, the time chosen to represent an estimate of time of incubation of the particle in the pulmonary alveolar hypophase before phagocytosis. Following incubation, surface analysis demonstrated the existence of aluminosilicate coating on quartz particles. Thus, relatively insoluble clay occlusion would be expected to persist at least until phagocytosis of a particle respired into the alveolar region of the lung. Longer term persistance under conditions of residence in interstitial tissue or the lymphatics is an open question. Longer persistance is likely a function of the mineral nature of the occluding material; therefore, the time of onset and nature of toxic activity could be a function of the specific mineralogy of the particle surface.

Additional research is needed to detail the nature of such occluded particle surfaces, the geological and processing factors which affect such occlusion, and the durability of such particles in tissue. Analyses of additional samples are needed to determine if surface occlusion is a factor in relationships of coal rank and quartz content of coal mine dust exposures and prevalence patterns for pneumoconioses and fibroses and to determine mining situations or conditions which affect the fractional distribution of occluded silica particles.

REFERENCES

1. **Walton, W. H., Dodgson, J., Hadden, G. G., and Jacobsen, M.,** The effect of quartz and other non-coal dusts in coalworkers' pneumoconioses, in *Inhaled Particles IV,* Vol. 2, Walton, W.H., Ed., Pergamon Press, Oxford, 1971, 669–689.
2. **Hurley, J. F., Burns, J., Copland, L., Dodgson, J., and Jacobsen, M.,** Coal workers simple pneumoconiosis and exposure to dust at 10 British coal mines, *Br. J. Ind. Med.,* 39, 120–127, 1982.
3. **Robock, K. and Bauer, H. D.,** Investigations into the specific fibrogenicity of mine dusts in hardcoal mines of countries in the European Community, in Proc. of the VIIth International Pneumoconioses Conference, Pittsburgh, 1988, DHHS (NIOSH) Publ. No. 90–108 Part 1, 208–283, 1990.
4. **Attfield, M. D. and Morring, K.,** An investigation into the relationship between coal workers' pneumoconiosis and dust exposure in U.S. coal mines, *Am. Indust. Hyg. Assoc. J.,* 53(8), 486–492 1992.
5. **Kriegseis, W. and Scharmann, A.,** Specific harmfulness of respirable dusts from West German coal mines V: influence of mineral surface properties, *Ann. Occup. Hyg.,* 26, 511–525, 1982.
6. **LeBouffant, L., Daniel, H., Martin, J. C., and Bruyere, S.,** Effect of impurities and associated minerals on quartz toxicity, *Ann. Occup. Hyg.,* 26, 625–634, 1982.

7. **Wallace, W. E., Harrison, J., Keane, M. J., Bolsaitis, P., Eppelsheimer, D., Poston, J., and Page, S. J.,** Clay occlusion of respirable quartz particles detected by low voltage scanning electron microscopy-X-Ray Analysis, *Ann. Occup. Hyg.*, 34(2), 195–204, 1990.
8. **Wallace, W. E. and Keane, M. J.,** Differential Surface Composition Analysis by Multiple-Voltage Electron Beam X-Ray Microscopy, U.S. Patent 5,210,414, 1993.
9. **Cosslett, V. E. and Thomas, R. N.,** Multiple scattering of 5–30 keV electrons in evaporated metal films, *Br. J. Appl. Phys.*, 15, 883–907, 1944.
10. **Goldstein, J. I. and Yakowitz, H.,** *Practical scanning electron microscopy, electron and ion microprobe analysis,* Plenum Press, New York, 1975, 83.
11. **Heinrich, K. F. J.,** *Electron beam X-ray microanalysis,* Van Nostrand Reinhold, Scarborough, CA, 1981, 240.
12. **Veigele, W. J.,** Attenuation cross sections in cm^2/g at selected wavelengths for 94 elements, in *Handbook of Spectroscopy,* Vol. 1, Robinson, J.W., Ed., CRC Press, Boca Raton, FL, 1974, 202.
13. **Wallace, W. E., Vallyathan, V., Keane, M. J., and Robinson, V.,** *In vitro* biologic toxicity of native and surface-modified silica and kaolin, *J. Toxicol. Environ. Health,* 16, 424–425, 1985.

Section III
Pathogenesis of Silicosis: Current Theories

Section III
Chapter 1

QUESTIONS AND CONTROVERSIES ABOUT THE PATHOGENESIS OF SILICOSIS

Agnes B. Kane

CONTENTS

I. INTRODUCTION

Workers are exposed to crystalline silica particles, most commonly α quartz, under a wide range of occupational conditions. Prolonged inhalation of silica particles is associated with the development of acute and chronic lung diseases (for review, see Reference 1). The prototype of these diseases is chronic silicosis, a slowly progressive disorder characterized by multiple fibrotic nodules in the lung parenchyma that results in impaired pulmonary function, right-sided heart failure, increased susceptibility to certain infections, and premature death.[2] The pathogenesis of silicosis was reviewed most recently by Davis[3] in 1986, prior to the isolation and characterization of multiple cytokines and fibrogenic factors implicated as mediators of pulmonary inflammation and fibrosis. This chapter will focus on the pathogenesis of chronic silicosis with an emphasis on the cellular and biochemical mediators responsible for the development of this important occupational disease. The referenced papers will emphasize newer developments published after Davis' review in 1986. Precautions and caveats to be considered in interpretation of these newer developments and in reassessment of earlier observations will be discussed.

0-8493-4709-2/96/$0.00+$.50

II. MACROPHAGES ARE THE INITIAL TARGET CELL OF SILICA PARTICLES

Macrophages are the first defense mechanism against any particulates that reach the terminal respiratory tract and alveolar spaces.[4] The most hazardous silica particles for humans are less than 1 μm in diameter.[1] Particulates of this size range, regardless of their chemical content, deposit preferentially on the walls and branch points of the respiratory bronchioles in humans[5] and on the surfaces of the terminal bronchioles, alveolar ducts, and connecting alveolar duct bifurcations in rodents that lack respiratory bronchioles.[6] The earliest cellular responses to any particles deposited in the lungs of rodents have been described by scanning electron microscopy after short-term inhalation of silica or carbonyl iron.[6,7] A transient migration of inflammatory cells, neutrophils followed by macrophages, appears at sites of particle deposition.[7] This transient inflammatory reaction has also been described by examination of bronchoalveolar lavage fluids following direct intratracheal instillation of silica or carbon particles in mice.[8] The initial phase in particle clearance is phagocytosis by neutrophils and macrophages that are subsequently removed by mucociliary transport.[9] A small fraction of particles may penetrate into the interstitium by transepithelial migration across type 1 alveolar epithelial cells.[10] These particles may be removed directly by lymphatic channels that terminate in the walls of the respiratory bronchioles or phagocytized by macrophages located in the interstitium.[8]

Although the initial sites of deposition do not depend on the biologic reactivity of the inhaled particle, the rates and routes of subsequent translocation and clearance may be different for equal numbers of nontoxic or toxic particles.[11] Warheit et al.[7] have recently observed delayed clearance of silica particles from bronchoalveolar junctions, while macrophages containing nontoxic carbonyl iron particles were seen on the surfaces of the terminal bronchioles as early as 48 hours after inhalation. The mechanisms responsible for delayed clearance of toxic particles such as silica will be explored in the next section. Autopsy examination of workers who have repeated exposure to toxic silica particles revealed focal accumulations of dust-containing macrophages at sites of lymphatics in the lung parenchyma and within their hilar lymph nodes.[1,12] It is hypothesized that impaired lymphatic clearance associated with fibrotic nodules in the hilar lymph nodes increases accumulation of silica particles in the interstitium. The close proximity of interstitial macrophages containing silica particles to fibroblasts is postulated to be an important factor predisposing to the development of pulmonary fibrosis.[12] In support of this hypothesis, exposure of rodents to high doses of nontoxic particles or depletion of inflammatory cells, enhanced particle deposition in the interstitium and hilar lymph nodes and increased fibrosis after instillation of silica. Increased deposition of large numbers of nontoxic particles in the interstitium of the lungs with excess particles in alveolar spaces and macrophages is termed the "overload phenomenon."[8] It is not known whether silica exposure produces an analogous situation as a result of impaired clearance of these toxic particles.

III. MECHANISTIC CLUES FROM THE HISTOPATHOLOGY OF SILICOSIS

The morphologic response to aggregates of macrophages containing silica particles in the pulmonary lymphatics and hilar lymph nodes is formation of collagenized nodules surrounded by fibroblasts and inflammatory cells. The earliest lesion identified morphologically in workers exposed chronically to silica particles is a *simple silicotic nodule or islet* less than 1 cm in diameter. These lesions occur more commonly in the upper lobes of the lung, in contrast to diffuse interstitial fibrosis characteristic of asbestosis that is more pronounced in the lower lobes. The simple silicotic nodule is composed of a central, hyalinized core of dense, acellular collagen surrounded concentrically by fibroblasts and whorled collagen fibers with dust-laden macrophages, lymphocytes, and randomly-oriented collagen fibers around the periphery (Figure 1). With longer periods of exposure to silica particles, these silicotic nodules gradually enlarge and coalesce, replacing adjacent lung parenchyma. These larger lesions characterize *conglomerate silicosis;* rarely, the fibrotic lesions progress rapidly and extensively as *progressive massive fibrosis.*[1]

The classic histopathologic lesion of early chronic silicosis, the simple silicotic nodule, is unique and should not be confused with a granuloma or diffuse interstitial pulmonary fibrosis that characterizes asbestosis. This unique histopathologic lesion provides important clues to the pathogenesis of chronic

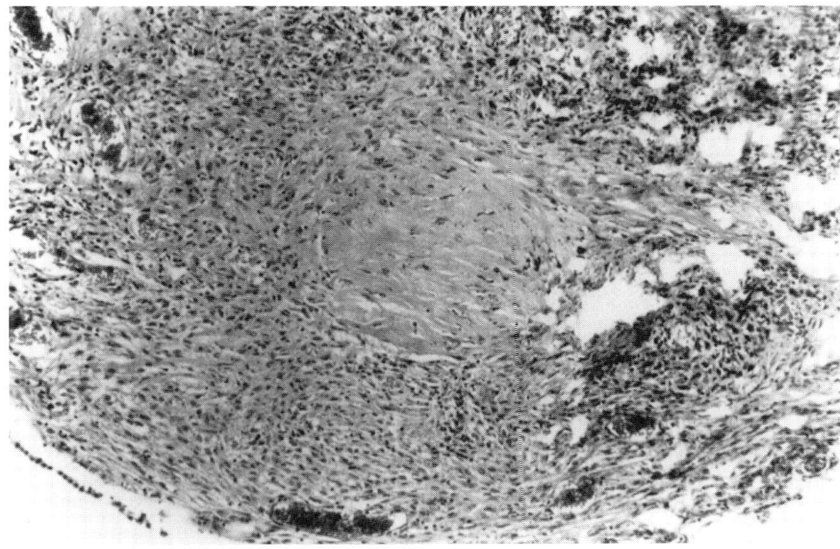

FIGURE 1 Photomicrograph of a human silicotic nodule within the lung parenchyma. A central mass of acellular collagen is surrounded by a rim of fibroblasts and inflammatory cells. Stained with hematoxylin and eosin; original magnification 250×.

silicosis, i.e., the mechanisms leading to the development of this lesion are most likely different, either qualitatively or quantitatively, from the mechanisms responsible for formation of a granuloma or diffuse interstitial pulmonary fibrosis. The simple silicotic nodule of early chronic silicosis is also distinct, both clinically and pathologically, from the disease acute silicosis or alveolar proteinosis that is caused by acute exposure to high levels of silica dust. Unfortunately, in many short-term animal models of silicosis, high levels of silica (10 to 100 mg/m^3 by inhalation or up to 50 mg by intratracheal instillation) are used. In these models, areas of nodular fibrosis that resemble the simple silicotic nodule seen in humans do develop, usually in combination with accumulation of foamy or lipid-laden alveolar macrophages and evidence of type 2 cell proliferation (see, for example, References 13 and 14). In addition, direct intratracheal installation may also produce the "bolus effect" or a local "overload phenomenon" associated with uneven deposition of large numbers of particles that is associated with a granulomatous inflammatory reaction and numerous multinucleated, foreign-body giant cells. Multinucleated giant cells and epithelioid cells occur rarely in chronic silicosis in humans, even in those people with superimposed tuberculosis.[1] The paucity of multinucleated giant cells and epithelioid cells in the tissue reactions to silica particles, even in the presence of *Mycobacterium tuberculosis* that usually provokes a vigorous granulomatous inflammatory response, provides another clue supporting a unique reaction of macrophages to silica particles. The spectrum of acute macrophage responses to these toxic particles will be discussed next.

IV. ACUTE COMPLICATIONS OF SILICA EXPOSURE

A. MACROPHAGE INJURY OR MACROPHAGE ACTIVATION?

While the importance of pulmonary macrophages as the initial target cell of inhaled silica particles is undisputed, the subsequent effect of these phagocytized particles on the functions of macrophages is controversial. Numerous *in vitro* studies (e.g., Reference 15) reported that addition of silica particles to cultured macrophages was acutely cytotoxic. It was hypothesized that silica particles ruptured lysosomes following fusion with the phagocytic vacuole allowing extracellular release of hydrolytic enzymes and local tissue destruction that was repaired by fibrosis.[16] Morphologic evidence of injury to alveolar macrophages after *in vivo* exposure to silica was also reported.[17,18] However, in 1984, Schmidt et al.[19] noted that silica particles stimulated release of the cytokine interleukin-1 (IL-1) from cultured monocytes. In addition, there were conflicting observations about the viability and function of macrophages obtained by bronchoalveolar lavage after acute or subchronic exposure to silica particles in different model systems (reviewed in Reference 3). The current hypothesis proposes that macrophages are activated, not injured, by exposure to silica particles to release increased levels of cytokines, such as IL-1, that stimulate fibrosis.[3]

What factors are responsible for the conflicting observations made in these different *in vitro* and *in vivo* models? Most investigators agree that *in vitro* exposure of cultured macrophages to mineral particles bypasses any protective (or deleterious) effect of the alveolar lining fluid[20,21] and exposes cells to high doses of particles over a short period of time.[3] The reasons for different observations in different animal models are more complex. Some of these discrepancies may be due to the route of exposure (intratracheal instillation vs. inhalation), different species (rat, mouse, guinea pig, or hamster), dose and source of particles (e.g., cristobalite is far more toxic than alpha quartz or silica), and different exposure times. With one exception, all of these animal models assessed the viability and function of macrophages collected by bronchoalveolar lavage. Because particulates are cleared from the alveolar spaces quite rapidly, a more appropriate target cell population would be macrophages in the interstitium and regional lymphatics. Interstitial macrophages have different properties in comparison to free alveolar macrophages.[4,22] In fact, Sjöstrand et al.[23] compared release of a lysosomal enzyme and fibroblast growth stimulating factors from rat alveolar macrophages collected by bronchoalveolar lavage and collagenase digestion to obtain adherent and interstitial macrophage after eight days of cristobalite inhalation. Lysosomal enzyme release from the lavaged alveolar macrophage population was increased with inconsistent release of fibroblast growth stimulatory activity from this subpopulation. In contrast, the adherent and interstitial macrophage subpopulation showed increased release of fibroblast growth stimulatory activity and decreased lysosomal enzyme release. These assays were carried out on media collected from macrophage subpopulations cultured *in vitro* for 24 hours. This short period of *in vitro* culture may not reflect the metabolic activity of these macrophage subpopulations *in situ*. Few *in situ* studies of pulmonary reactions to silica have been published (except for the pleural response to injection of 20 mg of silica into the pleural space of rats[24]). With the rapid development of immunohistochemical assays to detect expression of surface markers and cytokines and *in situ* hybridization to detect mRNA expression, such studies are now feasible and should help to resolve these conflicting observations.

Pending application of these new *in situ* techniques to these animal models, the majority of short-term bioassays have observed similar changes in cellular and biochemical parameters of bronchoalveolar lavage fluid after instillation or inhalation of silica particles (for example, see References 7, 13, 14 and 25–29). In these short-term bioassays, silica consistently produces the following cellular and biochemical changes in a dose-dependent manner: increased neutrophils, increased total protein and albumin, and increased levels of lactate dehydrogenase and lysosomal enzyme activities. These various cellular and biochemical changes in the bronchoalveolar lavage constituents serve as biomarkers for pulmonary injury induced by toxic particles. What do these cellular and biochemical changes tell us about the acute interaction between macrophages and silica particles? Lactate dehydrogenase and lysosomal enzymes could be released from several different lung cell populations. However, in their short-term bioassay using intratracheal instillation of silica in hamsters, Beck et al.[30] measured lactate dehydrogenase isoenzyme patterns and discovered that most of the lactate dehydrogenase activity measured in bronchoalveolar lavage fluid is released from neutrophils and macrophages. Increased neutrophils and albumin are also consistent markers of pulmonary inflammation and increased permeability of the alveolar-capillary barrier that accompany acute silica-induced pulmonary toxicity. The potential of this inflammatory response to amplify acute silica toxicity will be discussed in section IV.D.

In summary, these biochemical markers of pulmonary toxicity and morphologic evidence of macrophage injury[17,18] support the hypothesis that silica causes acute injury to alveolar macrophages accompanied by extracellular release of the cytoplasmic enzyme lactate dehydrogenase and lysosomal enzymes. It is not known whether macrophages in the interstitium and lymphatics experience the same toxic effects of silica particles. The biochemical mechanisms responsible for acute cytotoxicity of silica particles and the functional consequences of this injury will be discussed next.

B. BIOCHEMICAL MECHANISMS OF MACROPHAGE INJURY

The interaction between silica particles and macrophages is fundamental to understanding the early events that initiate silicosis and is a useful model for toxic cell injury in general. Earlier studies focused on lysosomal rupture by silica particles that resulted in death of the macrophage and injury to surrounding tissues.[15,16] Subsequent investigations revealed that silica-induced damage is not limited to the lysosomal membrane but disrupts the electrical potential gradient across the mitochondrial and plasma membranes as well.[31] The nature of the chemical interaction between the surface of silica particles and cellular membranes is uncertain. Recent studies by Wiessner et al.[32] comparing the hemolytic activity and fibrogenicity of chemically-modified silica preparations suggest that surface electrostatic interactions, rather than hydrogen bonding, determine the biologic reactivity of silica particles. The potential of silica particles to generate oxygen-derived free radicals was discussed in detail in Section II, Chapter 3; these by-products may also contribute to macrophage toxicity and lung injury.

What are the consequences of generalized membrane injury to the macrophage? A series of experiments using an *in vitro* model system has led to the conclusion that disruption of the integrity of either the lysosomal membrane[33] or the mitochondrial membrane is not in itself sufficient to kill the macrophage.[31] Additional metabolic derangements accompany disruption of these intracellular membranes. Macrophages exposed to silica particles, but not to nontoxic titanium dioxide particles, also show a reduction in ATP content accompanied by purine catabolism and extracellular release of inosine, hypoxanthine, xanthine, and uric acid.[34] Reduced ATP content produced by specific metabolic inhibitors is not in itself sufficient to kill the macrophage.[35] Other models of cell injury point to disruption of plasma membrane integrity leading to intracellular calcium accumulation as a common mediator of toxic cell death. Silica toxicity to macrophages is accompanied by increased free cytosolic calcium and increased membrane-associated calcium.[31,36] Exposure to lower doses of silica particles may cause sublethal injury to macrophages accompanied by a transient elevation of free cytosolic calcium. This transient calcium elevation may trigger synthesis and release of cytokines that will be discussed in the next section. Exposure to higher doses of silica particles results in a persistent elevation of free cytosolic calcium and increased calcium binding to cellular membranes. Persistent elevation of calcium may activate cellular proteases, phospholipases, and nucleases and produce irreversible cell injury. Thus, altered calcium homeostasis is postulated as a key biochemical event in the initiation of silicosis.

Inflammatory cells have recently been shown to undergo a different pathway leading to cell death: programmed cell death or apoptosis. This is a physiologic mechanism that occurs during embryogenesis and wound healing resulting in shrinkage, nuclear condensation, and removal of cells without provoking an inflammatory response. Mangan and Wahl[37] hypothesize that monocytes recruited to sites of inflammation undergo apoptosis as the levels of cytokines wane. In an *in vitro* model they discovered that the continued presence of tumor necrosis factor-α (TNF-α) and IL-1β prevented apoptosis in cultured human monocytes. Since macrophages are a major source of these cytokines at sites of inflammation, autocrine production or local paracrine secretion of TNF-α and IL-1β may promote the survival of macrophages and sustain the inflammatory response. It is possible that this cytokine network is perturbed by the interaction of silica particles with macrophages resulting in a prolonged inflammatory response and fibrogenesis. Alternatively, decreased production of TNF-α and IL-1β may result in death of macrophages by apoptosis, not as a result of direct silica cytotoxicity. These alternatives can be tested experimentally. The effects of silica on the synthesis and release of cytokines by macrophages is an important topic that will be considered next.

C. MECHANISMS LEADING TO RELEASE OF CYTOKINES

Macrophages are an important source of multiple inflammatory mediators, including cytokines, that modulate inflammation, immune responses, and wound healing.[38,39] Synthesis and release of cytokines are carefully timed and regulated such that in most inflammatory reactions to invading micro-organisms, tissue injury is limited and there is little or no permanent damage to the lung parenchyma.[39] In contrast, the interaction between macrophages and silica particles leads to chronic, progressive nodular fibrosis of the lung parenchyma and hilar lymph nodes. It is hypothesized that silica particles provoke continued release of cytokines and other fibrogenic factors from macrophages.[3] The following cytokines have been implicated in the development of silicosis: IL-1, TNF-α, and bombesin. This discussion will focus on potential mechanisms responsible for increased synthesis and release of cytokines from macrophages following acute exposure to silica particles. The complex interplay between release of cytokines and other mediators, amplification of the inflammatory response, and stimulation of fibrosis will be discussed in section V.

The first clue that silica particles may modulate synthesis and release of cytokines from macrophages was reported by Schmidt et al. in 1984.[19] Adherent human peripheral blood monocytes were directly exposed to 0, 25, 50 or 100 μg/ml of silica for 24 hours. A nonfibrogenic sample of diamond dust was used as a nontoxic particle control. The conditioned media were tested for IL-1 activity using fibroblast and thymocyte proliferation assays. Doses of 50–100 μg/ml of silica, but not diamond dust, caused a 5 to 10 fold increase in release of IL-1 activity; these doses did not decrease cell viability under these conditions. These data suggest that one of the fibroblast-stimulating factors released from macrophages exposed to silica *in vitro* as originally described by Heppelston and Stiles[40] is IL-1. Subsequent experiments have not consistently confirmed that direct exposure of rat alveolar macrophages to silica *in vitro* stimulates release of IL-1 (for example, see Reference 41); however, when alveolar macrophages were collected from rats 1 to 28 days after direct intratracheal instillation of silica particles and cultured for 24 hours, increased levels of IL-1 were released. In contrast, instillation of titanium dioxide particles did not result in increased IL-1 release from alveolar macrophages. Thus, increased release of IL-1 from alveolar macrophages after exposure to silica particles *in vivo* suggests that this cytokine may mediate the inflammatory and fibrotic effects of silica.

The experiments reported by Driscoll et al.[41] suggest that silica particles may not cause secretion of IL-1 by direct physical interaction. No one has shown directly that the macrophages containing silica particles are the source of secreted IL-1. Macrophages secrete IL-1 and other cytokines in many types of inflammatory reactions; therefore, it is possible that the increased release of IL-1 from macrophages demonstrated in these models may be secondary to the ongoing inflammatory response produced by toxic mineral particles. The mechanism responsible for increased release of IL-1 from macrophages in these model systems is unknown. Adherence to plastic *in vitro* rapidly induces synthesis of IL-1 and expression of membrane-associated IL-1 activity in normal mouse peritoneal macrophages.[42] This observation complicates the interpretation of those experiments that describe increased release of IL-1 from alveolar macrophages cultured on plastic for 24 hours. Two forms of IL-1 are produced by rodent and human macrophages: IL-1α and IL-1β. Both forms are synthesized as a large precursor of 31 to 33 kilodaltons (kDa). Suttles et al.[43] have suggested that elevated intracellular calcium stimulates rapid processing and secretion of IL-1α. Sublethal toxicity to macrophages exposed to silica particles may be associated with a transient increase in free cytosolic calcium and increased IL-1α release by this novel mechanism. Finally, Hogquist et al.[44] have recently reported release of both IL-1α and IL-1β from mouse peritoneal macrophages injured *in vitro*. Measurable quantities of IL-1 were detected from cultured monocytes that represented 10% of the total IL-1 content and corresponded to release of 14% of lactate dehydrogenase activity. Therefore, it is possible that a small percentage of dying macrophages could be responsible for the observed IL-1 released after exposure to silica. In Hogquist's model of lytic injury induced by scraping, H_2O_2 or saponin, processing and release of active IL-1α occurred, while unprocessed IL-1β was also released. In contrast, in their model of apoptosis, both forms of IL-1 were processed and released. One or both of these mechanisms may contribute to direct release of IL-1 from macrophages exposed to toxic silica particles *in vitro;* additional experiments are required to determine whether any of these mechanisms resulting in increased IL-1 synthesis, processing, and release occur after exposure to silica particles *in vivo*.

A second cytokine implicated in the development of silicosis is the neuropeptide bombesin. This cytokine is also chemotactic for monocytes and stimulates proliferation of fibroblasts. Wiedermann et al.[45] exposed rats to 10 mg of silica by direct intratracheal instillation and analyzed bronchoalveolar lavage fluid and macrophages for bombesin using a radioimmunoassay. Carbon dust was used as a nonfibrogenic control particle. No elevations in bombesin were detected in bronchoalveolar lavage fluids or in freshly isolated alveolar macrophages. However, when macrophages were cultured for four hours *in vitro,* 50% more bombesin was secreted from macrophages obtained from rats six weeks after instillation of silica. At this time, silica-injected rats had increased content of hydroxyproline in their lungs that indicates early fibrosis. Direct exposure of alveolar macrophages to carbon dust or silica *in vitro* did not increase bombesin release.

At this time, multiple lines of evidence support an important role for the cytokine TNF-α in the pathogenesis of silicosis. TNF-α and IL-1 have similar, often synergistic effects, including activation of immune cells, increased adherence of inflammatory cells to blood vessel walls in the early stages of acute inflammation, and stimulation of fibroblast proliferation. Systemic release of TNF-α and IL-1 can induce fever, cachexia, and endotoxic shock.[39] These cytokines are hypothesized to play a central role in formation of granulomas as demonstrated by production of pulmonary granulomas after direct intratracheal injection of agarose beads coupled with IL-1 or TNF-α, but not α-interferon or IL-2.[46] Two caveats must be introduced in interpretation of experimental studies with TNF-α. First, induction of TNF-α is extremely sensitive to low levels of contaminating endotoxin. Therefore, all *in vitro* studies should include precautions and controls to preclude artifactual TNF-α release. Second, while there is strong support for a role of TNF-α and IL-1 in granulomatous inflammation (reviewed in Reference 47), the silicotic nodules characteristic of human chronic silicosis are not granulomas. Altered release of these cytokines or other as yet unidentified mediators must be responsible for producing the unique morphologic lesion characteristic of chronic silicosis.

Despite these caveats, at least three independent studies demonstrated increased TNF-α production or release from macrophages after exposure to silica particles.[41,48,49] The study by Piguet et al.[49] is especially important, because it demonstrates expression of TNF-α mRNA and protein directly within silicotic nodules using *in situ* hybridization and immunohistochemistry. Another cytokine frequently involved in the early stages of acute inflammation, IL-6,[50] was also detected in silicotic nodules. At the level of mRNA expression in the total lung, some mice showed increased TNF-α mRNA expression 7, 15 or 70 days after direct intratracheal injection of 20 mg of silica; no increased levels of IL-1 or transforming growth factor-β (TGF-β, another important mediator of pulmonary fibrosis) mRNA expression were detected. Treatment with rabbit anti-mouse TNF-α or exogenous recombinant TNF-α for 15 days reduced or augmented, respectively, fibrosis in the silicotic nodules as determined by lung hydroxyproline content. Paradoxically, direct addition of TNF-α to fibroblasts *in vitro* inhibits collagen synthesis.[51] Therefore, TNF-α appears to stimulate early fibrosis in this model system indirectly, perhaps by amplifying the acute inflammatory response. This will be discussed in detail in section IV.D.

Piguet et al.[49] also assessed whether there was local or systemic release of these cytokines. No TNF-α or IL-6 activity was detected in the sera of silica-exposed mice. This observation is in agreement with the clinical features of human chronic silicosis which is not accompanied by fever, cachexia, or secondary amyloidosis — clinical symptoms produced by systemic release of these cytokines.[50] However, in another interesting model of chronic silicosis in the rat that develops four to nine months after inhalation of silica, no direct release of TNF-α from alveolar macrophages was reported, even though many of these cells contained silica particles. Mohr et al.[52] did discover that alveolar macrophages, as well as peritoneal macrophages, obtained after chronic inhalation of silica were "primed;" they were stimulated to secrete TNF-α after exposure to endotoxin *in vitro*. Driscoll et al.[41] also reported that alveolar macrophages obtained within one month after direct intratracheal instillation of silica or TiO_2 were "primed;" increased amounts of both IL-1 and TNF-α were released from alveolar macrophages collected from mice exposed to silica. Driscoll et al.[41] reported dose-dependent stimulation of TNF-α release from rat alveolar macrophages by direct exposure to silica *in vitro* but not to titanium dioxide. In contrast, Bissonnette and Rola-Pleszczynski[48] reported inhibition of spontaneous TNF-α release from mouse alveolar macrophages by direct exposure to silica particles *in vitro*.

The mechanisms responsible for induction of TNF-α mRNA and protein and its extracellular release after *in vitro* exposure to silica particles are unknown. Differences in response are noted after acute (less than one month) and chronic exposures and may reflect a greater role for TNF-α, as well as IL-1, in the early inflammatory response to silica as suggested by Driscoll et al.[41] Nonetheless, *in situ* demonstration of TNF-α and IL-6 within developing silicotic nodules and the inhibitory effect of anti-TNF-α antibody on collagen formation are strong pieces of evidence for a central role for TNF-α, at least during the early stages in the development of silicotic nodules.[49] Stimulation of release of TNF-α and other fibrogenic factors (for example, release of a platelet-derived growth factor (PDGF) homologue[53] from alveolar macrophages by direct exposure to inert particles such as titanium dioxide or carbonyl iron *in vitro*) suggests that any phagocytic stimulus may trigger a transient release of cytokines from macrophages. It is hypothesized that exposure of macrophages to toxic particles such as silica or asbestos provokes a sustained release of cytokines and fibrogenic factors leading to fibrosis. The role of other fibrogenic factors (PDGF, TGF-β, or insulin-like growth factors (IGF-1)[54]) in silicosis has not yet been explored.

D. WHAT ARE THE FUNCTIONAL CONSEQUENCES OF MACROPHAGE INJURY?

1. Impaired Particle Clearance

Three different investigators using short-term bioassays have reported that alveolar macrophages collected by bronchoalveolar lavage after inhalation[7,27] or intratracheal instillation[55] show impaired adherence *in vitro*, depressed motility, reduced chemotaxis, and decreased rates of phagocytosis. These observations led Warheit et al. (1991), to conclude: "silica inhibits macrophage clearance functions and consequently, limits its own removal from the lung."[7] Impaired macrophage phagocytosis and mobility would theoretically reduce the efficiency of removal via the mucociliary escalator that is the major route of clearance of particles from the distal respiratory tract and alveolar spaces. This impaired clearance might allow more silica particles to penetrate into the interstitium and lymphatics to initiate formation of the early silicotic nodule. Once these toxic particles reach the interstitium, it is hypothesized that there are repeated cycles of macrophage injury and particle release. Impaired clearance of interstitial silica particles, particularly in the setting of continued exposure, could account for the gradual enlargement of early silicotic nodules observed in an autopsy series of granite workers from Vermont.[1]

2. Increased Susceptibility to Mycobacterial and Fungal Infections

Workers with silicosis are vulnerable to serious pulmonary infections caused by mycobacteria and fungal organisms.[2] This increased susceptibility to infection appears to be limited to this class of pathogens. Mice exposed to silica dusts do not have altered resistance to influenza virus.[56] Macrophages are important in the defense against intracellular pathogens such as mycobacteria (reviewed in Reference 57). *In vitro,* macrophages do not kill mycobacteria as efficiently in the presence of silica.[58] Workers with silicosis frequently develop cavitary lesions when infected with *Mycobacterium tuberculosis.*[1] Histopathologic analysis reveals few epithelioid cells or multinucleated giant cells that are the histologic hallmark of the macrophage defense against persistent intracellular infections. Therefore, the *in vitro* studies and histopathologic evidence point to impaired macrophage defense mechanisms against these intracellular pathogens.

What is responsible for this impaired defense reaction? On the basis of the *in vitro* studies on the biochemical mechanisms of acute silica toxicity, it is possible that decreased energy metabolism could account for loss of many of the specialized functions of macrophages.[35] In addition, exposure to silica may perturb production and release of cytokines and other inflammatory signals from macrophages, thereby compromising their response to mycobacteria. On the basis of recent *in vitro* studies of normal human macrophages infected with *Mycobacterium avium-intracellulare,* the cytokines TNF-α and IL-6 appear to be important in the response to this intracellular pathogen. In their study, Newman et al.[59] discovered that macrophages responded to infection with these mycobacteria by induction of mRNA and protein for TNF-α and IL-6. Upregulation of these cytokines (but not IL-1β) correlated with increased survival *in vitro* after infection. Macrophages that did not induce these cytokines died. It is intriguing to speculate that exposure to silica directly or indirectly impairs induction of these cytokines during intracellular infection with mycobacteria, leading to macrophage death and inability to limit this type of infection. With the newer techniques available for *in situ* detection and modulation of cytokines, this hypothesis could be tested experimentally.

3. Extracellular Release of Proteases and Hydrolytic Enzymes

Exposure to silica causes acute toxicity to alveolar macrophages accompanied by extracellular release of lysosomal enzymes and neutral proteases,[60] including elastase[26] in a variety of animal models. These enzymes, elastase in particular, especially in the presence of the oxidized inhibitor, α-1-antitrypsin, have the potential to damage the delicate type 1 alveolar lining cells and the underlying basement membrane. This damage is reflected by increased leakage of serum proteins into alveolar spaces that has also been observed in short-term bioassays of silica toxicity. Damage to the alveolar epithelial lining, even if it is transient, is important because it may allow more silica particles to reach the interstitium. In addition, damage to the epithelial lining would also allow cytokines and growth factors released from alveolar macrophages and other inflammatory cells to penetrate into the interstitium and stimulate fibrosis. The evidence for alveolar epithelial cell injury in these animal model systems and in human silicosis will be discussed next.

E. WHAT IS THE ROLE OF ALVEOLAR EPITHELIAL CELL INJURY?

Damage to the alveolar-capillary permeability barrier manifested by increased protein and albumin content of bronchoalveolar lavage fluid is a common feature of short-term animal models of silicosis (see, for example, References 13, 29, 41, and 61). This increased permeability could be the result of direct toxicity to type 1 alveolar lining cells and/or secondary to an acute inflammatory response. Some investigators have directly observed acute necrosis of type 1 alveolar epithelial cells,[61] followed by proliferation and hypertrophy of type 2 alveolar cells.[7,28,29] Depletion of circulating leukocytes by injection of rabbit antibody into rats prior to intratracheal instillation of silica prevented an influx of neutrophils into the alveoli and decreased many of the markers of acute inflammation and cytotoxicity. In contrast, neutrophil depletion did not prevent hypertrophy of type 2 cells.[29] This observation in an acute model of silica toxicity provides substantial evidence for neutrophil-mediated injury to the alveolar-capillary permeability barrier. The mechanism leading to recruitment of neutrophils into the lungs after exposure to silica particles is unknown. In contrast to other types of mineral particles, activation of complement is not involved in the inflammatory response to silica.[62] Alveolar macrophages have been shown to release IL-8, which is a recently-characterized peptide chemotactic for neutrophils. TNF-α, IL-1β, and endotoxin induce expression of IL-8 by macrophages.[63] Since there is considerable evidence for the roles of TNF-α and IL-1 in silicosis, sequential induction of these three cytokines may contribute to the inflammatory response to silica particles. A second potential source of chemotactic factors is metabolism of arachidonic acid. Exposure of alveolar macrophages to silica particles stimulated arachidonic acid metabolism,[65] although similar metabolites are produced by phagocytosis of nontoxic carbonyl iron particles *in vitro*.[65]

In a chronic model of silicosis in rats[3] and in workers with silicosis,[67] an increased percentage of neutrophils as well as macrophages are recovered in bronchoalveolar lavage fluid. In addition, in humans with silicosis, lung uptake of ^{67}Ga is focally increased, especially in areas of conglomeration of silicotic nodules.[67] Therefore, this sensitive *in situ* technique reveals focal regions of active inflammation around evolving silicotic lesions. It is not known whether there is ongoing injury to type 1 alveolar epithelial cells adjacent to these foci of inflammation. However, evidence of repair of this epithelial cell injury manifest by hypertrophied type 2 cells is rare in chronic silicosis in humans.[3] In contrast, in acute silicosis or alveolar proteinosis occurring in humans, there is extensive injury to type 1 epithelial cells, followed by proliferation and hypertrophy of type 2 cells.[1]

In summary, injury to alveolar epithelial cells and damage to the alveolar-capillary permeability barrier secondary to an influx of neutrophils into the alveolar spaces is a common feature of acute silicosis in humans and in short-term animal models. In most of the animal models, the high doses of silica administered produce a persistent acute inflammatory response together with nodular fibrotic lesions.[7,14] These models combine the features of acute silicosis (alveolar proteinosis) and chronic silicosis that develop simultaneously. While this does not invalidate these short-term inhalation or instillation models as extremely useful for screening potentially toxic particulates using silica as a well-established positive control, the simultaneous development of two different diseases (although both may share some common mediators) limits their utility to study the pathogenesis of chronic silicosis. The use of chronic, slowly-progressive models developed by Davis[3] or Reiser and Last[68] are necessary to identify the complex sequence of events culminating in nodular pulmonary fibrosis. In chronic silicosis in humans, epithelial cell injury and the acute inflammatory response is less prominent, while the nodular fibrotic lesions gradually enlarge and coalesce over a period of many years. The ^{67}Ga uptake studies indicate, however, that active inflammation persists in areas of silicotic nodules throughout all stages in the evolution of chronic silicosis.[67] Therefore, it is likely that this localized inflammatory response amplifies and contributes to the progressive fibrosis. The role of these inflammatory mediators, in addition to other cytokines and fibrogenic factors derived from macrophages, in the chronic stages of silicosis will be discussed next.

V. CHRONIC COMPLICATIONS OF SILICA EXPOSURE: SILICOSIS

A. FIBROBLAST MIGRATION, PROLIFERATION, AND ACTIVATION

Formation of a fibrotic scar is a complex series of events that is tightly regulated at multiple steps. The first step is attraction of local fibroblasts to the site of injury. This process is called chemotaxis and is mediated by cytokines such as TGF-β released from neutrophils and macrophages and by extracellular matrix components such as fibronectin. Fibronectin release from macrophages has been demonstrated after intratracheal instillation of silica.[14,69] Fibronectin has also been demonstrated directly in silicotic nodules.[70] Within these nodules, fibronectin may serve to facilitate attachment of fibroblasts to the extracellular matrix and to stimulate their proliferation. Additional fibrogenic growth factors that may act in concert with fibronectin include PDGF, IGF-1, and TGF-β; macrophages are also potential sources of these growth factors.[39] During fibrosis, subpopulations of fibroblasts may accumulate that synthesize different quantities or subtypes of collagen. In various models of pulmonary fibrosis, increased rates of collagen synthesis are found reflecting increased transcription and increased steady-state mRNA levels for type I collagen. The growth factors TGF-β and IGF-1 stimulate collagen gene expression, while other inflammatory mediators, PGE_2 and γ-interferon, inhibit collagen gene expression. Following its synthesis, collagen molecules may be degraded intracellularly or released extracellularly. Additional posttranslational modifications in the collagen molecule occur prior to the formation of a mature, cross-linked collagen helix. Extracellular collagen is susceptible to degradation by the metalloproteinases collagenase (secreted by neutrophils and macrophages) and transin/stromelysin. TIMP-1 is an inhibitor of these metalloproteinases; TGF-β and IL-6 increase activity of TIMP-1 (reviewed by Goldstein, 1991[51]).

As discussed earlier in section IV, macrophages exposed to silica have been shown to release a variety of cytokines, as well as fibronectin, that modulate several of these steps in the formation of a collagen scar. The end result of the interaction between these released cytokines and interstitial fibroblasts is accumulation of collagen in the lung that has unique biochemical properties.[71] The biochemical characteristics of collagen deposited during the development of silicosis will be reviewed next.

B. CONNECTIVE TISSUE METABOLISM DURING THE DEVELOPMENT OF SILICOSIS

The total content, anatomic distribution, and biochemistry of collagen are altered in chronic silicosis. Direct intratracheal instillation or inhalation of silica in chronic animal models causes a progressive increase in total lung collagen content up to sixfold (reviewed in Reference 71). As described earlier, increased collagen accumulates in the center of early silicotic nodules that slowly expand and conglomerate as the disease progresses. Although there are at least 13 different collagen proteins, a collagen scar consists largely of collagen types I and III. The ratio of types I:III in normal lung is 2:1; this ratio is maintained in silicosis. In contrast, in animal models of diffuse interstitial fibrosis that develop acutely after exposure to bleomycin, paraquat, or ozone, the ratio is 5 to 6:1. In these models, in contrast to chronic silicosis, increased collagen content plateaus after several weeks and does not progress. In the bleomycin model, increased mRNA expression for several connective tissue components (type I collagen, fibronectin, and elastin) occurs coordinately and it is speculated that this is regulated by one or a few DNA binding proteins that increase transcription of these genes (reviewed in Reference 51). In chronic silicosis, the genes for both types I and III collagen are activated, with increased steady-state type III mRNA appearing before increased steady-state type I mRNA.[22] In contrast to silicosis, the distribution of collagen deposition in the bleomycin model is more diffuse and characterized by collapse of alveoli and chemotaxis of fibroblasts into air spaces.[73] Therefore, there are important differences in the temporal changes in collagen accumulation, regulation of connective tissue mRNA expression, and anatomic distribution of these connective tissue molecules between chronic silicosis and the bleomycin model of diffuse interstitial fibrosis. Although the regulation of connective tissue metabolism at the level of transcription has not yet been studied in chronic silicosis, it is likely that different regulatory mechanisms will be identified in silicosis.

Additional posttranslational modifications in collagen are characteristic of the animal models of chronic silicosis. These modifications are produced by cross-linking of the collagen chains by covalent bonding at lysine or hydroxylysine residues. Last and colleagues[71] have discovered that increased cross-linked hydroxypyridinium occurs at the time of formation of the mature silicotic nodule that is characterized by formation of a central, dense, acellular collagenous scar. Last speculates that this cross-linked collagen may be more resistant to degradation by collagenases. Thus, chronic silicosis is the summation of increased collagen synthesis plus decreased extracellular collagen degradation. This is one logical explanation for the somewhat paradoxical accumulation of collagen within silicotic nodules surrounded by inflammatory cells that are a rich source of collagenase and other proteases.

Some of the biochemical steps leading to formation of cross-linked collagen have been identified. Collagen in developing silicotic lungs shows a temporal sequence of biochemical modifications: increased content of hydroxylysine, increased ratio of dihydroxylysinonorleucine to hydroxylysinonorleucine, followed by increased formation of cross-linked hydroxypyridinium that is derived from condensation of three hydroxylysine residues. Altered regulation of the enzymes responsible for these posttranslational modifications during the development of silicosis is under active investigation.[71]

In summary, the biochemical regulation of increased collagen synthesis, deposition, and cross-linking that is characterized morphologically by the mature silicotic nodule is very complex. In the early stages in the development of a silicotic nodule, cytokines, fibronectin, and other mediators released from inflammatory cells trigger fibroblast chemotaxis, proliferation, and increased collagen synthesis at sites of focal aggregates of macrophages containing silica particles in the interstitium and lymphatics. Because the ratio of collagen types I:III in silicosis differs from this ratio in other models of pulmonary fibrosis, different fibroblast subpopulations or different transcriptional regulatory elements may be activated in silicosis. As the early silicotic nodule matures, local deposition of fibronectin may serve as a framework for focal deposition of collagen molecules with increased cross-links resistant to extracellular degradation by collagenases.

C. THE CYTOKINE-CYTOKINE INHIBITOR NETWORK

Are macrophage-derived cytokines the driving force responsible for these alterations in collagen metabolism? Numerous *in vitro* studies demonstrated that supernatants of cultured macrophages exposed to silica *in vitro* or *in vivo* stimulated proliferation of pulmonary fibroblasts.[74] After acute exposures to silica, alveolar macrophages released a fibroblast-inhibitory factor subsequently identified as PGE_2.[76] Type 2 alveolar epithelial cells were also shown to release PGE_2 after exposure to 50 to 200 μg/ml of silica for 24 hours.[77] This observation emphasizes the importance of mediators released from other lung cell populations besides inflammatory cells that could modify the development of fibrosis. These experiments also demonstrate the need to consider the net effect of multiple stimulatory and inhibitory factors in studying the pathogenesis of pulmonary fibrosis.[78] Unfortunately, the complex interaction between multiple cytokines and other inflammatory mediators has not yet been studied in the development of chronic silicosis.

A new group of factors that inhibits the action or production of the cytokines implicated in the development of silicosis has just been described. Cytokines mediate their effects by binding to specific receptors on the surface of the target cell to trigger the intracellular signals that lead to a specific response.[79] This new group of inhibitory factors operates by binding to or breaking down specific cytokine receptors; they are called cytokine receptor inhibitors. So far, cytokine receptor inhibitors have been described for IL-1, IL-6, TNF-α, and γ-interferon.[79] The IL-1 receptor antagonist binds directly to IL-1α and IL-1β receptors but does not induce any biologic response.[80] The other cytokine receptor inhibitors are hypothesized to induce proteolysis of surface cytokines or of the receptor itself.[79] Human alveolar macrophages have been shown to secrete IL-1 inhibitory activity.[82] Additional experiments are necessary to determine whether silica particles directly or indirectly perturb release of cytokines, as well as release of cytokine receptor inhibitors.

A new cytokine has been described that inhibits synthesis of the cytokines implicated in the development of silicosis, including IL-1α, IL-6, and TNF-α.[82] This inhibitory cytokine, IL-10, was shown to be produced by human monocytes. Therefore, it is hypothesized that activated mononuclear phagocytes produce endogenous inhibitors that down-regulate the synthesis and release of inflammatory and fibrogenic cytokines in an autocrine fashion.[83] The effects of exposure to silica particles on this autoregulatory network is unknown. Conceivably, phagocytosis of any mineral particle will trigger release of early inflammatory mediators (e.g., IL-1, TNF-α, and IL-6) from macrophages. After phagocytosis of nontoxic particles, subsequent synthesis of IL-10 by macrophages would down-regulate synthesis of these mediators so that they would be expressed only transiently and would not trigger prolonged inflammation and fibrosis. In contrast, after phagocytosis of toxic silica particles, subsequent synthesis of IL-10 may be impaired leading to prolonged release of cytokines, sustained inflammation, and fibrosis.

Finally, once cytokines are released extracellularly, there is a second line of defense against their unregulated activity. Extracellular carriers or binding proteins are present in serum and may accumulate at sites of tissue injury and inflammation. The antiprotease α_2-macroglobulin can bind multiple cytokines, including those relevant to silicosis (IL-1β, TNF-α, and IL-6). Circulating α_2-macroglobulin may carry cytokines in an active form or deliver them to cells with α_2-macroglobulin receptors for clearance. The importance of this cytokine clearance mechanism in disease, including silicosis, has yet to be evaluated.[84]

In summary, the hypothesis that silicosis is triggered by sustained release of cytokines, such as IL-1, from macrophages must be reevaluated. The effects of other inhibitory cytokines, receptor antagonists, and scavenger proteins must be considered in the complex interaction between silica particles, macrophages, and other target cell populations in the lung that participated in the development of chronic silicosis.

D. MODULATION OF FIBROSIS BY THE IMMUNE SYSTEM

Workers with silicosis frequently show evidence of increased immunoglobulin production: circulating immune complexes, antinuclear antibodies, and rheumatoid factor. In a small percentage of patients, rheumatoid arthritis exacerbates silicosis. Davis[3] hypothesizes that nonspecific activation of the immune system is triggered by release of IL-1 from macrophages exposed to silica. This cytokine would activate T-helper inducer cells to stimulate B cell growth and maturation. Activated T-helper cells also release cytokines such as γ-interferon that further activate macrophages. Hubbard[85] tested this hypothesis directly by exposing congenitally T-cell deficient and wild-type mice to silica delivered by intratracheal instillation. After 60 days, there was no difference in collagen deposition as determined by total hydroxyproline content between the two groups. Neutrophils persisted in the lungs over the duration of the experiment in the T-cell deficient group; this persistent inflammatory response may have exacerbated the fibrosis by mechanisms described earlier.

In summary, there is evidence for activation of the humoral immune system in silicosis although it is likely that this occurs secondarily and is not a primary factor in the pathogenesis of this disease. Cell-mediated immunity appears uncompromised in patients with silicosis.[3] Although Davis' hypothesis that T-cell activation contributes to the perpetuation of fibrosis in this disease is intriguing, it is not consistent with two other observations. First, T-cell activation and release of γ-interferon are important in the cell-mediated immune response to mycobacteria. Paradoxically, patients with silicosis have decreased defenses against mycobacteria most likely secondary to impaired macrophage function. Second, γ-interferon down-regulates collagen synthesis,[51] while there is biochemical evidence for increased collagen synthesis in silicosis.[71] Therefore, T-cell activation is probably not a primary factor in the pathogenesis of silicosis. It is possible, however, that individual variations in cellular or humoral immune responses may secondarily modulate the severity or rate of progression of silicosis.

VI. WORKING HYPOTHESIS

On the basis of the newer information about cytokines and other mediators implicated in the development of pulmonary fibrosis, a modification of Davis' hypothesis[3] is outlined in Figure 2. The initial encounter between macrophages and silica particles leads to a transient, local release of inflammatory mediators, soluble IL-1 and TNF-α, that attract additional macrophages to the site of particle deposition. Mucociliary clearance of toxic silica particles is impaired, leading to translocation of macrophages and free silica particles to the interstitium and lymphatics located around the terminal respiratory bronchioles. Focal aggregates of macrophages containing silica particles accumulate at these anatomic sites. Focal injury to macrophages also occurs at these sites, secondary to direct particle toxicity or apoptosis, leading to particle release and repeated triggering of this localized inflammatory reaction. Alternatively, toxic silica particles may impair down-regulation of pro-inflammatory cytokines resulting in their sustained release. Collagen deposition is hypothesized to be triggered by proteolytic damage to adjacent lung parenchyma, expression of surface IL-1 by macrophages, and local secretion of fibronectin by macrophages. Additional post-translational modifications of collagen occur that render it less susceptible to degradation by proteases. In contrast to injury leading to diffuse interstitial fibrosis, the sequence of events leading to formation of a silicotic nodule must be localized or limited anatomically. The end result is a dense, nodular, collagen scar surrounded by macrophages and fibroblasts that sustain a slowly progressive, expanding fibrotic reaction.

It is hoped that this hypothesis will stimulate new experimental approaches to test this proposed sequence of events and lead to the discovery of new mechanisms responsible for the development of chronic silicosis.

ACKNOWLEDGMENTS

The research presented from the author's laboratory was supported by grant R01 ES03189 from the National Institutes of Health. I would like to thank Dr. Charles Kuhn, III for his inspiring discussions and Ms. Carol White for preparation of the manuscript.

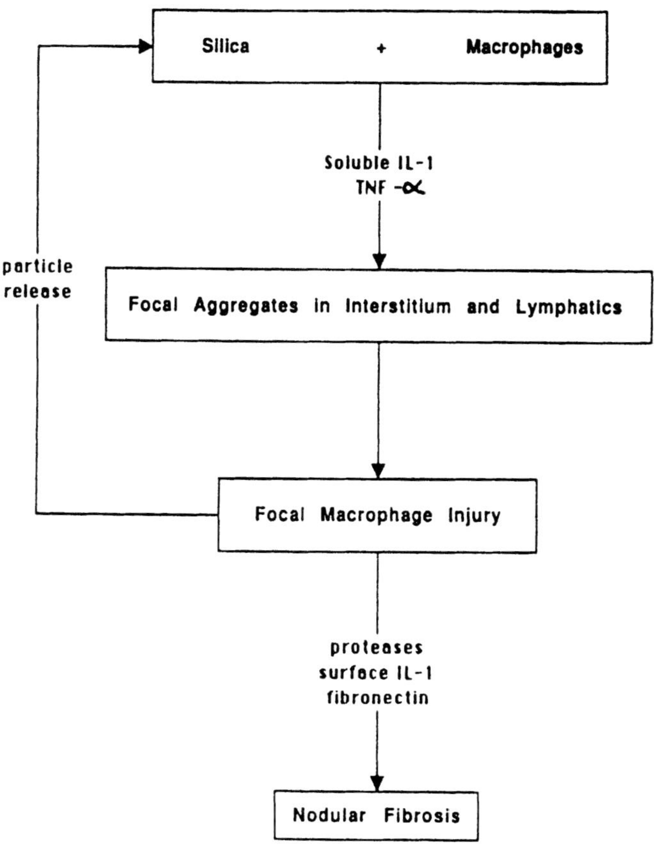

FIGURE 2 Working hypothesis describing the cells and mediators responsible for the development of chronic silicosis.

REFERENCES

1. Silicosis and Silicate Disease Committee, Diseases associated with exposure to silica and nonfibrous silicate minerals, *Arch. Pathol. Lab. Med.*, 112, 673, 1988.
2. **Ziskind, M., Jones, R. N., and Weill, H.,** Silicosis, *Am. Rev. Respir. Dis.*, 113, 643, 1976.
3. **Davis, G. S.,** The pathogenesis of silicosis: state of the art, *Chest*, 89, 166, 1986.
4. **Brain, J. D.,** Lung macrophages: how many kinds are there? What do they do? *Am. Rev. Respir. Dis.*, 137, 507, 1988.
5. **Churg, A., Wright, J. L., Wiggs, B., Paré, P. D., and Lazar, N.,** Small airways disease and mineral dust exposure, *Am. Rev. Respir. Dis.*, 131, 139, 1985.
6. **Brody, A. R. and Roe, M. W.,** Deposition pattern of inorganic particles at the alveolar level in the lungs of rats and mice, *Am. Rev. Respir. Dis.*, 128, 724, 1983.
7. **Warheit, D. B., Hansen, J. F., and Hartsky, M. A.,** Physiological and pathophysiological pulmonary responses to inhaled nuisance-like or fibrogenic dusts, *Anat. Rec.*, 231, 107, 1991.
8. **Adamson, I. Y. R.,** Cellular responses and translocation of particles following deposition in the lung, *J. Aerosol Med.*, 3, S-31, 1990.
9. **Lippmann, M., Yeates, D. B., and Albert, R. I.,** Deposition, retention, and clearance of inhaled particles, *Br. J. Ind. Med.*, 37, 337, 1980.

10. **Brody, A. R., Roe, M. W., Evans, J. N., and Davis, G. S.,** Deposition and translocation of inhaled silica in rats, *Lab. Invest.*, 47, 533, 1982.
11. **Vincent, J. H. and Donaldson, K.,** A dosimetric approach for relating the biological response of the lung to the accumulation of inhaled mineral dust, *Br. J. Ind. Med.*, 47, 302, 1990.
12. **Murrary, J., Webster, I., Reid, G., and Kielkowski, D.,** The relation between fibrosis of hilar lymph glands and the development of parenchymal silicosis, *Br. J. Ind. Med.*, 48, 267, 1991.
13. **Warheit, D. B., Carakostas, M. D., Hartsky, M. A., and Hansen, J. F.,** Development of a short-term inhalation bioassay to assess pulmonary toxicity of inhaled particles: comparisons of pulmonary responses to carbonyl iron and silica, *Toxicol. Appl. Pharmacol.*, 197, 350, 1991.
14. **Driscoll, K. E., Maurer, J. K., Lindenschmidt, R. C., Romberger, D., Rennard, S. I., and Crosby, L.,** Respiratory tract responses to dust: relationships between dust burden, lung injury, alveolar macrophage fibronectin release, and the development of pulmonary fibrosis, *Toxicol. Appl. Pharmacol.*, 106, 88, 1990.
15. **Allison, A. C., Harington, J. S., and Birbeck, M.,** An examination of the cytotoxic effects of silica on macrophages, *J. Exp. Med.*, 124, 141, 1966.
16. **Nadler, S. and Goldfischer, S.,** The intracellular release of lysosomal contents in macrophages that have ingested silica, *J. Histochem. Cytochem.*, 18, 368, 1970.
17. **Miller, K. and Kagan, E.,** The *in vivo* effects of quartz on alveolar macrophage membrane topography and on the characteristics of the intrapulmonary cell population, *J. Retic. Soc.*, 21, 307, 1977.
18. **Miller, K., Webster, I., Handfield, R. I. M., and Skikne, M. I.,** Ultrastructure of the lung in the rat following exposure to crocidolite asbestos and quartz, *J. Pathol.*, 124, 39, 1978.
19. **Schmidt, J. A., Oliver, C. N., Lepe-Zuniga, J. L., Green, I., and Gery, I.,** Silica-stimulated monocytes release fibroblast proliferation factors identical to interleukin 1, *J. Clin. Invest.*, 73, 1462, 1984.
20. **Wallace, W. E., Keane, M. J., Vallyathan, V., Hathaway, P., Regad, E. D., Castranova, V., and Green, F. H. Y.,** Suppression of inhaled particle cytotoxicity by pulmonary surfactant and re-toxification by phospholipase: distinguishing properties of quartz and kaolin, *Ann. Occup. Hyg.*, 32, 291, 1988.
21. **Khan, M. F., Gallagher, J. E., and Brody, A. R.,** Effects of proteins and lipids of the alveolar lining layer on particle binding and phagocytosis, *Toxicol. In Vitro,* 4, 93, 1990.
22. **Lehnert, B. E., Valdez, Y. E., and Holland, L. M.,** Pulmonary macrophages: alveolar and interstitial populations, *Exp. Lung Res.*, 9, 177, 1985.
23. **Sjöstrand, M., Absher, P. M., Hemenway, D. R., Trombley, L., and Baldor, L. C.,** Comparison of lung alveolar and tissue cells in silica-induced inflammation, *Am. Rev. Respir. Dis.*, 143, 47, 1991.
24. **Edwards, R. E., Wagner, M. M. F., and Moncrieff, C. B.,** Cell population and histochemistry of asbestos related lesions of rat pleural cavity after injection of various inorganic dusts, *Br. J. Ind. Med.*, 41, 506, 1984.
25. **Dauber, J. H., Rossman, M. D., Pietra, G. G., Jimenez, S. A., and Daniele, R. P.,** Experimental silicosis. Morphologic and biochemical abnormalities produced by intratracheal instillation of quartz into guinea pig lungs, *Am. J. Pathol.*, 101, 595, 1980.
26. **Beck, B. D., Brain, J. D., and Bohannon, D. E.,** An *in vivo* hamster bioassay to assess the toxicity of particulates for the lung, *Toxicol. Appl. Pharmacol.*, 66, 9, 1982.
27. **Fogelmark, B., Sjöstrand, M., Bergström, R., and Rylander, R.,** Pulmonary macrophage phagocytosis and enzyme production after *in vivo* exposure to silica dust, *Toxicol. Appl. Pharmacol.*, 68, 152, 1983.
28. **Adamson, I. Y. R. and Bowden, D. H.,** Role of polymorphonuclear leukocytes in silica-induced pulmonary fibrosis, *Am. J. Pathol.*, 117, 37, 1984.
29. **Henderson, R. F., Harkema, J. R., Hotchkiss, J. A., and Boehme, D. S.,** Effect of blood leucocyte depletion on the inflammatory response of the lung to quartz, *Toxicol. Appl. Pharmacol.*, 109, 127, 1991.
30. **Beck, B. D., Gerson, B., Feldman, H. A., and Brain, J. D.,** Lactate dehydrogenase isoenzymes in hamster lung lavage fluid after lung injury, *Toxicol. Appl. Pharmacol.*, 71, 59, 1983.
31. **Gleva, G. F., Goodglick, L. A., and Kane, A. B.,** Altered calcium homeostasis in irreversibly injured $P388D_1$ macrophages, *Am. J. Pathol.*, 137, 43, 1990.
32. **Wiessner, J. H., Mandel, N. S., Sohnle, P. G., Hasegawa, A., and Mandel, G. S.,** The effect of chemical modification of quartz surfaces on particulate-induced pulmonary inflammation and fibrosis in the mouse, *Am. Rev. Respir. Dis.*, 141, 111, 1990.
33. **Kane, A. B., Stanton, R. P., Raymond, E. G., Dobson, M. E., Knafelc, M. E., and Farber, J. L.,** Dissociation of intracellular lysosomal rupture from the cell death caused by silica, *J. Cell Biol.*, 87, 643, 1980.
34. **Dobson, M. E., Stern, R. O., and Kane, A. B.,** Selective purine release from $P388D_1$ macrophages injured by silica, *J. Cell. Physiol.*, 135, 244, 1988.
35. **Kane, A. B., Petrovich, D. R., Stern, R. O., and Farber, J. L.,** ATP depletion and loss of cell integrity in anoxic hepatocytes and silica-treated $P388D_1$ macrophages, *Am. J. Physiol.*, 249, C256, 1985.
36. **Chen, J., Armstrong, L. C., Liu, S., Gerriets, J. E., and Last, J. A.,** Silica increases cytosolic free calcium ion concentration of alveolar macrophages *in vitro, Toxicol. Appl. Pharm.*, 111, 211, 1991.
37. **Mangan, D. F. and Wahl, S. M.,** Differential regulation of human monocyte programmed cell death (apoptosis) by chemotactic factors and pro-inflammatory cytokines, *J. Immunol.*, 147, 3408, 1991.

38. **Sibille, Y. and Reynolds, H. Y.,** Macrophages and polymorphonuclear neutrophils in lung defense and injury, *Am. Rev. Respir. Dis.*, 141, 471, 1990.
39. **Kelley, J.,** Cytokines of the lung, *Am. Rev. Respir. Dis.*, 141, 765, 1990.
40. **Heppleston, A. G. and Stiles, J. A.,** Activity of a macrophage factor in collagen formation by silica, *Nature (London)*, 214, 521, 1967.
41. **Driscoll, K. E., Lindenschmidt, R. C., Maurer, J. K., Higgins, J. M., and Ridder, G.,** Pulmonary response to silica or titanium dioxide: inflammatory cells, alveolar macrophage-derived cytokines, and histopathology, *Am. J. Respir. Cell Mol. Biol.*, 2, 381, 1990.
42. **Labadia, M., Faanes, R. B., and Rothlein, R.,** Role of adherence vs. spreading in the induction of membrane-associated interleukin-1 on mouse peritoneal macrophages, *J. Leuk. Biol.*, 48, 420, 1990.
43. **Suttles, J., Giri, J. G., and Mizel, S. B.,** IL-1 secretion by macrophages, *J. Immunol.*, 144, 175, 1990.
44. **Hogquist, K. A., Nett, M. A., Unanue, E. R., and Chaplin, D. D.,** Interleukin 1 is processed and released during apoptosis, *Proc. Natl. Acad. Sci. U.S.A.*, 88, 8485, 1991.
45. **Wiedermann, C. J., Adamson, I. Y. R., Pert, C. B., and Bowden, D. H.,** Enhanced secretion of immunoreactive bombesin by alveolar macrophages exposed to silica, *J. Leuk. Biol.*, 43, 99, 1988.
46. **Shikama, Y., Kobayashi, K., Kasahara, K., Kaga, S., Hashimoto, M., Yoneya, I., Hosoda, S., Soejima, K., Ide, H., and Takahashi, T.,** Granuloma formation by artificial microparticles *in vitro*, *Am. J. Pathol.*, 134, 1189, 1989.
47. **Kunkel, S. L., Chensue, S. W., Strieter, R. M., Lynch, J. P., and Remick, D. G.,** Cellular and molecular aspects of granulomatous inflammation, *Am. J. Respir. Cell Mol. Biol.*, 1, 439, 1989.
48. **Bissonnette, E. and Rola-Pleszczynski, M.,** Pulmonary inflammation and fibrosis in a murine model of asbestosis and silicosis, *Inflammation*, 13, 329, 1989.
49. **Piguet, P. F., Collart, M. A., Grau, G. E., Sappino, A.-P., and Vassalli, P.,** Requirement of tumour necrosis factor for development of silica-induced pulmonary fibrosis, *Nature*, 344, 245, 1990.
50. **Heinrich, P. C., Castell, J. V., and Andus, T.,** Interleukin-6 and the acute phase response, *Biochem. J.*, 265, 621, 1990.
51. **Goldstein, R. H.,** Control of type I collagen formation in the lung, *Am. J. Physiol.*, 261, L29, 1991.
52. **Mohr, C., Gemsa, D., Graebner, C., Hemenway, D. R., Leslie, K. O., Absher, P. M., and Davis, G. S.,** Systemic macrophage stimulation in rats with silicosis: enhanced release of tumor necrosis factor-α from alveolar and peritoneal macrophages, *Am. J. Respir. Cell Mol. Biol.*, 5, 395, 1991.
53. **Bauman, M. D., Jetten, A. M., Bonner, J. C., Kumar, R. K., Bennett, R. A., and Brody, A. R.,** Secretion of a platelet-derived growth factor homologue by rat alveolar macrophages exposed to particulates *in vitro*, *Eur. J. Cell Biol.*, 51, 327, 1990.
54. **Rom, W. N., Bassett, P., Fells, G. A., Nukiwa, T., Trapnell, B. C., and Crystal, R. G.,** Alveolar macrophages release an insulin-like growth factor 1-type molecule, *J. Clin. Invest.*, 82, 1685, 1988.
55. **Dauber, J. H., Rossman, M. D., and Daniele, R. P.,** Pulmonary fibrosis: bronchoalveolar cell types and impaired function of alveolar macrophages in experimental silicosis, *Environ. Res.*, 27, 266, 1982.
56. **Zarkower, A., Scheuchenzuber, W. J., and Burns, C. A.,** Effects of silica dust inhalation on the susceptibility of mice to influenza infection, *Arch. Environ. Health*, Sept./Oct., 372, 1979.
57. **Dannenberg, A. M., Jr.,** Cellular hypersensitivity and cellular immunity in the pathogenesis of tuberculosis: specificity, systemic and local nature, and associated macrophage enzymes, *Bacteriol. Rev.*, 32, 85, 1968.
58. **Allison, A. C. and Hart, P. D.,** Potentiation by silica of the growth of *Mycobacterium tuberculosis* in macrophage cultures, *Br. J. Exp. Pathol.*, 69, 465, 1968.
59. **Newman, G. W., Gan, H. X., McCarthy, P. L., Jr., and Remold, H. G.,** Survival of human macrophages infected with *Mycobacterium avium intracellulare* correlates with increased production of tumor necrosis factor-α and IL-6, *J. Immunol.*, 147, 3942, 1991.
60. **Brown, G. M., Brown, D. M., Slight, J., and Donaldson, K.,** Persistent biological reactivity of quartz in the lung: raised protease burden compared with a non-pathogenic mineral dust and microbial particles, *Br. J. Ind. Med.*, 48, 61, 1991.
61. **Bowden, D. H. and Adamson, I. Y. R.,** The role of cell injury and the continuing inflammatory response in the generation of silicotic pulmonary fibrosis, *J. Pathol.*, 144, 149, 1984.
62. **Warheit, D. B., Carakostos, M. D., Bamberger, J. R., and Hartsky, M. A.,** Complement facilitates macrophage phagocytosis of inhaled iron particles but has little effect in mediating silica-induced lung inflammatory and clearance responses, *Environ. Res.*, 56, 186, 1991.
63. **Strieter, R. M., Chensue, S. W., Basha, M. A., Standiford, T. J., Lynch, J. P., Baggiolini, M., and Kunkel, S. L.,** Human alveolar macrophage gene expression of interleukin-8 by tumor necrosis factor-α, lipopolysaccharide, and interleukin-1β, *Am. J. Respir. Cell Mol. Biol.*, 2, 321, 1990.
64. **Holtzman, M. J.,** Arachidonic acid metabolism, *Am. Rev. Respir. Dis.*, 43, 188, 1991.
65. **Englen, M. D., Taylor, S. M., Laegreid, W. W., Liggitt, H. D., Silflow, R. M., Breeze, R. G., and Leid, R. W.,** Stimulation of arachidonic acid metabolism in silica-exposed alveolar macrophages, *Exp. Lung Res.*, 15, 511, 1989.
66. **Kouzan, S., Brody, A. R., Nettesheim, P., and Eling, T.,** Production of arachidonic acid metabolites by macrophages exposed *in vitro* to asbestos, carbonyl iron particles, or calcium ionophore, *Am. Rev. Respir. Dis.*, 131, 624, 1985.

67. **Bégin, R. O., Cantin, A. M., Boileau, R. D., and Bisson, G. Y.,** Spectrum of alveolitis in quartz-exposed human subjects, *Chest,* 92, 1061, 1987.
68. **Reiser, K. M. and Last, J. A.,** Collagen cross-linking in lungs of rats with experimental silicosis, *Collagen Related Res.,* 6, 313, 1986.
69. **Davies, R. and Erdogdu, G.,** Secretion of fibronectin by mineral dust-derived alveolar macrophages and activated peritoneal macrophages, *Exp. Lung Res.,* 15, 285, 1989.
70. **Wagner, J. C., Burns, J., Munday, D. E., and McGee, J.,** Presence of fibronectin in pneumoconiotic lesions, *Thorax,* 37, 54, 1982.
71. **Last, J. A., Wu, R., Chen, J., Gelzleichter, T., Sun, W.-M., and Armstrong, L. G.,** Particle-cell interactions: lung fibrogenesis, *J. Aerosol Med.,* 3, S-61, 1990.
72. **Vuorio, E. I., Makela, J. K., Vuorio, T. K., Poole, A., and Wagner, J. C.,** Characterization of excessive collagen production during development of pulmonary fibrosis induced by chronic silica inhalation in rats, *Br. J. Exp. Pathol.,* 70, 305, 1989.
73. **Lazenby, A. J., Crouch, E. C., McDonald, J. A., and Kuhn, C.,** Remodeling of the lung in bleomycin-induced pulmonary fibrosis in the rat, *Am. Rev. Respir. Dis.,* 142, 206, 1990.
74. **Brown, G. P., Monick, M., and Hunninghake, G. W.,** Fibroblast proliferation induced by silica-exposed human alveolar macrophages, *Am. Rev. Respir. Dis.,* 138, 85, 1988.
75. **Lugano, E. M., Dauber, J. H., Elias, J. A., Bashey, R. I., Jimenez, S. A., and Daniel, R. P.,** The regulation of lung fibroblast proliferation by alveolar macrophages in experimental silicosis, *Am. Rev. Respir. Dis.,* 129, 767, 1984.
76. **Elias, J. A., Rossman, M. D., Zurier, R. B., and Daniel, R. P.,** Human alveolar macrophage inhibition of lung fibroblast growth, *Am. Rev. Respir. Dis.,* 131, 94, 1985.
77. **Klein, J. H. and Adamson, I. Y. R.,** Fibroblast inhibition and prostaglandin secretion by alveolar epithelial cells exposed to silica, *Lab. Invest.,* 60, 808, 1989.
78. **Elias, J. A., Freudlich, B., Kern, J. A., and Rosenbloom, J.,** Cytokine networks in the regulation of inflammation and fibrosis in the lung. *Chest,* 97, 1439, 1990.
79. **Shepherd, V. L.,** Cytokine receptors of the lung, *Am. J. Respir. Cell Mol. Biol.,* 5, 403, 1991.
80. **Arend, W. P.,** Interleukin 1 receptor antagonist, *J. Clin. Invest.,* 88, 1445, 1991.
81. **Galve-de Rochemonteix, B., Nicod, L. P., Junod, A. F., and Dayer, J.-M.,** Characterization of a specific 20- to 25-kd interleukin-1 inhibitor from cultured human lung macrophages, *Am. J. Respir. Cell Mol. Biol.,* 3, 355, 1990.
82. **Fiorentino, D. F., Zlotnik, A., Mosmann, T. R., Howard, M., and O'Garra, A.,** IL-10 inhibits cytokine production by activated macrophages, *J. Immunol.,* 147, 3815, 1991.
83. **de Waal Malefyt, R., Abrams, J., Bennett, B., Figdor, C. G., and deVries, J. E.,** Interleukin 10 (IL-10) inhibits cytokine synthesis by human monocytes: an autoregulatory role of IL-10 produced by monocytes, *J. Exp. Med.,* 174, 1209, 1991.
84. **LaMarre, J., Wollenberg, G. K., Gonias, S. L., and Hayes, M. A.,** Cytokine binding and clearance properties of proteinase-activated α_2-macroglobulins, *Lab. Invest.,* 65, 3, 1991.
85. **Hubbard, A. K.,** Role for T lymphocytes in silica-induced pulmonary inflammation, *Lab. Invest.,* 61, 46, 1989.

Section III
Chapter 2

POTENTIAL INTRACELLULAR MESSENGERS INVOLVED IN SILICA STIMULATION OF ALVEOLAR MACROPHAGES

Abdallah J. Jabbour, Rashi Iyer, Ronald K. Scheule, and Andrij Holian

CONTENTS

I. INTRODUCTION

Crystalline silica is a ubiquitous environmental mineral that can cause chronic inflammation and fibrotic lung disease termed silicosis. Silicosis is characterized by so-called "silicotic nodules," that are composed of a central hyalinized core surrounded by layers of cellular collagenous capsules containing macrophages and fibroblasts.[1] Epidemiological and animal studies have shown that the severity of silicosis depends on many factors, such as silica dose, duration of exposure, nature and composition of the dust, subject variability, and other complicating diseases.[2–6] While fibrosis resulting from silica exposure is relatively well-described on an anatomical level, there is, as yet, no comprehensive understanding of the molecular and cellular events that lead to fibrosis as a consequence of the interaction of silica and lung cells.[2]

The first step in determining the mechanism of action of any toxic agent is to identify the primary target cell that is injured or whose function is altered. There is probably little argument in the case of silica-induced lung injury that the alveolar macrophage is the primary target cell and that, as a consequence of this interaction, an inflammatory response ensues. What is more debatable is the mechanism(s) by which the alveolar macrophage participates in an inflammatory response that leads to fibrosis of the lung. At least two overall cellular mechanisms may be involved. In one, phagocytosis of silica by the alveolar macrophage may be cytotoxic and cause the release of "factors" from the dying macrophage that may modulate or damage surrounding cells, e.g., epithelial cells, and initiate an inflammatory response. This inflammatory response may become chronic due to the release of silica particles from lysing macrophages and the subsequent phagocytosis of silica by functional macrophages, continuing the lytic cycle. In a second model, silica may interact with the alveolar macrophage in a nonlytic manner, activating one or more intracellular signalling pathways that lead to the release of inflammatory "mediators."

0-8493-4709-2/96/$0.00+$.50

It should be noted that these two cellular models are not mutually exclusive, i.e., either or both may be active at a given stage of the inflammatory response.

In this chapter, we hypothesize that the binding of silica to some membrane receptor(s) induces signal transduction through specific second messengers that in turn activate cellular kinases followed by nuclear transcription for various cytokines and other events (e.g., arachidonic acid metabolism) associated with macrophage activation by silica. Furthermore, the final outcome of the interaction of silica with alveolar macrophages depends on the dose of silica, as well as other factors, including extracellular conditions.

Unfortunately, there is limited information on the signal transduction pathway that is activated in the alveolar macrophage by silica. Current evidence supports a potential role for calcium as a second messenger in silica-induced alveolar macrophage activation and cytotoxicity. Additionally, we have shown recently that a tyrosine kinase pathway may be a potential target for silica's effect on the alveolar macrophage leading to cytokine production.

The purpose of this review is to describe the intracellular signalling pathways that may be involved in silica-induced alterations of alveolar macrophage function. Therefore, we will first discuss the two models of the potential outcome of the interaction of silica with the alveolar macrophage. Second, we will review the two major intracellular signalling pathways of the alveolar macrophage for which there is good evidence of involvement with silica. Third, we will review the data on silica alteration of these intracellular signalling pathways in alveolar macrophages.

II. CYTOTOXICITY OR CELL STIMULATION

As described earlier, there are at least two general outcomes that might occur when an alveolar macrophage encounters silica (Figure 1). First, silica may cause nonspecific damage to the macrophage cell membrane leading to cell lysis and death by necrosis. Second, silica may interact directly or indirectly with macrophage receptors to trigger specific intracellular pathways, leading to release of inflammatory products. The occurrence of either phenomenon may depend on the amount of silica that comes in contact with alveolar macrophages. In fact, both outcomes are probably correct and are dependent on dose (cell stimulation <100 μg/ml > cytotoxicity), composition of *in vitro* culture conditions (microenvironment) and the preexisting state of the alveolar macrophage. For example, the process of adherence has been shown to activate macrophages.[7] Alternatively, the two models could be combined to propose that silica could initiate cell death by an apoptotic mechanism involving some intracellular pathway.

It has been well described that *in vitro* silica can cause alveolar macrophage cytotoxicity and necrosis.[8–11] These observations usually occur at high concentrations of silica or high ratios of silica to macrophages.[12] However, most of these *in vitro* studies are not representative of physiological conditions, i.e., adherent macrophages in the absence of proteins and lipids that are normally present in lung lining fluid. Therefore, under certain conditions, silica can cause macrophage injury *in vitro*. However, the role of overt, silica-induced cytotoxicity in the pathogenesis of silicosis remains inconclusive. It is possible that, due to a heterogenous distribution of silica in the lung, there may be regions of high doses of silica causing direct cell injury. The potential mechanisms of cell injury may well involve free radicals and are covered in detail in Section II, Chapters 2 and 3.

In contrast, there is strong evidence that *in vivo* silica exposure either directly or indirectly leads to alveolar macrophage activation. Several reports have described that macrophages recovered by bronchoalveolar lavage from silica-exposed humans or rats exhibit increased release of a number of mediators, such as a wide variety of cytokines, prostaglandins, and oxygen radicals, capable of modulating the immune system of the lung as well as causing damage to surrounding lung tissue.[2,5,6,13–19] Chronic inflammation due to the persistent retention of silica dust, hence chronic release of inflammatory mediators in the lung, may eventually lead to silicosis. The observations that silica-induced collagen deposition in a mouse model was abolished by an anti TNF-α (tumor necrosis factor) antibody and significantly increased by infusion of mouse recombinant TNF-α, strongly suggest that cytokine production *in vivo* is involved in the development of silicosis.[20] Since alveolar macrophages are the most likely source of TNF-α in the lung, these findings suggest a determinant role for alveolar macrophage activation rather than silica-induced cytotoxicity in the development of fibrosis. Therefore, in the context of the existing evidence, the present report will adopt the hypothesis that it is the functional modulation of alveolar macrophages by silica rather than overt silica-induced cytotoxicity that leads to chronic lung inflammation and silicosis.

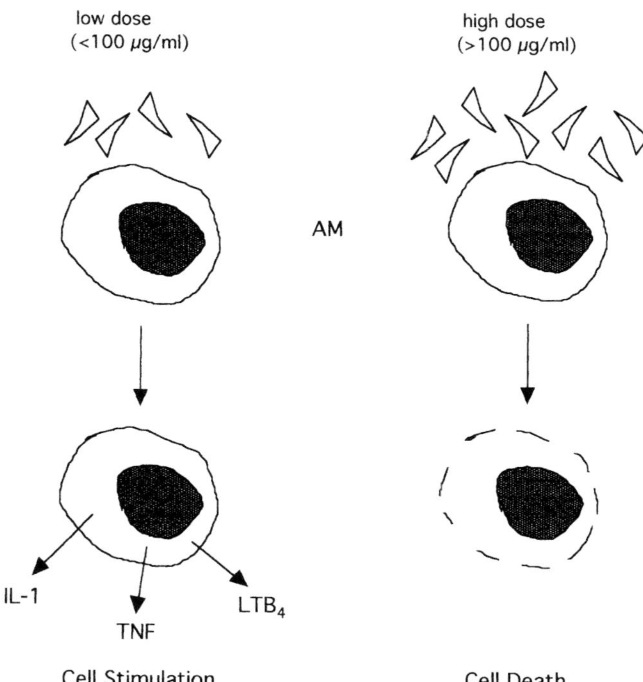

FIGURE 1 Silica exposure may cause cytotoxicity and/or cell stimulation. At concentrations of <100 µg/ml, silica favors stimulation of alveolar macrophages (AM) leading to release of inflammatory mediators. However, silica concentrations >100 µg/ml are more likely to cause irreversible damage to cell membranes and cell lysis.

Recent *in vitro* studies support the hypothesis that low doses of silica can cause alveolar macrophage stimulation. For example, silica has been shown to elicit interleukin-1 (IL-1) activity from normal rabbit and rat alveolar macrophages.[21–23] In our laboratory we have examined the release of IL-1 and TNF-α from human alveolar macrophages isolated from normal volunteers using cells in suspension culture. When these human cells were cultured in Medium 199 without added serum, silica did not stimulate any cytokine release; doses of silica such as 133 µg/ml were highly cytotoxic and were accompanied with rapid and sustained elevation of intracellular calcium. In contrast, in the presence of 10% fetal bovine serum, 133 µg/ml silica was minimally cytotoxic and did not cause elevation of intracellular calcium, but stimulated the release of these cytokines.[24] These findings support other reports that low doses of silica can cause macrophage activation and release of fibrogenic factors without significant cytotoxicity and that the culture conditions can determine the outcome.

Alternatively, it could be speculated that silica could induce macrophage injury by stimulating programmed cell death or apoptosis. In this model, silica could stimulate apoptosis that usually culminates in elevation of intracellular calcium, activation of endonuclease, and DNA fragmentation into characteristic 180–200 base pair fragments. Apoptosis has been observed in many cells including macrophages,[25] thymocytes,[26] endothelial cells,[27] and neutrophils[28] and provides a mechanism of cellular removal without the release of intracellular contents to the surrounding tissue. We have observed increased macrophage apoptosis by hydrogen peroxide, ozone, bleomycin, and heat (manuscripts in preparation). Therefore, we investigated whether silica could be inducing cell death by apoptosis in human alveolar macrophages. Apoptosis was detected as DNA fragmentation by the *in situ* DNA labelling technique[29] at 24 hours after 133 µg/ml of silica. Significant DNA fragmentation was detected. Therefore, human alveolar macrophages can be stimulated to undergo apoptosis by silica.

In summary, we have described two possible models through which silica might be acting, independently or together, to cause silicosis. Silica can be cytotoxic to lung cells causing cell death and tissue injury. This could be important in exposures to doses of silica that result in an acute disease. Alternatively, silica may activate alveolar macrophages to secrete various inflammatory mediators leading to chronic inflammation and lung fibrosis. The significance of these two models is that the type of intracellular pathways affected by silica might be different depending on the dose of silica used in the analysis.

III. INTRACELLULAR SIGNALLING PATHWAYS

A. INTRODUCTION

As described above, silica can stimulate alveolar macrophages to release a number of fibrogenic mediators. In order to do so, it must stimulate one or more signal transduction pathways leading to effector release. The mechanism by which silica stimulates effector release has been the focus of research in a number of laboratories, including our own. We have examined a number of potential pathways that silica may be affecting and ruled some out. Although asbestos stimulates phosphatidylinositol turnover and protein kinase C activation leading to superoxide anion production in alveolar macrophages,[30] we have found no evidence that silica activates this pathway. Furthermore, silica does not cause early (<60 min) changes in cyclic-adenosine monophosphate or -guanosine monophosphate levels in human alveolar macrophages, implying that these mediators are not involved in the primary signal transduction pathway. However, it does appear that two other signal transduction pathways may be involved in the early events following silica interaction with the alveolar macrophage. These pathways are intracellular calcium and activation of a tyrosine kinase pathway. Therefore, the next sections will briefly review these signal transduction events, followed by a review of the evidence of the role of these events in silica stimulation of macrophage effector release.

B. ELEVATION OF CYTOSOLIC CALCIUM

In contrast to the tyrosine kinases that will be covered later, intracellular calcium has long been recognized as a key regulator/modulator of many intracellular proteins. This protein regulation is accomplished by calcium binding to one or more sites on these proteins, thereby modifying their conformation and physiological function. Key examples of this in signal transduction include calcium binding to calmodulin,[31] which modulates a number of downstream kinases (e.g., calmodulin kinase) and protein kinase C.[32] Cells accomplish the task of using calcium in signal transduction by maintaining free (ionized) cytosolic calcium at approximately 100 n*M*[30,31,33] against an extracellular gradient in excess of 1 m*M*[34] by a number of mechanisms that also allow for rapid and transient changes in intracellular calcium.

The ability to utilize calcium in rapid signal transduction can be achieved by two primary mechanisms that can transiently raise cytosolic calcium sufficiently to modify effector protein function (diagrammed in Figure 2). The first mechanism includes the opening of one or more calcium channels. The alveolar macrophage probably has a number of these channels, including voltage-operated and receptor-operated.[35] For example, verapamil has been found to block both concanavalin A-[36] and zymosan-[37] stimulated superoxide anion production by rat alveolar macrophages; and both verapamil and nifedipine have been shown to block calcium entry into mouse peritoneal macrophages and the resulting cell activation.[38] The second mechanism is through the release of calcium sequestered in the endoplasmic reticulum. In this mechanism, inositol 1,4,5-trisphosphate is liberated by phospholipase C-β-mediated (activated by a receptor-G protein mechanism or phospholipase Cγ activation by tyrosine phosphorylation) hydrolysis of phosphatidylinositol-4,5-bisphosphate.[39] Liberated 1,4,5-trisphosphate binds to its receptor on the endoplasmic reticulum (opening a calcium channel) allowing the sequestered calcium to enter the cytosol.[39] We have previously shown that the fibrous particulate, asbestos, elevates cytosolic calcium by both mechanisms with the release of sequestered calcium causing a transient calcium elevation imposed on a more sustained calcium elevation by a verapamil sensitive calcium channel in alveolar macrophages that directly modified macrophage superoxide anion production.[40]

Once calcium is elevated, it can return to basal levels by a number of mechanisms that require energy expenditure usually in the form of ATP hydrolysis. These mechanisms include extracellular extrusion by

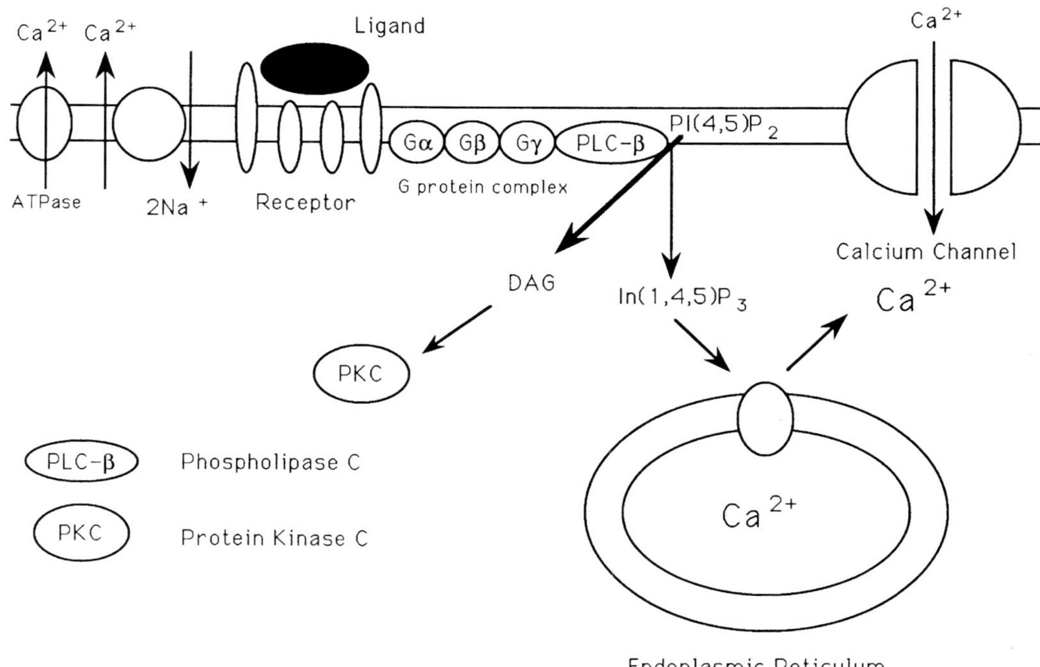

FIGURE 2 Schematic diagram of pathways for regulating intracellular calcium. The primary mechanisms for elevation of intracellular calcium are through calcium channels and release from the endoplasmic reticulum. Elevated intracellular calcium is either transferred to the extracellular space by calcium exchangers and pumps or removed from the cytosol by resequestration into the endoplasmic reticulum. DAG, Diacylglycerol; In(1,4,5)P_3, Inositol-1,4,5-trisphosphate; Pl(4,5)P_2, Phosphatidylinositol-4,5-bisphosphate.

a Na^+/Ca^{++} antiport or a Ca^{++} ATPase.[41] In addition, a number of other mechanisms may also be involved. All of these operate to rapidly decrease cytosolic calcium to basal levels in the absence of some mechanism(s) causing prolonged elevation and/or entry of extracellular calcium.

The signal transduction cascade following the elevation of cytosolic calcium can continue, leading to a number of downstream events including increased gene transcription.[42–45] Elevation of intracellular calcium is important in regulating the alveolar macrophage responses and is consistent with the variety of macrophage functions that have been shown to be regulated by changes in cytosolic calcium.[44,46–49] In contrast, when intracellular calcium is markedly elevated over a protracted period it can lead to irreversible cell injury by mechanisms that include depletion of energy stores resulting in disruption in ionic gradients and activation of intracellular proteases (e.g., calpain) and endonucleases.[50] The distinction of events and extent of calcium elevation between signal transduction leading to effector release from the macrophage and cell death is not entirely clear.

Intracellular calcium activates several enzymes resulting in either cell stimulation or cytotoxicity. Therefore, several effects of silica on alveolar macrophages including cytokine release might be mediated by elevation of intracellular calcium. Increases in intracellular calcium may also lead to several cellular events,[51,52] including the activation of phospholipase A_2 and the calcium-sensitive 5-lipoxygenase,[53–55] the release of proteases that can act on several membrane and cytoskeletal proteins,[56–59] and the activation of endonucleases.[50] Thus, the elevation of intracellular calcium by silica could lead to cytotoxicity by the calcium-dependent activation of proteinases and endonucleases acting on cellular proteins and DNA.

In summary, intracellular calcium has well defined roles in regulating intracellular events and cell death. In addition, a disruption of cytosolic calcium regulation can occur by:

1. inhibition of one or more of the calcium sequestration mechanisms or depletion of energy store;
2. a stimulated release of calcium from a storage pool;
3. opening of a divalent ion channel; or
4. generalized membrane injury resulting in calcium leakage that can not be compensated for by the normal regulatory mechanisms.

C. PROTEIN TYROSINE KINASES

Protein tyrosine kinases specifically catalyze the phosphorylation of proteins on tyrosine residues. Protein tyrosine kinases have been shown to be intrinsic to the oncogene products of certain retroviruses and to receptors of several mitogenic polypeptide growth factors including Epidermal Growth Factor, Insulin Receptor, and Platelet Derived Growth Factor.[60] The latter group, known as "Receptor protein tyrosine kinases" are characterized by having extracellular ligand binding as well as transmembrane and cytoplasmic catalytic domains. Ligand binding to the extracellular domain activates the tyrosine kinase in the cytoplasmic domain which leads to downstream activation of a number of common signalling molecules such as Phospholipase C γ, GTPase-activating protein, pp60c-src, p21ras, and erk1 and erk2 kinases (also known as MAP kinases).[61] Activation of these signaling pathways results in changes in gene expression and phenotypic changes of the cell. Nonreceptor protein tyrosine kinases represent a collection of cellular enzymes that are grouped together because of their lack of extracellular sequences.[62] They are devoid of transmembrane domains and are associated with the cytoplasmic face of the plasma membrane. A number of the nonreceptor protein tyrosine kinases have been found to be associated with other cell surface proteins (generally lacking endogenous enzyme activity) and are capable of facilitating cell surface initiated signal transduction much like the receptor protein tyrosine kinases.[62]

Nonreceptor protein tyrosine kinases include the oncogene products of several retroviruses, their normal cellular homologues, and normal tissue protein tyrosine kinases.[63] There appear to be at least eight distinct families of nonreceptor protein tyrosine kinases. These include src, abl, and fps families, as well as the focal adhesion kinase (fak), c-src kinases (csk), Janus kinases (JAK1, JAK2, and tyk2), spleen tyrosine kinase (syk), and interleukin-2-inducible T cell kinase (itk).[64–66] This list excludes protein kinases that have demonstrable multiple specificity, i.e., ability to phosphorylate tyrosine, threonine/serine residues, such as esk; MAP kinases, erk1 and erk2; and the MAP kinase kinase (MEK). It is likely that all the nonreceptor protein tyrosine kinases are directly or indirectly involved in some type of signalling pathway that modulates growth, differentiation and mature cell function.

The src-related enzymes represent the largest known family of nonreceptor protein tyrosine kinases.[64] The involvement of src kinases in several pathways has been clearly established (Figure 3(3)). These kinases are activated through a diverse group of cell surface receptors for soluble, as well as cell-associated, ligands. The src family contains nine members: src, yes, fyn, lyn, lck, hck, fgr, blk, and yrk.[64] Src, yes, fyn, and lyn are expressed in a variety of cell types, whereas lck, hck, fgr, and blk proteins are expressed primarily in hemopoietic cells.[67] The SH2 domains of these proteins bind tyrosine phosphorylated peptides implicated in normal signalling and cellular transformation.[68] Much of the analysis of the src protein tyrosine kinases has centered on their role as signalling components of multichain immune recognition receptors. Src family kinases have also been shown to associate with a variety of hemopoietic surface proteins such as CD4 and CD8, which function to enhance the signaling potential of other receptors.[67]

Another family of proteins, encoded by ras genes, serve as essential transducers of diverse physiological signals. Normal ras genes are critical regulators of physiological functions such as cell growth and differentiation. Activated c-ras (cellular genes) have repeatedly been implicated in many types of human cancer.[69,70] Activation of ras triggers a series of events which ultimately leads to the downstream activation of a number of kinases.[71] It has been suggested that binding of a ligand to receptor results in activation of the tyrosine kinase activity of the receptor and phosphorylation of GRB2-SOS.[72] The phosphorylated GRB2-SOS forms a complex with ras resulting in ras activation, which then activates raf-1 kinase (Figure 3(1)).[73,74] Activated raf-1 kinase activates MAP kinase (MAPK) by phosphorylation at tyrosine/threonine residues.[75]

MAP kinases are serine/threonine protein kinases activated via phosphorylation of both their tyrosine and threonine residues.[75] They function as key molecules in signalling processes stimulated by several mitogenic factors. At least four distinct MAP kinases have been identified and purified, they are, $p42^{mapk}$, $p44^{erk1}$, p54 and $p44^{mpk}$.[75] As described above MAP kinases are activated via the p21ras, p74raf1, and

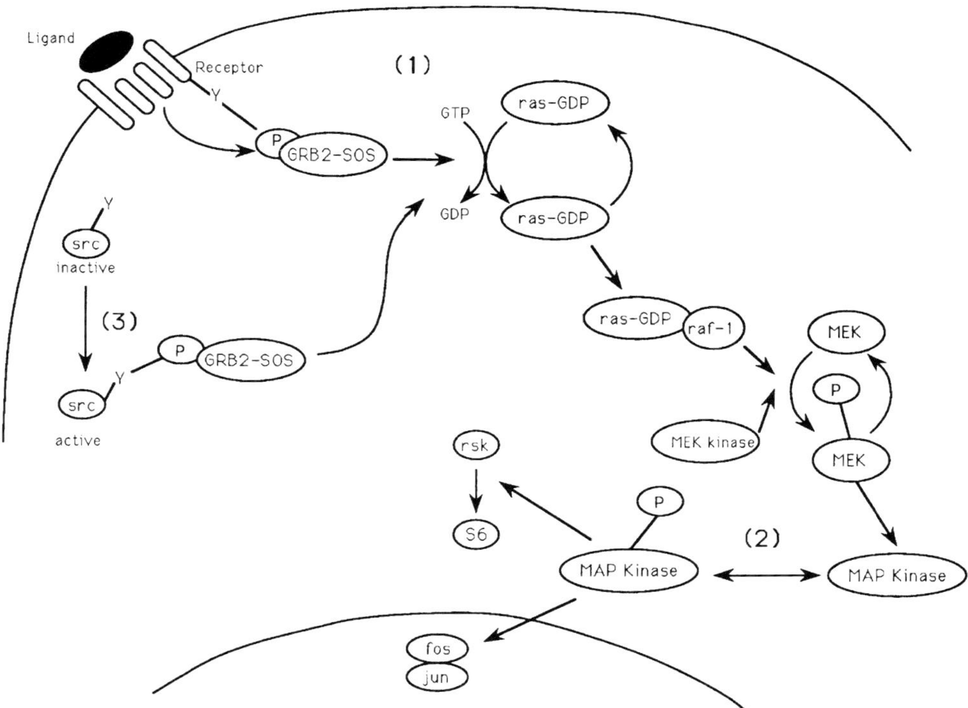

FIGURE 3 Schematic diagram of intracellular protein tyrosine kinase signalling pathways. (1) Receptor-ligand interaction results in the phosphorylation of tyrosine (Y) residues on the receptor, followed by the subsequent phosphorylation of the GRB2-SOS complex. This activated complex stimulates ras activity which further activates raf-1. (2) Raf-1 phosphorylates and activates MEK, which then stimulates MAP kinase activity. (3) Interaction of inactive src with phosphorylated peptides results in the activation of src and its subsequent stimulatory effects on ras, ultimately resulting in the activation of MAP kinase.

MAPK pathways. MAPKs phosphorylate and regulate the activity of various enzymes and transcription factors including the EGF receptor,[76] Rsk90,[77] c-myc,[78] and c-jun. With particular relevance to this discussion the MAPKs appear to integrate multiple intracellular signals transmitted by various second messengers (Figure 3*(2)*).

As is evident from the above discussion there is a high degree of interaction and overlap among the tyrosine kinase pathways. They appear to function as integrated components of a complex network of regulatory proteins, making it difficult to dissociate them from one another. In the next section we will attempt to integrate the various components of the tyrosine kinase pathways that may be involved in silica-stimulated signal transduction.

IV. EFFECTS OF SILICA ON SIGNALLING PATHWAYS IN ALVEOLAR MACROPHAGES

A. ELEVATION OF CYTOSOLIC CALCIUM

Recent studies have demonstrated that silica elicits a rapid, dose- and time-dependent elevation of intracellular calcium in rat alveolar macrophages[12,79] and human alveolar macrophages (as stated earlier, this effect is dependent on the absence of serum).[24] Rojanasakul and colleagues[79] have also reported that extracellular calcium chelators blocked the elevation of intracellular calcium induced by silica at low doses. The calcium channel blocker nifedipine inhibited silica-induced intracellular calcium increases at low doses of silica but not at high doses. The authors concluded from these results that elevation of intracellular calcium induced by silica involves at least two mechanisms. First, low doses of silica may cause an influx of extracellular calcium through specific calcium channels. Second, cytotoxic doses of silica may cause nonspecific membrane damage leading to increased calcium permeability. In addition, the authors have been able to demonstrate that the increase in intracellular calcium at high silica dose was completely abolished by catalase (H_2O_2 scavenger) but not by superoxide dismutase (O_2^- scavenger).[79] These results suggest that the elevation of intracellular calcium may be mediated by H_2O_2 and hydroxyl radicals.

Chelation of extracellular calcium partially inhibits silica-induced cytotoxicity to rat alveolar macrophages as measured by LDH release.[12] The increase of cytosolic calcium concentrations preceded LDH release, indicating that increased cytosolic calcium concentrations may contribute to silica cytotoxicity. Also, silica-induced cytotoxicity to P388D_1 macrophages has been shown to be dependent on the presence of extracellular calcium.[10] Cytotoxicity might be related to the influx of calcium leading to the disruption of cell functions by mechanisms described earlier.[9]

Silica-induced cytotoxicity also has been shown to correlate with the ability of silica to induce the secretion of leukotrienes from bovine alveolar macrophages.[80] The surface modification of silica with polyvinylpyridine-N-oxide has been shown to reduce silica cytotoxicity and to induce preferentially the stimulation of the cyclooxygenase pathway of arachidonic acid metabolism while inhibiting the lipoxygenase pathway, resulting in a decreased secretion of leukotrienes.[15] Interestingly, elevation of intracellular calcium has been shown to enhance selectively the secretion leukotriene C_4 in mouse peritoneal macrophages.[81]

In summary, recent studies have shown that silica can induce elevations of cytosolic calcium that appear to involve calcium channels. Furthermore, these effects are dose dependent, since at higher doses the increase in cytosolic calcium appears to be nonspecific and may involve a free radical mechanism by which the plasma membrane is injured. Finally, the effects of silica also appear to be dependent on the *in vitro* culture conditions since the opening of calcium channels in human alveolar macrophages did not occur in the presence of serum.

B. ACTIVATION OF MAP KINASE

As described earlier the interaction between silica dust and alveolar macrophages results in the release of inflammatory, chemotactic, and growth mediators from the alveolar macrophage that cause both local and systemic effects. Here, we will discuss the possible involvement and interaction of some of the intracellular tyrosine kinase pathways that may play a role in silica-stimulated macrophage activation.

It can be speculated that interaction of silica with the alveolar macrophage and its subsequent activation may be either receptor or nonreceptor mediated. This silica-stimulated alveolar macrophage activation may possibly be mediated by the activation of the ras protein. It is possible that the silica-macrophage interaction via a yet unknown receptor may lead to phosphorylation and activation of a receptor tyrosine kinase, followed by phosphorylation of GRB2-SOS by this activated receptor. This would subsequently result in the formation of an active GRB2-SOS-ras complex which further binds to and activates raf-1. Alternatively, silica-macrophage interaction may result in a nonreceptor mediated activation of GAP, leading to the binding of GTP to ras protein, thus increasing the abundance of the active GTP-bound form of ras. While GTP bound, the activated ras interacts with target proteins such as raf-1 resulting in its activation and phosphorylation. The mammalian serine/threonine protein kinase raf-1 phosphorylates and activates MEK[82,83] which results in activation of MAPK.[84,85] Therefore, raf-1 may activate MAPK in response to stimulation of membrane-associated tyrosine kinases. Additionally, nonreceptor tyrosine kinases, such as src-family kinase p56lck, may be activated by binding of tyrosine phosphorylated peptides, such as GRB2-SOS.[86] As discussed above, the GRB2-SOS complex may be phosphorylated by receptor tyrosine kinases activated by interaction of silica with these receptors. This activated lck kinase can then phosphorylate and stimulate MAPK activity.

As described earlier MAPKs are involved in the integration of various intracellular signal transducing pathways. It also appears to be a major focal point of convergence in several tyrosine kinase pathways. Therefore, we investigated the possible involvement of MAPK in intracellular events initiated by silica in alveolar macrophages (Figure 4). We measured MAPK activity in silica-treated human alveolar macrophages. In these preliminary studies, silica induced a rapid increase in MAPK activity at around 2 min, followed by an equally rapid decrease in MAPK activity within 15 min.

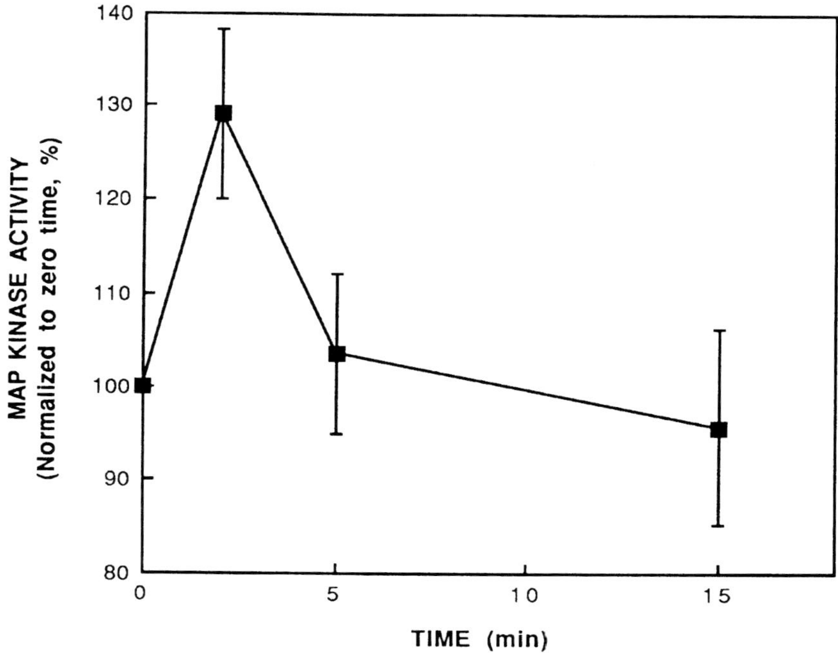

FIGURE 4 MAP kinase activity in human alveolar macrophages stimulated by 133 μg/ml silica. MAP kinase activity was measured following immunoprecipitation of MAP kinase and binding to Protein A agarose beads and by [γ-32P]ATP labelling of a peptide substrate (APRTPGGRR, purchased from UBI) in a similar manner as previously described.[87] Data are expressed as the mean ± SEM for five experiments.

Therefore, these studies established that, by some mechanism silica is transiently activating MAPK. Earlier experiments in our laboratory have demonstrated an increase in fos/jun expression in silica-treated alveolar macrophages. An increase in MAPK activity has often been associated with increased c-jun expression. The observed increase in c-jun expression further implicates the possible role of MAPKs in silica-stimulated signal transduction and possibly the activation of alveolar macrophages. However, the pathway by which MAP kinase is stimulated remains to be determined.

It is evident from the above that any or all of the kinase families may be involved in the intracellular signal transduction pathways stimulated by silica. From studies in our laboratory, we have confirmed that silica stimulates MAPK activity. The implications of this increased activity, that is, the earlier transduction events involved in this observed increase and the latter events that may occur due to this increase, have yet to be elucidated. Future studies may help to elucidate the intracellular events triggered by silica which ultimately result in the release of cytokines, proteases, and other factors by activated alveolar macrophages.

V. SUMMARY AND FUTURE RESEARCH NEEDS

The detailed mechanism by which silica exposure results in lung fibrosis is not yet understood. A large body of evidence implicates the involvement of alveolar macrophages, at some level, in the etiology of silicosis. From the data, it is clear that silica can cause macrophage injury by a necrotic mechanism that could cause an inflammatory response that could progress into chronic inflammation. Macrophage injury can be observed *in vitro;* however, it requires relatively high doses of silica and the absence of proteins and/or lipids that are normally present in lung lining fluid. Furthermore, it is clear that silica can cause macrophage stimulation that can be observed at lower doses of silica and in the presence of a matrix that may more closely simulate the lung environment. It is possible, that at any given time, both macrophage injury and stimulation are taking place in a heterogenous environment. Therefore, the *in vivo* reality of the relative contribution of both events remains to be established. Although animal models of silicosis are important research tools to understand mechanisms, it must be kept in mind that the human disease (that is chronic) may have a different mechanism.

Current evidence suggests that two intracellular signalling pathways may be involved in macrophage stimulation by silica. Silica can cause the opening of a calcium channel resulting in elevation of cytosolic calcium, and silica can stimulate a tyrosine kinase pathway detected as a transient increase in MAPK activity. Both pathways can result in downstream effects at the gene level resulting in cytokine expression. There are many unanswered questions about both pathways. First, the exact participation of both pathways needs to be substantiated and the optimal culture conditions need to be evaluated (dose of silica, non-human vs. human macrophages, adherent vs. suspension culture, presence of serum, and factors from lung lining fluid). Second, it is not clear whether silica acts through some receptor mechanism, production of free radicals causing local membrane changes, or some other physical mechanism. Third, the pathway by which MAPK is activated and the downstream events following either pathway needs to be described. Each of these areas is complicated, but they are current gaps in our knowledge of the mechanism by which silica causes lung injury.

ACKNOWLEDGMENTS

This work was supported by NIEHS Grant ES-04804 and NIH Grant M01-RR-02558.

REFERENCES

1. **Begin, R., Cantin, A., and Masse, S.,** Recent advances in the pathogenesis and clinical assessment of mineral dust pneumoconioses: asbestosis, silicosis and coal pneumoconiosis, *Eur. Respir. J.*, 2, 988, 1989.
2. **Davis, G. S.,** Pathogenesis of silicosis: current concepts and hypotheses, *Lung*, 164, 139, 1986.
3. **deShazo, R. D.,** Current concepts about the pathogenesis of silicosis and asbestosis, *J. Allergy Clin. Immunol.*, 70, 41, 1982.
4. **Lowrie, D. B.,** What goes wrong with the macrophage in silicosis? *Eur. J. Respir. Dis.*, 63, 180, 1982.
5. **Rom, W. N.,** Relationship of inflammatory cell cytokines to disease severity in individuals with occupational inorganic dust exposure, *Am. J. Ind. Med.*, 19, 15, 1991.
6. **Driscoll, K. E., Maurer, J. K., Lindenschmidt, R. C., Romberger, D., Rennard, S. I., and Crosby, L.,** Respiratory tract responses to dust: relationships between dust burden, lung injury, alveolar macrophage fibronectin release, and the development of pulmonary fibrosis, *Toxicol. Appl. Pharmacol.*, 106, 88, 1990.
7. **Hasahara, K., Strieter, R. M., Chensue, S. W., Standiford, T. J., and Kunkel, S. L.,** Mononuclear cell adherence induces neutrophil chemotactic factor/interleukin-8 gene expression, *J. Leukoc. Biol.*, 50, 287, 1991.
8. **Dobson, M. E., Stern, R. O., and Kane, A. B.,** Selective purine release from P338D1 macrophages injured by silica, *J. Cell. Physiol.*, 135, 244, 1988.
9. **Gleva, G. F., Goodglick, L. E., and Kane, A. B.,** Altered calcium homeostasis in irreversibly injured P338D1 macrophages, *Am. J. Pathol.*, 137, 43, 1990.
10. **Kane, A. B., Stanton, R. P., Raymond, E. G., Dobson, M. E., Knafelc, M. E., and Farber, J. L.,** Dissociation of intracellular lysosomal rupture from the cell death caused by silica, *J. Cell Biol.*, 87, 643, 1980.
11. **Nolan, R. P., Langer, A. M., Harington, J. S., Oster, G., and Selikoff, I. J.,** Quartz hemolysis as related to surface functionalities, *Environ. Res.*, 26, 503, 1981.
12. **Chen, J., Armstrong, L. C., Liu, S. J., Gerriets, J. E., and Last, J. A.,** Silica increases cytosolic free calcium ion concentration of alveolar macrophages *in vitro*, *Toxicol. Appl. Pharmacol.*, 111, 211, 1991.
13. **Cantin, A., Dubois, F., and Begin, R.,** Lung exposure to mineral dusts enhances the capacity of lung inflammatory cells to release superoxide anion, *J. Leukoc. Biol.*, 43, 299, 1988.
14. **Dubois, C. M., Bissonnette, E., and Rola-Pleszczynski, M.,** Asbestos fibers and silica particles stimulate rat alveolar macrophages to release tumor necrosis factor. Autoregulatory role of leukotriene B4, *Am. Rev. Respir. Dis.*, 139, 1257, 1989.
15. **Englen, M. D., Taylor, W. W., Laegreid, R. M., Silflow, R. M., and Leid, R. W.,** Diminished arachidonic acid metabolite release by bovine alveolar macrophages exposed to surface-modified silica, *Am. J. Respir. Cell Mol. Biol.*, 6, 527, 1992.

16. **Mohr, C., Davis, G. S., Graebner, C., Hemenway, D. R., and Gemsa, D.,** Enhanced release of prostaglandin E2 from macrophages of rats with silicosis, *Am. J. Respir. Cell. Mol. Biol.*, 6, 390, 1992.
17. **Rom, W. N., Bitterman, P. B., Rennard, S. I., Cantin, A., and Crystal, R. G.,** Characterization of the lower respiratory inflammation of nonsmoking individuals with interstitial lung disease associated chronic inhalation of inorganic dusts, *Am. Rev. Respir. Dis.*, 136, 1429, 1987.
18. **Souvannavong, V. and Adam, A.,** Macrophages from C3H/HeJ mice require an additional step to produce monokines: synergistic effects of silica and poly (I:C) in the release of interleukin 1, *J. Leukoc. Biol.*, 48, 183, 1990.
19. **Takemura, T., Rom, W. N., Ferrans, V. J., and Crystal, R. G.,** Morphologic characterization of alveolar macrophages from subjects with occupational exposure to inorganic particles, *Am. Rev. Respir. Dis.*, 140, 1674, 1989.
20. **Piguet, P. F., Collart, M. A., Grau, G. E., Sappino, A. P., and Vassalli, P.,** Requirement of tumour necrosis factor for development of silica-induced pulmonary fibrosis, *Nature*, 344, 245, 1990.
21. **Oghiso, Y. and Kubota, Y.,** Enhanced interleukin 1 production by alveolar macrophages and increase in la-positive lung cells in silica-exposed rats, *Microbiol. Immunol.*, 30, 1189, 1986.
22. **Oghiso, Y. and Kubota, Y.,** Interleukin 1 production and accessory cell function of rat alveolar macrophages exposed to mineral dust particles, *Microbiol. Immunol.*, 31, 275, 1987.
23. **Schmidt, J. A., Oliver, C. N., Lepe-Zuniga, J. L., Green, I., and Grey, I.,** Silica-stimulated monocytes release fibroblast proliferation factors identical to interleukin-1. A potential role for interleukin-1 in the pathogenesis of silicosis, *J. Clin. Invest.*, 73, 1462, 1984.
24. **Holian, A., Kelley, K., and Hamilton, R. F.,** Mechanisms associated with human alveolar macrophage stimulation by particulates, *Environ. Health Perspect.*, (in press).
25. **Van Bruggen, I., Robertson, T. A., and Papadimitriou, J. M.,** The effect of mild hyperthermia on the morphology and function of murine resident macrophages, *Exp. Mol. Pathol.*, 55, 119, 1991.
26. **Mosser, D. D., Duchaine, J., Bourget, L., and Martin, L. H.,** Changes in heat shock protein synthesis and heat sensitivity during mouse thymocyte development, *Dev. Genet.*, 14, 148, 1993.
27. **Buchman, T. G., Abello, P. A., Smith, E. H., and Bulkley, G. B.,** Induction of heat shock response leads to apoptosis in endothelial cells previously exposed to endotoxin, *Am. J. Physiol.*, 265, H165, 1993.
28. **Cox, G., Oberley, L. W., and Hunninghake, G. W.,** Manganese superoxide dismutase and heat shock protein 70 are not necessary for suppression of apoptosis in human peripheral blood neutrophils, *Am. J. Respir. Cell Mol. Biol.*, 10, 493, 1994.
29. **Wijsman, J. H., Jonker, R. R., Keijzer, R., Van De Velde, C. J. H., Cornelisse, C. J., and Van Dierendonck, J.,** A new method to detect apoptosis in paraffin sections: *in situ* End-labelling of fragmented DNA, *J. Histochem. Cytochem.*, 41, 7, 1993.
30. **Roney, P. L. and Holian, A.,** Possible mechanism of chrysotile asbestos-stimulated superoxide production in the guinea pig alveolar macrophage, *Toxicol. Appl. Pharmacol.*, 100, 132, 1989.
31. **Putney, J. W., Jr.,** Excitement about calcium signaling in inexcitable cells, *Science*, 262, 676, 1993.
32. **Nishizuka, Y.,** Intracellular signalling by hydrolysis of phospholipids and activation of protein kinase C, *Science*, 258, 607, 1993.
33. **Smith, M. W., Ambudkar, I. S., Phelps, P. C., Regec, A. L., and Trump, B. F.,** $HgCl_2$-induced changes in cytosolic Ca^{2+} of cultured rabbit renal tubular cells, *Biochem. Biophys. Acta*, 931, 130, 1987.
34. **Levine, B. A. and Williams, R. J. P.,** Calcium binding to proteins and other large biological anion centers, in *Calcium and Cell Function*, Cheung, W.Y., Ed., Vol. II, Academic Press, New York, 1–38.
35. **Hurwitz, L.,** Pharmacology of calcium channels and smooth muscle, *Annu. Rev. Pharmacol. Toxicol.*, 26, 225, 1986.
36. **Forman, J. H. and Nelson, J.,** Effect of extracellular calcium on superoxide release by rat alveolar macrophages, *J. Appl. Physiol.*, 54, 1249, 1983.
37. **Sweeny, T. D., Castranova, V., Bowman, L., and Miles, P. R.,** Factors which affect superoxide anion release from rat alveolar macrophages, *Exp. Lung Res.*, 2, 85, 1981.
38. **Wright, B., Zeidman, I., Greig, R., and Poste, G.,** Inhibition of macrophage activation by calcium channel blockers and calmodulin antagonists, *Cell. Immunol.*, 95, 46, 1985.
39. **Berridge, M. J.,** A tale of two messengers, *Nature*, 365, 388, 1993.
40. **Kalla, B., Hamilton, R. F., Scheule, R. K., and Holian, A.,** Role of extracellular calcium in chrysotile asbestos stimulation of alveolar macrophages, *Toxicol. Appl. Pharmacol.*, 104, 130, 1990.
41. **Schatzman, H. J.,** Calcium extrusion across the plasma membrane by the Ca^{2+}-pump and Ca^{2+}–Na^{+} exchange system, in *Cell Calcium, and Physiology* Marme, D., Ed., Springer-Verlag, New York, 18–52, 1985.
42. **Somers, S. D., Weiel, J. E., Hamilton, T. A., and Adams, D. O.,** Biochemical mechanism of macrophage activation: phorbol esters and calcium ionophore act synergistically to prime macrophages for tumor destruction, *J. Immunol.*, 136, 4199, 1986.
43. **Klein, J. B., Schepers, T. M., Dean, W. L., Sonnenfeld, G., and McLeish, K.,** Role of intracellular calcium concentration and protein kinase c activation in IFNγ stimulation of U937 cells, *J. Immunol.*, 144, 4305, 1990.
44. **Buchmuller-Rouiller, Y. and Mauel, J.,** Macrophage activation for intracellular killing as induced by calcium ionophore. Correlation with biologic and biochemical events, *J. Immunol.*, 146, 217, 1991.
45. **Hunter, T. and Karin, M.,** The regulation of transcription by phosphorylation, *Cell*, 70, 375, 1992.

46. **Collart, M. A., Belin, D., Briottet, C., Thorens, B., Vassalli, J. D., and Vassalli, P.,** Receptor-mediated phagocytosis by macrophages induces a calcium-dependent transient increase in c-fos transcription, *Oncogene,* 4, 237, 1989.
47. **Collart, M. A., Tourkine, N., Belin, D., Vassali, P., Jeanteur, P., and Blanchard, J. M.,** c-fos gene transcription in murine macrophages is modulated by a calcium-dependent block to elongation in intron 1, *Mol. Cell. Biol.,* 11, 2826, 1991.
48. **Finkel, T. H., Pabst, M. J., Suzuki, H., Guthrie, L. A., Forehand, J. R., Phillips, W. A., and Johnston, R. B., Jr.,** Priming of neutrophils and macrophages for enhanced release of superoxide anion by the calcium ionophore ionomycin. Implications for regulation of the respiratory burst, *J. Biol. Chem.,* 262, 1258, 1987.
49. **Suttles, J., Giri, J. G., and Mizel, S. B.,** IL-1 secretion by macrophages. Enhancement of IL-1 secretion and processing by calcium ionophores, *J. Immunol.,* 144, 175, 1990.
50. **McConkey, D. J., Hartzell, P., Duddy, S. K., Hakansson, H., and Orrenius, S.,** 2,3,7,8-tetrachlorodibenzo-p-dioxin kills immature thymocytes by Ca^{2+}-mediated endonuclease activation, *Science,* 242, 256, 1988.
51. **Nicotera, P., Bellomo, G., and Orrenius, S.,** The role of calcium in cell killing, *Chem. Res. Toxicol.,* 3, 484, 1990.
52. **Orrenius, S., McConkey, D. J., Bellemo, G., and Nicotera, P.,** Role of calcium in toxic cell killing, *Trends Pharmacol. Sci.,* 10, 281, 1989.
53. **Aharony, D. and Stein, R. L.,** Kinetic mechanism of guinea pig neutrophil 5-lipoxygenase, *J. Biol. Chem.,* 261, 11512, 1986.
54. **Van Den Bosch, H.,** Intracellular phospholipases A, *Biochim. Biophys. Acta,* 604, 191, 1980.
55. **Van Kuijk, F. J. G. M. M., Sevaniam, A., Handelman, G. J., and Dratz, E. A.,** A new role of phospholipase A2: protection of membrane from lipid peroxidation damage, *Trends Biochem. Sci.,* 12, 31, 1987.
56. **Hinshaw, D. B., Sklar, L. A., Bohl, B., Schraufstatter, I. U., Hyslop, P. A., Rossi, M. W., Sprag, R. G., and Cochrane, C. G.,** Cytoskeletal and morphological impact of cellular oxidant injury, *Am. J. Pathol.,* 123, 454, 1986.
57. **Jewell, S. A., Bellemo, G., Thor, H., Orrenius, S., and Smith, M. T.,** Bleb formation in hepatocytes during metabolism is caused by disturbances in thiol and calcium ion homeostasis, *Science,* 217, 1257, 1982.
58. **Kajikawa, N., Kishimoto, A., Shiota, M., and Nishizuka, Y.,** Ca^{2+}-dependent neutral protease and proteolytic activation of Ca^{2+}-activated, phospholipid dependent protein kinase, in *Methods in Enzymology,* Jakoby, W. B., Ed., 1983, 279.
59. **Mellgren, R. L.,** Calcium-dependent proteases: an enzyme system active at cellular membrane? *FASEB J.,* 1, 110, 1987.
60. **Hanks, S. K., Quinn, A. M., and Hunter, T.,** The protein kinase family: conserved features and deduced phylogeny of the catalytic domain, *Science,* 241, 42–52, 1990.
61. **Ullrich, A. and Schlessinger, J.,** Signal transduction by receptors with tyrosine kinase activity, *Cell,* 61, 203, 1990.
62. **Lavan, B. E., Kuhne, M. R., Garner, C. W., Anderson, D., Reedijk, M., Pawson, T., and Lienhard, G. E.,** The association of insulin-elicited phosphotyrosine protein with src homology 2 domains, *J. Biol. Chem.,* 267, 11631, 1992.
63. **Cantley, L. C., Auger, K. R., Carpenter, C., Duckworth, B., Graziani, A., Kapeller, R., and Soltoff, S.,** Oncogenes and signal transduction, *Cell,* 64, 281, 1991.
64. **Toyoshima, K., Yamanashi, Y., Inoue, K., Semba, K., Yamamoto, T., and Akiyama, T.,** Protein tyrosine kinases belonging to the src family, *Ciba Symposium on Interactions Among Cell Signal Systems,* 164, 240, 1992.
65. **Kono, T., Minami, Y., and Taniguchi, T.,** The interleukin-2 receptor complex and signal transduction: role of beta-chain, *Semin. Immunol.,* 5, 299, 1993.
66. **Wang, J. Y.,** Ab1 tyrosine kinase in signal transduction and cell cycle regulation, *Curr. Opinions Genet. Dev.,* 3, 35, 1993.
67. **Tsygankov, A. and Bolen, J.,** The src family of tyrosine protein kinases in hemopoietic signal transduction, *Stem Cells,* 11, 371, 1993.
68. **Pawson, T. and Gish, G. D.,** SH2 and SH3 domains: from structure to function, *Cell,* 71, 359, 1992.
69. **Bos, J. L.,** Ras oncogenes in human cancer, *Cancer Res.,* 49, 4682, 1989.
70. **Rodenhuis, S.,** Ras and human tumors, *Semin. Cancer Biol.,* 3, 241, 1992.
71. **Lowy, D. R. and Willumsen, B. M.,** Function and regulation of ras, *Annu. Rev. Biochem.,* 62, 851, 1993.
72. **Lowenstein, E. J., Daly, R. J., Batzer, A. G., Li, W., Margolis, B., Lammers, R., Ullrich, A., Skolnik, E. Y., Bar-Sagi, D., and Schlesinger, J.,** The SH2 and SH3 domain-containing protein GRB2 links receptor tyrosine kinases to ras signalling, *Cell,* 70, 431–442, 1992.
73. **Moodie, S. A., Willumsen, B. M., Weber, M. J., and Wolfman, A.,** Complexes of Ras-GTP with Raf-1 and mitogen-activated protein kinase kinase, *Science,* 260, 1658, 1993.
74. **Skolnik, E. Y., Batzer, A., Li, N., Lee, C. H., Lowenstein, E., Mohammadi, M., Margolis, B., and Schlesinger, J.,** The function of GRB2 in linking the insulin receptor to Ras signaling pathways, *Science,* 260, 1953, 1993.
75. **Pelech, S. and Sanghera, J.,** Mitogen-activated protein kinases: versatile transducers for cell signaling, *Trends Biochem. Sci.,* 1, 233, 1992.
76. **Northwood, I. C., Gonzalez, G. A., Wartmann, M., Raden, D. L., and Davis, R. J.,** Isolation and characterization of two growth factor-stimulated protein kinases that phosphorylate the epidermis growth factor receptor at threonine 669, *J. Biol. Chem.,* 266, 15266, 1991.

77. **Chung, J., Pelech, S. L., and Blenis, J.,** Mitogen-activated swiss mouse 3T3 RSK kinases I and II are related to pp44mpk from sea star oocytes and participate in the regulation of pp90rsk activity, *Proc. Natl. Acad. Sci. U.S.A.*, 88, 4981, 1991.
78. **Seth, A., Alvarez, E., Gupta, S., and Davis, R. J.,** A phosphorylation site located in the NH2-terminal domain of c-Myc increases transactivation of gene expression, *J. Biol. Chem.*, 266, 23521, 1991.
79. **Rojanasakul, Y., Wang, L. Y., Banks, D. E., and Ma, J. H. K.,** Role of intracellular calcium in silica and oxygen radical induced injury in lung macrophages, Abstract, 1992.
80. **Englen, M. D., Taylor, S. M., Laegreid, W. W., Silflow, R. M., and Leid, R. W.,** The effects of different silicas on arachidonic acid metabolism in alveolar macrophages, *Exp. Lung Res.*, 16, 691, 1990.
81. **Kaever, V., Pfannkuche, H. J., Wessel, K., and Resch, K.,** The ratio of macrophage prostaglandin and leukotriene synthesis is determined by the intracellular free calcium levels, *Biochem. Pharmacol.*, 39, 1313, 1990.
82. **Cobb, M. H., Boulton, T. G., and Robbins, D. T.,** Extracellular signal-regulated kinases: ERKs in progress, *Cell Regul.*, 2, 965, 1991.
83. **Ray, L. B. and Sturgill, T. W.,** Insulin-stimulated microtubule-associated protein kinases is phosphorylated on tyrosine and threonine *in vivo, Proc. Natl. Acad. Sci. U.S.A.*, 85, 3753, 1988.
84. **Dent, P., Jelnik, T., Woljman, A., Weber, M. J., and Sturgle, T. W.,** Activation of mitogen-activated protein kinase kinase by v-Raf in HIH 3T3 cells and *in vitro, Science*, 257, 1404, 1992.
85. **Kyriakis, J. M., App, H., Zhang, X. F., Banerjee, P., Brautigan, D. L., Rapp, U. R., and Avruch, J.,** Raf-1 activates MAP kinase-kinase, *Nature*, 358, 417, 1992.
86. **Penninger, J. M., Wallace, V. A., Kishihara, K., and Mak, T. W.,** The role of p56lck and p59fyn tyrosine kinase and CD45 protein tyrosine phosphatase in T cell development and clonal selection, *Immunol. Rev.*, 135, 183, 1993.
87. **Clark-Lewis, I., Sanghera, J. S., and Pelech, S. L.,** Definition of a consensus sequence for peptide substrate recognition by p44mpk, the meiosis-activated myelin basic protein kinase, *J. Biol. Chem.*, 266, 15180, 1991.

Section III
Chapter 3

CALCIUM-MEDIATED SILICA CYTOTOXICITY

Yongyut Rojanasakul, Vincent Castranova, Daniel E. Banks, and Joseph K.H. Ma

CONTENTS

I. ABSTRACT

There is evidence that cytotoxic injury that occurs following phagocytic activation of alveolar macrophages (AMs) by silica particles may be caused by the alteration of intracellular calcium $[Ca^{2+}]_i$ homeostasis, as well as the generation of reactive oxygen radicals (ORs). Until recently, however, the relationship between these two mechanisms of injury has not been directly addressed. In the case of reactive oxygen species, there is almost universal agreement that oxygen radicals can cause lipid peroxidation of unsaturated fatty acids within membranes leading to disruption of membrane functions and destruction of cells. As for calcium, the perturbation of its cellular control mechanisms, which leads to sustained accumulation of $[Ca^{2+}]_i$, has long been recognized as the major determinative factor leading to irreversible cell injury. Several recent studies have indicated that silica can induce a rise in $[Ca^{2+}]_i$ as well as the generation of ORs, and that the inhibition of these cellular processes by calcium chelators or OR scavengers can prevent cell death. The perturbation of $[Ca^{2-}]_i$ homeostasis by silica has been shown to activate several degradative enzymes such as phospholipases, proteases, and endonucleases and cause disruptions of cytoskeletal and other structural proteins. The present report will review existing evidence for the involvement of calcium in these cellular processes and its relationship to ORs in silica toxicity. Attempts will also be made to elucidate potential mechanisms involved in these cytotoxic processes.

II. INTRODUCTION

The concept of cell injury is fundamental to the study of the pathogenesis of disease. Cell injury occurs as a consequence of alterations of physiologic functions and the morphologic organization of cells. Thus, the pathogenesis of disease must be understood in terms of those biologic events by which physiology and morphology of the cells are altered. Such an understanding entails determining which cells are affected and how they are changed under pathological conditions. Then, the pathogenesis of such cellular alterations must be understood in terms of the mechanisms responsible. Among the possible mechanisms

0-8493-4709-2/96/$0.00+$.50

of injury, the alteration of $[Ca^{2+}]_i$ homeostasis and the generation of ORs have received the most attention. The involvement of calcium in the normal regulation of a large number of physiological processes is now well established. Yet, increasing evidence indicates that calcium may also play a determinant role in a variety of pathological and toxicological processes. It has been recognized for many years now that injured or dead cells accumulate calcium,[1,2] and subsequent work has revealed that a disruption of $[Ca^{2+}]_i$ homeostasis is frequently associated with the early development of cell injury.[3,4] This led to the hypothesis that disruption of the $[Ca^{2+}]_i$ homeostasis may be a common process in the development of cytotoxicity.[3] During the past several years, it has become progressively clear that sustained increases in $[Ca^{2+}]_i$ caused by a wide variety of toxicants can activate cytotoxic mechanisms associated with irreversible injury in various cell systems, including phagocytes,[5,6] epithelial cells,[7] hepatocytes,[8,9] cardiac myocytes,[10,11] and renal cells.[12] In the lungs, most studies on the mechanisms of cell injury, particularly those associated with silicosis, have focused mainly on the role of toxic ORs and the degradative products of phospholipases, although several recent studies have also indicated the involvement of calcium and its potential linkage to these known cellular products of silicotic cell injury.

III. ROLE OF CALCIUM AND OXYGEN RADICALS

One of the most prominent features of acute silicosis is the widespread injury of various lung cells, particularly the parenchymal epithelial cells and the AMs. The alveolar epithelial cells form a protective barrier that serves to prevent direct contact of the dust particles and activated AMs with the interstitial connective tissue cells. Such contact could result in accelerated fibroblast proliferation and secretion of extracellular matrix macromolecules leading to fibrosis. Previous studies have indicated that the development of pulmonary fibrosis requires severe epithelial barrier damage with associated disruption of the epithelial basement membrane, allowing migration of connective tissue cells into the airspace.[13] In some cases, the activation of fibroblasts appears to be reversible after cessation of cell injury and re-epithelialization.[13] The alveolar wall consists of a specialized epithelium and closely apposed network of capillaries supported by a delicate fibroelastic matrix. The alveolus is populated by several different cell types that vary in their susceptibility to injury and replicative potential. Nearly 95% of the alveolar surface area is covered by a single layer of flattened type I epithelial pneumocytes. These terminally differentiated cells are vulnerable to a variety of injuries and have little, if any, regenerative or replicative potential. In contrast, type II cells, the progenitors of type I cells, have the capacity to proliferate or repopulate the alveolar surface after injury.[14] The ability of type II pneumocytes to regenerate appears to depend on the magnitude of insults. Exposure of type II cells to low-dose silica dust (2.5–20 μg/ml) stimulates replication, growth activity, and repair, whereas silica, at high doses (10–250 μg/ml), causes a dose-dependent irreversible cell injury.[15] In the normal adult lung, the alveolar epithelium, and to a lesser extent the vascular endothelium, presents the major protective barrier to the invasion of toxic substances.[16] The barrier property of the epithelium is primarily attributed to the apical tight junctions, where the membranes of adjacent cells join to obliterate the intercellular space. Recent studies[17] have indicated that silica can directly disrupt the tight junction barrier of alveolar epithelial monolayers in cultured alveolar epithelial systems. In these experiments, however, the epithelial cells did not appear to be damaged by their contact with particles. While it has not yet been firmly established, the effect of silica on the epithelial barrier is believed to be more dramatic *in vivo* due to enhanced generation of reactive ORs and other cytotoxic metabolites resulting from the interaction of AMs with silica particles. In animal studies, necrosis of type I cells was observed following the intratracheal instillation of silica.[18,19] The mechanisms by which silica affects the epithelial cells remain unclear, but several studies have linked silica toxicity with the radical formation and the alteration of phospholipase activity.[7,17] The former is of particular importance since a large number of inhaled oxidants and fibrogenic agents, such as paraquat, bleomycin, and radiation, are known to exert a direct cytotoxic effect on lung epithelial cells through the generation of free radicals.[20] The alteration of phospholipase activity and its degradative products have been reported to be associated with various forms of toxicant-induced cell injury.[21,22] In alveolar epithelial cells, certain phospholipase products, particularly lysophosphatides and free fatty acids, have been shown to be toxic toward type I cells.[23] Subsequent studies by the same group[20,24] further indicate that the toxicity of these degradative products is highly selective to type I cells but has less severe effects on endothelial and other lung cells. The role of phospholipases in silica-induced lung cell injury will be discussed in greater detail in a subsequent section.

Most of our knowledge of silica-induced lung cell injury has been obtained from the studies using AMs. The AM is the principal target for inhaled toxicants and its role in scavenging and detoxifying these agents has been well recognized.[13,25] Upon contact with these agents, the AM becomes activated and releases various reactive oxygen species (the so-called "respiratory burst" process) which can be toxic to the cells. In this process, oxygen is taken up by the cell and enzymatically converted to superoxide anion (O_2^-), which leads to the formation of H_2O_2 and other reactive peroxides.[26,27] H_2O_2, if not reduced, can further lead to the formation of the very reactive $OH^{\cdot}$ and lipid hydroperoxides that can damage membranes, nucleic acids, and proteins and alter their functions.[28] Under normal circumstances, however, these OR products are eliminated by numerous cellular enzymatic and chemical mechanisms, most notably the glutathione redox cycle.[28] Impairment of these protective mechanisms by toxic chemicals or by excessive exposure of the cells to these oxidative products can lead to cell injury and death.[28] Interestingly, several recent studies indicate that the ability of the reactive oxygen products to cause cell injury may be associated with changes in $[Ca^{2+}]_i$ homeostasis. Exposure of cells to reactive peroxides and several other chemicals has been shown to induce a rise in $[Ca^{2+}]_i$ and subsequently cell death in a wide variety of cell systems including cardiac myocytes,[11] hepatocytes,[29] and alveolar macrophages.[5] Addition of antioxidants such as α-tocopherol or N,N′-diphenyl-p-phenylenediamine, and the calcium chelator, EDTA, protects the cells from injury.[30] The severity of cell injury caused by peroxides has also been demonstrated to depend on iron and the formation of more potent oxidizing species, namely $OH^{\cdot}$ and alkoxyl radicals.[29] Interestingly, however, removal of cellular iron by deferoxamine prevents the formation of these radicals and reduces oxidant damage without having any protective effect on $[Ca^{2+}]_i$ levels.[29] These results appear to suggest that oxidative cell injury, in contrary to the general belief, is not associated with the $[Ca^{2+}]_i$ perturbation. Further studies by the same group[31] latter elucidated that oxidative stress induced by peroxides causes a sequential change in intracellular calcium response, i.e., an initial transient $[Ca^{2+}]_i$ rise followed by a more pronounced and sustained $[Ca^{2+}]_i$ elevation. Depletion of cellular iron by deferoxamine had no effect on the initial $[Ca^{2+}]_i$ rise but greatly reduced the rise of the late $[Ca^{2+}]_i$ response. Whether this latter change in $[Ca^{2+}]_i$ response is associated with cell injury and the formation of reactive oxygen radicals has yet to be confirmed. Several inhaled toxic substances such as crystalline silica and asbestos have been shown to generate reactive oxygen radicals and induce lipid peroxidation leading to membrane damage.[32,33] In their recent studies using ESR spectroscopy, Vallyathan et al.[33] show that there is a direct relationship between the degree of cell toxicity and the amount of ORs generated during silica- or asbestos-induced phagocytosis by AMs or neutrophils. Addition of radical scavengers, such as catalase, dimethyl sulfoxide, dimethyl thiourea, sodium benzoate, and mannitol, prevents the accumulation of radicals. In contrast, addition of carmustine, a glutathione reductase-glutathione peroxidase inhibitor, causes a 5-fold increase in radical generation. Exposure of phagocytes to these OR-generating particles has also been shown to induce a rise in $[Ca^{2+}]_i$ in a dose dependent manner.[34–36] In cultured rat AMs, silica significantly increases $[Ca^{2+}]_i$ from its basal level of 107 ± 14 n*M* to 142 ± 19 n*M* at a concentration of 0.01 mg/ml and by up to 4 fold (418 ± 24 n*M*) at a silica concentration of 1 mg/ml (Figure 1). The silica effect on $[Ca^{2+}]_i$ is transient at low doses (<0.1 mg/ml) and becomes sustained and more pronounced at high doses (>0.1 mg/ml).[35] Cell injury occurs only at high doses of silica (>0.1 mg/ml) and is associated with prolonged and sustained elevations of $[Ca^{2+}]_i$ (Figure 2). The potential linkage between OR generation and altered calcium homeostasis in silica-induced AM injury is further investigated with the use of OR scavengers, such as catalase and superoxide dismutase (SOD). Catalase completely inhibits the silica-induced rise in $[Ca^{2+}]_i$, whereas SOD exhibits no inhibitory effect (Figure 3). These data suggest a definitive role of H_2O_2 and possibly its reactive metabolite, $OH^{\cdot}$, in silica-induced calcium toxicity.

IV. ROLE OF CALCIUM AND PHOSPHOLIPID ALTERATIONS

In addition to ORs, the functional and structural derangements of the cells following silica exposure may also be attributed to the alterations in membrane phospholipids.[6,37] Niewoehner et al.[37] showed that exposure of isolated perfused lungs to phospholipases and certain of their degradative products caused large increases in lung permeability and injury. Since many intracellular phospholipases are susceptible to activation by an increase in $[Ca^{2+}]_i$, it is conceivable that subtle derangements in calcium homeostasis may be involved in the activation of membrane-associated phospholipases with subsequent accelerated phospholipid degradation, leading to cell damage. Indeed, experimental observations of isolated perfused

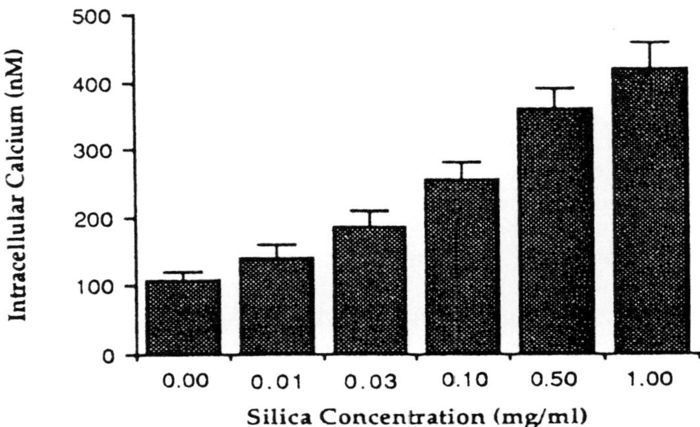

FIGURE 1 Dose-response effect of silica on intracellular calcium in cultured rat alveolar macrophages. Cells (1×10^6/ml) were pre-incubated with 1 μ*M* Fura-2 AM for 30 min at 37°C and then treated with various concentrations of silica in HEPES-buffered medium containing 1 m*M* Ca^{2+}. Intracellular Ca^{2+} values given are maximum levels obtained within minutes of silica addition. (From Rojanasakul, Y. et al., *J. Cell. Physiol.,* 154, 310, 1993.)

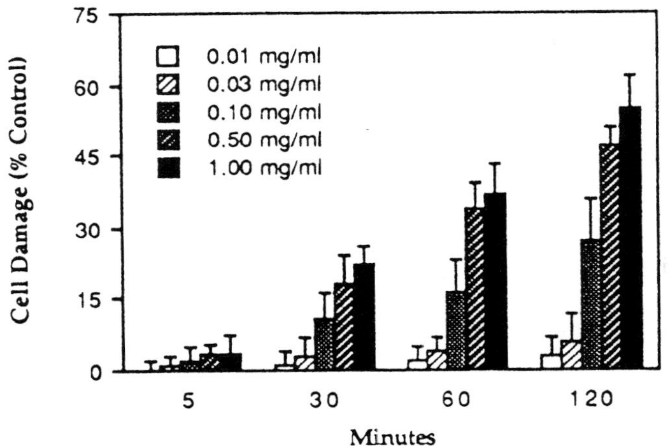

FIGURE 2 Dose effect of silica on cellular damage in alveolar macrophages as a function of time. Cell damage was calculated from nuclear fluorescence emitted from silica-exposed cells in the presence of the membrane integrity indicator propidium iodide (1 μ*M*) and was plotted as percent of controls at indicated times. Triton X-100 was used to establish maximum fluorescence response. (From Rojanasakul, Y. et al., *J. Cell. Physiol.,* 154, 310, 1993.)

lungs exposed to calcium ionophores showed the wide spread lysis of various lung cells, particularly alveolar epithelial cells.[37] This effect was found to be dose- and time-dependent and associated with the liberation of phospholipid degradative products in reactions catalyzed by phospholipase C and A.[7] The effect of the ionophores is specific for the presence of extracellular calcium, as the cells are protected when exposed to ionophores in Ca^{2+}-free medium. Thus, the ionophores appear to act by accelerating the flux of Ca^{2+} across the plasma membrane and into the cytoplasm, which in turn triggers intracellular processes leading to cell lysis. Evidence for the role of phospholipid alterations in silica-induced cytotoxicity were reported by numerous investigators.[38–42] In these studies, silica was found to be a potent stimulator of arachidonic acid (AA) metabolism. Since AA is normally stored in membrane phospholipids, elevation of free arachidonate serves as a marker of accelerated phospholipid degradation. In AMs,

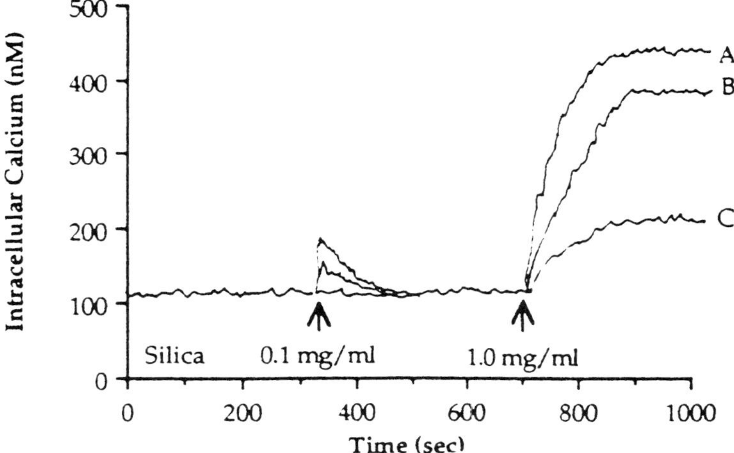

FIGURE 3 Effect of various oxygen radical scavengers on silica-induced $[Ca^{2+}]_i$ rise in rat alveolar macrophages. Trace (A) represents $[Ca^{2+}]_i$ change of cells in response to silica stimulation in HEPES-buffered medium containing 1 m*M* Ca^{2+}. (B) and (C) represent $[Ca^{2+}]_i$ response of cells pretreated with SOD (100 μg/ml) or catalase (1,000 U/ml) in the same medium respectively.

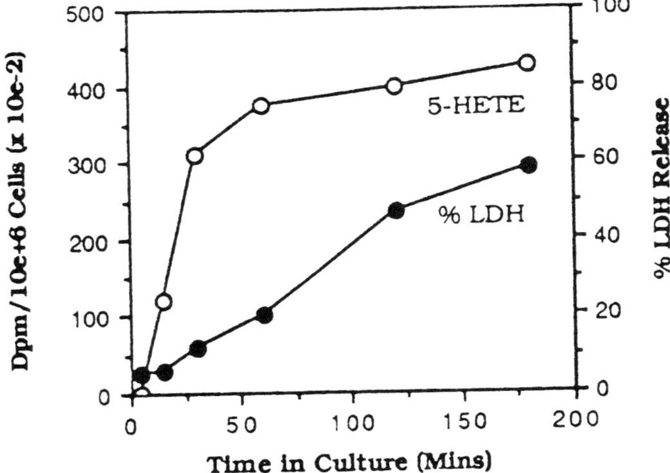

FIGURE 4 Comparison of the kinetics of 5-HETE and LDH release by ^{3}H-AA-labeled bovine AM incubated with 3.0 mg silica. 5-HETE was quantitated from HPLC radiograms and is expressed as dpm/10^6 cells. LDH release is expressed as a percentage of the absorbance recorded for saponin-solubilized AM positive-control cultures in the LDH assay. (From Englen, M.D. et al., *Exp. Lung Res.*, 15, 511, 1989.)

silica selectively stimulates the lipoxygenase pathway with 5-hydroxyeicosatetraenoic acid (5-HETE) as a major AA metabolite, and inhibits the cycloxygenase pathway as the dose of silica increases.[38] This rapid alteration in AA metabolism precedes and correlates well with the degree of cell toxicity, as measured by the LDH release assay (Figure 4). Altered AA metabolism caused by silica depends on its surface charge characteristic, since its modification by treating the particles with polyvinylpyridine-N-oxide or aluminum lactate inhibits AA metabolism as well as cell injury.[40] Klein and Adamson[42] showed, in alveolar epithelial cells, that silica alters eicosanoid production by alveolar type II cells in primary culture in a concentration-dependent manner and results in a 6-fold increase in PGE_2 secretion. *In vivo* studies conducted by Panos et al.[41] also demonstrated an increased basal production of PGE_2 and PGI_2 by hypertropic type II cells isolated after silica-induced lung injury. This increase in eicosanoid production was attributed to the increases in AA availability and prostacyclin synthetase activity of the cells. Stimulation of AA metabolism by silica may result from an influx of extracellular calcium due to membrane damage or disruption caused by contact with silica particles. The dose-dependent elevation of $[Ca^{2+}]_i$ resulting from extracellular sources might be expected to increase the activity of Ca^{2+}-dependent phospholipases, which would be consistent with the observed increase in the dose-dependent generation and release of AA metabolites by silica- or ionophore-exposed AMs.[38–42] Indeed, as has been shown by Kane et al.,[43] cell death in macrophages exposed to silica could be prevented by eliminating calcium from the culture medium.

V. OTHER MECHANISMS OF CALCIUM-MEDIATED SILICA TOXICITY

Other mechanisms have been postulated to contribute to the progression of membrane and cellular injury caused by silica. One such mechanism involves the alterations of cytoskeletal structures. It has been known for some time that one of the early signs of macrophage injury caused by a variety of toxic agents is the impairment of its migratory and phagocytic functions.[44,45] Although other mechanisms may also contribute to these cellular changes, it is generally accepted that perturbation of cytoskeletal organization and the interaction between the cytoskeleton and the plasma membrane play important roles in regulating cell functions. Cytoskeletal alterations have been implicated in the immobilization and cessation of alveolar clearance of particle-laden macrophages following excessive dust exposure.[44] Disruption and dissociation of microfilaments and microtubules from plasma membrane were observed in AMs during oxidative cell injury or following AM exposure to cytoskeleton-active agents, such as cytochalasin B and colchicine.[44,46] The cytoskeletal complex consists of a three-dimensional network of filaments and associated proteins. Microfilaments, the predominant cytoskeletal element in macrophage cortical cytoplasm, are mainly composed of actin and several actin-binding proteins.[47] Many of these actin binding proteins require calcium in order to interact with other cytoskeletal constituents. Typical examples include gelsolin and severin which serve to regulate actin polymerization.[47] Calcium also regulates the function of other actin-binding proteins which are directly involved in the association of microfilaments with the plasma membrane. Among these proteins, α-actinin is involved in the normal organization of actin filaments into regular, parallel arrays. However, in the presence of micromolar Ca^{2+} concentrations, α-actinin dissociates from the actin filaments.[48] The other actin-binding protein (ABP) is a substrate for Ca^{2+}-dependent proteases.[49] Thus, an increase in $[Ca^{2+}]_i$ to micromolar levels (e.g., after exposure of cells to Ca^{2+} ionophores) results in the proteolysis of the protein. Further evidence on the role of calcium in the toxic alterations of actin filaments is demonstrated by the experiments which indicate that the dissociation of α-actinin and proteolysis of ABP by oxidants can be prevented by preloading the cells with intracellular Ca^{2+} chelators.[50] In addition to actin filaments, the organization of microtubules is also reported to be controlled by Ca^{2+}. For example, studies by Gaskin et al.[51] demonstrated that the polymerization of GTP-dependent microtubules can be abolished in the presence of micromolar Ca^{2+} concentrations. In addition, the activity of microtubule-associated proteins (MAPs), which control the turnover and the distribution of microtubules, is modulated by phosphorylation catalyzed by a Ca^{2+}- and calmodulin-dependent protein kinase.[52] Although the depolymerization of microtubules during toxic cell injury has been reported,[50,53] the possible involvement of Ca^{2+} in this process has not been clarified.

Other potential mechanisms of cell toxicity involve catabolic effects of Ca^{2+}-dependent degradative enzymes on phospholipids, proteins, and nucleic acids. Unlike phospholipases which are previously described, the role of proteases and endonucleases on degenerative cell injury is less understood, although both of these enzymes can be similarly activated by a sustained increase in $[Ca^{2+}]_i$. Ca^{2+}-dependent proteases or calpains are known to be present in virtually all mammalian cells.[54] Studies from several laboratories have suggested the involvement of Ca^{2+}-activated proteases in the toxicity of certain agents in various cell types.[55,56] Although the substrates for protease activity during cell injury remain largely unidentified, it appears that cytoskeletal and membrane integral proteins may be the major targets for Ca^{2+}-activated proteases during cell toxicity.[49,50,57] Ca^{2+} overload can also trigger endonuclease activation, which has been implicated as an important factor in damage to macrophages caused by oxidative stress[58] and in cell killing by bacterial toxins.[59] Ca^{2+} overload caused by oxidative stress[58] can also stimulate other enzymatic processes that result in DNA damage, this process can be prevented by intracellular Ca^{2+} chelators.[60]

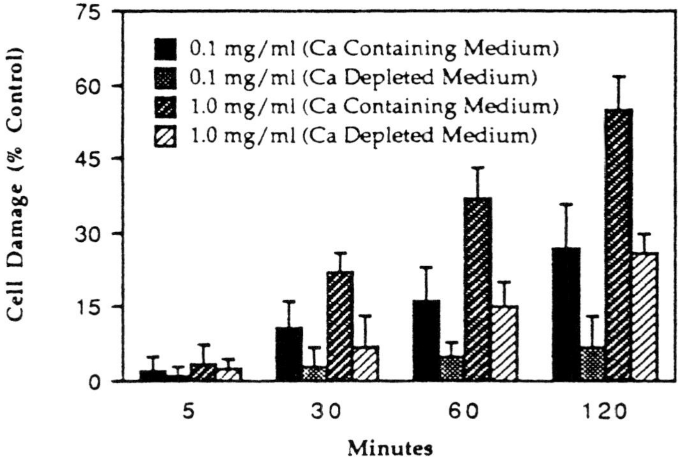

FIGURE 5 Effect of extracellular calcium depletion on silica-induced cell damage in alveolar macrophages. Cells were incubated either in HEPES-buffered medium containing 1 m*M* Ca^{2+} or in the same buffer but without Ca^{2+} (+100 μ*M* EGTA). Silica concentrations used for *in vitro* exposure are given in the figure. (From Rojanasakul, Y. et al., *J. Cell. Physiol.*, 154, 310, 1993.)

VI. MECHANISMS OF ALTERED CALCIUM HOMEOSTASIS BY SILICA

The aforementioned studies provide pertinent evidence for the role of Ca^{2+} overload in cell toxicity. This section focuses on the mechanisms of $[Ca^{2+}]_i$ alterations induced by toxic silica particles in AMs. Like most other cell types, the AM maintains its $[Ca^{2+}]_i$ level in the range of 100–200 n*M*.[34,35] This is in contrast to a much higher calcium concentration of approximately 1–2 m*M* present in the extracellular bathing fluids. Consequently, there is a concentration gradient of about four orders of magnitude between the extracellular and intracellular compartments. Maintenance of this remarkably high calcium gradient is vital to cell viability. Thus, considerable attention has been focused on identifying and understanding the cellular mechanisms which serve to control cellular calcium fluxes. Normally, $[Ca^{2+}]_i$ homeostasis is maintained by the concert operation of various cellular transport and compartmentalization systems including active calcium efflux by Ca^{2+}-ATPase pumps and the Na^+/Ca^{2+} exchanger, transport via voltage-and receptor-dependent membrane ion channels, and intracellular sequestration by calcium regulating proteins and organelles, such as endoplasmic recticulum, mitochondria, and nuclear membranes.[30] For silica-induced cell injury, a number of mechanisms have been proposed as potential causes of silica-induced calcium overloading: 1) non-specific membrane damage, i.e. due to lipid peroxidation, with subsequent leakage of calcium through membrane holes, 2) calcium influx through specific calcium channels, 3) internal calcium release from intracellular stores, i.e., mitochondria and endoplasmic recticulum, 4) ATP depletion which impairs Ca^{2+}-ATPase pumps and restricts calcium efflux, and 5) Ca^{2+} leakage during phagocytosis. By using the extracellular Ca^{2+} chelator, EGTA, it was first established that the induction of a $[Ca^{2+}]_i$ rise by silica (0.1 mg/ml) can be greatly inhibited (≈90%) by EGTA.[35] This suggests that Ca^{2+} influx from an extracellular source is a major mechanism for Ca^{2+} overload. EGTA also results in a significant decrease of silica-induced cell damage (Figure 5). These observations are consistent with earlier findings by Kane et al.,[43] who demonstrated the inhibition of silica-induced LDH release upon removal of extracellular Ca^{2+}. At a higher dose of silica (1.0 mg/ml), however, a moderate increase in cell damage was observed (Figure 5). The result suggests that additional mechanism(s) of injury, e.g., lipid peroxidation which was previously reported to induce hemolysis in AMs,[61,62] may also be operative at high silica doses. The effect of silica-induced Ca^{2+} influx was further substantiated by experiments using Ca^{2+} channel blockers. In these experiments, it was found that the rate of Ca^{2+} uptake following silica exposure, particularly at low doses, was greatly inhibited in cells pretreated with the Ca^{2+} channel blocker nifedipine (Figure 6).

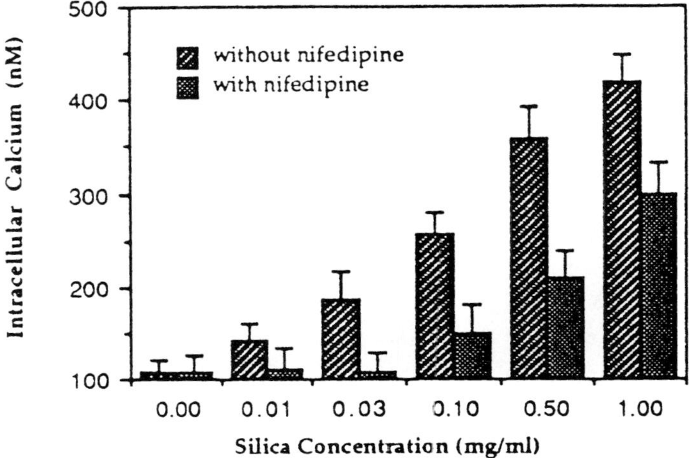

FIGURE 6 Effect of nifedipine on silica-induced $[Ca^{2+}]_i$ rise in alveolar macrophages. Cells were incubated in HEPES-buffered medium containing 1 m*M* Ca^{2+} in the absence or presence of 1 μ*M* nifedipine. (From Rojanasakul, Y. et al., *J. Cell. Physiol.*, 154, 310, 1993.)

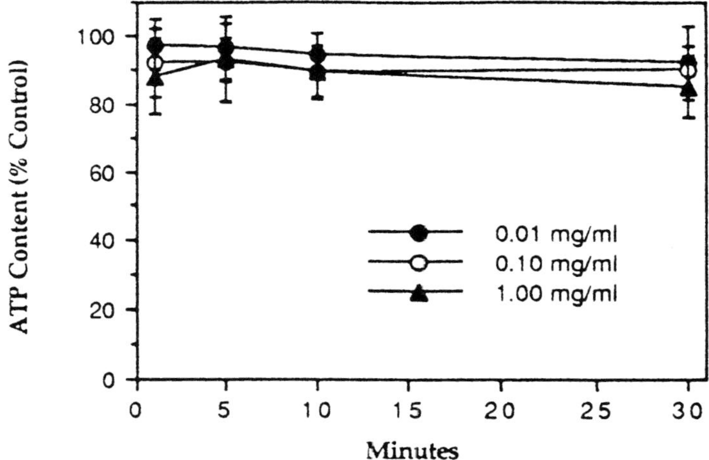

FIGURE 7 Cellular ATP content in alveolar macrophages as a function of time after the addition of various concentrations of silica. Alveolar macrophages (1×10^6/ml) were incubated with and without silica (control) in HEPES-buffered medium, and the ATP levels were determined by the firefly luciferase assay at various time points. Mean control ATP value = 1.08 ± 0.12 nmoles/10^6 cells. (From Rojanasakul, Y. et al., *J. Cell. Physiol.*, 154, 310, 1993.)

Because the maintenance of the $[Ca^{2+}]_i$ at a physiological level depends on energy-dependent transport systems, there was a possibility that the observed rise in $[Ca^{2+}]_i$ caused by silica may have been due to energy depletion. ATP depletion was reported to occur following Ca^{2+} overloading in other cell systems.[11,63] In silica-exposed AM systems, however, no significant reduction in cellular ATP content was observed at silica concentrations of 0.01–1.0 mg/ml, well after the time period that the $[Ca^{2+}]_i$ and membrane integrity changes had occurred (Figure 7). The possibility that Ca^{2+} overload may result from Ca^{2+} intake during phagocytosis or from the release of the internalized silica-bound Ca^{2+} was also ruled out. This is evidenced by the inability of the phagocytic inhibitor cytochalasin B (0.1 m*M*) to inhibit the silica-induced $[Ca^{2+}]_i$ rise.[35] Thus, it is concluded that silica-induced $[Ca^{2+}]_i$ rise was not associated with either ATP depletion or Ca^{2+} leakage during phagocytosis.

VII. CONCLUSIONS

The results presented here suggest that the disturbance of intracellular Ca^{2+} homeostasis by silica is closely associated with cell injury in AMs. The mechanisms responsible for the early events of this silica-induced $[Ca^{2+}]_i$ rise appear to involve at least two different mechanisms and are dose-dependent: a) Ca^{2+} influx through specific Ca^{2+} channels which results in a transient $[Ca^{2+}]_i$ increase at low doses of silica and b) non-specific membrane damage with sustained $[Ca^{2+}]_i$ rise at high silica doses. The low dose effect, which excludes consequences resulting from non-specific cell damage by high dose of silica, is of interest in further elucidation of the Ca^{2+}-mediated cytotoxicity. Alveolar macrophage is an active cell type which interacts and modulates cellular activities of other lung cells. Alterations in its Ca^{2+} homeostasis could mediate several Ca^{2+}-dependent cellular events including activation of phospholipases, proteases, endonucleases, and oxidases which catalyze the degradation of membrane phospholipids and cytoskeletal and membrane proteins. All of these responses may directly or indirectly impair cellular physiological functions and cause cellular injury of not only the macrophage itself but other effector cells as well.

REFERENCES

1. **Fleckenstein, A., Frey, M., and Fleckenstein-Grun, G.,** Cellular injury by cytosolic calcium overload and its prevention by calcium agonists — a new principle of tissue protection, in: *Mechanisms of Hepatocyte Injury and Death*, D. Keppler, H. Popper, L. Bianchi, and W. Reutter, Eds., MTP Press, Lancaster, 1983, 321–335.
2. **Schanne, F. A. X., Kane, A. B., Young, E. E., and Farber, J. L.,** Calcium dependence of toxic cell death: a final common pathway, *Science*, 206, 700–702, 1979.
3. **Jewell, S. A., Bellomo, G., Thor, H., Orrenius, S., and Smith, M. T.,** Bleb formation in hepatocytes during drug metabolism is associated with alterations in intracellular thiol and calcium ion homeostasis, *Science*, 217, 1257–1259, 1982.
4. **Starke, P. E., Hoek, J., and Farber, J. L.,** Calcium-dependent and calcium-independent mechanisms of irreversible cell injury in cultured rat hepatocytes, *J. Biol. Chem.*, 261, 3006–3011, 1986.
5. **Forman, H. J., Dorio, R. J., and Skelton, D. C.,** Hydroperoxide-induced damage to alveolar macrophage function and membrane integrity: alterations in intracellular-free Ca^{2+} and membrane potential, *Arch. Biochem. Biophys.*, 259, 457–465, 1987.
6. **Gleva, G. F., Goodglick, L. A., and Kane, A. B.,** Altered calcium homeostasis in irreversibly injured P388D1 macrophages, *Am. J. Pathol.*, 137, 43–57, 1990.
7. **Rice, K. L., Duane, P. G., Mielke, G., Sinha, A. A., and Niewoehner, D. E.,** Calcium ionophore injure alveolar epithelial cells: relation to phospholipase activity, *Am. J. Physiol.*, 259, L439–L450, 1990.
8. **Moore, M., Thor, H., Moore, G., Nelson, S., Moldeus, P., and Orrenius, S.,** The toxicity of acetaminophen and N-acetyl-p-benzoquinoneimine in isolated hepatocytes is associated with thiol depletion and increased cytosolic Ca^{2+}, *J. Biol. Chem.*, 260, 13035–13040, 1985.
9. **Boobis, A. R., Seddon, C. E., Nasseri-Sina, P., and Davies, D. S.,** Evidence for a direct role of intracellular Ca^{2+} in paracetamol toxicity, *Biochem. Pharmacol.*, 39, 1277–1281, 1990.
10. **Tani, M.,** Mechanisms of Ca^{2+} overload in reperfused ischemic myocardium, *Annu. Rev. Physiol.*, 52, 543–559, 1990.
11. **Josephson, R. A., Silverman, H. S., Lakatta, E. G., Stern, M. D., and Zweier, J. L.,** Study of the mechanisms of hydrogen peroxide and hydroxyl free radical-induced cellular injury and calcium overload in cardiac myocytes, *J. Biol. Chem.*, 266, 2354–2361, 1991.
12. **Cotterill, L. A., Gower, J. D., Fuller, B. J., and Green, C. J.,** Oxidative damage to kidney membranes during cold ischemia: evidence of a role for calcium, *Transplantation*, 48, 745–751, 1989.
13. **Crouch, E.,** Pathobiology of pulmonary fibrosis, *Am. J. Physiol.*, 259, L159–L184, 1990.
14. **Bowden, D. H.,** Alveolar response to injury, *Thorax*, 36, 801–804, 1981.
15. **Lesur, O., Cantin, A. M., Tanswell, K., Melloni, B., Beaulieu, J. F., and Begin, R.,** Silica exposure induces cytotoxicity and proliferative activity of type II pneumocytes, *Exp. Lung Res.*, 18, 173–190, 1992.
16. **Weibel, E. R. and Gil, J.,** Electron microscopic demonstration of an extra-cellular duplex lining layer of alveoli, *Respir. Physiol.*, 4, 42–57, 1968.
17. **Merchant, R. K., Peterson, M. W., and Hunninghake, G. W.,** Silica directly increases permeability of alveolar epithelial cells, *J. Appl. Physiol.*, 68, 1354–1359, 1990.
18. **Bowden, D. H. and Adamson, I. Y. R.,** The role of cell injury and the continuing inflammatory response in the generation of silicotic pulmonary fibrosis, *J. Pathol.*, 144, 149–161, 1984.

19. **Adamson, I. Y. R. and Bowden, D. H.,** Role of polymorphonuclear leukocytes in silica-induced pulmonary fibrosis, *Am. J. Pathol.,* 117, 37–43, 1984.
20. **Johnson, K. G., Fantone, J. C., III, Kaplan, J., and Ward, P. A.,** *In vivo* damage of rat lungs by oxygen metabolites, *J. Clin. Invest.,* 67, 983–993, 1981.
21. **Van Kuijk, F. J. G. M., Sevanian, A., Handelman, G. J., and Dratz, E. A.,** A new role of phospholipase A_2: Protection of membranes from lipid peroxidation damage, *Trends Biochem. Sci.,* 12, 31–34, 1987.
22. **Glende, E. A., Jr. and Pushpendran, K. C.,** Activation of phospholipase A_2 by carbon tetrachloride in isolated rat hepatocytes, *Biochem. Pharmacol.,* 35, 3301–3307, 1986.
23. **Niewoehner, D. E., Rice, K., Sinha, A. A., and Wangensteen, D.,** Injurious effects of lysophosphatidylcholine on barrier properties of alveolar epithelium, *J. Appl. Physiol.,* 63, 1979–1986, 1987.
24. **Niewoehner, D. E., Sinha, A. A., Rice, K., Cadman, S., and Wangensteen, D.,** Effects of proteolytic enzymes upon transepithelial solute transport, *J. Appl. Physiol.,* 61, 1418–1430, 1986.
25. **Brody, A. R. and Davis, G. S.,** Alveolar macrophage toxicology, in: *Mechanisms in Respiratory Toxicology,* Witschi, H. and Nettesheim, P., Eds., Vol. II, CRC Press Inc., Boca Raton, 1982, 3–12.
26. **Johnson, R. B., Jr. and Kitagawa, S.,** Molecular basis for the enhanced respiratory burst of activated macrophages, *Fed. Proc.,* 44, 2927–2932, 1985.
27. **Takemura, R. and Werb, Z.,** Secretory products of macrophages and their physiological functions, *Am. J. Physiol.,* 246, C1–C8, 1984.
28. **Reed, D. J.,** Regulation of reductive processes by glutathione, *Biochem. Pharmacol.,* 35, 7–13, 1986.
29. **Masaki, N., Kyle, M. E., and Farber, J. L.,** Tert-butyl hydroperoxide kills cultured hepatocytes by peroxidizing membrane lipids, *Arch. Biochem. Biophys.,* 270, 390–399, 1989.
30. **Reed, D. J.,** Review of the current status of calcium and thiols in cellular injury, *Chem. Res. Toxicol.,* 3, 495–502, 1990.
31. **Sakaida, I., Thomas, A. P., and Farber, J. L.,** Increases in cytosolic calcium ion concentration can be dissociated from killing of cultured hepatocytes by tert-butyl hydroperoxide, *J. Biol. Chem.,* (in press).
32. **Shi, X., Dalal, N. S., and Vallyathan, V.,** ESR evidence for the hydroxyl radical formation in aqueous suspension of quartz particles and its possible significance to lipid peroxidation in silicosis, *J. Toxicol. Environ. Health,* 25, 237–245, 1988.
33. **Vallyathan, V., Mega, J. F., Shi, X., and Dalal, N. S.,** Enhanced generation of free radicals from phagocytes induced by mineral dusts, *Am. J. Respir. Cell Mol. Biol.,* 6, 404–413, 1992.
34. **Chen, J., Armstrong, L. C., Liu, S., Gerriets, J. E., and Last, J. A.,** Silica increases cytosolic free calcium ion concentration of alveolar macrophages *in vitro, Toxicol. Appl. Pharmacol.,* 111, 211–220, 1991.
35. **Rojanasakul, Y., Wang, L. Y., Malanga, C. J., Ma, J. Y. C., Banks, D. E., and Ma, J. K. H.,** Altered calcium homeostasis and cell injury in silica-exposed alveolar macrophages, *J. Cell. Physiol.,* 154, 310–316, 1993.
36. **Roney, P. L. and Holian, A.,** Possible mechanism of chrysotile asbestos-stimulated superoxide anion production in guinea pig alveolar macrophages, *Toxicol. Appl. Pharmacol.,* 100, 132–144, 1989.
37. **Niewoehner, D. E., Rice, K., Duane, P., Sinha, A., Gebhard, R., and Wangensteen, D.,** Induction of alveolar epithelial injury by phospholipase A_2, *J. Appl. Physiol.,* 66, 261–267, 1989.
38. **Englen, M. D., Taylor, S. M., Laegreid, W. W., Liggitt, H. D., Silflow, R. M., Breeze, R. G., and Leid, R. W.,** Stimulation of arachidonic acid metabolism in silica-exposed alveolar macrophages, *Exp. Lung Res.,* 15, 511–526, 1989.
39. **Englen, M. D., Taylor, S. M., Laegreid, W. W., Silflow, R. M., and Leid, R. W.,** The effects of different silicas on arachidonic acid metabolism in alveolar macrophages, *Exp. Lung Res.,* 16, 691–709, 1990.
40. **Englen, M. D., Taylor, S. M., Laegreid, W. W., Silflow, R. M., and Leid, R. W.,** Diminished arachidonic acid metabolite release by bovine alveolar macrophages exposed to surface-modified silica, *Am. J. Respir. Cell Mol. Biol.,* 6, 527–534, 1992.
41. **Panos, R. J., Voelkel, N. F., Cott, G. R., Mason, R. J., and Westcott, J. Y.,** Alterations in eicosanoid production by rat alveolar type II cells after silica-induced lung injury, *Am. J. Respir. Cell Mol. Biol.,* 6, 430–438, 1992.
42. **Klein, J. H. and Adamson, I. Y. R.,** Fibroblast inhibition and prostaglandin secretion by alveolar epithelial cells exposed to silica, *Lab. Invest.,* 60, 808–813, 1989.
43. **Kane, A. B., Stanton, R. P., Raymond, E. G., Dobson, M. E., Knafeic, M. E., and Farber, J. L.,** Dissociation of intracellular lysosomal rupture from the cell death caused by silica, *J. Cell Biol.,* 87, 643–651, 1980.
44. **Morrow, P. E.,** Possible mechanisms to explain dust overloading of the lungs, *Fundam. Appl. Toxicol.,* 10, 369–384, 1988.
45. **Rister, M. and Vollmering, M.,** Concanavalin A distribution in polymorphonuclear leukocytes and alveolar macrophages during hyperoxia, *Virchows Arch.,* 43, 179–187, 1983.
46. **Rister, M.,** The toxic effect of oxygen on alveolar macrophages and granulocytes, *Fortschr. Med.,* 100, 1247–1250, 1982.
47. **Hartwig, J. H.,** Actin filament architecture and movements in macrophage cytoplasm, in, *Biochemistry of Macrophages,* Evered, D., Nugent, J., and O'Connor, M. Eds., Pitman, London (Ciba Foundation Symposium 118), 1986, 42–53.

48. **Bennett, J. P., Zaner, K. S., and Stossel, T. P.,** Isolation and some properties of macrophages alpha-actinin: evidence that it is not an actin gelling protein, *Biochem.,* 23, 5081–5186, 1984.
49. **Dayton, W. R., Shollmayer, J., Lepley, R. A., and Cortes, L. R.,** A calcium-activated protease possibly involved in myofibrillar protein turnover. Isolation of a low calcium-requiring form of the protease, *Biochim. Biophys. Acta,* 659, 48–61, 1981.
50. **Mirabelli, F., Salis, A., Vairetti, M., Bellomo, G., Thor, H., and Orrenius, S.,** Cytoskeletal alterations in human platelets exposed to oxidative stress are modulated by oxidative and Ca^{2+}-dependent mechanisms, *Arch. Biochem. Biophys.,* 270, 478–488, 1989.
51. **Gaskin, F., Cantor, C. R., and Shelanski, M. R.,** Turbidimetric studies of the *in vitro* assembly and diassembly of porcine neurotubules, *J. Mol. Biol.,* 89, 737–758, 1974.
52. **Olmsted, J. B.,** Microtubule-associated proteins, *Annu. Rev. Cell Biol.,* 2, 421–457, 1986.
53. **Bellomo, G., Mirabelli, F., Vairetti, M., Iosi, F., and Malorni, W.,** Cytoskeleton as a target in menadione-induced oxidative stress in cultured mammalian cells. Biochemical and immunocytochemical features, *J. Cell Physiol.,* 143, 118–128, 1990.
54. **Nicotera, P., McConkey, D. J., Svensson, S. A., Bellomo, G., and Orrenius, S.,** Correlation between cytosolic Ca^{2+} concentration and cytotoxicity in hepatocytes exposed to oxidative stress, *Toxicology,* 52, 55–63, 1988.
55. **Nicotera, P., Hartzell, P., Baldi, C., Svensson, S. A., Bellomo, G., and Orrenius, S.,** Cystamine induces toxicity in hepatocytes through the elevation of cytosolic Ca^{2+} and the stimulation of a non-lysosomal proteolytic system, *J. Biol. Chem.,* 261, 14628–35, 1986.
56. **Tzeng, W. F. and Chen, Y. H.,** Suppression of snake-venom cardiomyocyte degeneration by blockage of Ca^{2+} influx or inhibition of non-lysosomal proteinases, *Biochem. J.,* 256, 89–95, 1988.
57. **Mellgren, R. L.,** Calcium-dependent proteases: an enzyme system active at cellular membrane? *FASEB J.,* 1, 110–115, 1987.
58. **Waring, P., Eichner, R. D., Mullbacher, A., and Sjaarda, A.,** Gliotoxin induces apoptosis in macrophages unrelated to its antiphagocytic properties, *Sciences,* 263, 18493–18499, 1988.
59. **Chang, M. P., Baldwin, R. L., Bruce, C., and Wisnieski, B. J.,** Second cytotoxic pathway of diphteria toxin suggested by nuclease activity, *Science,* 1165–1168, 1989.
60. **Dypbukt, J. M., Thor, H., and Nicotera, P.,** Intracellular calcium chelators prevent DNA damage and protect hepatoma 1c1c7 cells from quinone-induced cell killing, *Free Radical Res. Commun.,* 8, 347–354, 1990.
61. **Vallyathan, V., Shi, X., Dalal, N. S., Irr, W., and Castranova, V.,** Generation of free radicals from freshly fractured silica dust: potential role in acute silica-induced lung injury, *Am. Rev. Respir. Dis.,* 138, 1213–1219, 1988.
62. **Depasse, J.,** Mechanisms of the hemolysis by colloidal silica, in *The In Vivo Effects of Mineral Dusts,* Brown, M., Chamberlin, M., Davies, R., and Gormley, I.P., Eds., Academic Press, London, 1980, 125–130.
63. **Albano, E., Bellomo, G., Parola, M., Carini, R., and Dianzani, M. U.,** Stimulation of lipid peroxidation increases the intracellular calcium content of isolated hepatocytes, *Biochim. Biophys. Acta,* 1091, 310–316, 1991.

Section III
Chapter 4

THE ROLE OF INTERLEUKIN-1 AND TUMOR NECROSIS FACTOR α IN THE LUNG'S RESPONSE TO SILICA

Kevin E. Driscoll

CONTENTS

I. INTRODUCTION

Interleukin-1 (IL-1) and tumor necrosis factor α (TNFα) are members of a class of molecules called cytokines which are essential polypeptide mediators of cell to cell communication and play key roles in physiologic and pathophysiologic processes. In particular, IL-1 and TNFα are recognized to be important mediators of host defense, being effectors of inflammatory and immune responses. IL-1 and TNFα also are involved in cell growth and differentiation and can influence normal tissue homeostasis as well as tissue repair and regeneration following injury. There is increasing evidence that IL-1 and TNFα play important roles in the pathogenesis of silicosis, a chronic interstitial lung disease resulting from inhalation of crystalline forms of silica and characterized by a persistent inflammatory response, immune cell activation, and fibroproliferation. This chapter will briefly review selected aspects of IL-1 and TNFα biology and then discuss the current understanding of their role in the lung's response to silica.

0-8493-4709-2/96/$0.00+$.50

II. INTERLEUKIN-1

A. HISTORY

IL-1 was first described in the 1940s for its ability to produce fever and was known as endogenous pyrogen.[1] Endogenous pyrogen was subsequently revealed to be a protein associated with the febrile response to a variety of infectious or inflammatory stimuli.[2] In the 1960s, a phagocyte-derived factor called leukocyte endogenous mediator (LEM) was identified which stimulated aspects of the hepatic acute-phase response such as increased synthesis of fibrinogen, haptoglobin, C-reactive protein, and $\alpha 2$ macroglobin. LEM was later shown to be indistinguishable from endogenous pyrogen.[3] In 1972, Gery and co-workers[4] described a macrophage-derived soluble product, lymphocyte activating factor (LAF), which potentiated the proliferative response of T-lymphocytes to mitogenic or antigenic stimuli. Subsequent studies demonstrated endogenous pyrogen, LEM, and LAF to be the same factor,[5–7] and, in 1979, the term IL-1 was recommended to describe this protein mediator.[8]

B. MOLECULAR BIOLOGY

IL-1 exists in two structurally related but biochemically distinct forms called IL-1α and IL-1β.[9–11] Each form is encoded by a separate gene located on the long arm of chromosome 2 in both humans and mice.[12,13] The mature IL-1α and β proteins have molecular weights of ~17 kiloDaltons (kDa), with isoelectric points of 5.0 and 7.0 for the α and β forms, respectively.[13,14] Both IL-1α and β are recognized equally by IL-1 receptors, and both molecules appear to possess the same spectrum of biological activities. However, there is only 26% homology in amino acid sequence between the two proteins.[12–15]

IL-1 is translated as a propeptide of approximately 270 amino acids and, although IL-1 is released by cells, the molecule lacks the typical hydrophobic signal peptide found on most secreted proteins. The IL-1 precursor molecule can be processed by a specific IL-1 converting enzyme (ICE) which is a cysteine protease[16] or by serine proteases such as elastin and plasmin.[17,18] In addition to the mature ~17 kd extracellular form of IL-1, a 31 kDa precursor and an intermediate ~22 kDa IL-1 molecule have been identified in association with the cell membrane of macrophages, monocytes, dendritic cells, and fibroblasts.[18–20] Membrane bound IL-1 participates in antigen presentation and may be particularly significant in local immunostimulatory responses occurring in lymphoid tissue.[14] A significant portion of IL-1 activity found extracellularly is IL-1β while membrane-associated IL-1 consists primarily of IL-1α.[14] Although IL-1 production was primarily associated with mononuclear phagocytes in earlier studies, other cell types known to produce this cytokine include polymorphonuclear leukocytes, keratinocytes, Langerhans cells, vascular endothelial cells, smooth muscle cells, fibroblasts, and natural killer cells.[21–26]

III. TUMOR NECROSIS FACTOR α

A. HISTORY

In the late 1800s reduction of tumor mass and hemorrhagic necrosis of tumors in cancer patients treated with live bacteria or bacterial broths was reported by William Coley, a New York surgeon.[27] It is believed the responses Coley observed were, at least in part, due to the actions of TNFα. Later studies demonstrated treatment of mice with endotoxin, a lipolysaccharide (LPS) component of bacterial cell walls, caused necrosis of transplanted tumors.[28] In 1975, Carswell and colleagues[29] described a protein, "Tumor Necrosis Factor," in the serum of Bacillus-Calmette-Guerin (BCG) and LPS treated animals which produced hemorrhagic necrosis of tumors *in vivo* and was cytostatic or cytotoxic for tumor cells *in vitro*. Subsequently, several groups reported on the isolation and purification of a protein mediating this tumor necrotizing activity and ultimately the cloning and expression of the human and murine TNFα genes.[30–33]

Research to understand cachexia, a wasting syndrome associated with infectious disease, independently led to the isolation and characterization of TNFα. Rabbits infected with Trypanosoma *brucei* were shown to exhibit a cachexia-like response which included a marked hypertriglyceridemia associated with suppressed lipoprotein lipase activity.[34] In 1985, Beutler and co-workers[35] isolated a 17 kDa peptide from mice which exhibited lipoprotein lipase suppressing activity; the protein was named cachectin. Cachectin was demonstrated by N-terminal sequencing to be identical to TNFα.[36]

B. MOLECULAR AND PROTEIN BIOLOGY

In humans the gene for TNFα is located on the short arm of chromosome 6 and is linked to genes coding for the Major Histocompatability Complex (MHC) class I antigens and the major heat shock protein, hsp 70.[37,38] In mice the TNFα gene is also associated with MHC genes and is located on chromosome 17.[33,39] The human gene codes for a 233 amino acid, 26 kDa precursor protein devoid of N-glycosylation sites,[31,32,40] while the mouse gene codes for a 235 amino acid precursor protein with a single N-glycosylation site.[33,39] There is approximately 80% amino acid homology between the human and mouse TNFα proteins. In both humans and mice, the TNFα gene is associated with the gene for a closely related cytokine, TNFβ (also called lymphotoxin).[30] TNFβ binds to the same receptors as TNFα and exhibits many of the same bioactivities[41] but appears to be synthesized primarily by lymphocytes and has only 28% amino acid sequence homology with TNFα.[30,42]

TNFα is produced by a variety of phagocytic and nonphagocytic cell types including: macrophages, monocytes, polymorphonuclear leukocytes, lymphocytes, smooth muscle cells, and mast cells.[34,35,43–45] The TNFα propeptide is processed to a mature 17 kd secreted form which consists of 157 amino acids, has a isoelectric point of 5.3, and contains two cysteine residues involved in a single intramolecular disulfide bond.[30] Unlike most other well characterized cytokines, but similar to IL-1, TNFα lacks the typical 20–30 amino acid hydrophobic signal sequence characteristic of secretory proteins. Recent studies indicate that monocytes express a membrane-associated form of TNFα which appears to be the 26 kD propeptide and possesses cytotoxic activity for tumor cells.[46–48] Secreted TNFα exists as oligomers of the 17 kd protein ranging in molecular weight from 34 to 140 kDa. X-ray crystallographic studies demonstrate TNFα forms trimers of 17-kd protein sub-units.[49,50] The TNFα trimer binds with significantly greater avidity to the TNFα receptor and possesses greater cytotoxicity for tumor cells than monomeric TNFα.[51]

IV. BIOACTIVITIES OF IL-1 AND TNFα

Both TNFα and IL-1 are pleiotropic cytokines and share a wide range of biologic activities in a variety of *in vitro* and *in vivo* systems. The activities of TNFα and IL-1 have been the subject of several detailed reviews.[52–54] The discussion below focuses on the role of these cytokines in recruitment and activation of inflammatory cells, proliferation of cells, and synthesis of connective tissue, i.e., activities having potential significance to the lung's response to silica and other mineral dusts.

A. INFLAMMATORY CELL RECRUITMENT AND ACTIVATION

TNFα and IL-1 are thought to play key roles in host defense by mediating the recruitment and activation of inflammatory cells. Table 1 summarizes some of the cellular processes influenced by these cytokines which are of particular relevance to inflammation. Direct evidence that TNFα and IL-1 are involved in cell recruitment has come from studies demonstrating intradermal injection of these cytokines results in localized accumulation of inflammatory cells.[55–58] More recent studies demonstrated that intratracheal administration of IL-1 and TNFα results in a pulmonary inflammation characterized by a transient increase in neutrophils.[59] Although IL-1 is directly chemotactic for T-lymphocytes,[60] neither IL-1 nor TNFα is chemotactic for inflammatory cells such as neutrophils and monocytes. In recent years, significant progress has been made in understanding the mechanisms by which IL-1 and TNFα facilitate inflammatory cell recruitment. In this respect, the ability of IL-1 and TNFα to stimulate both the adhesion of leukocytes to post-capillary venules and the elaboration of specific chemotactic cytokines by several cell types contributes to their role in inflammation.

1. Adhesion Molecule Expression

For inflammatory cells to leave the peripheral blood and move to sites of infection or injury they must migrate and adhere to vascular endothelial cells. *In vitro,* studies demonstrated that TNFα or IL-1 stimulate the adherence of neutrophils to endothelial cells and that this interaction requires the expression of IL-1 and TNFα-inducible proteins on the surface of endothelial cells and leukocytes.[61–66] It is now known that IL-1 and TNFα increase expression of at least three different adhesion proteins on endothelial cells: intercellular adhesion molecule 1 (ICAM-1), endothelial leukocyte adhesion molecule-1 (ELAM-1), and vascular cell adhesion molecule-1 (VCAM-1).[63,66–68] These adhesion proteins serve as ligands for

TABLE 1
Inflammatory and Immune Processes Stimulated by IL-1 or TNFα

Process	TNFα	IL-1	Ref.
Expression of adhesion molecules, ELAM, ICAM, VCAM	+	–	62–66
Integrin expression on Leukocytes	+	?	61,69,70
T and B Lymphocyte proliferation	+/–	+	4,5,52,53,115–118
Chemotactic protein (Chemokine) expression	+	+	81–87,91
Prostaglandin, prostacyclin and platelet activating factor biosynthesis	+	+	100–104
Neutrophil oxidative burst and degranulation	+	+	22,105–108,111,112
Expression of IL-1, TNF, IL-6, and GM-CSF	+	+	13,96–99
Induction of procoagulant activity from endothelial cells	+	+	64,65
Acute phase protein response	+	+	7,90

complementary molecules, called integrins, on leukocytes.[69] *In vitro,* ELAM-1 expression is rapidly but transiently upregulated on endothelial cells by IL-1 and TNFα and is thought to be of importance in mediating early neutrophil responses.[70] ICAM-1, which is expressed by several cell types including endothelial cells, fibroblasts, and lymphocytes, is involved in a variety of cell:cell interactions including adherence of neutrophils and lymphocytes to endothelium.[70] The receptor on leukocytes which interacts with ICAM-1 is lymphocyte function-associated antigen (LFA-1), also called CD-11a/CD-18.[71–73] VCAM-1 appears to play a role in adherence and recruitment of T and B lymphocytes as well as monocytes.[67] The leukocyte receptor for VCAM-1 is the integrin, VLA-4.[67,74,75]

2. Chemokine Expression

In addition to cell adherence, recruitment of inflammatory cells involves emigration of these cells into tissues in response to local chemotactic gradients. In this respect, IL-1 and TNFα stimulate production of several structurally related cytokines, called chemokines, which possess chemotactic activity for inflammatory and immunocompetent cells (Table 2). Chemokines are believed to be key mediators of inflammatory cell recruitment in a variety of tissues including lung.[76] Members of the chemokine family bind heparin, range in molecular weight from ~8 to 10 kDa, and possess a conserved 4 cysteine motif in their mature protein sequence.[77,78] The chemokine family can be subdivided into two groups based on the spacing of these cysteine residues. In one group, which includes interleukin-8 (IL-8), a neutrophil, and lymphocyte chemotaxin, the amino-terminal cysteines are separated by a single amino acid (CxC proteins). In the other group, which includes monocyte chemotactic peptide 1 (MCP-1), the two amino-terminal cysteines are adjacent (CC proteins). Chemokines are secreted by a variety of cell types in response to IL-1 and TNFα. For example, IL-1 and TNFα stimulate production of IL-8 by epithelial cells, fibroblasts, and endothelial cells as well as macrophages and neutrophils[78–84] and MCP-1 secretion by fibroblasts, endothelial cells, and epithelial cells.[85–87]

3. Cell Activation

In addition to inducing chemokine expression, IL-1 and TNFα stimulate release of other mediators relevant to inflammatory cell recruitment and activation. For example, IL-1 and TNFα induce secretion of interleukin-6, a cytokine which stimulates acute phase protein synthesis and immunoglobulin secretion by B lymphocytes and participates in the activation and differentiation of T-lymphocytes.[13,96] In addition, IL-1 and TNFα can induce their own expression, as well as the expression of each other,[97–99] suggesting a mechanism for autostimulatory or co-stimulatory regulatory loops. IL-1 and TNFα also stimulate eicosanoid biosynthesis, including the production of prostacyclin and platelet activating factor by endothelial cells,[100,101] prostaglandin E2 (PGE2) by fibroblasts,[103] and leukotriene B4 (LTB4) by

TABLE 2
Chemokine Cytokines Shown to be Induced by IL-1 and/or TNFα

Chemokine	Species	Cell Source	Function	Ref.
Interleukin 8 (IL-8)	Human	Macrophage/monocyte fibroblast, epithelial cell endothelial cell, keratinocyte neutrophil	Neutrophil and lymphocyte chemotaxin; neutrophil activating factor	78,80–82,84
ENA-78	Human	Lung epithelial cell line	Neutrophil chemotaxis and activation	189
Gro/MDSA	Human	Endothelial cell	Neutrophil chemotaxis, growth factor	95
Macrophage Activating & Chemotactic Factor/ Monocyte Chemotactic Peptide (MACF/MCP)	Human Rat, mouse	Monocyte, smooth muscle cell, fibroblast, epithelial cell, endothelial cell, lymphocyte	Monocyte chemotactic factor; activation of macrophage cytotoxicity	85–90
Macrophage Inflammatory Protein 2 (MIP-2)	Rat, mouse	Macrophage, epithelial cell, fibroblast	Neutrophil chemotaxin	77,91,92
Macrophage Inflammatory Protein 1α (MIP-1α)	Rat, mouse	Macrophage, T-cell, epithelial cell, fibroblast	Neutrophil chemokenesis & activation; monocyte chemotaxin; pyrogen	77,91,93
Cytokine-Induced Neutrophil Chemoattractant (CINC)	Rat	Kidney cell line	Neutrophil chemotaxin	94

neutrophils.[104] These lipid mediators can cause vasodilation and directly elicit inflammatory cell infiltration and activation. Inflammatory and immunocompetent cells can be activated by IL-1 and TNFα to release mediators important to the inactivation of pathogens such as reactive oxygen species, hydrolytic enzymes, lysozyme, and lactoferrin.[105–115] Importantly, while the recruitment and activation of inflammatory cells constitutes an important host defense mechanism, this response can contribute to tissue injury through excessive or persistent release of tissue-damaging mediators such as oxidents and protealytic enzymes.

B. CELL PROLIFERATION

One of the first bioactivities attributed to IL-1 was its ability to lower the threshold for mitogen or antigen-induced T-lymphocyte proliferation.[4,114,115] This effect is now known to result, at least in part, from IL-1 induced IL-2 (T-cell growth factor) release and IL-2 receptor expression by T lymphocytes. More recently, TNFα has also been shown to increase T-lymphocyte IL-2 receptor expression and enhance proliferative responses to IL-2.[116,117] TNFα and IL-1 also increase IL-2-induced B cell proliferation and immunoglobulin secretion.[118] In addition to immunocompetent cells, IL-1 and TNFα have been shown to affect the proliferation of tissue structural cells such as fibroblasts, epithelial cells, endothelial cells, and smooth muscle cells. For example, treatment of fibroblasts *in vitro* with IL-1 has been shown to both stimulate and inhibit cell proliferation depending on the assay conditions and the specific target cells being studied.[119–121] While early studies demonstrated TNFα exerts a growth-inhibitory effect on some transformed cell lines, more recent studies indicate this cytokine can stimulate proliferation of normal fibroblasts from a variety of tissues.[122] Thus, in addition to modulating the immune response, IL-1 and TNFα have the potential to contribute to wound healing by influencing proliferation of cells critical to tissue repair and regeneration.

Table 3 summarizes several recent studies characterizing the effects of IL-1 and TNFα on growth of tissue structural cells. In addition to fibroblasts, TNFα and/or IL-1 can stimulate the proliferation of smooth muscle cells, chondrocytes, and astrocytes.[123–126] The growth promoting or inhibiting activity of IL-1 and TNFα appears to be, at least in part, mediated indirectly. For example, culture of human foreskin fibroblasts in the presence of TNFα results in increased expression of epidermal growth factor (EGF) receptors.[127,128] The dose-related pattern of TNFα-induced EGF receptor expression is similar to the concentration dependent mitogenic effects of TNFα on the fibroblasts. These results suggest the effect of TNFα on proliferation *in vitro* may be due to increasing the responsiveness to serum EGF. Studies by Hajjar and co-workers[129] demonstrate an additional mechanism by which TNFα may increase cell proliferation. These investigators demonstrated that TNFα induces expression of the platelet derived

TABLE 3
Effect of TNFα and IL-1 on Proliferation of Tissue Structural Cells

Cell Type/Line	Cytokine	Response	Ref.
Human dermal fibroblasts	IL-1	Highly purified human and murine IL-1 stimulated 3-H thymidine incorporation.	119
Human smooth muscle cells	IL-1	IL-1 inhibited growth of smooth muscle cells in short-term (2 d) cultures by a prostaglandin mediated mechanism. IL-1 stimulated growth in longer-term (≥7 d) cultures.	123
Human dermal fibroblasts and aortic smooth muscle cells	IL-1	IL-1 increased expression of PDGF gene and secretion of PDGF protein. Antibody to PDGF blocked IL-1 stimulated growth of fibroblasts and smooth muscle cells.	130
Mouse fibroblasts and endothelial cells *in vivo*	IL-1	Sustained subcutaneous release of IL-1 resulted in neovascularization and fibrosis.	135
Human astrocytoma	IL-1, TNFα	Both IL-1 and TNFα stimulated 3-H thymidine incorporation into an astrocytoma cell line.	125
Human endothelial cells	IL-1, TNFα	TNFα or IL-1 stimulated release of platelet-derived growth factor from endothelial cells.	129
Rat chondrocytes	IL-1, TNFα	TNFα but not IL-1 stimulated 3-H thymidine incorporation in confluent and subconfluent cultures.	124
Human lung fibroblasts	IL-1, TNFα	IL-1 and TNFα inhibited proliferation of fibroblasts by a prostaglandin dependent mechanism. The inhibitory effect required both IL-1 and TNF. IL-1 alone stimulated growth.	120,121,131
Human and mouse fibroblasts, epithelial cells	TNFα	*In vitro* response was cell type dependent. TNFα increased, decreased, or had no effect on proliferation.	122
Human fibroblasts	TNFα	TNFα increased number of epidermal growth factor (EGF) receptors on fibroblasts. Dose-related effects on EGF receptor corresponded to TNF effects on fibroblast proliferation.	127
Human smooth muscle cells (SMC), fibroblasts, endothelial cells	TNFα	TNF and TNFβ stimulated proliferation of SMC and fibroblasts but inhibited growth of endothelial cells.	126
Balb C 3T3 fibroblasts	TNFα	TNFα stimulated proliferation of density arrested cultures but was cytostatic or cytotoxic for rapidly proliferating cells. The TNF stimulation was attenuated by a phospholipase inhibitor.	128
Mouse fibroblasts and endothelial cells *in vivo*	TNFα	Sustained subcutaneous administration of TNFα resulted in increased fibroblasts, collagen, and capillaries.	136

growth factor (PDGF) gene in endothelial cells and that mitogenic activity present in supernatants from these cells could be blocked by antibodies to PDGF. Similar to what was demonstrated for TNFα, Raines and colleagues[130] have shown the mitogenic effect of IL-1 on fibroblasts and smooth muscle cells is, at least in part, mediated through induction of PDGF A-chain synthesis and secretion. Interestingly, an indirect effect of IL-1 on fibroblast growth is consistent with the action of this cytokine on the proliferation of T cells in which the lymphocytes response is ultimately mediated by release of IL-2.

Under certain *in vitro* conditions, IL-1 and TNFα have been shown to inhibit proliferation of cells such as fibroblasts. Elias and colleagues[120,121,131] reported that combined exposure to IL-1 and TNFα inhibited fibroblast proliferation. However, when fibroblasts were treated with IL-1 or TNFα, alone or together, in the presence of indomethacin, stimulation of fibroblast proliferation occurred. These results suggest the

TABLE 4
Effect of TNFα and IL-1 on Synthesis of Extracellular Matrix Proteins

Cell Type/Line	Cytokine	Response	Ref.
Human chondrocytes	IL-1	IL-1 suppressed synthesis of type II collagen but stimulated expression of both type I and III collagen when prostaglandin E2 synthesis was inhibited with indomethacin.	134
Human chondrocytes, synovial and foreskin fibroblasts	IL-1	IL-1 decreased collagen and fibronectin. IL-1 + indomethacin stimulated collagen and fibronectin synthesis. In foreskin fibroblasts with a low innate PGE2 production, IL-1 stimulated collagen synthesis.	133
Rat lung fibroblasts	IL-1	IL-1 decreased elastin and type I collagen synthesis. This effect was inhibited by indomethacin.	139
Human vascular smooth muscle cells	IL-1	IL-1 increased synthesis of types I and III collagens. γ interferon inhibited IL-1 induced collagen synthesis.	140
Rat chondrocytes	IL-1, TNF	IL-1 and TNF inhibited synthesis of glycosaminoglycans.	124
Human dermal fibroblasts	IL-1, TNF	IL-1 increased procollagen mRNA but decreased collagen synthesis. TNF decreased collagen gene expression and protein synthesis.	141,142
Human skin fibroblasts	IL-1, TNF	IL-1 and TNF increased type IV collagen gene expression, but not expression of several other basement membrane proteins.	143
Human fetal fibroblasts	TNF	TNF inhibited collagen synthesis and expression type I procollagen mRNA.	144
Human lung fibroblasts	TNF	TNF stimulated glycosaminoglycan production. Hyaluronic acid constituted a major component of the increased GAG and was associated with increased hyaluronate synthetase activity.	131,132
Rat hepatic lipocytes	IL-1, TNF	IL-1 and TNF inhibited procollagen synthesis	145

growth inhibitory effects of combined IL-1 and TNFα treatment may be due to the synergistic effect of these cytokines on fibroblast PGE2 synthesis, PGE2 being growth inhibitory to these cells.[131] These *in vitro* studies indicate the microenvironment of the target cell *in vivo* may be critical to the type of proliferative response elicited by IL-1 and TNFα with the ultimate effect observed, stimulation or inhibition of growth, depending on the relative concentrations of IL-1 and TNFα as well as other regulatory factors such as PGE2, EGF, or PDGF.

C. SYNTHESIS OF EXTRACELLULAR MATRIX PROTEINS

Synthesis and accumulation of connective tissue protein plays a key role in development, tissue homeostasis,and wound healing. IL-1 and TNFα have been reported to both increase and decrease connective tissue protein synthesis *in vitro* (Table 4). Elias and colleagues[131,132] demonstrated that under serum-free conditions IL-1 and TNFα increased synthesis of collagen types I and III by human lung fibroblasts, a response associated with increased procollagen mRNA transcription. However, when fibroblasts were cultured with serum, individually, IL-1 or TNFα had no effect on collagen synthesis, but when combined, they inhibited collagen synthesis. Studies by Goldring and Krane[133,134] also indicated the presence of serum influences the *in vitro* effect of IL-1 and TNFα on collagen synthesis. These investigators reported exposure of chrondrocytes or synovial fibroblasts to IL-1 in serum containing medium inhibited expression of types I and II procollagen mRNA. However, if PGE2 synthesis was inhibited by indomethacin (PGE2 can inhibit collagen synthesis), IL-1 stimulated collagen production. In this respect, IL-1 treatment of human foreskin fibroblasts which produce only low levels of PGE2 increases collagen synthesis by these cells.

Although *in vitro* studies have reported IL-1 and TNFα can stimulate or inhibit fibroblast proliferation and collagen synthesis, *in vivo* studies demonstrate an association between these cytokines and increased cellular proliferation and connective tissue accumulation. Two recent studies characterized the tissue response to IL-1 and TNFα under conditions in which their release was local and sustained. Dunn and co-workers[135] administered IL-1 subcutaneously to mice in a slow release ethylene vinyl acetate co-polymer and reported that IL-1 treatment elicited inflammation, neovascularization, and fibrosis. Similarly, TNFα administered to mice subcutaneously via an osmotic minipump produced local accumulation of neutrophils followed by formation of a tissue mass consisting of fibroblasts, collagen, and capillaries.[136] Passive immunization studies demonstrated treatment of mice with anti-TNFα antibodies markedly attenuated collagen accumulation in bleomycin and silica models of pulmonary fibrosis.[137,138] These *in vivo* studies demonstrate that IL-1 or TNFα can increase cell proliferation and collagen deposition; however, whether these cytokines are acting directly or indirectly, for example, by stimulating release of, or responsiveness to other mediators, is not certain.

V. ROLE OF IL-1 AND TNFα IN THE LUNG'S RESPONSE TO SILICA

The response of the lung to crystalline forms of silica includes an inflammatory response comprised of increased numbers of macrophages, neutrophils, and lymphocytes.[149] Evidence exists indicating lung injury associated with silica inhalation results, at least in part, from the inherent cytotoxic properties of silica as well as the release of mediators (i.e., proteases and oxidants) by inflammatory cells.[146–148] Silica exposure can result in activation of tissue repair processes involving epithelial and fibroblast proliferation and accumulation of connective tissue, often resulting in pulmonary fibrosis. Silica exposure can also result in a granulomatous response, consisting of compact collections of activated macrophages in association with lymphocytes, fibroblasts, and collagen.[149] Given the bioactivities of IL-1 and TNFα discussed in the preceding section, it is clear these multifunctional cytokines have the potential to play a role in the types of responses to silica described above. To date, however, only a limited number of studies have directly investigated involvement of these cytokines in silica-induced lung injury. Available data indicate both IL-1 and TNFα contribute to the lung's response to silica as well as other mineral dusts. Below is a brief review of the data base demonstrating silica can activate TNFα and IL-1 release by macrophages, followed by a discussion of recent findings supporting a role for these cytokines in specific aspects of the lung's response to this mineral dust.

A. SILICA EXPOSURE AND IL-1 AND TNFα RELEASE

Macrophages are known to be sources of inflammatory and growth regulatory factors and are one of the first cells to respond to inhaled particles in the lung. Several studies have investigated effects of silica on IL-1 and TNFα production by macrophages (Table 5). Both silica and asbestos stimulate production of TNFα by rat alveolar macrophages *in vitro*.[150–153] In contrast, exposure of these cells to relatively innocuous particles such as titanium dioxide or latex beads has no effect on TNFα production.[150–152] Preliminary results using a myelomonocytic cell line transfected with a CAT reporter construct indicate silica-induced increases in TNFα result from increased gene transcription.[153] DuBois and co-workers[152] demonstrated that silica-induced macrophage TNFα production can be influenced by other mediators. These investigators stimulated alveolar macrophages *in vitro* with silica or asbestos and found they produced both TNFα and LTB4. When LTB4 synthesis was inhibited, dust-induced TNFα production was markedly reduced, while co-exposure of macrophages to silica and exogeneous LTB4 increased TNFα release above that elicited by the mineral dusts alone. LTB4 has been previously shown to enhance the production of IL-1, IL-2, and γ interferon.[154–156] It is possible that the marked inflammatory activity of silica and asbestos is due to their ability to stimulate both TNFα and LTB4 release.

Exposure to silica *in vitro* has been shown to stimulate human monocytes as well as peritoneal macrophages from mouse or rabbit to produce IL-1.[4,17,157–159] However, the ability of silica to stimulate alveolar macrophage release of IL-1 is less clear. Some studies have reported increased IL-1-like bioactivity in conditioned media from silica exposed rat alveolar macrophages.[160–162] However, in other studies using silica preparations treated to remove endotoxin (a potent stimulator of macrophage IL-1

TABLE 5
***In Vitro* Effects of Crystalline Silica on Production of IL-1 or TNFα**

Target Cell	Response	Ref.
Human monocytes	Silica (50 μg/ml) stimulated release of IL-1 like activity.	17
Human monocytes	Silica (25–100 μg/ml) stimulated dose related increases in release of IL-1 activity; treatment of monocytes with nonfibrogenic diamond particles did not. A factor released by monocytes which stimulated fibroblast growth appeared identical to IL-1.	157
Mouse peritoneal macrophages	Silica (60 μg/ml) increased extracellular IL-1-like activity and to a lesser extent intracellular IL-1 activity. A positive correlation was observed between cell damage and release of IL-1 activity. Combination of LPS (20 mg/ml) and silica was synergistic for IL-1 release.	4
Mouse peritoneal macrophages	Silica and chrysotile asbestos (50 and 100 μg/ml) stimulated release of IL-1 like activity. Treatment of cells with the relatively innocuous dust, titanium dioxide, did not stimulate release of IL-1-like activity.	159
Rabbit peritoneal macrophages	Oil elicited, LPS stimulated macrophages released increased amounts of IL-1-like activity when stimulated with 50 μg/ml silica.	158
Human alveolar macrophages	Exposure to coal dust stimulated release of TNF and IL-6 but not IL-1. Silica (100 μg/ml) stimulated TNF release, but to a lesser extent than coal. Silica did not stimulate IL-6 release. Titanium dioxide had a minimal effect on TNF and IL-6 release. Mineral dust did not stimulate release of IL-1 protein.	150
Rat alveolar macrophages	Silica, chrysotile, and crocidolite (~250 μg/ml) stimulated release of IL-1-like activity and fibroblasts proliferation activity. Combining mineral dust exposure with LPS resulted in a synergistic increase in IL-1 activity.	160
Rat alveolar macrophages	Silica and asbestos stimulated release of IL-1-like activity from unfractionated and density fractionated macrophages. Titanium dioxide did not stimulate release of IL-1 activity.	161
Rat alveolar macrophages	Silica and crocidolite asbestos (10–300 μg/ml) stimulated release of TNF but not IL-1. Treatment with similar doses of titanium dioxide or aluminum oxide did not stimulate TNF or IL-1 release.	151
Rat alveolar macrophages	Silica and asbestos (20–100 μg/ml) stimulated release of TNF and leukotriene B4 (LTB4); latex beads did not stimulate this response. Inhibition of LTB4 release attenuated mineral dust-induced TNF release.	152
Rat alveolar macrophages	Silica stimulated release of IL-1-like activity. Release of IL-1 was attenuated by the antifibrotic drug tetrandrine.	162
THP-1 cells (myelomonocytic cell line)	Silica (100 and 1000 μg/ml) stimulated TNF gene transcription and release of TNF protein.	153

release), rat or human alveolar macrophage production of TNFα, but not IL-1, was increased.[150,151] That silica may be more effective in activating alveolar macrophages to release TNFα compared to IL-1 is not entirely surprising considering studies on the relative expression of these cytokines by monocytes and macrophages.[163–166,190,191] *In vitro* LPS stimulates monocytes to produce large amounts of IL-1 and relatively low levels of TNFα and the IL-1 receptor antagonist protein (IRAP). In contrast, activated alveolar macrophages release high levels of TNFα and IRAP but relatively little IL-1. *In vitro* when monocytes are made to differentiate into macrophage-like cells their IL-1 and IRAP releasing profiles become more like that of alveolar macrophages.[166] Recently it was demonstrated that the inability of alveolar macrophages to release IL-1 may be due to impaired processing of the IL-1 precursor protein.[167] Overall, these studies suggest alveolar macrophages may be more responsive to silica by releasing TNFα than IL-1. However, after silica exposure *in vivo* there is a significant recruitment of monocytes to the lung and these recruited cells may then be important sources of IL-1 in silicosis.

Research characterizing responses to silica *in vivo* has demonstrated increased TNFα and/or IL-1 expression in lung tissue or by lung cells. Using a murine model of silicosis, Piguet and co-workers[137] reported that instillation of 2 mg silica increased steady-state levels of TNFα mRNA in lung. However, they detected no change in IL-1 gene expression. Studies in our laboratory have demonstrated that intratracheal instillation of rats with silica increased macrophage TNFα and IL-1 production, whereas, exposure to relatively innocuous dusts, such as titanium dioxide, has no (IL-1) or minimal effect (TNFα) on release of these cytokines.[168] More recently we demonstrated that, in addition to acute instillation exposure, subchronic inhalation of 1 mg/m^3 cristobalite silica increased steady-state levels of TNFα mRNA in rat lung.[169] Several other studies using shorter-term silica inhalation exposures demonstrated rat alveolar macrophages are "primed" to release increased amounts of IL-1 and TNFα upon subsequent *ex vivo* stimulation with LPS.[170–173] The ability of silica exposure to prime macrophages for cytokine release clearly indicates a change in the lung macrophage population; however, the implications of this response for involvement of IL-1 and TNFα in silica elicited lung effects are not clear.

In toto, *in vitro* and *in vivo* studies demonstrate silica increases release of TNFα and IL-1 in the lung. The TNFα response results, at least in part, from a direct effect of silica on the macrophages, and macrophage responsiveness may be influenced by mediators such as LTB4. Silica may also directly stimulate alveolar macrophages to release IL-1; however, because of the relatively greater capacity of monocytes to release this cytokine, silica increases in IL-1 *in vivo* may be dependent on recruitment of monocytes.

B. SILICA-INDUCED FIBROSIS

A study by Piguet and co-workers[137] has provided compelling evidence that TNFα plays an important role in silica-induced fibrosis. These investigators passively immunized mice with an anti-TNFα IgG (control animals were treated with saline or a nonimmune IgG) and then intratracheally instilled silica. Control animals developed silicosis characterized histologically by the presence of fibrotic nodules and biochemically by increased lung hydroxyproline, a marker of collagen. Using this model the development of silicosis was associated with increased expression of TNFα mRNA in lung. Pretreatment of silica exposed mice with anti-TNFα IgG prevented the increase in lung collagen. Using a similar approach these same investigators demonstrated that passive immunization of mice with anti-TNFα IgG attenuates bleomycin-induced pulmonary fibrosis.[138] These findings indicate a causal relationship between increased TNFα and fibrosis in this murine model of silicosis. While there is a paucity of information on TNFα expression in humans with silicosis, recent studies indicate that alveolar macrophages from individuals with asbestosis or coal workers pneumoconiosis are activated to release increased amounts of TNFα.[175,176]

Based on the bioactivities of TNFα one can postulate several mechanisms by which this cytokine contributes to silica-induced fibrosis. As suggested by Piguet and co-workers,[137] TNFα may act directly on fibroblasts, stimulating their proliferation and collagen deposition. This possibility is supported, at least in part, by *in vitro* data demonstrating TNFα under some conditions can stimulate proliferation of fibroblasts from a number of species including mouse (see Table 3). In addition, while *in vitro* studies have suggested TNFα may have an inhibitory effect on collagen synthesis (see Table 4), *in vivo* studies indicate TNFα increased collagen deposition. The discrepancy between the *in vitro* and *in vivo* observations suggest TNFα may affect collagen deposition *in vivo* indirectly, potentially by stimulating release of other cytokines or recruitment of cells which are more proximate effectors of increased collagen synthesis. In this respect, there is evidence that TNFα can stimulate recruitment of inflammatory cells, and recent studies suggest that blocking inflammatory cell infiltration significantly attenuates adverse pulmonary responses to silica including fibrosis.[148,177]

C. INFLAMMATORY CELL RECRUITMENT

Neutrophils have been proposed to play an important role in the pathogenesis of interstitial lung disease through their ability to release a variety of mediators such as reactive oxygen species and proteolytic enzymes which can damage lung tissue.[178,179] More recently, neutrophils have been recognized as potentially important sources of cytokines and growth factors.[43,180,181] A recent study by Henderson and co-workers[148] provided evidence that neutrophils play an important role in lung injury after silica exposure. These investigators depleted rats of neutrophils using a specific anti-sera and exposed neutrophil

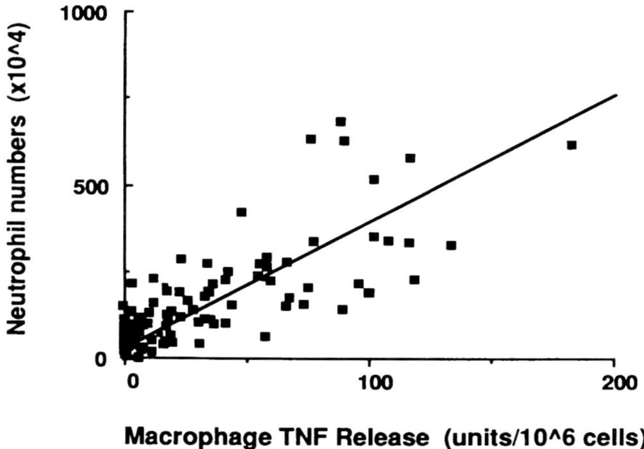

FIGURE 1 Correlation between mineral dust-induced neutrophil recruitment and alveolar macrophage TNFα release. F344 rats were intratracheally instilled with crystalline silica (α quartz) or titanium dioxide at doses of 5, 10, 50, and 100 mg dust/kg body weight. Animals were killed at 1, 7, 14, and 28 d after exposure, bronchoalveolar lavage (BAL) performed, and lavage cell number and type determined. Alveolar macrophages obtained by BAL were cultured for 24 h and spontaneous release of TNFα determined. Regression analysis of BAL neutrophil number vs. *ex vivo* macrophage TNFα release demonstrated a significant positive correlation ($P < 0.001$) with a correlation coefficient of 0.81. (Modified from Driscoll, K.E., et al., *Am. J. Respir. Cell Mol. Biol.,* 2, 381, 1990.)

depleted and nondepleted animals to silica. In neutrophil depleted animals there was no significant neutrophilic inflammation and a reduced cytotoxic response to silica as compared to non-neutrophil depleted rats. Along these same lines, results from a recent study demonstrated that blocking inflammatory cell recruitment in silica exposed mice by treatment with anti-CD11 antibodies attenuates development of silicosis.[177] These studies indicate that inflammatory cells play an important role in the pathogenesis of silicosis.

1. TNFα and Neutrophil Recruitment

As mentioned above, intratracheal instillation of silica increases TNFα production by alveolar macrophages.[137,168] Figure 1 summarizes some of our results,[168,182] demonstrating a positive correlation between neutrophilic inflammation in the lung and increased alveolar macrophage TNFα production after exposure of rats to silica or titanium dioxide. Given the bioactivities of TNFα (i.e., increased adhesion molecule expression and chemokine release), this correlation suggested TNFα was involved in the neutrophilic response to silica. In subsequent studies we have obtained additional evidence that the correlation between macrophage TNFα production and the presence of neutrophils reflects a cause and effect relationship. Briefly, rats were passively immunized with anti-TNFα antibody followed by acute inhalation exposure to silica. Twenty-four hours after silica, neutrophil recruitment was assessed by analysis of bronchoalveolar lavage fluid. As shown in Figure 2, the silica-induced neutrophil response was markedly attenuated by passive immunization with anti-TNFα; treatment with a nonimmune antisera did not attenuate this response. These findings indicate that TNFα is responsible, at least in part, for silica-induced neutrophil recruitment. It is noteworthy that passive immunization against TNFα did not completely abrogate the neutrophil response suggesting that additional, non-TNFα mediated mechanisms are also active in silica-induced inflammatory cell recruitment.

The above studies demonstrate TNFα is an important factor in mineral dust-induced inflammation. However, the mechanism by which TNFα facilitates this response is presently unknown. TNFα can increase expression of leukocyte adhesion proteins on endothelial cells as well as stimulate release of specific chemotactic factors for inflammatory cells (summarized in section III). To better understand the mechanisms of TNFα-induced neutrophil recruitment, we investigated the role of the chemokines, macrophage inflammatory protein 1α (MIP-1α), and macrophage inflammatory protein 2 (MIP-2), in lung inflammation after silica.[183] MIP-1α and MIP-2 are TNFα-inducible cytokines previously identified in the rat and mouse.[77,91,93] *In vitro,* MIP-2 and MIP-1α are chemotactic for neutrophils.[77,92] *In vivo* administration of either cytokine is associated with a localized neutrophilic response and in the case of

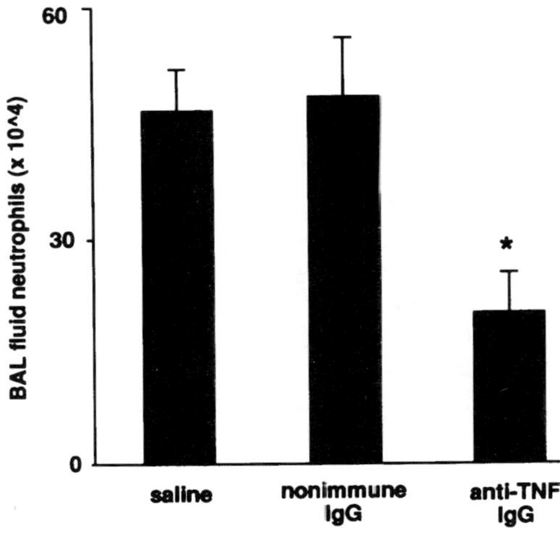

FIGURE 2 Passive immunization with anti-TNF IgG attenuates silica-induced neutrophil recruitment. Groups of six F344 rats were injected via the tail vein with either 400 µl of saline, a non-immune IgG (750 µg), or an anti-murine TNF IgG (750 µg) (Genzyme). Eighteen hours later, three animals with each pretreatment were exposed to air (control) or 100 mg/m^3 silica for 6 h. Twenty-four hours after silica or air-sham inhalation exposure, animals were killed, the lungs lavaged, and the number of neutrophils in the bronchoalveolar lavage fluid determined. No increase in neutrophils was observed for the air control groups. Silica exposure resulted in a marked increase in BAL neutrophils; however, pretreatment with anti-TNF IgG significantly attenuated this response; $p < 0.01$.

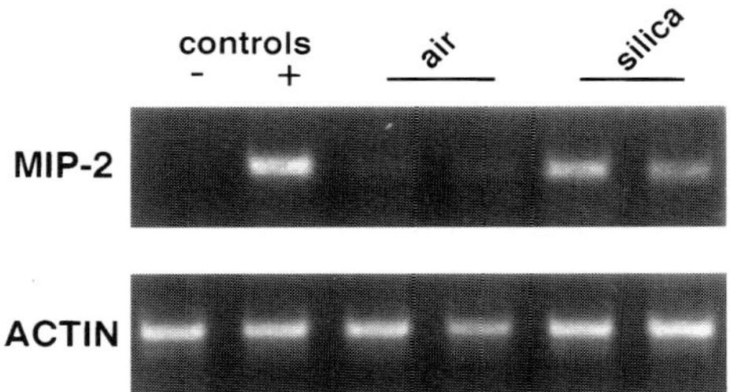

FIGURE 3 Subchronic silica inhalation increases MIP-2 expression in rat lung. Ethidium bromide stained gels showing MIP-2 and β-actin PCR products (N = 2 rats) amplified from 1 µg RNA from the lungs of rats after a 13 week inhalation exposure to air or cristobalite silica (see Reference 184 for details). (+) and (–) control lanes represent MIP expression detected in total lung RNA from LPS instilled and normal rats, respectively. PCR analysis for MIP-2 was performed as described previously by Driscoll and coworkers.[183] Silica inhalation increased levels of MIP-2 mRNA expression in lung tissue. No changes in β-actin mRNA expression were detected.

MIP-1α, also a monocytic response.[77,92,93] Our studies demonstrated that expression of MIP-1α and MIP-2 mRNA is increased in rat lung after intratracheal instillation of silica and titanium dioxide at doses which stimulate TNFα release.[183] We observed a similar relationship between silica exposure, TNFα production, and MIP mRNA expression with longer-term silica inhalation.[169] As shown in Plate 1* a and b, inhalation of 1 mg/m^3 cristobalite silica (6 h/d × 5 d/week × 13 weeks) resulted in increased pulmonary expression of immunoreactive TNF in lung tissue with minimal TNF detected in lungs from air exposed control animals. Lung tissue from identically exposed animals demonstrated increased expression of MIP-2 mRNA after silica exposure relative to air control animals (Figure 3).

Previous studies have shown that MIP-1α is expressed by macrophages in response to TNFα but not by fibroblasts or epithelial cells; in contrast, MIP-2 is expressed by all three of these cell types.[183] These results suggest that tissue structural cells may act as effectors of inflammation through release of MIP-2.

* Plate 1 follows page 178.

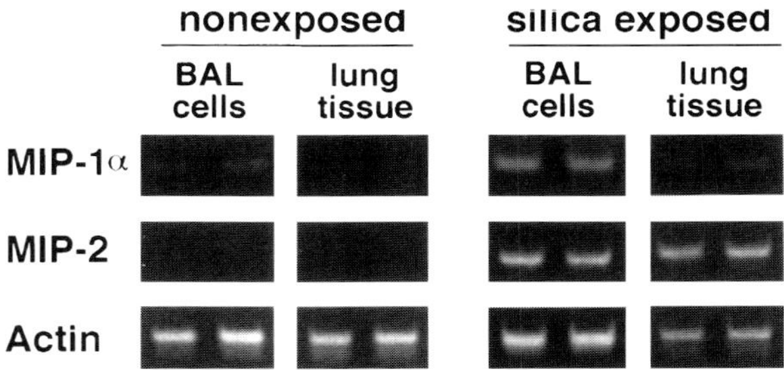

FIGURE 4 MIP-1α and MIP-2 mRNA expression in BAL cells and lavaged lungs tissue after silica. Ethidium bromide stained gels showing MIP-1α, MIP-2, and β-actin PCR products (N = 2 rats) amplified from 1 μg RNA obtained from either bronchoalveolar lavage (BAL) cells, lavaged lung tissue from nonexposed control rats, or from rats 6 h after intratracheal instillation of 10 mg/kg body weight silica (α quartz). Minimal (MIP-1α) or no (MIP-2) mRNA expression was detected in BAL cells or lung tissue from nonexposed control animals. After silica, increased MIP-1α mRNA expression was associated primarily with BAL cells. In contrast to MIP-1α, increased MIP-2 mRNA expression was similar for BAL cells and lavaged lung tissue after silica. (Modified from Driscoll, K.E., et al., *Am. J. Respir. Cell. Mol. Biol.*, 8, 311, 1993.)

Studies summarized in Figure 4, support a role for tissue structural cells as a source of chemokines in silica-induced inflammation. Briefly, after instillation of rats with silica, increased MIP-1α expression was detected in BAL cells and not lung tissue which was lavaged extensively to remove free macrophages and other inflammatory cells. In contrast, MIP-2 expression was elevated in both BAL cells and extensively lavaged lung. This pattern of response indicates that MIP-2 is expressed by cells not removed by lavage and not expressing MIP-1α (e.g., fibroblasts and epithelial cells), suggesting tissue structural cells are contributing to MIP-2 expression in silica exposed rat lungs. In summary, the studies on silica, TNFα, and MIP cytokines indicate that silica elicits recruitment of neutrophils and likely other inflammatory cells, at least partly, by stimulating macrophages to release TNFα (Figure 5). TNFα then may act via autocrine and paracrine pathways to stimulate release of chemotactic cytokines like MIP-1α and MIP-2 and, in conjunction with increased adhesion molecules expression, results in an infiltration of inflammatory cells into lung tissue.

2. Granulomatous Inflammation

A prominent feature of silica exposure is development of a granulomatous response characterized by compact focal collections of macrophages typically in close association with lymphocytes, fibroblasts, and collagen.[149,168] Recent studies provide experimental support for a role of IL-1 and TNFα in the granulomatous response to silica.[168] We demonstrated prominent pulmonary granulomas in rats occurred only at silica exposure levels which result in a persistent stimulation of IL-1 and TNFα release. That IL-1 and TNFα contribute to the pathogenesis of granulomatous inflammation is supported by a number of studies.[135,185–188] In addition to silica, increased IL-1 and/or TNFα in lung has been associated with granulomas induced by Sephadex beads,[185] antigen coated beads,[186] and Schistosome eggs.[187] Dunn and co-workers[135] provided direct evidence for a role of IL-1 and TNFα in granuloma formation. These investigators demonstrated that intradermal injection of recombinant IL-1 in slow release ethylene vinyl acetate copolymer resulted in a localized granulomatous response. Using a similar approach, Kasahara and colleagues[185,188] showed that intratracheal injection of sepharose beads coated with recombinant IL-1 or TNFα, but not IL-2 or γ interferon, produced large pulmonary granulomas. In the silica exposed lung, it is likely that the activation of macrophages and monocytes to release TNFα and IL-1 at sites of silica deposition, combined with the inability of the macrophages to effectively clear the silica particles, results in high focal concentrations of IL-1 and TNFα. Given IL-1 is chemotactic for T-helper lymphocytes and TNFα and IL-1 can activate a variety of processes (see Tables 1 and 2) that would facilitate recruitment of lymphocytes and monocytes, it is not unexpected that these cytokines play a role in silica-induced granulomas.

VI. SUMMARY

IL-1 and TNFα are multifunctional cytokines which play a key role in many physiologic and pathophysiologic processes. Several studies have demonstrated that crystalline silica *in vitro* and/or *in*

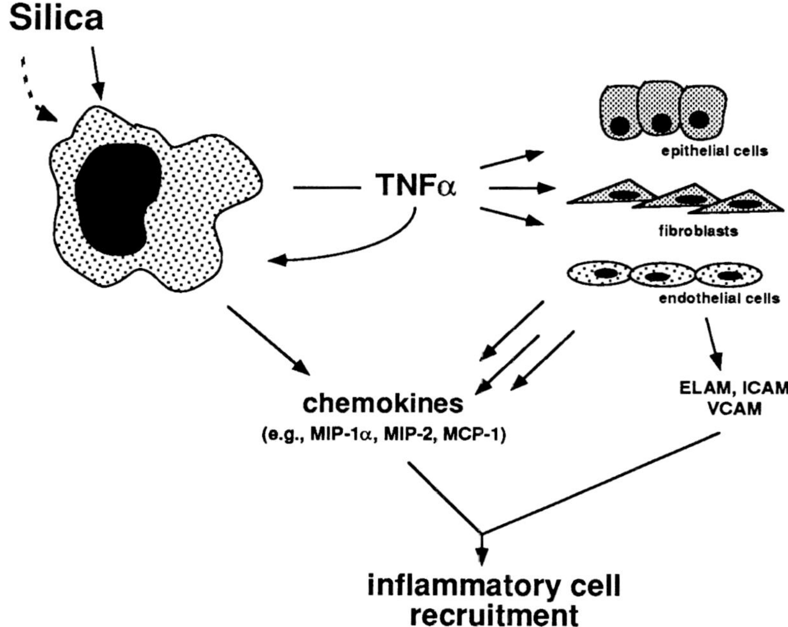

FIGURE 5 Role of TNFα in silica-induced inflammatory cell recruitment. Silica particles activate alveolar macrophages to release TNFα. TNFα acts via paracrine and autocrine pathways to stimulate release of chemokines by tissue structural cells (i.e., epithelial cells, fibroblasts, and endothelial cells) and macrophages, as well as increase expression of adhesion molecules (i.e., ELAM, ICAM, and VCAM) on endothelial cells. Inflammatory cells interact with adhesion molecules on vascular endothelium and migrate along chemotactic gradients into the lung interstitium and airspaces.

vivo can stimulate release of TNFα and IL-1 by lung cells. There is convincing evidence that TNFα contributes to collagen accumulation following silica exposure. However, the exact mechanism by which TNF is influencing the fibrotic response is not yet clear. TNFα could increase collagen accumulation by multiple mechanisms including acting directly to stimulate proliferation and/or collagen synthesis by fibroblasts, or TNFα could act indirectly by stimulating the release of other mediators or the recruitment of cells more directly responsible for development of the fibrotic lesion. In respect to the latter, TNFα has been shown to play an important role in the recruitment of neutrophils to the lung after silica exposure. Here the effect of TNFα likely results from a network of cell:cell interactions involving, at least in part, TNFα-induced production of potent chemotactic peptides by macrophages and tissue structural cells in the lung. It is likely that IL-1 and TNFα also contribute to increased lymphocytes, macrophages, and ultimately to granulomatous inflammation resulting from silica exposure. IL-1 is directly chemotactic for T-cells, the predominant lymphocyte type increased by silica, and both IL-1 and TNFα can induce expression of other lymphocyte or monocyte chemotactic cytokines such as IL-8, MCP-1, and MIP-1α. Several investigators have provided direct evidence that IL-1 and TNFα are key to the pathogenesis of granulomatous inflammation. Recent studies demonstrating an association between silica-induced granuloma formation and IL-1 and TNFα production provide experimental support that these cytokines also contribute to this aspect of the lung's response to silica.

REFERENCES

1. **Atkins, E.,** Pathogenesis of fever, *Physiol. Rev.,* 40, 580, 1960.
2. **Dinarello, C. A. and Wolff, S. M.,** Molecular basis of fever in humans, *Am. J. Med.,* 72, 799, 1982.
3. **Kampschmidt, R. F.,** *Infection: The physiological and metabolic responses of the Host,* Powanda, M.C. and Canonico, P.G., Eds., Elsevier/North-Holland, Amsterdam, 1982, 55.

4. **Gery, I., Davies, P., Derr, I., Krett, N., and Barranger, J. A.,** Relationship between production and release of lymphocyte-activating factor (interleukin 1) by murine macrophages. Effects of various agents, *Cell. Immunol.*, 64, 293, 1981.
5. **Rosenwasser, L. J., Dinarello, C. A., and Rosenthal, A. S.,** Adherent cell function in murine T-lymphocyte antigen recognition. IV. Enhancement of murine T-cell antigen recognition by human leukocytic pyrogen, *J. Exp. Med.*, 150, 709, 1979.
6. **Murphy, P. A., Simon, P. L., and Willoughby, W. F.,** Endogenous pyrogens made by rabbit peritoneal exudate cells are identical with lymphocyte-activating factors made by rabbit alveolar macrophages, *J. Immunol.*, 124, 2498, 1980.
7. **Stein, M. B., Vogel, S. N., Sipe, J. D., Murphy, P. A., Mizel, S. B., Oppenheim, O. J. J., and Rosenstreich, D. L.,** The role of macrophages in the acute-phase response: SAA inducer is closely related to lymphocyte activating factor and endogenous pyrogen, *Cell. Immunol.*, 63, 164, 1981.
8. **Aarden, L. A., Brunner, T. K., Cerottini, J.-C., Dayer, J.-M., deWeck, A. L., Dinarello, C. A., DiSabato, G., Farrar, J. J., Gery, I., Gillis, S., Handschumacher, R. E., Henney, C. S., Hoffmann, M. K., Koopman, W. J., Krane, S. M., Lachman, L. B., Lefkowits, I., Mishell, R. I., Mizel, S. B., Oppenheim, J. J., Paetkau, V., Plate, J., Röllinghoff, M., Rosenstreich, D., Rosenthal, A. S., Rosenwasser, L. J., Schimpl, A., Shim, H. S., Simon, P. L., Smith, K. A., Wagner, H., Watson, J. D., Wecker, E., and Wood, D. D.,** Revised nomenclature for antigen-non-specific T-cell proliferation and helper factors [letter], *J. Immunol.*, 123, 2928, 1979.
9. **Auron, P. E., Webb, A. C., Rosenwasserr, L. J., Mucci, S. F., Rich, A., Wolfe, S. M., and Dinarello, C. A.,** Nucleotide sequence of human monocyte interleukin 1 precursor cDNA, *Proc. Natl. Acad. Sci. U.S.A.*, 81, 7907, 1984.
10. **Lomedico, P. T., Gubler, U., Hellmann, C., Kukovich, M., Giri, J. G., Pan, Y.-C. E., Collier, K., Semionow, R., Chua, A. O., and Mizel, S. B.,** Cloning and expression of murine interleukin-1 cDNA in *Escherichia coli, Nature,* 312, 438, 1984.
11. **Cameron, P. M., Limjuco, G. A., Chin, J., Silberstein, L., and Schmidt, J. A.,** Purification to homogeneity and amino acid sequence analysis of two anionic species of human interleukin 1, *J. Exp. Med.*, 164, 237, 1986.
12. **March, C. J., Mosley, B., Larsen, A., Cerretti, D. P., Braedt, G., Price, V., Gillis, S., Henney, C. S., Kronheim, S. R., Grabstein, K., Conlon, P. J., Hopp, T. P., and Cosman, D.,** Cloning, sequence and expression of two distinct human interleukin-1 complementary cDNAs, *Nature,* 315, 641, 1985.
13. **Akira, S., Hirano, T., Taga, T., and Kishimoto, T.,** Biology of multifunctional cytokines: IL 6 and related molecules (IL 1 and TNF), *FASEB J.*, 4, 2862, 1990.
14. **Dinarello, C. A.,** Biology of interleukin 1, *FASEB J.*, 2, 108, 1988.
15. **Gubler, U., Chua, A. O., Stern, A. S., Hellmann, C. P., Vitek, M. P., Dechiara, T. M., Benjamin, W. R., Collier, K. J., Dukovich, M., Familletti, P. C., Fiedler-Nagy, C., Jenson, J., Kaffka, K., Kilian, P. L., Stremlo, D., Wittreich, B. H., Woehle, D., Mizel, S. B., and Lomedico, P. T.,** Recombinant human interleukin 1α: purification and biological characterization, *Immunology,* 136, 2492, 1986.
16. **Thornberry, N. A., Bull, H. G., Calaycay, J. R., Chapman, K. T., Howard, A. D., Kostura, M. J., Miller, D. K., Molineaux, S. M., Weidner, J. R., Aunins, J., Elliston, K. O., Ayala, J. M., Casano, F. J., Chin, J., Ding, G. J. F., Egger, L. A., Gaffney, E. P., Limjuco, G., Palyha, O. C., Raju, S. M., Rolando, A. M., Salley, J. P., Yamin, T.-T., Lee, T. D., Shively, J. E., MacCross, M., Mumford, R. A., Schmidt, J. A., and Tocci, M. J.,** A novel heretodimeric cysteine protease is required for interleukin-1β processing in monocytes, *Nature,* 356, 768, 1992.
17. **Lepe-Zuniga, J. L. and Gery, I.,** Production of intra- and extracellular interleukin-1 (IL-1) by human monocytes, *Clin. Immunol. Immunopathol.*, 31, 222, 1984.
18. **Matsushima, K., Taguchi, M., Kovacs, E. J., Young, H. A., and Oppenheim, J. J.,** Intracellular localization of human monocyte associated interleukin 1 (IL 1) activity and release of biologically active IL 1 from monocytes by trypsin and plasmin, *J. Immunol.*, 136, 2883, 1986.
19. **Kurt-Jones, E. A., Beller, D. I., Mizel, S. B., and Unanue, E. R.,** Identification of a membrane-associated interleukin 1, *Proc. Natl. Acad. Sci. U.S.A.*, 82, 1204, 1985.
20. **Nagelkerken, L. M., and van Breda Vriesman, P. J. C.,** Membrane-associated IL 1-like activity on rat dendritic cells, *J. Immunol.*, 6, 2164, 1986.
21. **Tiku, K., Tiku, M. L., and Skosey, J. L.,** Interleukin-1 production by human polymorphonuclear neutrophils, *J. Immunol.*, 136, 3677, 1986.
22. **Sauder, D. N.,** Epidermal-derived cytokines: properties of epidermal-derived thymocyte activating factor, *Lymphokine Res.*, 3, 145, 1985.
23. **Libby, R., Ordovas, J. M., Auger, K. R., Robbins, A. H., Birinyl, L. K., and Dinarello, C. A.,** Inducible interleukin-1 gene expression in vascular smooth muscle cells, *J. Clin. Invest.*, 78, 1432, 1986.
24. **Libby, R., Ordovas, J. M., Auger, K. R., Robbins, A. H., Birinyl, L. K., and Dinarello, C. A.,** Endotoxin and tumor necrosis factor induce interleukin-1 gene expression in adult human vascular endothelial cells, *Am. J. Pathol.*, 124, 179, 1986.
25. **Akahosi, T., Oppenheim, J. J., and Matsushima, K.,** Interleukin-1 stimulates its own receptor expression on human fibroblasts through the endogenous production of prostaglandin(s), *J. Clin. Invest.*, 82, 1219, 1988.
26. **Scala, G., Allavena, P., Djeu, et al.,** Human large granular lymphocytes are potent producers of interleukin-1, *Nature,* 309, 56, 1984.

27. **Coley, W. B.,** Late results of the treatment of inoperable sarcoma by the mixed toxins of erysipelas and Bacillus prodigious, *Am. J. Med. Sci.,* 131, 487, 1906.
28. **Shear, M. J.,** Chemical treatment of tumors. IX. Reactions of mice with primary subcutaneous tumors to injections of a hemorrhage-producing bacterial polysaccharide, *J. Natl. Cancer Inst.,* 4, 461, 1944.
29. **Carswell, E. A., Old, L. J., Kassel, R. L., Green, S., Fiore, N., and Williamson, B.,** An endotoxin-induced serum factor that causes necrosis of tumors, *Proc. Natl. Acad. Sci. U.S.A.,* 72, 3666, 1975.
30. **Pennica, D., Nedwin, G. E., Hayflick, J. S., Seeburg, P. H., Derynck, R., Palladino, M. A., Kohr, W. J., Aggarwal, B. B., and Goeddel, D. V.,** Human tumor necrosis factor: precursor structure, expression and homology to lymphotoxin, *Nature,* 312, 724, 1984.
31. **Marmenout, A., Fransen, L., Tavernier, J., Van der Heyden, J., Tizard, R., Kawashima, E., Shaw, A., Johnson, M. J., Semon, D., Muller, R., Ruysschaert, M. R., Van Vliet, A., and Fiers, W.,** Molecular cloning and expression of human tumor necrosis factor and comparison with mouse tumor necrosis factor, *Eur. J. Biochem.,* 152, 515, 1985.
32. **Shirai, T., Yamaguchi, H., Ito, H., Todd, C. W., and Wallace, R. B.,** Cloning and expression in *Escherichia coli* of the gene for human tumour necrosis factor, *Nature,* 313, 803, 1985.
33. **Fransen, L., Muller, R., Marmenout, A., Tavernier, J., Van der Heyden, J., Kawashima, E., Chollet, A., Tizard, R., Van Heuverswyn, H., Van Vliet, A., Ruysschaert, M. R., and Fiers, W.,** Molecular cloning of mouse tumour necrosis factor cDNA and its eukaryotic expression, *Nucleic Acids Res.,* 13, 4417, 1985.
34. **Kawakami, M., and Cerami, A.,** Studies of endotoxin-induced decrease in lipoprotein lipase activity, *J. Exp. Med.,* 154, 631, 1981.
35. **Beutler, B., Mahoney, J., LeTrang, N., Pekala, P., and Cerami, A.,** Purification of cachectin a lipoprotein lipase-suppressing hormone secreted by endotoxin-induced raw-264.7 cells, *J. Exp. Med.,* 161, 984, 1985.
36. **Beutler, B., Greenwald, D., Hulmes, J. D., Chang, M., Pan, Y.-C. E., Mathison, J., Ulvetich, R., and Cerami, A.,** Identity of tumor necrosis factor and the macrophage secreted factor cachectin, *Nature,* 316, 552, 1985.
37. **Carroll, M. C., Katzman, P., Alicot, E. M., Koller, B. H., Geraghty, D. E., Orr, H. T., Strominger, J. L., and Spies, T.,** Linkage map of the human major histocompatibility complex including the tumor necrosis factor genes, *Proc. Natl. Acad. Sci. U.S.A.,* 84, 8535, 1987.
38. **Sargent, C. A., Dunham, I., Trowsdae, J., and Cambell, R. D.,** Human major histocompatibility complex contains genes for the major heat shock protein HSP70, *Proc. Natl. Acad. Sci. U.S.A.,* 86, 1967, 1989.
39. **Muller, U., Jongeneel, C. V., Nedospasov, S. A., Lindahl, K. F., and Steinmetz, M.,** Tumour necrosis factor and lymphotoxin genes map close to H-2D in the mouse major histocompatibility complex, *Nature,* 325, 265, 1987.
40. **Wang, A. M., Creasey, A. A., Ladner, M. B., Lin, L. S., Strickler, J., Van Arsdell, J. N., Yamamoto, R., and Mark, D. F.,** Molecular cloning of the complementary DNA from human tumor necrosis factor, *Science,* 228, 149, 1985.
41. **Aggarwal, B. B., Eessalu, T. E., and Hass, P. E.,** Characterization of receptors for human tumor necrosis factor and their regulation by γ-interferon, *Nature,* 318, 665, 1985.
42. **Granger, G. A. and Kolb, W. P.,** Lymphocyte *in vitro* cytotoxicity: mechanisms of immune and non-immune small lymphocyte mediated target L cell destruction, *J. Immunol.,* 116, 111, 1988.
43. **Dubravec, D. B., Spriggs, D. R., Mannick, J. A., and Rodrick, M. L.,** Circulating human peripheral blood granulocytes synthesize and secrete tumor necrosis factor α, *Proc. Natl. Acad. Sci. U.S.A.,* 87, 6758, 1990.
44. **Young, J. D., Liu, C., Butler, G., Cohn, Z. A., and Galli, S. J.,** Identification, purification, and characterization of a mast cell-associated cytolytic factor related to tumor necrosis factor, *Proc. Natl. Acad. Sci. U.S.A.,* 84, 9175, 1987.
45. **Warner, S. J. C., and Liby, P.,** Human vascular smooth muscle cells. Target for and source of tumor necrosis factor, *J. Immunol.,* 142, 100, 1989.
46. **Kriegler, M., Perez, C., DeFay, K., Albert, I., and Lu, S. D.,** A novel form of TNF cachectin is a cell surface cytotoxic transmembrane protein: ramifications for the complex physiology of TNF, *Cell,* 53, 45, 1988.
47. **Decker, T., Lohmann-Matthews, M.-L., and Gifford, G. E.,** Cell-associated tumor necrosis factor (TNF) as a killing mechanism of activated cytotoxic macrophages, *J. Immunol.,* 138, 957, 1987.
48. **Espevik, T. and Nissen-Meyer, J. A.,** Tumor necrosis factor like activity on paraformaldehyde-fixed monocyte monolayers, *Immunology,* 61, 443, 1987.
49. **Eck, M. J., Beutler, B., Kuo, G., Merryweather, J. P., and Sprang, S. P.,** Crystallization of trimeric recombinant human tumor necrosis factor (cachectin), *J. Biol. Chem.,* 263, 12816, 1988.
50. **Jones, E. Y., Stuart, D. I., and Walker, N. P. C.,** Structure of tumour necrosis factor, *Nature,* 338, 225, 1989.
51. **Smith, R. A., and Baglioni, C.,** The active form of tumor necrosis factor is a trimer, *J. Biol. Chem.,* 262, 6951, 1987.
52. **Jaattela, M.,** Biology of disease: biologic activities and mechanisms of action of tumor necrosis factor-α/cachectin, *Lab. Invest.,* 64, 724, 1991.
53. **Le, J. and Vilcek, J.,** Biology of disease: tumor necrosis factor and interleukin 1: cytokines with multiple overlapping biological activities, *Lab. Invest.,* 56, 234, 1987.
54. **Sherry, B. and Cerami, A.,** Cachectin/Tumor necrosis factor exerts endocrine, paracrine, and autocrine control of inflammatory responses, *J. Cell. Biol.,* 107, 1269, 1988.
55. **Movat, H. Z.,** Tumor necrosis factor and interleukin-1: role in acute inflammation and microvascular injury, *J. Lab. Clin. Med.,* 110, 668, 1987.

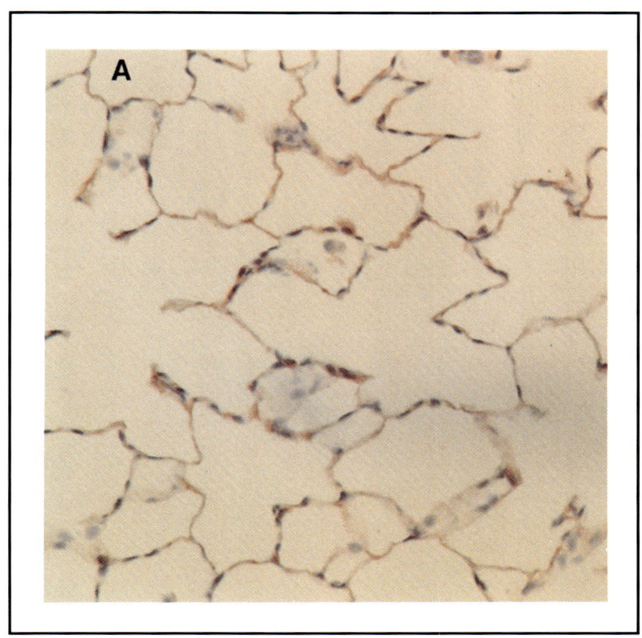

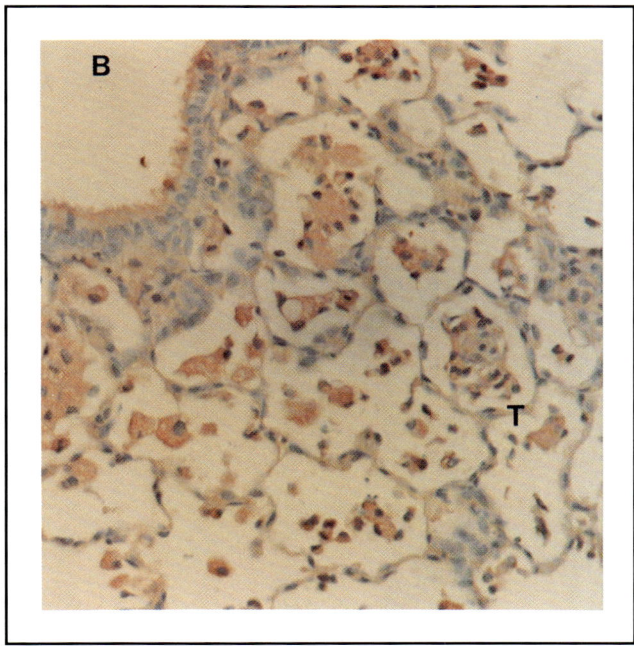

SECTION III, CHAPTER 4, PLATE 1A AND B

Increased TNFα Immunostaining in Lungs of Rats After Subchronic Inhalation of Silica.
F344 rats were exposed to air (control) or 1 mg/m^3 cristobalite silica (see ref. 169 for details), 6h/d × 5d/week for 13 weeks. The cells were identified by immunoperoxidase staining as described by Maurer and coworkers.[184] Aminoethylcarbazole was used as the peroxidase substrate resulting in a red color product; tissue sections are counterstained with hematoxylin and eosin; magnification 100×. (a) air control; (b) silica exposed. Increased immuno-reactive TNF can be seen after silica inhalation in macrophages, epithelial cells and neutrophils.

56. **Wankowicz, Z., Megyeri, P., and Issekutz, A.,** Synergy between tumour necrosis factor α and interleukin-1 in the induction of polymorphonuclear leukocyte migration during inflammation, *J. Leukocyte Biol.*, 43, 349, 1988.
57. **Issekutz, A. C., Megyeri, P., and Issekutz, T. B.,** Role for macrophage products in endotoxin-induced polymorphonuclear leukocyte accumulation during inflammation, *Lab. Invest.*, 56, 49, 1987.
58. **Sayers, T. J., Wiltrout, T. A., Bull, C. A., Denn, A. C., Pilaro, A. M., and Lokesh, B.,** Effects of cytokines on polymorphonuclear infiltration in the mouse, *J. Immunol.*, 141, 1670, 1988.
59. **Ulich, T. R., Watson, L. R., Yin, S., Guo, K., Wang, P., Thang, H., and del Castillo, J.,** The intratracheal administration of endotoxin and cytokines: 1. Characterization of LPS-induced IL-1 and TNF mRNA expression and the LPS-, IL-1-, and TNF-induced inflammatory infiltrate, *Am. J. Pathol.*, 138, 1485, 1991.
60. **Hunninghake, G. W., Glazier, A. J., Monick, M. M., and Dinarello, C. A.,** Interleukin-1 is a chemotactic factor for human T-lymphocytes, *Am. Rev. Respir. Dis.*, 135, 66, 1987.
61. **Gamble, J. R., Harlan, J. M., Klebanoff, S. J., and Vadas, M. A.,** Stimulation of the adherence of neutrophils to umbilical vein endothelium by human recombinant tumor necrosis factor, *Proc. Natl. Acad. Sci. U.S.A.*, 82, 8667, 1985.
62. **Bevilacqua, M. P., Pober, J. S., Wheeler, M. E., Cotran, R. S., and Gimbrone, M. A., Jr.,** Interleukin-1 acts on cultured human vascular endothelium to increase the adhesion of polymorphonuclear leukocytes, monocytes and related leukocytic cell lines, *J. Clin. Invest.*, 76, 2003, 1985.
63. **Bevilacqua, M. P., Stengelin, S., Gimbrone, M. A., Jr., and Seed, B.,** Endothelial leukocyte adhesion molecule 1: an inducible receptor for neutrophils related to complement regulatory proteins and lectins, *Science*, 243, 1160, 1989.
64. **Bevilacqua, M. P., Pober, J. S., Majeau, G. R., Fiers, W., Cotran, R. S., and Gimbrone, M. A.,** Recombinant tumor necrosis factor induces procoagulant activity in cultured human vascular endothelium: characterization and comparison with the actions of interleukin 1, *Proc. Natl. Acad. Sci. U.S.A.*, 83, 4533, 1986.
65. **Bevilacqua, M. P., Pober, J. S., Wheeler, M. E., Cotran, R. S., and Gimbrone, M. A.,** Interleukin-1 activation of vascular endothelium, effects on procoagulant activity and leukocyte adhesion, *Am. J. Pathol.*, 121, 393, 1985.
66. **Pober, J. S., Gimbrone, M. A., Jr., Lapierre, L. A., et al.,** Overlapping patterns of activation of human endothelial cells by interleukin-1, tumor necrosis factor and immune interferon, *J. Immunol.*, 137, 1893, 1986.
67. **Osborn, L., Hession, C., Tizard, R., Vassallo, C., Luhowskyl, S., Ghi-Rosso, G., and Lobb, R.,** Direct expression cloning of vascular cell adhesion molecule 1, a cytokine-induced endothelial protein that binds to lymphocytes, *Cell*, 59, 1203, 1989.
68. **Wallis, W. J., Beatty, P. G., Ochs, H. D., and Harlan, J. M.,** Human monocyte adherence to cultured vascular endothelium: monoclonal antibody-defined mechanisms, *J. Immunol.*, 135, 2323, 1985.
69. **Kishimoto, T. K., Larson, R. S., Corbi, A. L., Dustin, M. L., Staunton, D. E., and Springer, T. A.,** The leukocyte integrins, *Adv. Immunol.*, 46, 149, 1989.
70. **Cotran, R. S. and Pober, J. S.,** Cytokine-endothelial interactions in inflammation, immunity, and vascular injury, *J. Am. Soc. Nephrology*, 1, 225, 1990.
71. **Simmons, D., Makgoba, M. W., and Seed, B.,** ICAM, an adhesion ligand of LFA-1, is homologous to the neural cell adhesion molecule NCAM, *Nature*, 331, 624, 1988.
72. **Haskard, D., Cavender, D., Beatty, P., Springer, T., and Ziff, M.,** T lymphocyte adhesion to endothelial cells: mechanisms demonstrated by anti-LFA-1 monoclonal antibodies, *J. Immunol.*, 137, 2901, 1986.
73. **Dustin, M. L. and Springer, T. A.,** Lymphocyte function-associated antigen-1 (LFA-1) interaction with intercellular adhesion molecule-1 (ICAM-1) is one of at least three mechanisms for lymphocyte adhesion to cultured endothelial cells, *J. Cell Biol.*, 107, 321, 1988.
74. **Walsh, G. M., Mermod, J.-J., Hartnell, A., Kay, A. B., and Wardlaw, A. J.,** Human eosinophil, but not neutrophil, adherence to IL-1-stimulated human umbilical vascular endothelial cells is α4β1 (very late antigen-4) dependent, *J. Immunol.*, 146, 3419, 1991.
75. **Elices, M. J., Osborn, L., Takada, Y., et al.,** VCAM-1 on activated endothelium interacts with the leukocyte integrin VLA-4 at a site distinct from the VLA-4/Fibronectin binding site, *Cell*, 60, 577, 1990.
76. **Kunkel, S. L., Standiford, T., Kasahara, K., and Strieter, R. M.,** Interleukin-8 (IL-8): the major neutrophil chemotactic factor in the lung, *Exp. Lung Res.*, 17, 17, 1991.
77. **Wolpe, S. D. and Cerami, A.,** Macrophage inflammatory proteins 1 and 2: members of a novel superfamily of cytokines, *FASEB J.*, 3, 2565, 1989.
78. **Matsushima, K. and Oppenheim, J. J.,** Interleukin 8 and MCAF: novel inflammatory cytokines inducible by IL1 and TNF, *Cytokine*, 1, 2, 1989.
79. **Strieter, R. M., Kunkel, S. L., Showell, H. J., Remick, D. R., Phan, S. H., Ward, P. A., and Marks, R. M.,** Endothelial cell gene expression of a neutrophil chemotactic factor by TNFα, LPS, and IL-1β, *Science*, 243, 1467, 1989.
80. **Strieter, R. M., Chensue, S. W., Basha, M. A., Standiford, T. J., Lynch, J. P., III, Baggiolini, M., and Kunkel, S. L.,** Human alveolar macrophage expression of IL-8 by tumor necrosis factor-α, lipopolysaccharide, and interleukin-1β, *Am. J. Respir. Cell. Mol. Biol.*, 2, 321, 1990.
81. **Larsen, C. G., Anderson, A. O., Oppenheim, J. J., and Matsushima, K.,** Production of interleukin-8 by dermal fibroblasts and keratinocytes in response to interleukin-1 and tumour necrosis factor, *Immunology*, 68, 31, 1989.

82. **Nakamura, H., Yoshimura, K., Jaffe, H. A., and Crystal, R. G.,** Interleukin-8 gene expression in human bronchial epithelial cells, *J. Biol. Chem.*, 266, 19611, 1991.
83. **Bazzoni, F., Cassatella, M. A., Rossi, F., Ceska, M., Dewald, B., and Baggiolini, M.,** Phagocytosing neutrophils produce and release high amounts of the neutrophil-activating peptide/interleukin-8, *J. Exp. Med.*, 173, 771, 1991.
84. **Rolfe, M. W., Kunkel, S. L., Standiford, T. J., Chensue, S. W., Allen, R. M., Evanoff, H. L., Phan, S. H., and Strieter, R. M.,** Pulmonary fibroblast expression of interleukin-8: a model for alveolar macrophage-derived cytokine networking, *Am. J. Respir. Cell. Mol. Biol.*, 5, 493, 1991.
85. **Rollins, B. J., Morrison, E. D., and Stiles, C. D.,** Cloning and expression of JE, a gene inducible by platelet-derived growth factor and whose product has cytokine-like properties, *Proc. Natl. Acad. Sci. U.S.A.*, 85, 3738, 1988.
86. **Strieter, R. M., Wiggins, R., Phan, S. H., Wharram, B. L., Showell, H. L., Remick, D. G., Chensue, S. W., and Kunkel, S. L.,** Monocyte chemotactic protein gene expression by cytokine-treated human fibroblasts and endothelial cells, *Biochem. Biophys. Res. Commun.*, 162, 694, 1989.
87. **Elner, S. G., Streiter, R. M., Elner, V. M., Rollins, B. J., Del Monte, M. A., and Kunkel, S. L.,** Monocyte chemotactic protein gene expression by cytokine-treated human retinal pigment epithelial cells, *Lab. Invest.*, 64, 819, 1991.
88. **Yoshimura, T., Robinson, E. A., Tanaka, S., Appella, E., and Leonard, E. J.,** Purification and amino acid analysis of two human monocyte chemoattractants produced by phytohemagglutinin-stimulated human blood mononuclear leukocytes, *J. Immunol.*, 142, 1956, 1989.
89. **Yoshimura, T. and Leonard, E. J.,** Secretion by human fibroblasts of monocyte chemoattractant protein-1, the product of gene JE, *J. Immunol.*, 144, 2377, 1990.
90. **Koj, A., Magielska-Zero, D., Bereta, J., Kurdowska, A., Rokita, H., and Gauldie, J.,** The cascade of inflammatory cytokines regulating synthesis of acute phase proteins, *J. Exp. Clin. Med.*, 6, 255, 1988.
91. **Driscoll, K. E., Hassenbein, D., Carter, J., Poynter, J., Asquith, T., Grant, R. A., Whitten, J., Purdon, M., and Takigiku, R.,** Macrophage inflammatory proteins 1 and 2: expression by rat alveolar macrophages, fibroblasts and epithelial cells and in rat lung tissue after mineral dust exposure, *Am. J. Respir. Cell. Mol. Biol.*, 8, 311, 1993.
92. **Wolpe, S. D., Sherry, B., Juers, D., Davatelis, G., Yurt, R. W., and Cerami, A.,** Identification and characterization of macrophage inflammatory protein 2, *Proc. Natl. Acad. Sci. U.S.A.*, 86, 612, 1989.
93. **Davatelis, G., Tekamp-Olson, P., Wolpe, S. D., Hermsen, K., Luedke, C., Gallegos, C., Coit, D., Merryweather, J., and Cerami, A.,** Cloning and characterization of a cDNA for murine macrophage inflammatory protein (MIP), a novel monokine with inflammatory and chemokinetic properties, *J. Exp. Med.*, 167, 1939, 1988.
94. **Watanabe, K. and Nakagawa, H.,** Production of a chemotactic factor for polymorphonuclear leukocytes by epithelioid cells from rat renal glomeruli in culture, *Biochem. Biophys. Res. Commun.*, 149, 989, 1987.
95. **Wen, D., Rowland, A., and Derynck, R.,** Expression and secretion of gro/MGSA by stimulated human endothelial cells, *EMBO J.*, 8, 1761, 1989.
96. **Kohase, M., Henriksen-DeStefano, D., May, L. T., Vilcek, J., and Sehgal, P. B.,** Induction of β_2-interferon by tumor necrosis factor: a homeostatic mechanism in the control of cell proliferation, *Cell*, 45, 659, 1986.
97. **Dinarello, C. A., Cannon, J. G., Wolff, S. M., Bernheim, H. A., Beutler, B., Cerami, A., Figari, I. S., Palladino, M. A., Jr., and O'Connor, J. V.,** Tumor necrosis factor (cachectin) is an endogenous pyrogen and induces production of interleukin 1, *J. Exp. Med.*, 163, 1433, 1986.
98. **Philip, R. and Epstein, L. B.,** Tumour necrosis factor as immunomodulator and mediator of monocyte cytoxicity induced by itself, gamma-interferon and interleukin-1, *Nature*, 323, 86, 1986.
99. **Nawroth, P. P., Bank, I., Handley, D., Cassimeris, J., Chess, L., and Stern, D.,** Tumor necrosis factor/cachectin interacts with endothelial cell receptors to induce release of interleukin 1, *J. Exp. Med.*, 163, 1363, 1986.
100. **Camussi, G., Bussolino, F., Salvidio, G., and Baglioni, C.,** Tumor necrosis factor/cachectin stimulates peritoneal macrophages, polymorphonuclear neutrophils, and vascular endothelial cells to synthesize and release platelet-activating factor, *J. Exp. Med.*, 166, 1390, 1987.
101. **Bussolino, F., Camussi, G., and Baglioni, C.,** Synthesis and release of platelet-activating factor by human vascular endothelial cells treated with tumor necrosis factor or interleukin 1α, *J. Biol. Chem.*, 263, 11856, 1988.
102. **Kawakami, M., Hishibashi, S., Ogawa, H., Murase, T., Takaku, F., and Shibata, S.,** Cachectin/TNF as well as interleukin-1 induces prostacyclin synthesis in cultured vascular endothelial cells, *Biochem. Biophys. Res. Commun.*, 141, 482, 1986.
103. **Dayer, J.-M., Beutler, B., and Cerami, A.,** Cachectin/tumor necrosis factor: stimulates collagenase and prostaglandin E2 by human synovial cells and dermal fibroblasts, *J. Exp. Med.*, 162, 2163, 1985.
104. **Bussolino, F., Breviario, F., Tetta, C., Aglietta, M., Sanavio, F., Mantovani, A., and Dejana, E.,** Interleukin 1 stimulates platelet activating factor production in cultured human endothelial cells, *Pharmacol. Res. Commun.*, 18, 133, 1986.
105. **Klebanoff, S. J., Vadas, M. A., Harlan, J. M., Sparks, L. H., Gamble, J. R., Agosti, J. M., and Waltersdorph, A. M.,** Stimulation of neutrophils by tumor necrosis factor, *J. Immunol.*, 136, 4220, 1986.
106. **Klempner, M. S., Dinarello, C. A., and Gallin, J. I.,** Human leukocytic pyrogen induces release of specific granule contents from human neutrophils, *J. Clin. Invest.*, 61, 1330, 1978.

107. **Das, U. N., Padma, M., Sangeetha, A., Sagar, P., Ramesh, G., and Koratkar, R.,** Stimulation of free radical generation in human leukocytes by various agents including tumor necrosis factor is a calmodulin dependent process, *Biochem. Biophys. Res. Commun.*, 167, 1030, 1990.
108. **Hoffman, M. and Weinbert, J. B.,** Tumor necrosis factor-α induces increased hydrogen peroxide production and fc receptor expression, but not increased la antigen expression by peritoneal macrophages, *J. Leukocyte Biol.*, 42, 704, 1987.
109. **Ozaki, Y., Ohashi, T., and Kume, S.,** Potentiation of neutrophil function by recombinant DNA-produced interleukin 1α, *J. Leukocyte Biol.*, 42, 621, 1987.
110. **Schwartz, L. W., Yem, A. W., and Marshall, P. J.,** IL-1β induced alveolar macrophage production of LTB_4, *J. Cell Biochem.*, 14, 337, 1990.
111. **Tsujimoto, M., Yokota, S., Vilcek, J., Weissmann, G.,** Tumor necrosis factor provokes superoxide anion generation from neutrophils, *Biochem. Biophys. Res. Commun.*, 137, 1094, 1986.
112. **Warren, J. S., Kunkel, S. L., Cunningham, T. W., Johnson, K. J., and Ward, P. A.,** Macrophage-derived cytokines amplify immune complex-triggered O_2-responses by rat alveolar macrophages, *Am. J. Pathol.*, 130, 489, 1988.
113. **Richter, J., Andersson, T., and Olsson, I.,** Effect of tumor necrosis factor and granulocyte/macrophage colony-stimulating factor on neutrophil degranulation, *J. Immunol.*, 142, 3199, 1989.
114. **Gery, I., Gershon, R. K., and Waksman, B. H.,** Potentiation of the T-lymphocyte response to mitogens. I. The responding cell, *J. Exp. Med.*, 136, 128, 1972.
115. **Gery, I. and Lepe-Zuniga, J. L.,** Interleukin-1: uniqueness of its production and spectrum of activities, *Lymphokines*, 9, 109, 1984.
116. **Lee, J. C., Truneh, A., Smith, M. F., and Tsang, K. Y.,** Induction of interleukin 2 receptor (TAC) by tumor necrosis factor in YT cells, *J. Immunol.*, 139, 1935, 1987.
117. **Scheurich, P., Thoma, B., Ucer, U., and Pfizenmaier, K.,** Immunoregulatory activity of recombinant human tumor necrosis factor (TNF)-α: induction of TNF receptors on human T cells and TNF-α-mediated enhancement of T cell responses, *J. Immunol.*, 138, 1786, 1987.
118. **Jelinek, D. F. and Lipsky, P. E.,** Enhancement of human B cell proliferation and differentiation by tumor necrosis factor-α and interleukin, *J. Immunol.*, 139, 2970, 1987.
119. **Schmidt, J. A., Mizel, S. B., Cohen, D., and Green, I.,** Interleukin-1, a potential regulator of fibroblast proliferation, *J. Immunol.*, 128, 2177, 1982.
120. **Elias, J. A.,** Tumor necrosis factor interacts with interleukin-1 and interferons to inhibit fibroblast proliferation via fibroblast prostaglandin-dependent and -independent mechanisms, *Am. Rev. Respir. Dis.*, 138, 652, 1988.
121. **Elias, J. A., Gustilo, K., and Freundlich, B.,** Human alveolar macrophage and blood monocyte inhibition of fibroblast proliferation, *Am. Rev. Respir. Dis.*, 138, 1595, 1988.
122. **Sugarman, B. J., Aggarwal, B. B., Hass, P. E., Figari, I. S., Palladino, M. A., Jr., and Shepard, H. M.,** Recombinant human tumor necrosis factor-α: effects on proliferation of normal and transformed cells *in vitro*, *Science*, 230, 943, 1985.
123. **Libby, P., Warner, S. J. C., and Friedman, G. B.,** Interleukin 1: a mitogen for human vascular smooth muscle cells that induces the release of growth-inhibitory prostanoids, *J. Clin. Invest.*, 81, 487, 1988.
124. **Ikebe, T., Hirata, M., and Koga, T.,** Effects of human recombinant tumor necrosis factor-α and interleukin 1 on the synthesis of glycosaminoglycan and DNA in cultured rat costal chondrocytes, *J. Immunol.*, 140, 827, 1988.
125. **Lachman, L. B., Brown, D. C., and Dinarello, C. A.,** Growth-promoting effect of recombinant interleukin 1 and tumor necrosis factor for a human astrocytoma cell line, *J. Immunol.*, 138, 2913, 1987.
126. **Kahaleh, M. B., Smith, E. A., Soma, Y., and Leroy, E. C.,** Effect of lymphotoxin and tumor necrosis factor on endothelial and connective tissue cell growth and function, *Clin. Immunol. Immunopathol.*, 49, 261, 1988.
127. **Palombella, V. J., Yamashiro, D. J., Maxfield, F. R., Decker, S. J., and Vilcek, J.,** Tumor necrosis factor increases the number of epidermal growth factor receptors on human fibroblasts, *J. Biol. Chem.*, 262, 1950, 1987.
128. **Palombella, V. J. and Vilcek, J.,** Mitogenic and cytotoxic actions of tumor necrosis factor in BALB/c 3T3 cells, *J. Biol. Chem.*, 264, 18128, 1989.
129. **Hajjar, K. A., Hajjar, D. P., Silverstein, R. L., and Nachman, R. L.,** Tumor necrosis factor-mediated release from platelet-derived growth factor from cultured endothelial cells, *J. Exp. Med.*, 166, 235, 1987.
130. **Raines, E. W., Dower, S. K., and Ross, R.,** Interleukin-1 mitogenic activity for fibroblasts and smooth muscle cells is due to PDGF-AA, *Science*, 243, 393, 1989.
131. **Elias, J. A., Freundlich, B., Adams, S., and Rosenbloom, J.,** Regulation of human lung fibroblast collagen production by recombinant interleukin-1, tumor necrosis factor, and interferon-γ, *Ann. N.Y. Acad. Sci.*, 580, 233, 1990.
132. **Elias, J. A., Krol, R. C., Freundlich, B., and Sampson, P. M.,** Regulation of human lung fibroblast glycosaminoglycan production by recombinant interferons, tumor necrosis factor, and lymphotoxin, *J. Clin. Invest.*, 81, 325, 1988.
133. **Goldring, M. B. and Krane, S. M.,** Modulation by recombinant interleukin 1 of synthesis of types I and III collagens and associated procollagen mRNA levels in cultured human cells, *J. Biol. Chem.*, 262, 16724, 1987.

134. **Goldring, M. B., Birkhead, J., Sandell, L. J., Kimura, T., and Krane, S. M.,** Interleukin 1 suppresses expression of cartilage-specific types II and IX collagens and increases types I and III collagens in human chondrocytes, *J. Clin. Invest.*, 82, 2026, 1988.
135. **Dunn, C. J., Hardee, M. M., Gibbons, A. J., Staite, N. D., and Richard, K. A.,** Local pathological responses to slow-release recombinant interleukin-1, interleukin-2 and γ-interferon in the mouse and their relevance to chronic inflammatory disease, *Clin. Sci.*, 76, 261, 1989.
136. **Piguet, P. F., Grau, G. E., Vassalli, P.,** Subcutaneous perfusion of tumor necrosis factor induces local proliferation of fibroblasts, capillaries, and epidermal cells, or massive tissue necrosis, *Am. J. Pathol.*, 136, 103, 1990.
137. **Piguet, P. F., Collart, M. A., Grau, G. E., Sappino, A.-P., Vassalli, P.,** Requirement for tumour necrosis factor for development of silica-induced pulmonary fibrosis, *Nature*, 344, 245, 1990.
138. **Piguet, P. F., Collart, M. A., Grau, G. E., Kapanci, Y., and Vassalli, P.,** Tumor necrosis factor/cachectin plays a key role in bleomycin-induced pneumopathy and fibrosis, *J. Exp. Med.*, 170, 655, 1989.
139. **Berk, J. L., Franzblau, C., and Goldstein, R. H.,** Recombinant interleukin-1β inhibits elastin formation: a neonatal rat lung fibroblast subtype, *J. Biol. Chem.*, 266, 3192, 1991.
140. **Amento, E. P., Ehsani, N., Palmer, H., and Libby, P.,** Cytokines and growth factors positively and negatively regulate interstitial collagen gene expression in human vascular smooth muscle cells, *Arteriosclerosis Thrombosis*, 11, 1223, 1991.
141. **Mauviel, A., Redini, F., Hartmann, D. J., Pujol, J.-P., Evans, C. H.,** Modulation of human dermal fibroblast extracellular matrix metabolism by the lymphokine leukoregulin, *J. Cell Biol.*, 113, 1455, 1991.
142. **Mauviel, A., Heino, J., Kahari, V.-M., Hartmann, D.-J., Loyau, G., Pujol, J.-P., and Vuorio, E.,** Comparative effects of interleukin-1 and tumor necrosis factor-α on collagen production and corresponding procollagen mRNA levels in human dermal fibroblasts, *J. Invest. Dermatol.*, 96, 243, 1991.
143. **Lankat-Buttgereit, B., Kulozik, M., Hunzelmann, N., and Krieg, T.,** Cytokines alter mRNA steady state levels for basement membrane proteins in human skin fibroblasts, *J. Dermatol. Sci.*, 2, 300, 1991.
144. **Solis-Herruzo, J. A., Brenner, D. A., and Chojkier, M.,** Tumor necrosis factor α inhibits collagen gene transcription and collagen synthesis in cultured human fibroblasts, *J. Biol. Chem.*, 263, 5841, 1988.
145. **Armendariz-Borunda, J., Katayama, K., and Seyer, J. M.,** Transcriptional mechanisms of type I collagen gene expression are differentially regulated by interleukin-1β, tumor necrosis factor α, and transforming growth factor β in Ito cells, *J. Biol. Chem.*, 267, 14316, 1992.
146. **Allison, A. C., Harington, J. S., and Birbeck, M.,** An examination of the cytotoxic effects of silica on macrophages, *J. Exp. Med.*, 124, 141, 1966.
147. **Heppelston, A. G.,** Minerals, Fibrosis, and the Lung, *Environ. Health Persp.*, 94, 149, 1991.
148. **Henderson, R. F., Harkema, J. R., Hotchkiss, J. A., and Boehme, D. S.,** Effect of blood leukocyte and depletion on the inflammatory response of the lung to quartz, *Toxicol. Appl. Pharmacol.*, 109, 127, 1991.
149. **Seaton, A.,** Silicosis, *Occup. Lung Dis.*, 250, 1984.
150. **Gosset, P., Lassalle, P., Vanhee, D., Wallaert, B., Aerts, C., Voisin, C., and Tonnel, A.-B.,** Production of tumor necrosis factor-α and interleukin-6 by human alveolar macrophages exposed *in vitro* to coal mine dust, *Am. J. Respir. Cell Mol. Biol.*, 5, 431, 1991.
151. **Driscoll, K. E., Higgins, J. M., Leytart, M. J., and Crosby, L. L.,** Differential effects of mineral dusts on the *in vitro* activation of alveolar macrophage eicosanoid and cytokine release, *Toxicol. in Vitro*, 4, 284, 1990.
152. **DuBois, C. M., Bissonnette, E., and Rla-Pleszczynski, M.,** Asbestos fibers and silica particles stimulate rat alveolar macrophages to release tumor necrosis factor, *Am. Rev. Respir. Dis.*, 139, 1257, 1989.
153. **Savici, D., Geist, L. J., Monick, M. M., and Hunninghake, G. W.,** Silica increases release of tumor necrosis factor from mononuclear phagocytes, in part, by increasing expression of the tumor necrosis factor (TNF) gene, *Clin. Res.*, 40, 186A, 1992.
154. **Rola-Pleszczynski, M. and Lemaire, I.,** Leukotrienes augment interleukin 1 a production by human monocytes, *J. Immunol.*, 135, 3958, 1985.
155. **Rola-Pleszczynski, M., Chavaillaz, P.-A., and Lemaire, I.,** Stimulation of interleukin 2 and interferon-gamma production by leukotriene B_4 and human lymphocyte culture, *Prostaglandins Leukotrienes Med.*, 23, 207, 1986.
156. **Rola-Pleszczynski, M., Bouvrette, L., Gingras, D., and Girard, M.,** Identification of interferon γ as the lymphokine that mediates leukotriene B_4 induced immunoregulation, *J. Immunol.*, 139, 513, 1987.
157. **Schmidt, J. A., Oliver, C. N., Lepe-Zuniga, J. L., Green, I., and Gery, I.,** Silica-stimulated monocytes release fibroblast proliferation factors identical to interleukin 1: a potential role for interleukin 1 in the pathogenesis of silicosis, *J. Clin. Invest.*, 73, 1462, 1984.
158. **Kampschmidt, R. F., Worthington, M. L., and Mesecher, M. I.,** Release of interleukin-1 (IL-1) and IL-1-like factors from rabbit macrophages with silica, *J. Leukocyte Biol.*, 39, 123, 1986.
159. **Godelaine, D. and Beaufay, H.,** Comparative study of the effect of chrysotile, quartz and rutile on the release of lymphocyte-activating factor (interleukin 1) by murine peritoneal macrophages *in vitro*, *IARC Sci. Publ.*, 90, 149, 1989.
160. **Oghiso, Y. and Kubota, Y.,** Interleukin 1-like thymocyte and fibroblast activating factors from rat alveolar macrophages exposed to silica and asbestos particles, *Jpn. J. Vet. Sci.*, 48, 461, 1986.

161. **Oghiso, Y.,** Heterogeneity in immunologic functions of rat alveolar macrophages — their accessory cell function and IL-1 production, *Microbiol. Immunol.*, 31, 247, 1987.
162. **Kang, J. H., Lewis, D. M., Castranova, V., Rojanasakul, Y., Banks, D. E., Ma, J. Y. C., and Ma, J. K. H.,** Inhibitory action of tetrandrine on macrophage production of interleukin-1 (IL-1)-like activity and thymocyte proliferation, *Exp. Lung Res.*, 18, 715, 1992.
163. **Roux-Lombard, P., Modoux, C., and Dayer, J.-M.,** Production of interleukin-1 (IL-1) and a specific IL-1 inhibitor during human monocyte-macrophage differentiation: influence of GM-CSF, *Cytokine*, 1, 45, 1989.
164. **Elias, J. A., Schreiber, A. D., Gustilo, K., Chien, P., Rossman, M. D., Lammie, P. J., and Daniele, R. P.,** Differential interleukin 1 elaboration by unfractionated and density fractionated human alveolar macrophages and blood monocytes: relationship to cell maturity, *J. Immunol.*, 135, 3198, 1985.
165. **Moore, S. A., Strieter, R. M., Rolfe, M. W., Standiford, T. J., Burdick, M. D., and Kunkel, S. L.,** Expression and regulation of human alveolar macrophage-derived interleukin-1 receptor antagonist, *Am. J. Respir. Cell Mol. Biol.*, 6, 569, 1992.
166. **Jansen, R. W., Hance, K. R., and Arend, W. P.,** Production of IL-1 receptor antagonist by human *in vitro*-derived macrophages: effects of lipopolysaccharide and granulocyte-macrophage colony-stimulating factor, *J. Immunol.*, 147, 4218, 1991.
167. **Wewers, M. D., and Herzuk, D. J.,** Alveolar macrophages differ from blood monocytes in human IL-1β release, *J. Immunol.*, 143, 1635, 1989.
168. **Driscoll, K. E., Lindenschmidt, R. C., Maurer, J. K., Higgins, J. M., and Ridder, G.,** Pulmonary response to silica or titanium dioxide: inflammatory cells, alveolar macrophage-derived cytokines, and histopathology, *Am. J. Respir. Cell Mol. Biol.*, 2, 381, 1990.
169. **Driscoll, K. E., Strzelecki, J., Hassenbein, D., Janssen, Y. M. W., March, J. K., Oberdoerster, G., and Mossman, B. T.,** Tumor necrosis factor (TNF): Evidence for the role of TNF in increased expression of manganese superoxide dismutase after inhalation of mineral dusts, *Ann. Occup. Hyg.*, 38, 375, 1994.
170. **Oghiso, Y. and Kubota, Y.,** Enhanced interleukin 1 production by alveolar macrophages and increase in 1a-positive lung cells in silica-exposed rats, *Microbiol. Immunol.*, 30, 1189, 1986.
171. **Mohr, C., Gemsa, D., Graebner, C., Hemenway, D. R., Leslie, K. O., Absher, P. M., and Davis, G. S.,** Systemic macrophage stimulation in rats with silicosis: enhanced release of tumor necrosis factor-α from alveolar and peritoneal macrophages, *Am. J. Respir. Cell Mol. Biol.*, 5, 395, 1991.
172. **Struhar, D. J., Harbeck, R. J., Gegen, N., Kawada, H., and Mason, R. J.,** Increased expression of class II antigens of the major histocompatibility complex on alveolar macrophages and alveolar type II cells and interleukin-1 (IL-1) secretion from alveolar macrophages in an animal model of silicosis, *Clin. Exp. Immunol.*, 77, 281, 1989.
173. **Driscoll, K. E., Lindenschmidt, R. C., Maurer, J. K., Perkins, L., Perkins, M., and Higgins, J.,** Pulmonary response to inhaled silica or titanium dioxide, *Toxicol. Appl. Pharmacol.*, 111, 201, 1991.
174. **Lassalle, P., Gosset, P., Aerts, C., Fournier, E., Lafitte, J. J., Degreef, J. M., Wallaert, B., Tonnel, A. B., and Voisin, C.,** Abnormal secretion of interleukin-1 and tumor necrosis factor α by alveolar comparison between simple pneumoconiosis and progressive massive fibrosis, *Exp. Lung. Res.*, 16, 73, 1990.
175. **Zhang, Y., Lee, T. C., Guillemin, B., Yu, M.-C., and Rom, W. N.,** Enhanced expression of interleukin-1β and tumor necrosis factor-α genes in macrophages from idiopathic pulmonary fibrosis or following asbestos-exposure and accumulation of extracellular matrix, *Am. Rev. Respir. Dis.*, 145, A841, 1992.
176. **Borm, P. J. A., Meijers, J. M. M., and Swaen, G. M. H.,** Molecular epidemiology of coal worker's pneumoconiosis: application to risk assessment of oxidant and monokine generation by mineral dusts, *Exp. Lung Res.*, 16, 57, 1990.
177. **Piguet, P. F., Grau, G., Rosen, H., and Vesin, C.,** Antibody to the leukocyte integrins CD-11-a or b prevent or cure pulmonary fibrosis elicited in mice by bleomycin or silica, *Respir. Dis.*, 145, A190, 1992.
178. **Ward, P. A., Warren, J. S., and Johnson, K. J.,** Oxygen radicals, inflammation, and tissue injury, *Free Radical Biol. Med.*, 5, 403, 1988.
179. **Freeman, B. A. and Crapo, J. D.,** Biology of disease. Free radicals and tissue injury, *Lab. Invest.*, 47, 412, 1982.
180. **Djeu, J. Y., Serbousek, D., and Blanchard, D. K.,** Release of tumor necrosis factor by human polymorphonuclear leukocytes, *Blood*, 76, 1405, 1990.
181. **Lindemann, A., Riedel, D., Oster, W., Ziegler-Heitbrock, H. W. L., Mertelsman, R., and Herrman, F.,** Granulocyte-macrophage colony-stimulating factor induces cytokine secretion by human polymorphonuclear leukocytes, *J. Clin. Invest.*, 83, 1308, 1989.
182. **Driscoll, K. E. and Maurer, J. K.,** Cytokine and growth factor release by alveolar macrophages: potential biomarkers of pulmonary toxicity, *Toxicol. Pathol.*, 19, 398, 1991.
183. **Driscoll, K. E., Hassenbein, D. G., Carter, J., Poynter, J., Asquith, T. N., Grant, R. A., Whitten, J., Purdon, M. P., and Takigiku, R.,** Macrophage inflammatory proteins 1 and 2: expression by rat alveolar macrophages, fibroblasts, and epithelial cells and in rat lung after mineral dust exposure, *Am. J. Respir. Cell Mol. Biol.*, 8, 311, 1993.
184. **Driscoll, K. E., Maurer, J. K., Hassenben, D., Carter, J., Janssen, Y. M. W., Mossman, B. T., Osier, M., and Oberdorster, G.,** Contribution of Macrophage-derived Cytokines and Cytokine Networks to Mineral Dust-induced Lung Inflammation, in *Toxic and Carcinogenic Effects of Solid Particles in the Respiratory Tract*, Mohr, U., Mauderly, J., and Oberdorster, G., Eds., USI Press, Washington, D.C., 1994, 177–190.

185. **Kasahara, K., Kobayashi, K., Shikama, Y., Yoneya, K., Soezima, K., Ide, H., and Takahashi, T.,** Direct evidence for granuloma-inducing activity of interleukin-1, *Am. J. Pathol.,* 130, 629, 1988.
186. **Kobayashi, K., Allred, C., Cohen, S., and Yoshida, T.,** Role of interleukin-1 in experimental pulmonary granuloma in mice, *J. Immunol.,* 358, 358, 1985.
187. **Kunkel, S. L., Chensue, S. W., Strieter, R. M., Lynch, J. P., and Remick, D. G.,** Cellular and molecular aspects of granulomatous inflammation, *Am. J. Respir. Cell Mol. Biol.,* 1, 439, 1989.
188. **Kasahara, K., Kobayashi, K., Shikama, Y., et al.,** The role of monokines in granuloma formation in mice: the ability of interleukin 1 and tumor necrosis factor-α to include lung granulomas, *Clin. Immunol. Immunopathol.,* 51, 419, 1989.
189. **Walz, A., Burgener, R., Car, B., Baggiolini, M., Kunkel, S. L., and Strieter, R. M.,** Structure and neutrophil-activating properties of a novel inflammatory peptide (ENA-78) with homology to interleukin 8, *J. Exp. Med.,* 174, 1355, 1991.
190. **Strieter, R. M., Remick, D. G., Lynch, J. P., III, Spengler, R. N., and Kunkel, S. L.,** Interleukin-2-induced tumor necrosis factor-alpha (TNF-α) gene expression in human alveolar macrophages and blood monocytes, *Am. Rev. Respir. Dis.,* 139, 335, 1989.
191. **Rich, E. A., Panuska, J. R., Wallis, R. S., Wolf, C. B., Leonard, M. L., and Ellner, J. J.,** Dyscoordinate expression of tumor necrosis factor-alpha by human blood monocytes and alveolar macrophages,[1–3] *Am. Rev. Respir. Dis.,* 139, 1010, 1989.

Section III
Chapter 5

OXIDANT RELEASE FROM PULMONARY PHAGOCYTES

Vincent Castranova, James M. Antonini, Mark J. Reasor, Lixin Wu, and Knox Van Dyke

CONTENTS

I. INTRODUCTION

One of the proposed mechanisms involved in the pathogenesis of silicosis is that inhaled silica dust activates a "respiratory burst" in pulmonary phagocytes, such as macrophages and neutrophils. This increase in oxidative metabolism results in enhanced generation of reactive oxygen species which, if produced in excess, would overwhelm natural defense mechanisms and cause damage to the lung parenchyma. This damage would then result in scarring, fibrosis, and decreased gas exchange.

Weiss and LoBuglio[1] have listed several oxygen species produced by phagocytes which may be involved in cellular injury. These oxidants include superoxide anion, hydrogen, peroxide, hydroxyl radical, and hypochlorous acid. Superoxide anion ($O_2^{\bar{\cdot}}$) is generated from molecular oxygen by the plasma membrane bound enzyme NADPH oxidase according to the following reaction:

$$O_2 + NADPH \xrightarrow[\text{oxidase}]{\text{NADPH}} O_2^{\bar{\cdot}} + NADP + H^+$$

Once generated, superoxide anion can form hydrogen peroxide:

$$2\,O_2^{\bar{\cdot}} + O_2 + 2H^+ \longrightarrow H_2O_2 + 2\,O_2$$

In the presence of myeloperoxidase and halide, hydrogen peroxide can form hypochlorous acid:

$$H_2O_2 + Cl^- \xrightarrow[H^+]{\text{myeloperoxidase}} HOCl + H_2O$$

Superoxide and hydrogen peroxide can also form highly reactive hydroxyl radicals. Hydroxyl radicals can be generated slowly by the Haber-Weiss reaction:

$$O_2^{\cdot -} + H_2O_2 \longrightarrow OH^{\cdot} + OH^- + O_2$$

In addition, hydroxyl radical production can be catalyzed via the Fenton reaction:

$$O_2^{\cdot -} + Fe^{3+} \longrightarrow O_2 + Fe^{2+}$$

$$Fe^{2+} + H_2O_2 \longrightarrow Fe^{3+} + OH^{\cdot} + OH^-$$

Hydroxyl radicals can also be generated from the reaction of superoxide and hypochlorous acid as follows:

$$O_2^{\cdot -} + HOCl \longrightarrow OH^{\cdot} + Cl^- + O_2$$

Recent investigations suggest that, in addition to the reactive oxygen species discussed above, nitric oxide may be a potential mediator of silica-induced toxicity.[2–4] Nitric oxide ($NO^{\cdot}$) can be generated by the cytosolic enzyme nitric oxide synthase according to the following reaction:

$$L-\text{arginine} \xrightarrow[\text{NADPH} \quad \text{NADP}]{\text{NO synthase}} L-\text{citruline} + NO^{\cdot}$$

NO synthase exists in two forms, i.e., a constitutive, Ca^{2+}-calmodulin-dependent form and an inducible, Ca^{2+}-calmodulin-independent form. In pulmonary phagocytes, the activity of the constitutive form of NO synthase is low. However, NO synthase can be induced in macrophages and neutrophils by a variety of stimulants such as lipopolysaccharide, interferon γ, chemotactic peptide, platelet activating factor, or leukotriene B_4.[3,5]

Once generated, nitric oxide can combine with superoxide anion to form peroxynitrite as follows:

$$NO^{\cdot} + O_2^{\cdot -} \longrightarrow OONO^-$$

Peroxynitrite is a potent oxidizing agent. In addition, peroxynitrite can form peroxynitrous acid, which in turn can produce hydroxyl radical and nitrogen dioxide (all of which exhibit strong oxidizing potential) by the following reactions:

$$OONO^- + H^+ \longrightarrow HOONO$$

$$HOONO \longrightarrow OH^{\cdot} + NO_2$$

Oxygen metabolites have been shown to cause lung damage *in vivo*.[6] Such damage includes edema, leakiness of the alveolar endothelial/epithelial barriers, and airway constriction.[7] Superoxide and hydrogen peroxide have been associated with membrane damage and cell lysis.[8] These oxidants have also been associated with alteration of cytoskeletal structures at cell-cell junctions and elevation of transepithelial conductance in cultured monolayers.[9] Macrophages or neutrophils can be stimulated by bacteria or phorbol myristate acetate to produce sufficient oxidant levels to lyse lymphoma cells.[10] This cell killing is inhibited by catalase but is unaffected by superoxide dismutase, hydroxyl radical scavengers, or azide, i.e., an inhibitor of peroxidase. This implicates hydrogen peroxide as the active oxidant. Similarly, Weiss et al.[11] have reported that hydrogen peroxide is critical in the death of cultured endothelial cells due to neutrophil activation. In addition, hydroxyl radicals generated by monocytes have been associated with cell injury.[12] Lastly, peroxynitrite has been shown to oxidize sulfhydryl groups and to inactivate α-1-proteinase inhibitor making the lung more susceptible to damage caused by phagocytotic enzymes.[13] Therefore, a strong case can be made that activated pulmonary macrophages and neutrophils are capable of causing oxidant injury. This chapter presents *in vitro* and *in vivo* data indicating that silica is associated with the production of reactive oxygen species from these pulmonary phagocytes.

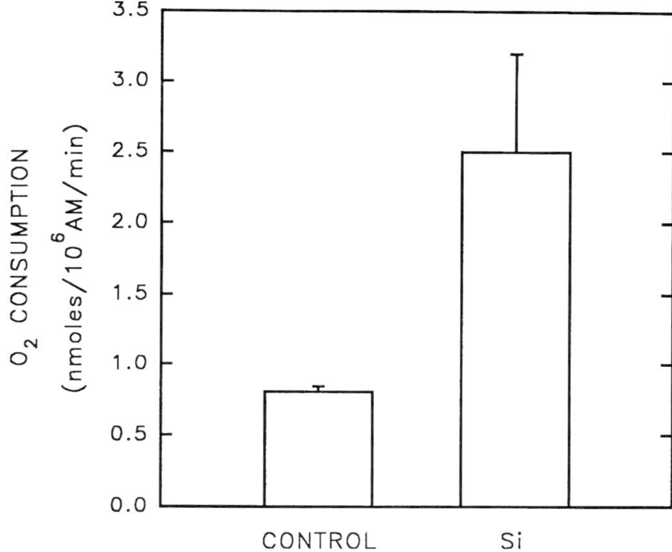

FIGURE 1 Induction of a respiratory burst in alveolar macrophages exposed to silica. Macrophages (4×10^6 cells) were exposed *in vitro* to 2 mg/ml silica. Oxygen consumption was monitored at 37°C before (control) and after silica exposure using a Clark electrode. Data are means ± SE of 3 experiments.

II. SILICA-INDUCED RELEASE OF OXIDANTS: *IN VITRO* STUDIES

A. STIMULATION OF OXIDANT PRODUCTION BY ALVEOLAR MACROPHAGES

Castranova et al.[14] have shown that crystalline silica is a potent stimulant of oxygen metabolism in alveolar macrophages. *In vitro* exposure of alveolar macrophages to 2 mg/ml silica increases oxygen consumption by 213% (Figure 1). Half maximal stimulation is observed at 0.56 mg/ml silica. This increase in oxygen consumption by alveolar macrophages is associated with an elevated production of reactive oxygen species. Data in Figure 2 show that 2 mg/ml silica stimulates superoxide production by 123%. The ED_{50} for this activation is 0.17 mg/ml silica. Furthermore, hydrogen peroxide release is increased by 313-fold in alveolar macrophages exposed to 1 mg/ml silica (Figure 3). The ED_{50} for silica-induced stimulation of hydrogen peroxide is 0.41 mg/ml silica. Similarly, chemiluminescence is increased by 961% after *in vitro* exposure of macrophages to 0.6 mg/ml silica (Figure 4) with an ED_{50} of 0.27 mg/ml. In each case, the stimulatory effect of silica on respiratory burst activity is apparent within 1 to 2 min of *in vitro* exposure.

B. STIMULATION OF OXIDANT PRODUCTION BY NEUTROPHILS

Silica is a potent, direct stimulant of oxygen metabolism in neutrophils.[15] *In vitro* exposure of neutrophils to 5 mg/ml silica results in an 815% increase in chemiluminescence (Figure 5). Silica is also an indirect stimulant of neutrophils; i.e., silica stimulates the release of platelet-activating factor (PAF) from alveolar macrophages.[16] This silica-induced release of PAF is shown in Figure 6. Note that *in vitro* exposure of macrophages to 10 mg/ml silica stimulates PAF release by 3750%. Activation of PAF release is significant 1 to 2 min after silica exposure and is maximal 10 min post-exposure. PAF is a potent chemoattractant for neutrophils.[17] Therefore, alveolar macrophage interaction with inhaled silica would result in infiltration of neutrophils into the airspaces. Once in the airspaces, macrophage-derived PAF can directly activate oxygen metabolism in these neutrophils. This activation is shown in Figure 7; i.e., *in vitro* treatment of neutrophils with 10^{-9}M PAF causes a significant increase in chemiluminescence. This stimulation occurs within minutes and is apparent at PAF concentrations as low as 10^{-10}M. PAF also potentiates the response of neutrophils to other stimulants; i.e., PAF increases chemiluminescence in response to n-formyl-leucyl-phenylalanine by 88%.[16]

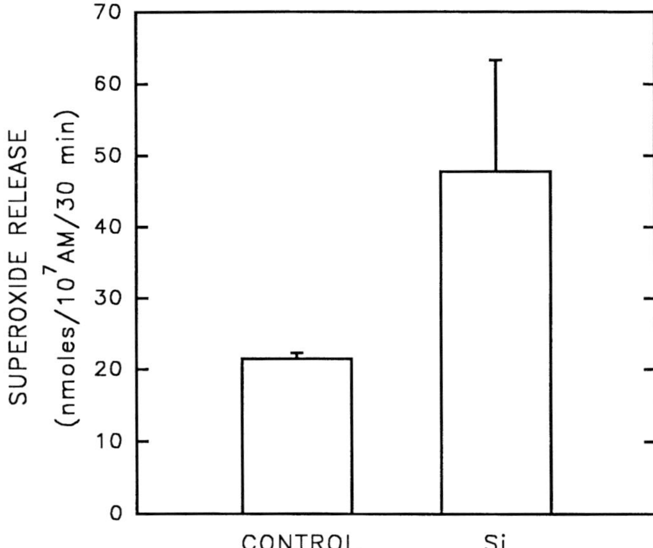

FIGURE 2 Stimulation of superoxide release from silica-exposed alveolar macrophages. Macrophages (3×10^6 cells) were exposed *in vitro* to 2 mg/ml silica. Cytochrome C reduction was monitored spectrophotometrically at 37°C before (control) and after silica exposure. Data are means ± SE of 3 experiments.

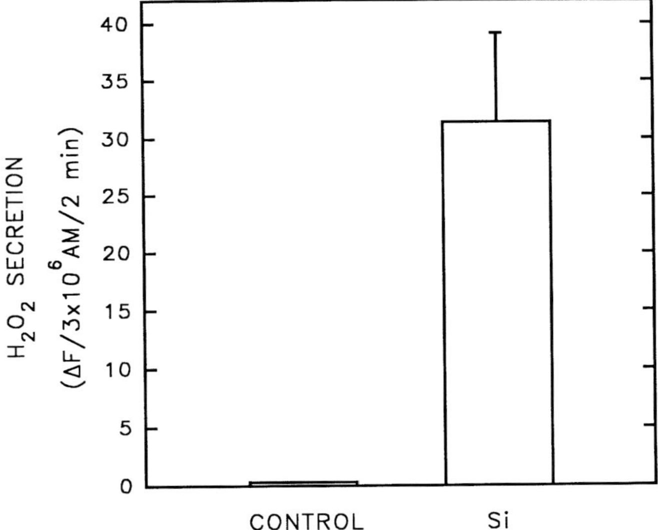

FIGURE 3 Stimulation of hydrogen peroxide secretion from silica-exposed alveolar macrophages. Macrophages (3×10^6 cells) were exposed *in vitro* to 1 mg/ml silica. Hydrogen peroxide was monitored by measuring the fluorescence of scopoletin at 37°C before (control) and after silica exposure. Data are means ± SE of 3 experiments.

III. SILICA-INDUCED RELEASE OF OXIDANTS: *IN VIVO* STUDIES

A. ANIMAL MODELS

Evidence indicates that *in vivo* exposure of rats to silica potentiates the activity of pulmonary phagocytes; i.e., oxygen metabolism in response to an *in vitro* stimulant is augmented in pulmonary phagocytes harvested from silica-exposed animals.[18,19] Figure 8 shows that zymosan-stimulated hydrogen

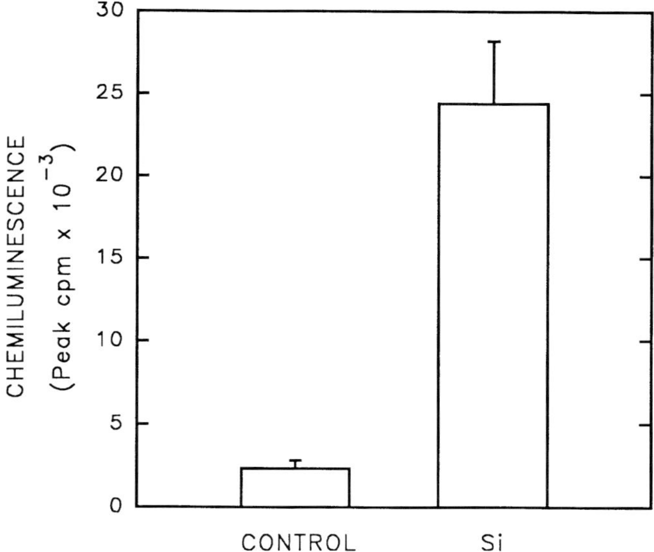

FIGURE 4 Stimulation of chemiluminescence generated from silica-exposed alveolar macrophages. Macrophages (5×10^6 cells) were exposed *in vitro* to 0.6 mg/ml silica. Chemiluminescence was monitored at 37°C before (control) and after silica exposure using a liquid scintillation counter. Data are means ± SE of 3 experiments.

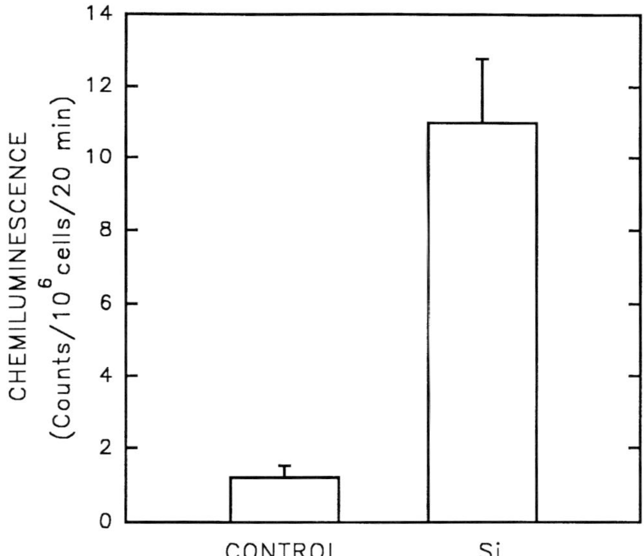

FIGURE 5 Silica-induced chemiluminescence generated from neutrophils. Neutrophils (10^6 cells) were exposed *in vitro* to 5 mg/ml silica and chemiluminescence monitored at 37°C in the presence of luminol (10^{-7} M) using a luminometer. Data are means ± SE of 9 experiments.

peroxide release is increased by 111% in phagocytes harvested from rats 30 days after a single intratracheal instillation of 40 mg silica. No change in resting levels of hydrogen peroxide release is observed. It should be noted that unopsonized zymosan was used in these experiments. Therefore, this response represents potentiation of alveolar macrophages, since neutrophils do not respond to unopsonized zymosan.

Priming of oxygen metabolism in alveolar macrophages is also noted four days after a 6-h inhalation of silica. Zymosan-stimulated oxygen consumption is increased by 44% (Figure 9), while zymosan-stimulated hydrogen peroxide release is elevated by 38% (Figure 10). In both cases, no change in resting

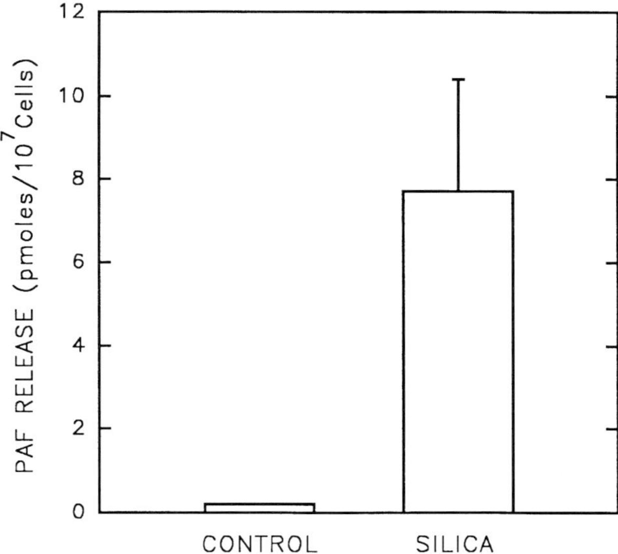

FIGURE 6 Silica-induced release of platelet-activating factor from alveolar macrophages. Macrophages (10^7 cells) were exposed *in vitro* to 10 mg/ml for 30 min at 37°C and PAF release monitored by measuring serotonin release from platelets in response to conditioned media from untreated (control) or silica-exposed macrophages. Data are means ± SE of 3 experiments.

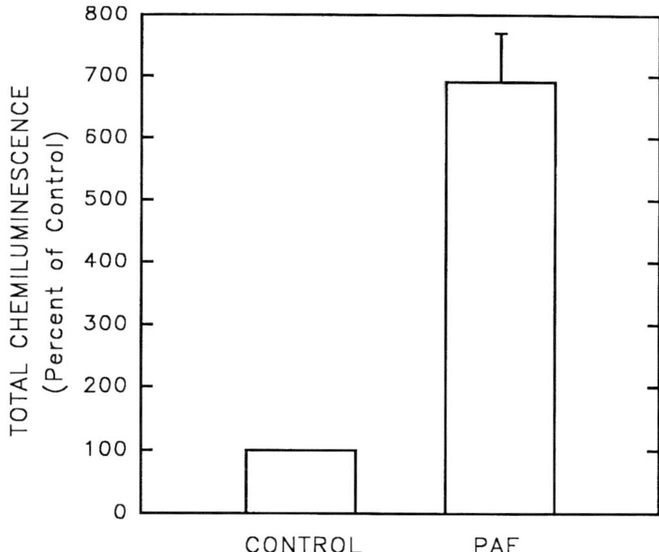

FIGURE 7 Chemiluminescence generated from PAF-treated neutrophils. Neutrophils were exposed *in vitro* to 10^{-9} PAF and the chemiluminescent response measured at 37°C for 30 min using a liquid scintillation counter. Data are means ± SE of 3 experiments.

(basal) levels is noted. This *in vivo* priming of alveolar macrophages is also supported by an increase in the surface activity of the phagocytes; i.e., cell spreading is increased by 62% four days after a 6-h inhalation of silica (Figure 11).

In addition to stimulation of oxygen metabolism, *in vivo* exposure to silica also causes an induction of NO synthase in lung cells. Figure 12 shows that chemiluminescence monitored from lung tissue is enhanced one day after an intratracheal instillation of silica (20 mg). Resting or basal chemiluminescence is increased by 91%, while PMA-stimulated generation of chemiluminescence is increased by 455% in silica-exposed

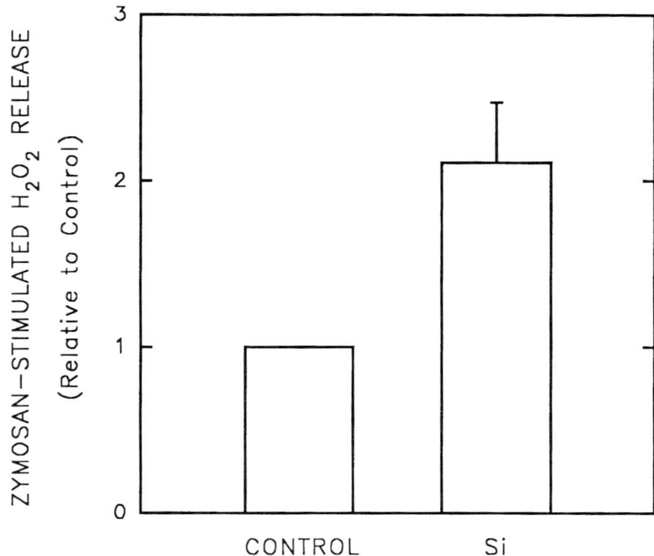

FIGURE 8 Enhancement of zymosan-stimulated hydrogen peroxide release by macrophages harvested from silica-exposed rats. Rats were intratracheally instilled with saline (control) or silica (40 mg) and alveolar macrophages harvested by bronchoalveolar lavage 30 days post-exposure. Macrophages were stimulated with zymosan (2 mg/ml) and hydrogen peroxide release measured at 37°C. Data are means ± SE of 3 experiments.

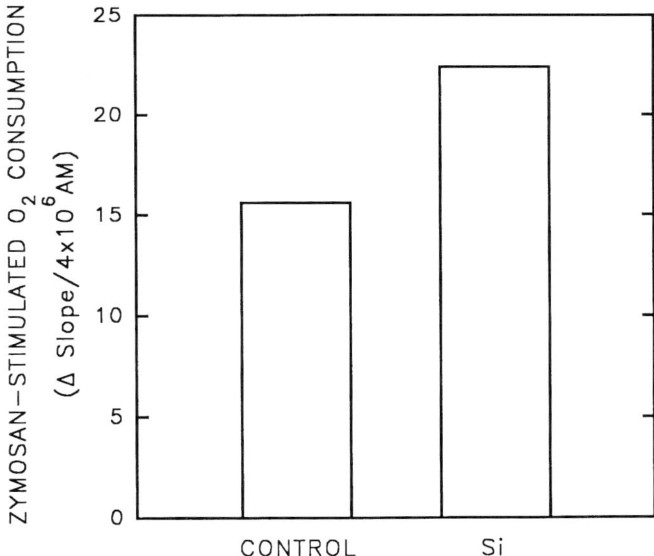

FIGURE 9 Enhancement of zymosan-stimulated oxygen consumption by macrophages harvested from silica-exposed rats. Rats were exposed by inhalation of silica (110 mg/m^3) for 6 h and alveolar macrophages harvested four days post-exposure. Macrophages were stimulated with zymosan (2 mg/ml) and oxygen consumption measured at 37°C. Data are means of 3 experiments.

lung tissue. A significant proportion of this silica-stimulated activity involves the induction of NO synthase and production of nitric oxide. Indeed, NO synthase-dependent activity, i.e., PMA-stimulated chemiluminescence inhibited by 1 mM L-NAME (Nω-Nitro-L-Arginine Methyl Ester), is increased by 993% in silica-exposed lung tissue. A similar activation can be demonstrated in alveolar macrophages isolated from lungs one day after intratracheal (IT) exposure to silica (Figure 13). Silica exposure does not alter resting

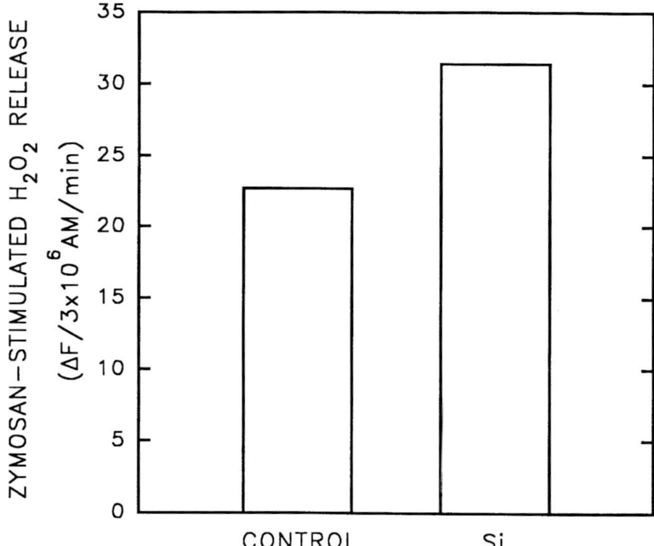

FIGURE 10 Enhancement of zymosan-stimulated hydrogen peroxide release from macrophages harvested from silica-exposed rats. Rats were exposed by inhalation of silica (110 mg/m^3) for 6 h and alveolar macrophages harvested four days post-exposure. Macrophages were stimulated with zymosan (2 mg/ml) and hydrogen peroxide monitored at 37°C by measuring the fluorescence of scopoletin. Data are means of 3 experiments.

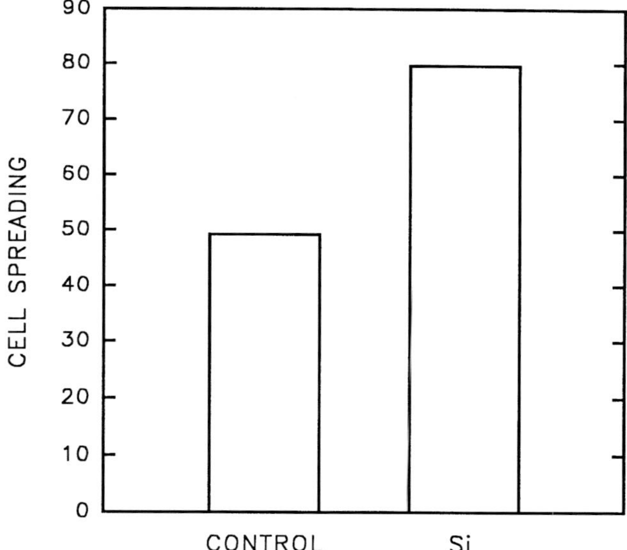

FIGURE 11 Enhanced surface activation of macrophages harvested from silica-exposed rats. Rats were exposed by inhalation of silica (110 mg/m^3) for 6 h and alveolar macrophages harvested four days post-exposure. Cell spreading was measured morphometrically under scanning electron microscopy. Data are means of 3 experiments.

chemiluminescence from pulmonary phagocytes. However, it does increase zymosan-stimulated chemiluminescence by 209% and induces NO synthase-dependent activity by 154% above the control.

B. SILICOTIC PATIENTS

Silica-induced stimulation of resting activity and potentiation of responses to other stimulants have also been noted in humans, i.e., with pulmonary phagocytes harvested by bronchoalveolar lavage of

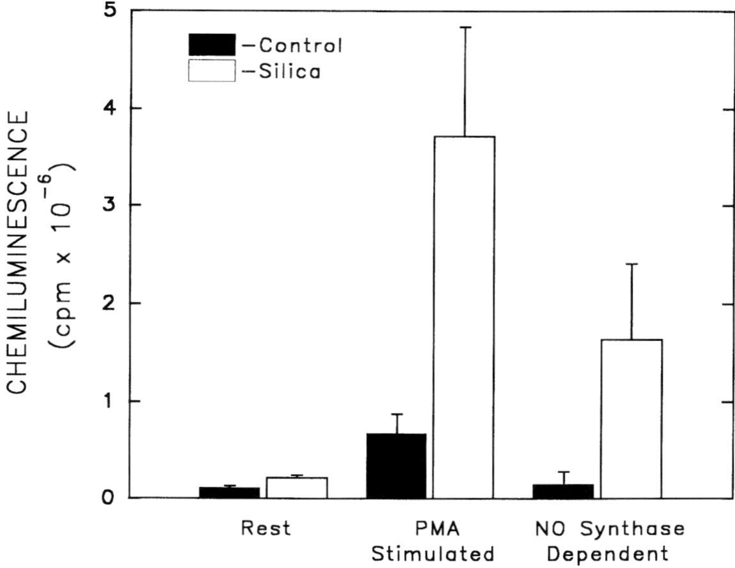

FIGURE 12 Chemiluminescence generated by lung tissue from control and silica-treated rats. Rats were exposed by intratracheal intubation to saline (control) or 20 mg silica (treated) one day prior to sacrifice. Chemiluminescence was monitored in the presence of luminol (10^{-7} M) using a luminometer. Chemiluminescence was determined at rest (no stimulant), after stimulation with 10^{-7} M PMA (PMA-stimulated), or in the presence of PMA plus 1 mM L-NAME (NO synthase-dependent). Data are means ± SE of 2 experiments.

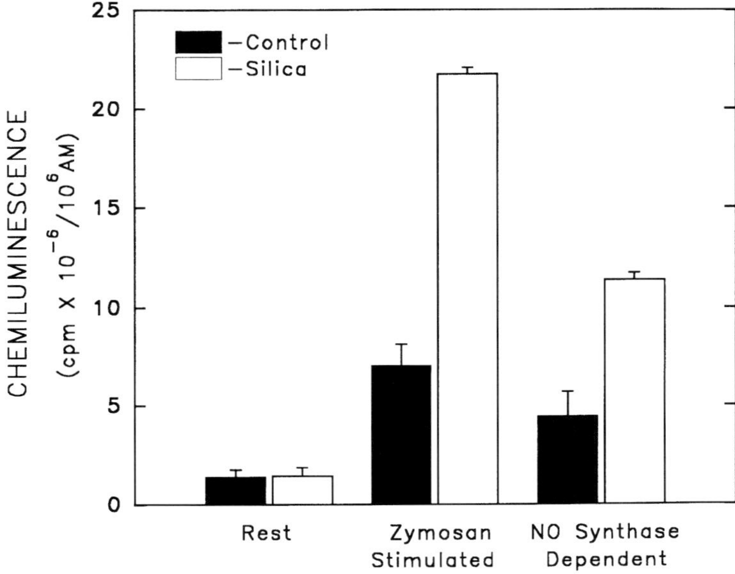

FIGURE 13 Chemiluminescence generated by pulmonary phagocytes harvested from control and silica-treated rats. Rats were exposed by intratracheal intubation to saline (control) or 20 mg silica (treated) one day prior to sacrifice. Chemiluminescence was monitored in the presence of luminol (10^{-7} M) using a luminometer. Chemiluminescence was determined at rest (no stimulant), after stimulation with 2 mg/ml unopsonized zymosan (zymosan-stimulated), or in the presence of zymosan plus 1 mM L-NAME (NO synthase-dependent). Data are means ± SE of 2 experiments.

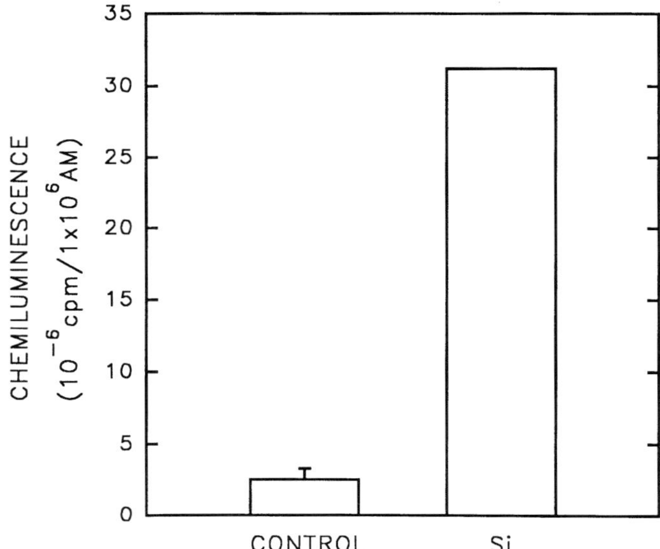

FIGURE 14 Enhanced resting chemiluminescence generated from pulmonary phagocytes harvested from a patient with acute silicosis. Chemiluminescence was measured with a liquid scintillation counter using cells harvested by bronchoalveolar lavage of normal volunteers (control) and an acute silicotic patient (Si).

patients with silicosis. Rom et al.[20] have reported that resting release of superoxide anion and hydrogen peroxide is elevated in patients with chronic silicosis. Similarly, our laboratory has reported elevated basal chemiluminescence in pulmonary phagocytes harvested from a rock driller with acute silicosis.[21] Resting chemiluminescence is increased by 1128% above levels generated by cells from healthy volunteers (Figure 14). Pulmonary phagocytes from this acute silicotic are also primed exhibiting a 267% increase in PMA-induced chemiluminescence and an 1129% increase in zymosan-induced chemiluminescence.

IV. SUMMARY

In conclusion, crystalline silica is a direct stimulant of oxygen metabolism and release of reactive oxidant species by both alveolar macrophages and neutrophils *in vitro*. In addition, *in vitro* exposure of macrophages to silica can induce the release of mediators, which are chemoattractants and activators of neutrophils. In animal models, *in vivo* exposure to silica acts to prime pulmonary phagocytes, i.e., potentiating oxidant release in response to stimulants. Thus far, the few studies of phagocytes obtained by bronchoalveolar lavage of silicotic patients indicate that silicosis is associated with increases in both basal and stimulant-induced production of reactive oxidants. The continuously elevated production of oxidants by pulmonary phagocytes in this disease state may be sufficient to overwhelm the native antioxidant defense systems of lung cells, thus resulting in parenchymal damage, scarring, and fibrosis that is characteristic of silicosis.

REFERENCES

1. **Weiss, S. J. and LoBuglio, A. F.,** Biology of disease: phagocyte-generated oxygen metabolites and cellular injury, *Lab. Invest.*, 47, 5–18, 1982.
2. **Stamler, J. S., Singel, D. J., and Loscalzo, J.,** Biochemistry of nitric oxide and its redox-activated forms, *Science,* 258, 1898–1902, 1992.

3. **Moncada, S., Palmer, R. M. J., and Higgs, E. A.,** Nitric oxide: physiology, pathophysiology, and pharmacology, *Pharmacol. Rev.,* 43, 109–141, 1991.
4. **Lancaster, J. R., Jr.,** Nitric oxide in cells, *Am. Sci.,* 80, 248–259, 1992.
5. **Schmidt, H. H. H. W., Seifert, R., and Böhme, E.,** Formation and release of nitric oxide from human neutrophils and HL-60 cells induced by a chemotactic peptide, platelet activating factor, and leukotriene B_4, *FEBS Lett.,* 244, 357–360, 1989.
6. **Johnson, K. J., Fantone, J. C., Kaplan, J., and Ward, P. A.,** *In vivo* damage of rat lungs by oxygen metabolites, *J. Clin. Invest.,* 67, 983–993, 1981.
7. **Tate, R. M., VanBenthuysen, K. M., Shasby, D. M., McMurtry, R. F., and Repine, J. E.,** Oxygen radical mediated permeability, edema, and vasoconstriction in isolated perfused rabbit lung, *Am. Rev. Respir. Dis.,* 126, 802–806, 1982.
8. **Kellogg, E. W. and Fridovich, I.,** Liposome oxidation and erythrocyte lysis by enzymatically generated superoxide and hydrogen peroxide, *J. Biol. Chem.,* 252, 6721–6726, 1977.
9. **Welsh, M. J., Shasby, D. M., and Husted, R. M.,** Oxidants increase paracellular permeability in a cultured epithelial cell line, *J. Clin. Invest.,* 76, 1155–1168, 1985.
10. **Nathan, C. F., Silverstein, S. C., Brukner, L. H., and Cohn, Z. A.,** Extracellular cytolysis by activated macrophages and granulocytes: II. Hydrogen peroxide as a mediator of cytotoxicity, *J. Exp. Med.,* 149, 100–113, 1979.
11. **Weiss, S. J., Young, J., LoBuglio, A. F., Slivka, A., and Nimeh, N. F.,** Role of hydrogen peroxide in neutrophil-mediated destruction of cultured endothelial cells, *J. Clin. Invest.,* 68, 714–721, 1981.
12. **Weiss, S. J., King, G. W., and LoBuglio, A. F.,** Evidence for hydroxyl radical formation by human monocytes, *J. Clin. Invest.,* 60, 370–376, 1977.
13. **Moreno, J. J. and Pryor, W. A.,** Inactivation of α-1-proteinase inhibitor by peroxynitrite, *Chem. Res. Toxicol.,* 5, 425–431, 1992.
14. **Castranova, V., Pailes, W. H., and Li, C.,** Effects of silica exposure on alveolar macrophages: action of tetrandrine, in *Proc. of the International Symposium on Pneumoconioses,* Li, Y., Yao, P., Schlipköter, H.W., Idel, H., and Rosenbruch, M., Eds., Stefan Walbers Velag, Düsseldorf, 256–260, 1990.
15. **Gutierrez, J.,** Selective inhibition of 5-lipoxygenase enzyme both in DMSO-differentiated HL-60 cells and neutrophils exposed to silica and asbestos, thesis, West Virginia University, 1991.
16. **Kang, J. H., Van Dyke, K., Pailes, W. H., and Castranova, V.,** Potential role of platelet-activating factor in development of occupational lung disease: action as an activator or potentiator of pulmonary phagocytes, *Proc. of Resp. Dusts in the Mineral Ind.,* Soc. of Mining, Metallurgy, and Exploration, 183–190, 1991.
17. **Czarnetzki, B. M. and Benveniste, J.,** Effect of 1–0-octadecyl-2–0-acetyl-sn-glycero-3-phosphocholine (PAF-acether) on leukocytes. I. Analysis of the *in vitro* migration of human neutrophils, *Chem. Phys. Lipids,* 29, 317–326, 1981.
18. **Castranova, V., Kang, J. H., Moore, M. D., Pailes, W. H., Frazer, D. G., and Schwegler-Berry, D.,** Inhibition of stimulant-induced activation of phagocytic cells with tetrandrine, *J. Leuk. Biol.,* 50, 412–422, 1991.
19. **Moore, M. D.,** Acute pulmonary responses to inhalation of silica: action of tetrandrine, thesis, West Virginia University, 1988.
20. **Rom, W. M., Bitterman, P. B., Rennard, S. I., Cantin, A., and Crystal, R. G.,** Characterization of the lower respiratory tract inflammation of non-smoking individuals with interstitial lung disease associated with chronic inhalation of inorganic dusts, *Am. Rev. Respir. Dis.,* 136, 1429–1434, 1987.
21. **Goodman, G. B., Kaplan, P. D., Stachura, I., Castranova, V., Pailes, W. H., and Lapp, N. L.,** Acute silicosis responding to corticosteroid therapy, *Chest,* 101, 366–370, 1992.

Section III
Chapter 6

LAVAGABLE BIOMARKERS OF EXPOSURE TO FIBROGENIC DUSTS

Theresa D. Sweeney and Joseph D. Brain

CONTENTS

I. INTRODUCTION

The mechanisms of fibrogenesis currently include an extensive list of potential mediators, growth factors, and cytokines; the ultimate culprit, if there is one, is not easily identifiable. One common response to an insult of a fibrogenic dust is increased number and/or activity of phagocytic cells [both polymorphonuclear neutrophils (PMNs) and alveolar macrophages (AMs)]. As these cells become increasingly active at the site of retention of a dust, they release oxygen radicals, lysosomal enzymes, and cytokines. The orchestration of the response is complex involving multiple cell types, time of arrival at the site, release of mediators, and response by various cell types. One approach to determine the magnitude of the response and the potential risk for a particular dust is through an *in vivo* bioassay. This has the advantage of a quick determination (days to weeks) and low cost; the bioassay can be calibrated for various dusts. We have used this method in the laboratory to compare the relative toxicity of a variety of dusts to assess their potential health risk to humans. The central theme common to this technique is bronchoalveolar lavage (BAL). In this review, we will discuss BAL and what it can and cannot tell you about lung injury. Then we will discuss how it is performed, the types of responses that can be measured, and how well BAL parameters predict fibrosis.

0-8493-4709-2/96/$0.00+$.50

A. BRONCHOALVEOLAR LAVAGE (BAL): WHAT IS IT?

BAL is a way to sample the extensive surface area of the respiratory tract by introducing saline via the airways and recovering the fluid for further analysis. Both cells and molecules present in the liquid lining layers of the lungs are harvested by this process. Normally the whole lung is sampled in small animals (rodents and rabbits). In humans and dogs, only a portion of the lung, usually a lung segment, is sampled. This is performed through a bronchoscope wedged in a third or fourth generation airway.

Like other global measures of whole lung function, e.g., FEV_1, identification of specific responses in a particular lung region is limited. Since the whole lung is sampled when fluid is instilled into the trachea, cells and molecules are collected from all regions of the respiratory tract. The majority of lung surface area (95%) resides in the parenchyma, so most of the sample represents the alveolar region. Airway components of the wash are diluted by the huge surface area of the lung periphery. This effect is smaller in segmental washes. It is possible to lavage only the trachea and mainstem bronchi, but sampling of intermediate and peripheral airways is impossible without some alveolar contamination.

B. FACTORS THAT AFFECT BAL INTERPRETATION

Does normal BAL evenly sample the entire respiratory surface? Brain et al.[1] instilled saline (0.15 cc/100 gm B.W.) containing Tc^{99m}-sulfur colloid particles into the lungs of rats and hamsters. Postinstillation, the distribution of the radioactivity throughout the lungs was determined. After a single instillation, the distribution was nonuniformly distributed throughout the lungs with preferential deposition in the gravity dependent lung lobes. Repeated instillations improved distribution. Fortunately, when larger volumes such as 2 cc/100 gm B.W. are used these nonuniformities largely disappear. Repeated lavages (usually at least six are recommended[2]) sample the entire lung surface and improve the consistency of cell recovery. Brain and Frank[3–5] found improved recovery of fluid and alveolar macrophages from animals with increasing lavage number and by using saline free of divalent cations. Washout patterns of various BAL components differ in normal and diseased lungs and vary with the component. For instance, the first lavage contains the fewer alveolar macrophages in normal animals than the third or fourth.[6,7] Brain and Frank[5] found that this is due to a divalent cation-dependent cell adhesiveness. Divalent cations are washed out of the lung with the first wash, and then cells are less adherent and more easily removed from lung surfaces. Some molecules (the lysosomal enzyme, β-N-acetylglucosaminidase, and ascorbic acid) are washed out of rodent lungs in a pattern reflecting a dilution model.[6,8] Other molecules (potassium and carbohydrates) exhibit a delayed washout,[9] suggesting that they may be more adherent to alveolar surfaces. Lung disease can also affect washout patterns. One obvious reason is that disease is often nonuniformly distributed throughout the lung. Diseased and nondiseased regions may not be equally sampled due to alterations in local surface forces and lung compliance.

How can one interpret BAL results? Many investigators have shown that the time course of injury or disease progression can be followed by BAL at periodic intervals.[10–14] However, the BAL procedure itself can elicit increased PMNs in the lung[15] and cause transient hypoxemia in sheep and humans.[11,14,16] The interpretation of response depends on controlled studies among groups of animals (for rodents) and within the same animal (for segmental lavages in dogs and humans). Proper controls, including positive and negative controls, are imperative for any meaningful interpretation.

Correlations have been made between the number and types of cells recovered by BAL and corresponding biopsy.[17] Experimental models of injury in animals have demonstrated close relationships between BAL and histopathology.[18–20] However if lesions are focal, BAL may not fairly represent these regions since it contains more cells and molecules from normal lung zones. It is also difficult to correlate anatomic changes to BAL since cellular and macromolecular changes precede anatomic changes. Since fibrosis occurs within the lung interstitium, BAL may not adequately represent the cellular and biochemical changes after the acute stage, since the fluid does not have access to interstitial spaces unless epithelial permeability in these regions is elevated.

One final difficulty in repeated segmental lavages in humans is the proper calibration of the response from lavage to lavage. It is impossible to know how much of the alveolar surface is sampled with a segmental lavage. This becomes more problematic when comparisons among animals are made. One attempt to control differences is to measure the urea content of the lavage fluid.[21] Since urea is freely permeable across alveolar surfaces, comparing the concentration in the lavage to that in blood will provide an estimate of the dilution of urea and hence the volume of the tissue sampled. This method has been challenged.[22] Effros,[23] Marcy,[24] and Kelly[25] noted that some urea diffuses into the lung during the

BAL procedure. Effros[23] devised a method where lungs were lavaged with isotonic mannitol. The results of Feng et al.[22] suggest that albumin or transferrin may more accurately estimate the dilution of epithelial lining fluid by BAL.

II. BAL: WHAT TO MEASURE, AND WHAT DO THESE MARKERS MEAN?

A. CELL NUMBER, TYPE, AND ACTIVITY

One of the major advantages of BAL is the acquisition of lung cells for study. The most prominent cell in the BAL fluid is the pulmonary macrophage. It comprises >90% of all lavaged cells in normal animals[3,6] and humans.[26] In laboratory animals, generally a greater proportion of recovered cells are macrophages. These include those from airways as well as alveoli.[27] In humans, lymphocytes comprise about 9% of the BAL fluid,[26,28] but this number is lower in animals.[29,30] Polymorphonuclear leukocytes (PMNs) are <2% of the BAL wash fluid.[6,26,28]

Changes in the total number of cells recovered and the type of cells are a first indication of lung injury and can reveal signs of chronic lung damage. For instance, inflammation is usually signaled by an influx of PMNs into the locally inflamed area, followed by an increase of macrophages in the region. In the lung exposed to fibrogenic dusts, increases in the number of PMNs signal acute lung injury, and their persistent presence in the lung signals continuing injury. This increase could also reflect an increase in vascular permeability.[31] Lung macrophage numbers can diminish (with damage to existing macrophage populations by the fibrogenic dusts) or can increase (with recruitment of macrophages to the sites of damage). These changes could lower lung defenses (by removing the primary defender of the lower respiratory tract[7,32]) or enhance the release of potentially damaging mediators into already damaged lung regions.

B. SIGNS OF DAMAGE TO THE AIR/BLOOD BARRIER

Vascular leakage of fluid into the alveolar space is one of the early signs of damage to epithelial and endothelial cells. Markers in the BAL that have been used to indicate these changes are the number of red blood cells (RBC) in the lavage fluid and the amount of albumin present in the BAL. RBCs are rarely present in normal BAL.[2,26] Their presence in the lavage fluid indicates rupture of capillaries. Albumin is a serum protein (MW 69000) that is synthesized solely in the liver. It is the most abundant protein in BAL from animals[33,34] and 30% of the total protein in humans.[26] An increase in the amount of albumin in the lavage serves as an indication of increased vascular permeability and alveolar edema.[2]

C. LYSOSOMAL ENZYMES

The two most commonly assayed lysosomal enzymes in BAL are β-N-acetyl glucosaminidase and peroxidase. β-N-acetyl glucosaminidase is an acid hydrolase that is found in the lysosomes of alveolar macrophages,[35] polymorphonuclear leukocytes,[36] and in type II epithelial cells.[37] It is probably nontoxic, but it is a good marker for increases in lysosomal enzyme release. Allison[38] originally had suggested that it could mediate chronic inflammation.

Peroxidase is an enzyme that catalyzes the oxidation of substrate using H_2O_2 as an electron acceptor. It is found in upper airway epithelial cells,[39] macrophages,[40] and PMNs.[41,42] PMN peroxidase can inactivate lung antiproteases[43] and lyse RBCs and platelets.[44] The presence of this enzyme in BAL fluid could thus enhance lung protease damage by inhibiting existing antiproteases as well as damaging cells directly.

D. PROTEINS AND PROTEASES

Lactate dehydrogenase (LDH) is a cytoplasmic enzyme involved in energy metabolism. Its presence in BAL fluid indicates cell damage.[45] Henderson et al.[46] showed that increased damage to the lungs of rats with Triton X-100 caused a dose-dependent increase in LDH release into BAL fluid (correlation factor = 0.98). Since LDH is a cytoplasmic enzyme present in all cells, the localization of damage to a particular cell type cannot be assessed simply by measuring its levels in BAL but can be addressed by measuring LDH isoenzyme patterns in BAL.[45,46]

Although not a strict lysosomal enzyme, alkaline phosphatase is a plasma membrane-associated enzyme that is present in BAL fluid.[47] Isoenzyme patterns show that the likely source is type 2 epithelial cells.[48] DeNicola et al.[49] suggest that increases in the amount of alkaline phosphatase in BAL could indicate type II injury or proliferation.

Both PMNs and macrophages secrete elastase.[50,51] BAL fluid contains elastase derived from each cell type.[52] The balance between elastases and antiproteases is important in the development of lung disease,[52] although its role in fibrotic lung disease is less certain. Frequently, increased elastase levels are complexed with endogenous inhibitors and are not enzymatically active.

Many other substances including large (immunoglobulins) and small (complement, interleukins, and tumor necrosis factors) proteins have been measured and observed in BAL fluid of animals or patients with fibrotic lung disease.[20,26,53,54] The existence and importance of soluble mediators have been addressed in other chapters of this book. Many have been included in reviews elsewhere[2] and will not be discussed further here.

III. HOW WELL DOES BAL PREDICT FIBROSIS?

In an effort to determine the key early events that lead to pulmonary fibrosis, investigators have frequently used BAL techniques. Isolated *in vitro* studies have been helpful in examining the effect of silica and other dusts on a particular cell type. Since the development of fibrosis involves the complex orchestration of events, BAL techniques have been used to sample the lung lining for inferences about the disease process with the hope of elucidating mechanisms and isolating factors that can predict the fibrogenicity of a particular dust or material.

Early studies on the effect of silica in isolated systems suggested that the early events, in fact the key events, that led to the development of fibrosis surrounded the effect of silica on the alveolar macrophage.[38,55,56] Exposing alveolar macrophages to quartz leads to cell death, lysosomal enzyme release, and overall diminished cell function. Investigators hypothesized that these cells then released fibroblast stimulating factors that activated fibroblast activity, increased collagen deposition, and eventually led to fibrosis.[19] Although it is clear that exposing cells directly to silica does cause cell damage, the extent to which this happens in the *in vivo* exposure is not as clear.

A. CELL RESPONSES

1. Instilled Silica

Morgan et al.[57] and Moores et al.[58] gave rats from 0.2 to 5 mg of silica by intratracheal instillation. They examined the effect of these varying doses at different times up to three months after dust exposure. BAL and histopathology (at three months) were used to evaluate the effect of silica on the lungs. They found a dose-dependent increase in PMN levels in the BAL 24 hours post silica, with a decrease in the number of macrophages. After seven days, the elevation in PMN numbers was persistent and was accompanied by an elevation of macrophage numbers. This persistent elevation of PMNs and macrophages in the lavage fluid was observed by others in rats,[54,59,60] by Beck et al.[6] in hamsters, by Dauber et al.[29] in guinea pigs, and by Bégin et al.[11,14] in sheep. The doses of quartz given to the animals varied, but when silica is given by intratracheal instillation, PMN numbers increase within 24 hours, persist up to three months post-instillation, and are accompanied by a persistent increase in macrophages. The number of macrophages at 24 hours was variable among the investigators, but the ultimate rise is consistent in all these studies.

How can we interpret elevation in cell numbers and their persistence? It seems clear that these types of elevations, and in particular the persistence of the elevation, may be crucial to the ultimate development of fibrosis. However, one way to evaluate these effects is to compare the cell response to quartz with another dust that is relatively inert. Beck et al.[6,61] have calibrated the response of hamsters to α-quartz with other non-toxic dusts such as iron oxide. When 3.75 mg of dust was instilled into the lungs, macrophage numbers were unchanged up to two weeks post instillation, but PMN numbers were significantly higher than control. The elevation in PMN number was half that of the response to quartz and diminished over time post instillation. Driscoll et al.[54] and Lindenschmidt et al.[60] compared instilled SiO_2 to TiO_2. Both studies found increased PMN numbers in rats given either 5 or 10 mg[54,60] TiO_2. This elevation was persistent but again was less than half of the PMN response to SiO_2 exposure. Macrophage numbers were also elevated only 24 hours post TiO_2. Then these numbers diminished over time. These studies together suggest that persistent elevation of both PMN and macrophage numbers may be important in distinguishing responses to fibrogenic and nonfibrogenic dusts.

2. Inhaled Silica

Other investigators argue that intratracheal instillation (IT) is an artificial way to deliver dust to the lungs. In humans, exposure to quartz is by aerosol. Responses in animals may differ if given by the inhalation route, especially since we know that aerosols produce a more uniform distribution of dust throughout the respiratory tract than instillation.[1] Yet instillation is much more convenient, rapid, and assures the delivery of the same amount of dust to each animal. With aerosols, the delivery to each animal may be more physiologic but takes longer, and the amount given to each individual animal is not as controlled.

How do the cellular responses to aerosolized quartz exposure compare to the responses described for IT quartz? It should be noted that the inhalation studies cannot be directly compared either to the intratracheal instillation studies or each other. As mentioned above, one cannot be assured of equivalent animal-to-animal dosing in inhalation studies nor can one compare studies since the conditions vary widely. For discussions of some of the issues that determine deposition in animal studies, see reviews by Brain and Valberg[62] and Sweeney.[63] In the following discussion we will only look at trends noted in each study and compare these trends with those observed in instillation studies.

Warheit et al.[20] exposed rats to concentrations up to 100 mg/m^3 SiO_2 for a single 6 h exposure or for 6 h on three consecutive days. The number of macrophages was not different, but PMN numbers were elevated within 24 hours post exposure and remained elevated for three months following exposure. Inhalation of 50 mg/m^3 for just 6 h resulted in a sustained PMN response. Rats exposed to similar concentrations and durations to a nontoxic dust, carbonyl iron, had similar macrophage and PMN numbers in their BAL fluid as sham controls at all times post exposure.

Other investigators have observed generally similar results as Warheit and colleagues.[20] Persistent PMN elevations in the BAL were found in guinea pigs (exposed to 28 mg/m^3 SiO_2 for three weeks[64]), rats (exposed to 100 mg/m^3 quartz for 6 h/d for 10 days[65]), and monkeys (exposed to 100 mg/m^3 quartz for 4 h/d for 18 weeks[66]). This elevation persisted up to nine months post-exposure.[65] When these elevations were compared with the response to relatively inert dusts, TiO_2, again PMN numbers in the lavage were no different than control.[64] The macrophage response was more variable; although in all studies, no persistent elevation in macrophage number was noted.

3. Summary

Whether exposed by intratracheal instillation or aerosol inhalation, a persistent elevation in PMN numbers in the BAL lavage fluid was consistently noted even up to nine months post exposure. These responses were either nonexistent (in aerosol exposed) or attenuated (in IT exposed) in animals given relatively nontoxic dusts. Variability in the number of macrophages in the BAL fluid occurred among the studies. Persistent increases were noted 48 h after instilled silica, but no persistent elevation was observed with inhaled silica. These differences may reflect the two exposure techniques. More important may be not how many macrophages were recovered in BAL, but how active these macrophages were. Were they activated? Inhibited? Mature? What cytokines do they produce?

If the results of these studies are based on function, rather than numbers, then some consistent results among the studies become clear. Beck et al.[6] measured *in vivo* phagocytic capability of macrophages. They found that exposure to quartz produced a dose-dependent depression of macrophage phagocytosis 24 hours after exposure but returned to normal by three days. Warheit et al.[20] found similar results in rats exposed to 100 mg/m^3 quartz for three days. Although the macrophage numbers were not different in aerosol-exposed animals, the population of macrophages in the lungs were younger in monkeys,[66] and the chemotactic ability of macrophages was reduced in quartz-exposed rat macrophages.[20,65] These data suggest that the population and activity of the resident macrophages in quartz-exposed lungs is different than in normal animal lungs.

B. PROTEINS AND ENZYMES IN BAL

Instilled silica causes a dose-dependent elevation of RBC and albumin in the BAL fluid 24 hours after instillation.[6] This response diminishes over time and returns to normal by 14 days post-instillation. Others have measured total protein in BAL and found it to have a dose-dependent increase[59,67] that is persistent beyond 14 days. Martin et al.[65] and Warheit et al.[20] also noted an increase in total protein in the BAL of rats exposed to aerosolized quartz.

Dethloff et al.[59] analyzed the protein in BAL and found that the increases could not be accounted for by damage to the blood/air barrier because many serum proteins were excluded from the lung; thus the lung maintained its selectivity despite quartz exposure. The source of these enhanced proteins may be other lung cells.

Another indicator of cell damage is the enzyme LDH. Beck and coworkers[6] noted a dose-dependent increase in LDH levels in BAL fluid 24 hours post instillation of silica. Similar results were obtained by Lindenschmidt et al.[60] This enhanced LDH level was persistent with time post lavage and diminished by 14 days in the hamster but was very prominent at 63 days in the rat.[6] Warheit et al.[20] and Sjostrand and Rylander[68] also noted increased LDH levels in the BAL of rats and guinea pigs exposed to aerosolized quartz.

Since LDH can come from a variety of sources including serum, macrophages, PMNs, RBCs, or other lung cells, Beck and coworkers[45] analyzed the LDH isoenzyme patterns following lung injury and found that the isoenzyme pattern following α-quartz exposure resembled damage to PMNs or macrophages. Moores et al.[58] suggested that PMN lysis may account for the increase in LDH levels, because LDH and PMN numbers correlated well. However the release of LDH from other lung cells cannot be excluded.

Lysosomal enzymes released into the BAL fluid indicate either enhanced release from cells or damage to cells. N-acetyl-glucosaminadase (NAG) levels were measured after instillation of quartz into the lungs of hamsters. The level of this enzyme in lung lavage fluid increased in a dose-dependent manner 24 hours after dust exposure and was persistent for two weeks after exposure.[6] Similar dose-dependent increases in NAG levels in BAL were found for rats.[59,60] In rats, the increased NAG levels persisted up to 63 days post exposure.[60] Exposure of rats[68] or guinea pigs[64] to aerosolized quartz also enhanced the levels of NAG in BAL fluid. Other enzymes measured include acid phosphatase, alkaline phosphatase, and peroxidase. The release of all of the enzymes into BAL fluid increased with exposure to α-quartz whether the animals were exposed by instillation[6,57–59] or by aerosol.[20,64,68]

C. CONCLUSIONS

Beck et al.[6] have tried to determine which parameter in BAL fluid would best predict subsequent disease by calibrating the assay with fibrogenic (α-quartz) compared with nonfibrogenic (iron oxide) exposures. When the ratio of the quartz to the iron oxide response was calculated for each parameter, some seemed more predictive if measured one day after exposure while others were more predictive at four days following exposure. At one day, albumin, peroxidase, NAG, and macrophage phagocytosis were the most important parameters. At four days, LDH levels and PMN and macrophage numbers were more predictive.

Dethloff and colleagues[59,67] also thought that the early events that occur after silica deposition in the lung may be key in understanding the mechanisms that lead to fibrosis. They examined how cellular and extracellular responses to silica related to each other. They suggested that since the amount of soluble protein in the BAL increases enormously after silica, silica may increase the rate at which these proteins cross the air/blood barrier due to leakage through a broken epithelial lining. Morphologically they observed damage to epithelial cells. Furthermore they found a correlation between the amount of phospholipid in BAL and the amount of soluble protein. They found no correlation between the amount of NAG or alkaline phosphatase in BAL and the amount of PMNs, suggesting that although PMNs make both proteins, these cells probably aren't the cause of their release. Since Type II epithelial cells make both,[69] these cells may be the primary source. These cells are also the source of the increased lipid they found in the lavage fluid and thus may play a role in the developing disease process.

Lindenschmidt and coworkers[60] compared the response to quartz with nonfibrogenic dusts (titanium dioxide and aluminum oxide). They observed animals for up to two months after dust exposure and found that the BAL parameters continued to increase for quartz-exposed animals but not for the other dusts. LDH, total protein, and NAG levels all were persistently elevated in quartz-exposed but not in the nonfibrogenic dust-exposed animals. PMN and lymphocyte numbers were the most sensitive of the cell changes to quartz exposure. Not only can the magnitude of the changes predict the toxic nature of the dust, but the persistence of these changes over time post exposure can as well.

IV. WHY ASSAY BY BAL?

As just discussed, there can be a large degree of variability in the pulmonary response to instilled or inhaled particles when lung lining fluid is assayed by BAL. Are the results worth pursuing? We think they are for a number of reasons. First, in animals, if properly calibrated, BAL can be used as a predictor of

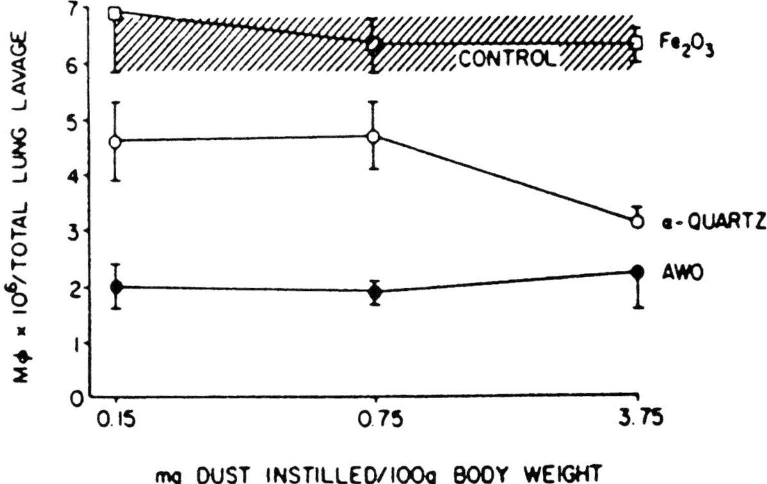

FIGURE 1 Dose response curve for macrophage numbers at day one post exposure. (From Beck et al., *Inhaled Particles VI,* Pergamon Press, Oxford, 1988, 257.)

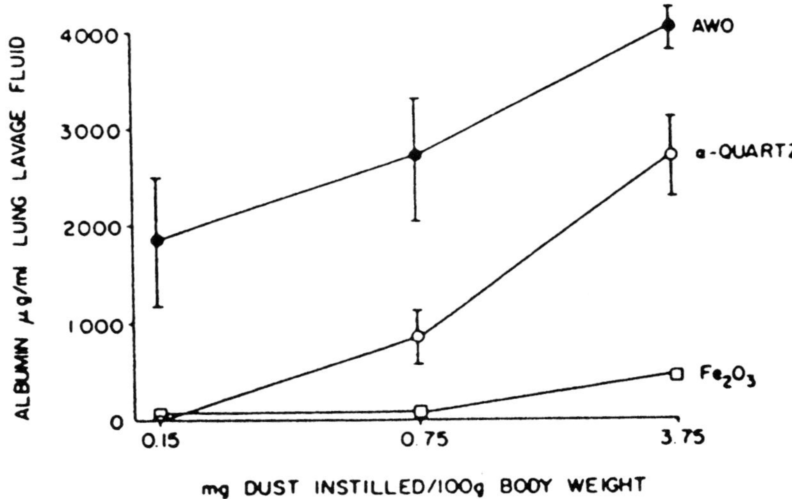

FIGURE 2 Dose response curve for albumin levels at day one post exposure. (From Beck et al., *Inhaled Particles VI,* Pergamon Press, Oxford, 1988, 257.)

potentially harmful dusts. Second, in humans, BAL offers the best method available to study the pathogenesis of pulmonary disease and to test therapeutic interventions. Third, BAL can be used to explore the mechanisms of disease in both animals and humans. Importantly, new techniques of molecular biology permit measurement of cytokines in BAL that may be involved in fibrogenesis, such as TGFB, TNF, PDGF, and other mediators.

Beck et al.[6,45,61,70] and Henderson et al.[15,46] have used BAL to predict the potential toxicity of unknown dusts. An example of these types of data are shown in Figures 1 and 2. Respirable particulates were collected from an air-atomizing oil space heater using automobile waste crankcase oil (AWO[70]). The responses in hamsters one day after instillation were compared to known fibrogenic dusts (α-quartz) and an inert dust (Fe_2O_3). Macrophage (M) numbers and activity were depressed, while albumin and glucosaminidase in the lavage fluid were elevated to levels equaling or exceeding known fibrogenic dusts.

These data suggest that AWO may be as toxic as α-quartz. Yet when BAL was analyzed 14 days after exposure, most indicators approached control values. Thus, the inflammation caused by AWO is not chronic and persistent, as it would be with a true fibrogenic dust. Comparisons such as these are useful when evaluating the potential toxicity of unknown dusts.

As reviewed by Daniele et al.[71] and Reynolds,[72] BAL has been increasingly used to evaluate patients with interstitial lung disease to help understand the pathogenesis of the disease. Cell types and soluble products recovered by lavage have been used to assess the inflammatory process in the lung. Cells in lung lavage fluid are similar to those found in lung biopsy of patients with pulmonary fibrosis.[17,73] Although interpretation of the data is complicated, as discussed in this review, several important insights have been observed using this technique.[71] Fibrotic lung disease is characterized by increases in both neutrophil and monocyte cell numbers. Cell activation may play a pivotal role in the pathogenesis of fibrosis,[74] and types of cell responses may differentiate types of interstitial lung disease. When soluble products in BAL can be quantified so that the exact amount can be compared from patient to patient, then mechanisms of fibrogenesis can better be explored.

V. SUMMARY AND FUTURE DIRECTIONS

Refining techniques for BAL in humans and developing better ways to quantify the constituents of lavage fluid from patient to patient will extend the usefulness of this technique from a diagnostic tool to a quantitative technique. BAL is of importance in evaluating the mechanisms and the therapeutic treatment of disease. In animal models, correlations between responses in animals to those in humans will help the interpretation of experimental results. Animal models provide the best way at present to explore disease mechanisms and pathogenesis.

REFERENCES

1. **Brain, J. D., Knudson, D. E., Sorokin, S. P., and Davis, M. A.,** Pulmonary distribution of particles given by intratracheal instillation or by aerosol inhalation, *Environ. Res.,* 11, 13–33, 1976.
2. **Brain, J. D. and Beck, B. D.,** Bronchoalveolar Lavage, in *Handbook of Experimental Pharmacology,* Witschi, H.P. and Brain, J.D., Eds., Vol. 75, Springer Verlag, Berlin, 1985, 203–226.
3. **Brain, J. D. and Frank, N. R.,** Recovery of free cells from rat lungs by repeated washings, *J. Appl. Physiol.,* 25, 63–69, 1968.
4. **Brain, J. D. and Frank, N. R.,** The relation of age to the number of lung free cells, lung weight, and body weight of rats, *J. Gerontol.,* 23, 58–62, 1968.
5. **Brain, J. D. and Frank, N. R.,** Alveolar macrophage adhesion: wash electrolyte composition and free cell yield, *J. Appl. Physiol.,* 34, 75–80, 1973.
6. **Beck, B. D., Brain, J. D., and Bohannon, D. E.,** An *in vivo* hamster bioassay to assess the toxicity of particulates for the lungs, *Toxicol. Appl. Pharmacol.,* 66, 9–29, 1982.
7. **Brain, J. D.,** Free cells in the lungs, *Arch. Intern. Med.,* 126, 477–487, 1970.
8. **Skoza, L., Snyder, A., and Kikkawa, Y.,** Ascorbic acid in bronchoalveolar wash, *Lung,* 161, 99–109, 1983.
9. **Davis, G. S., Giancola, M. S., Costanza, M. C., and Low, R. B.,** Analysis of sequential bronchoalveolar lavage samples from healthy human volunteers, *Am. Rev. Respir. Dis.,* 126, 611–616, 1982.
10. **Cohen, A. B. and Batra, G. K.,** Bronchoscopy and lung lavage induced bilateral pulmonary neutrophil influx and blood leukocytosis in dogs and monkeys, *Am. Rev. Respir. Dis.,* 122, 239–247, 1980.
11. **Bégin, R., Rola-Pleszczynski, M., Sirois, P., Masse, S., Nadeau, D., and Bureau, M. A.,** Sequential analysis of the bronchoalveolar milieu in conscious sheep, *J. Appl. Physiol.,* 50, 665–671, 1981.
12. **Strumpf, I. J., Feld, M. K., Cornelius, M. J., Keogh, B. A., and Crystal, R. G.,** Safety of fiberoptic bronchoalveolar lavage in evaluation of interstitial lung disease, *Chest,* 80, 268–271, 1981.
13. **Fahey, P. J., Utell, M. J., Mayewski, R. J., Wandtke, J. D., and Hyde, R. W.,** Early diagnosis of bleomycin pulmonary toxicity using bronchoalveolar lavage in dogs, *Am. Rev. Respir. Dis.,* 126, 126–130, 1982.
14. **Bégin, R., Dufresne, A., Cantin, A., Possmayer, F., and Sebastien, P.,** Quartz exposure, retention and early silicosis in sheep, *Exper. Lung Res.,* 15, 409–428, 1989.
15. **Henderson, R. F., Rebar, A. H., Pickrell, J. A., and Newton, G. J.,** Early damage indicators in the lung. III. Biochemical and cytological response of the lung to inhaled metal salts, *Toxicol. Appl. Pharm.,* 50, 123–136, 1979.

16. **Burns, D. M., Shure, D., Francoz, R., Kalafer, M., Harrell, J., Witztum, K., and Moser, K. M.,** The physiologic consequences of saline lobar lavage in healthy human adults, *Am. Rev. Respir. Dis.*, 127, 695–701, 1983.
17. **Hunninghake, G. W., Kawanami, O., Ferrans, V. J., Young, R. C., Roberts, W. C., and Crystal, R. G.,** Characterization of inflammatory and immune effector cells in the lung parenchyma of patients with interstitial lung disease, *Am. Rev. Respir. Dis.*, 123, 407–12, 1981.
18. **Kaelin, R. M., Center, D. M., Bernardo, J., Grant, M., and Snider, G. L.,** The role of macrophage-derived chemoattractant activities in the early inflammatory events of bleomycin-induced pulmonary injury, *Am. Rev. Respir. Dis.*, 128, 132–137, 1983.
19. **Lugano, E. M., Dauber, J. H., and Daniele, R. P.,** Acute experimental silicosis: Lung morphology, histology, and macrophage chemotaxin secretion, *Am. J. Pathol.*, 109, 27–36, 1984.
20. **Warheit, D. B., Carakostas, M. C., Hartsky, M. A., and Hansen, J. F.,** Development of a short-term inhalation bioassay to assess pulmonary toxicity of inhaled particles: comparisons of pulmonary responses to carbonyl iron and silica, *Toxicol. Appl. Pharmacol.*, 107, 350–368, 1991.
21. **Rennard, S. I., Basset, G., Lecossier, D., O'Donnell, K. M., Pinkston, P., Martin, P. G., and Crystal, R. G.,** Estimation of volume of epithelial lining fluid recovered by lavage using urea as marker of dilution, *J. Appl. Physiol.*, 60, 532–538, 1986.
22. **Feng, N. H., Hacker, A., and Effros, R. M.,** Solute exchange between the plasma and epithelial lining fluid of rat lungs, *J. Appl. Physiol.*, 72, 1081–1089, 1992.
23. **Effros, R. M., Feng, D., Mason, G., Sietsema, K., Silverman, P., and Hukkanen, J.,** Solute concentrations of the epithelial lining fluid in anesthetized rats, *J. Appl. Physiol.*, 68, 275–281, 1990.
24. **Marcy, T. W., Merrill, W. W., Rankin, J. A., and Reynolds, H. Y.,** Limitations of using urea to quantify epithelial lining fluid recovered by bronchoalveolar lavage, *Am. Rev. Respir. Dis.*, 135, 1276–1280, 1987.
25. **Kelly, C. A., Fenwick, J. D., Corris, P. A., Fleetwood, A., Hendrick, D. J., and Walters, E. H.,** Fluid dynamics during bronchoalveolar lavage, *Am. Rev. Respir. Dis.*, 138, 81–84, 1988.
26. **Young, K. R. and Reynolds, H. Y.,** Bronchoalveolar lavage in inhalation lung toxicity, in *Pathophysiology and Treatment of Inhalation Injuries*, Loke, J., Ed., Marcel Dekker, New York, 1988, 207–237.
27. **Brain, J. D.,** Lung macrophages. How many kinds are there and what do they do? *Am. Rev. Respir. Dis.*, 1988.
28. **Hunninghake, G. W., Gadek, J. E., Kawanami, O., Ferrans, V. J., and Crystal, R. G.,** Inflammatory and immune processes in the human lung in health and disease: evaluation by bronchoalveolar lavage, *Am. J. Pathol.*, 97, 149–206, 1979.
29. **Dauber, J. H., Rossman, M. D., and Daniele, R. P.,** Pulmonary fibrosis: bronchoalveolar cell types and impaired function of alveolar macrophages in experimental silicosis, *Environ. Res.*, 27, 226–236, 1982.
30. **Thrall, R. S., Phan, S. H., McCormick, J. R., and Ward, P. A.,** The development of bleomycin-induced pulmonary fibrosis in the neutrophil depleted and complement depleted rats, *Am. J. Pathol.*, 105, 76–81, 1981.
31. **Wedmore, C. V. and Williams, T. V.,** Control of vascular permeability by polymorphonuclear leukocytes in inflammation, *Nature*, 289, 646–650, 1981.
32. **Gardner, D. E., and Graham, J. A.,** Increased pulmonary disease mediated through altered bacterial defenses, in *Pulmonary Macrophages and Epithelial Cells*, Sanders, C.L., Schneider, R.P., Dagle, G.E., and Ragan, H.E., Eds., Technical Information Center, Springfield, VA, 1977, 1–21.
33. **Bell, D. Y., Haseman, J. A., Spock, A., McLennan, G., and Hook, G. E. R.,** Plasma proteins of the bronchoalveolar surface of the lungs of smokers and nonsmokers, *Am. Rev. Respir. Dis.*, 124, 72–79, 1981.
34. **Merrill, W., O'Hearn, E., Rankin, J., Naegel, G., Matthay, G., and Reynolds, H. Y.,** Kinetic analysis of respiratory tract proteins recovered during a sequential lavage protocol, *Am. Rev. Respir. Dis.*, 126, 617–620, 1982.
35. **Davies, P. and Bonney, R. J.,** The secretion of hydrolytic enzymes of mononuclear phagocytes, in *The Cell Biology of Inflammation*, Weissman, G., Ed., Elsevier, North Holland, NY, 1980, 497–542.
36. **Weissman, G., Smolin, J. E., and Korchak, H. M.,** Release of inflammatory mediators from stimulated neutrophils, *N. Engl. J. Med.*, 303, 27–39, 1980.
37. **Hook, G. E. R.,** Extracellular hydrolases of the lung, *Biochem.*, 17, 520–528, 1979.
38. **Allison, A. C.,** Mechanism of macrophage damage in relation to the pathogenesis of some lung diseases, in *Respiratory Defense Mechanisms*, Brain, J.D., Proctor, D.F., and Reid, L.M., Eds., Marcel Dekker, New York, 1977, 1075–1102.
39. **Christensen, T. G. and Hayes, H. A.,** Endogenous peroxidase in the conducting airways of hamsters, *Am. Rev. Respir. Dis.*, 125, 341–346, 1982.
40. **Daems, T., Roos, D., vanBerkel, T. J. C., and Van der Rhee, H. H.,** The subcellular distribution and biochemical properties of peroxidase in monocytes and macrophages, in, *Lysosomes in Applied Biology and Therapeutics*, Dingle, J.T., Jacques, P.J., and Shaw, I.H., Eds., North Holland, New York, 1979, 463–514.
41. **Klebanoff, S. J., Clem, W. H., and Leubke, R. G.,** The peroxidase-thiocyanate-hydrogen peroxide antimicrobial system, *Biochim. Biophys. Acta*, 117, 63–72, 1966.
42. **Klebanoff, S. H.,** Oxygen metabolism and the toxic properties of phagocytes, *Ann. Intern. Med.*, 93, 480–488, 1980.
43. **Matheson, N. R., Wong, P. S., Schuyler, M., and Travis, J.,** Interaction of alpha-1-proteinase inhibitor with neutrophil myeloperoxidase, *Biochem.*, 20, 331–336, 1981.

44. **Weiss, S. J. and LoBuglio, A. F.,** Biology of disease. Phagocytic-generated oxygen metabolites and cellular injury, *Lab. Invest.*, 47, 5–18, 1982.
45. **Beck, B. D., Gerson, B., Feldman, H. A., and Brain, J. D.,** Lactate dehydrogenase isoenzymes in hamster lung lavage fluid after lung injury, *Toxicol. Appl. Pharmacol.*, 71, 59–71, 1983.
46. **Henderson, R. F., Damon, E. G., and Henderson, T. R.,** Early damage indicators in the lung. I. Lactate dehydrogenase activity in the airways, *Toxicol. Appl. Pharmacol.*, 44, 291–297, 1978.
47. **Reasor, M. J., Nadeau, D., and Hook, G. E. R.,** Extracellular alkaline phosphatase in the rabbit lung, *Lung,* 155, 321–335, 1978.
48. **DiAugustine, R. P.,** Lung concentric laminar organelle. Hydrolase activity and compositional analysis, *J. Biol. Chem.*, 249, 584–593, 1974.
49. **DeNicola, D. B., Rebar, A. H., and Henderson, R. F.,** Early damage indicators in the lung. V. Biochemical and cytological response to NO_2 inhalation, *Toxicol. Appl. Pharmacol.*, 60, 301–312, 1981.
50. **Ohlsson, K. and Olsson, I.,** The neutral proteases of human granulocytes: isolation and partial characterization of granulocyte elastase, *Eur. J. Biochem.*, 42, 519, 1974.
51. **Hinman, L. J., Stevens, C., Matthay, R. A., and Gee, J. B. L.,** Elastase and lysozyme activities in human alveolar macrophages, *Am. Rev. Respir. Dis.*, 121, 263–271, 1980.
52. **Janoff, A., Raju, L., and Dearing, R.,** Levels of elastase activity in bronchoalveolar lavage fluids of healthy smokers and nonsmokers, *Am. Rev. Respir. Dis.*, 127, 540–544, 1983.
53. **Phan, S. H., Varani, J., and Smith, D.,** Rat lung fibroblast collagen metabolism in bleomycin-induced pulmonary fibrosis, *J. Clin. Invest.*, 76, 241–247, 1985.
54. **Driscoll, K. E., Linderschmidt, R. C., Maurer, J. K., Higgins, J. M., and Ridder, G.,** Pulmonary response to silica or titanium dioxide: inflammatory cells, alveolar macrophage-derived cytokines, and histopathology, *Am. J. Respir. Cell Mol. Biol.*, 2, 381–390, 1990.
55. **Miller, K. and Kagan, E.,** The *in vivo* effects of quartz on alveolar macrophage membrane topography and on the characteristics of the intrapulmonary cell population, *J. Reticuloendothel. Soc.*, 21, 307–316, 1977.
56. **Reiser, K. M. and Last, J. A.,** Silicosis and fibrogenesis-fact and artifact, *Toxicology,* 13, 51–72, 1979.
57. **Morgan, A., Moores, S. R., Holmes, A., Evans, J. C., Evans, N. H., and Black, A.,** The effect of quartz, administered by intratracheal instillation, on the rat lung. I. The cellular response, *Environ. Res.*, 22, 1–12, 1980.
58. **Moores, S. R., Black, A., Evans, J. C., Evans, N. H., Holmes, A., and Morgan, A.,** The effect of quartz, administered by intratracheal instillation, on the rat lung. II. The short-term biochemical response, *Environ. Res.*, 24, 275–285, 1981.
59. **Dethloff, L. A., Gilmore, L. B., Gladen, B. C., George, G., Chhabra, R. S., and Hook, G. E. R.,** Effects of silica on the composition of the pulmonary extracellular lining, *Toxicol. Appl. Pharmacol.*, 84, 66–83, 1986.
60. **Lindenschmidt, R. C., Driscoll, K. E., Perkins, M. A., Higgins, J. M., Maurer, J. K., and Belfiore, K. A.,** The comparison of a fibrogenic and two nonfibrogenic dusts by bronchoalveolar lavage, *Toxicol. Appl. Pharmacol.*, 102, 268–281, 1990.
61. **Beck, B. D. and Brain, J. D.,** Predicting the pulmonary toxicity of particulates using damage indicators in lung lavage fluid, in *Health Issues Related to Metal and Nonmetallic Mining,* Wagner, W.L., Rom, W.N., and Merchant, J.A., Eds., Butterworth, Boston, 1983, 83–103.
62. **Brain, J. D. and Valberg, P. A.,** Deposition of aerosol in the respiratory tract, *Am. Rev. Respir. Dis.*, 120, 1325–1373, 1979.
63. **Sweeney, T. D.,** Exposing animals to aerosols: considerations that influence regional lung deposition, *J. Aerosol Med.*, 3, 169–186, 1990.
64. **Fogelmark, B., Sjostrand, M., Bergstrom, R., and Rylander, R.,** Pulmonary macrophage phagocytosis and enzyme production after *in vivo* exposure to silica dust, *Toxicol. Appl. Pharmacol.*, 68, 152–160, 1983.
65. **Martin, T. R., Chi, E. Y., Covert, D. S., Hodson, W. A., Kessler, D. E., Moore, W. E., Altman, L. C., and Butler, J.,** Comparative effects of inhaled volcanic ash and quartz in rats, *Am. Rev. Respir. Dis.*, 128, 144–152, 1983.
66. **Hannothiaux, M. H., Scharfman, A., Wastiaux, A., Cornu, L., Van Brussel, E., Lafitte, J. J., Sebastien, P., and Roussel, P.,** An attempt to evaluate lung aggression in monkey silicosis: hydrolases, peroxidase and antiproteases activities in serial bronchoalveolar lavages, *Eur. Respir. J.*, 4, 191–204, 1991.
67. **Dethloff, L. A., Gladon, B. C., Gilmore, L. B., and Hook, G. E. R.,** Quantitation of cellular and extracellular constituents of the pulmonary lining in rats by using bronchoalveolar lavage. Effects of silica-induced pulmonary inflammation, *Am. Rev. Respir. Dis.*, 136, 899–907, 1987.
68. **Sjostrand, M. and Rylander, R.,** Enzymes in lung lavage fluid after inhalation exposure to silica dust, *Environ. Res.*, 33, 307–311, 1984.
69. **Hook, G. E. R. and Gilmore, L. B.,** Hydrolases of pulmonary lysosomes and lamellar bodies, *J. Biol. Chem.*, 257, 9211–9220, 1982.
70. **Beck, B. D., Brain, J. D., and Wolfthal, S. F.,** Assessment of lung injury produced by particulate emissions of space heaters burning automobile waste oil, in *Inhaled Particles VI,* Dodgson, J., McCallum, R.I., Bailey, M.R., and Fisher, D.R., Eds., Pergamon Press, Oxford, 1988, 257.

71. **Daniele, R. P., Elias, J. A., Epstein, P. E., and Rossman, M. D.,** Bronchoalveolar lavage: role in the pathogenesis, diagnosis, and management of interstitial lung disease, *Ann. Intern. Med.,* 102, 93–108, 1985.
72. **Reynolds, H. Y.,** Bronchoalveolar lavage, *Am. Rev. Respir. Dis.,* 135, 250–263, 1987.
73. **Haslam, P. L., Turton, C. W. G., Heard, B., et al.,** Bronchoalveolar lavage in pulmonary fibrosis: comparison of cells obtained with lung biopsy and clinical features, *Thorax,* 35, 9–18, 1980.
74. **Crystal, R. G., Bitterman, P. B., Rennard, S. I., Hance, A. J., and Keogh, B. A.,** Interstitial lung diseases of unknown cause: disorders characterized by chronic inflammation of the lower respiratory tract. Part 1, *New Engl. J. Med.,* 94, 73–94, 1981.

Section III
Chapter 7

EARLY ROLE OF LIPID INFLAMMATORY MEDIATORS IN SILICA TOXICITY: POSSIBLE METHODS TO DETOXIFY SILICA

Knox Van Dyke, Jaime Gutierrez, Christopher Van Dyke, and Lixin Wu

CONTENTS

0-8493-4709-2/96/$0.00+$.50

I. INTRODUCTION (SILICA, THE LUNG, INFLAMMATION, AND FIBROSIS)

Inhalation of respirable-size silica (0.1 to 5 μm in diameter) deposits the particles in the deep spaces of the lung where oxygen is exchanged. The resulting pattern of inflammation is substantially different compared to that observed from other inhaled substances such as carbon, polystyrene, titanium dioxide, etc.[1] Following the inflammatory reaction, the body attempts to isolate the damage by walling off the area via fibrosis.[2] The unique nature of the inflammatory response to silica makes it logical to infer that fibrosis is a later-stage manifestation of the initial inflammatory damage. In addition to the inflammation, extensive lysis and cellular death, particularly to macrophages and neutrophils, can occur, depending on the dose of silica.[3] The ingestion of significant amounts of silica by macrophages and neutrophils produces an inflammatory sequence which activates the lipoxygenase pathway of arachidonic acid metabolism and produces platelet activating factor (PAF) and leukotrienes (LT).[4,5]

II. CALCIUM IONOPHORE MIMICS SILICA TOXICITY *IN VITRO*

Phagocytic cells exposed to silica *in vitro* produce PAF and LT. This response is reminiscent of phagocytic cells exposed to the calcium ionophore (A23187) in the presence of ionic calcium.[6–8] A23187 forms a complex with free, ionic calcium which passes through cellular membranes, thus transporting calcium inside the cell. The increased intracellular calcium concentration triggers the production of small amounts of prostaglandins, large amounts of LT, PAF, and, depending on dose, cellular death (see Figure 1). Could silica cause LT production and cellular death by a similar mechanism? How could silica — an inert solid — act in a similar fashion as a soluble stimulant? Clearly, the negative SiO_2^- and OH^- surface of silica can bind calcium ions[9] and therefore could theoretically act as a solid-state ionophore releasing bound calcium inside of cells following phagocytosis.

III. METABOLISM OF ARACHIDONIC ACID AND PAF PRODUCTION

Several pathways exist for the metabolism of arachidonic acid. First, at low intracellular calcium concentration, the cyclooxygenase pathway predominates, resulting in the production of prostaglandins, prostacyclin, and thromboxanes.[10] Secondly, under certain conditions, arachidonic acid can react with oxygen to produce lipoxins. Finally, at high concentrations of intracellular calcium, arachidonic acid is

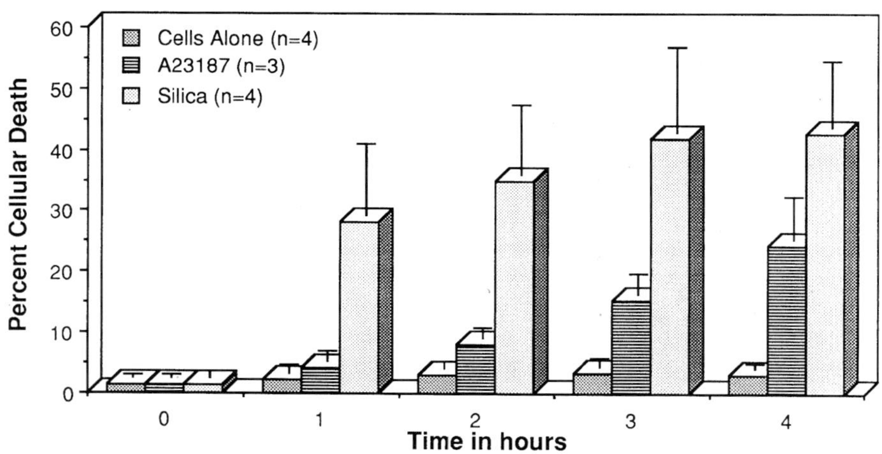

FIGURE 1 Flow cytometry of human neutrophils either exposed to silica or calcium ionophore (A23187) vs. time at room temperature. Note that both silica and A23187 cause significant cellular death as compared to the sample containing only cells as measured propidium iodide assay (see Methods for details).

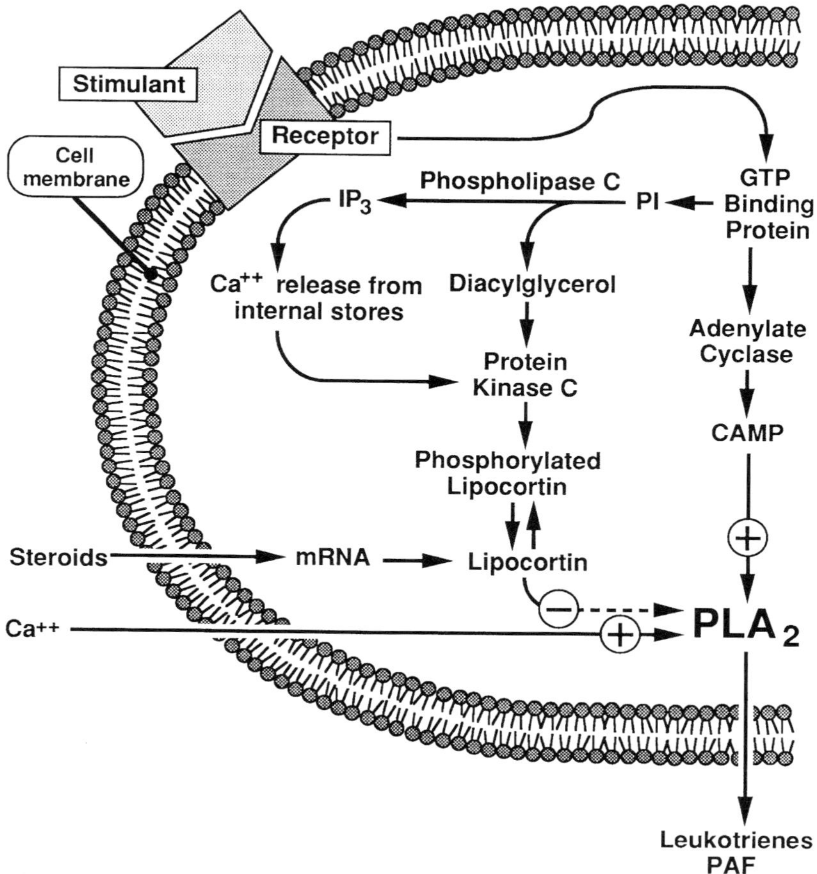

FIGURE 2 A schematic representation of the activation of phospholipase A_2 (PLA_2). PLA_2 may be activated by either a stimulant/receptor mechanism activating a guanosine 5′-triphosphate (GTP) binding protein and initiating a cascade of events or via increased intracellular calcium. The addition of steroids interferes with PLA_2. Notice that ionic calcium acts directly to activate PLA_2, bypassing the normal negative feedback.

predominantly metabolized by lipoxygenase.[11] Note that intracellular calcium concentrations are normally around 10^{-7} *M,* while concentrations in extracellular fluids are 10^{-3} *M;* therefore, relatively small amounts of external calcium can be toxic if carried into a cell.

Following activation of the lipoxygenase pathway, arachidonic acid which is esterified in the C_2 position of the glycerol backbone in phospholipids is released. The phospholipid could be an etherated type (1–0 alkyl 2-arachidonyl-glycero phosphocholine) or an esterified type (1-alkyl 2-arachidonyl glycero phosphocholine). In either case, arachidonic acid is made available by the action of calcium on phospholipase activating protein (PLAP) located in the membrane of phagocytes, and phospholipase A_2 (PLA_2), a docking enzyme from the cytoplasm (see Figure 2).[12,13] The arachidonic acid then reacts with activated 5′ lipoxygenase in the presence of 5′ lipoxygenase activating protein (FLAP), ionic calcium, adenosine 5′ triphosphate, and oxygen (see Figure 3).[14] The above reaction produces LTA_4, which can further react with oxygen to produce LTB_4 or react with glutathione to produce LTC_4. LTC_4 degrades to LTD_4 and then to LTE_4 (see Figure 4). LTC_4, LTD_4, and LTE_4 are known as slow-reacting substances of anaphylaxsis. The LTB_4 is a tremendously active chemotactic substance for neutrophils, the cell type which dominates the lavage fluid of silicotics.[15]

Both silica and the calcium ionophore cause a large increase in intracellular calcium concentration, which results in the domination of the lipoxygenase pathway of arachidonic acid metabolism. While the mechanism by which A23187 raises intracellular calcium levels is known, the mechanism of silica is not entirely understood. Silica, in the presence of extracellular calcium, may bind calcium which is released

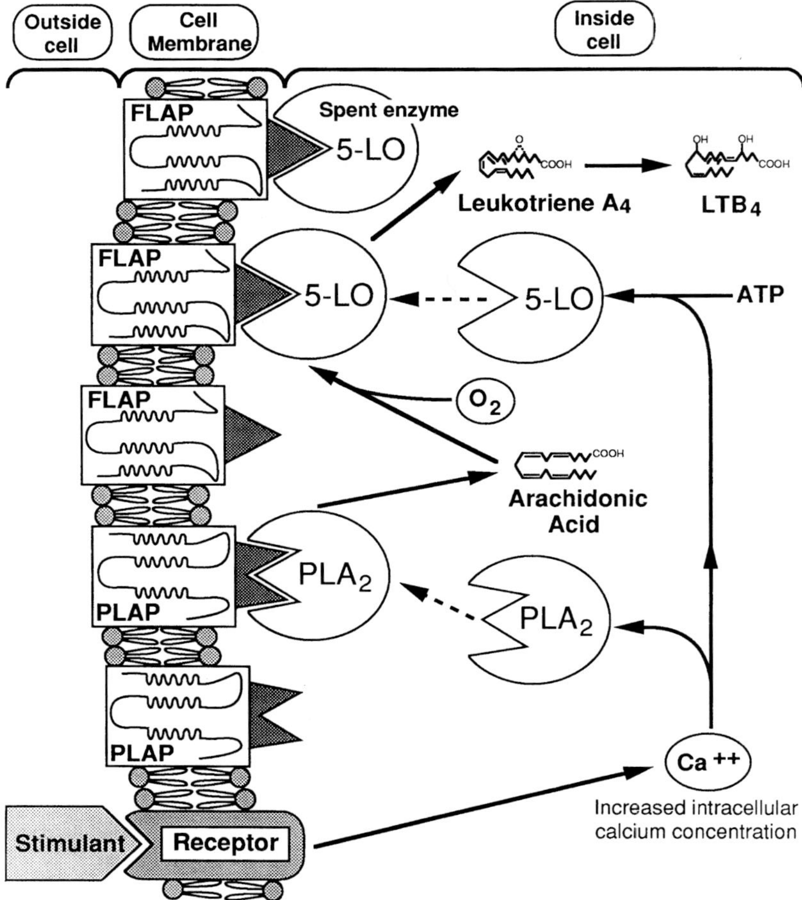

FIGURE 3 A schematic representation showing the activation and docking of phospholipase A_2 (PLA_2) and 5-lipoxygenase (5-LO), resulting in the production of leukotrienes A_4 and B_4. Following increased intracellular calcium concentration, PLA_2 docks on PLA_2 activating protein (PLAP) located in the cell membrane, resulting in the production of arachidonic acid. Increased calcium concentration also triggers 5-LO to dock to 5-LO activating protein (FLAP). With the addition of ATP and oxygen, arachidonic acid is converted by the activated 5-LO to leukotrienes, most notably LTB_4, a potent chemotatic agent. Following the production of leukotrienes, the spent enzyme stays attached to FLAP.

inside the cell following phagocytosis. In this fashion, silica may act as a calcium carrier (see Figure 5).[16] The ingestion of silica may also cause membrane damage and allow calcium to leak into the cell (see Figure 6).[17] A final possibility is that silica somehow causes the release of ionic calcium from intracellular stores.[18] Regardless of whether the above possibilities occur singly or in combination, it is clear that calcium plays a key role in the activation of the lipoxygenase metabolism of arachidonic acid, production of PAF, and cellular death. If the intracellular calcium is chelated using INDO-1AM (which is metabolized to an active chelator inside the cell), death in neutrophils exposed to silica is prevented from occurring so rapidly (see Figure 16).

IV. SURFACE CHARACTERISTICS OF SILICA AND METAL BINDING

Silica has the molecular formula SiO_2 and occurs naturally in a variety of crystalline and amorphous states; some common examples include quartz, sand, and glass. Given the biologically inert nature of these examples, why should silica create massive, acute inflammatory reactions and tremendous cyclic

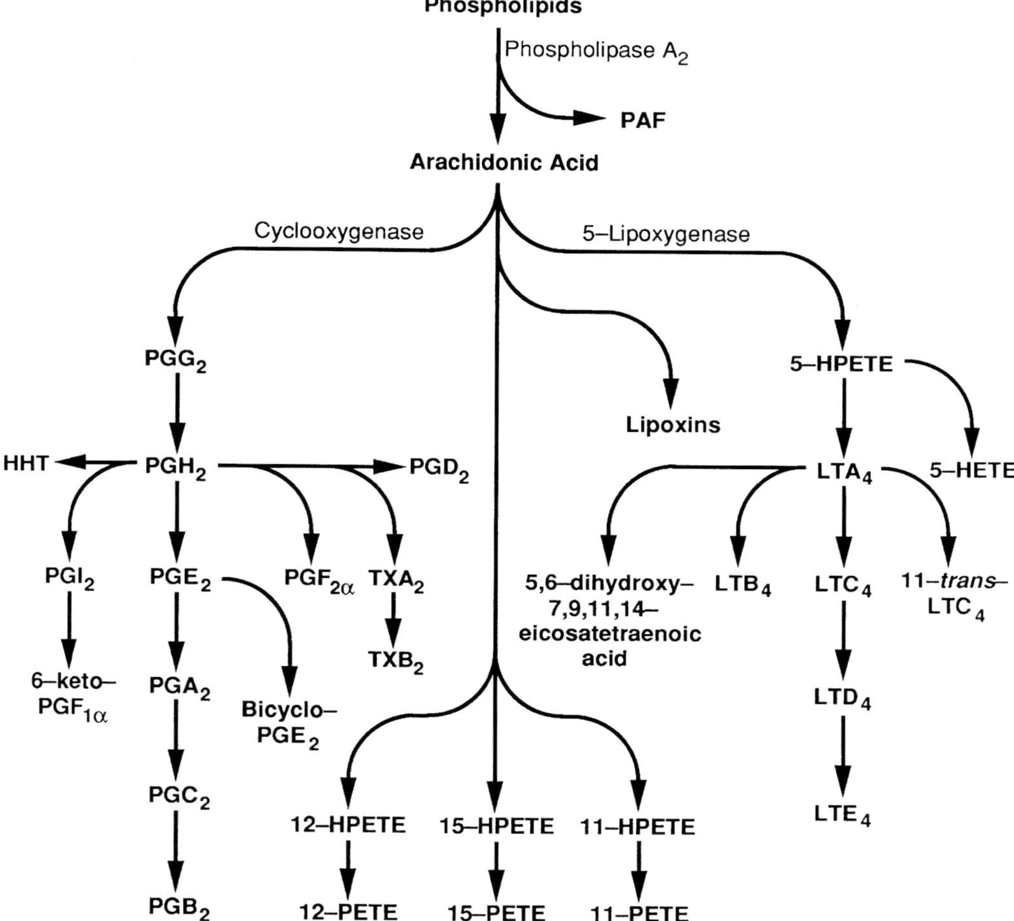

FIGURE 4 The arachidonic acid cascade in neutrophils. Once arachidonic acid is produced from phospholipids, it can be metabolized by various pathways based on conditions in the intracellular environment. Metabolism via cyclooxygenase results in the production of various prostaglandins (PG) and thromboxanes (TX), while metabolism via 5-lipoxygenase results in the production of leukotrienes. Arachidonic acid metabolism may also result in the production of lipoxins or slow-reacting substances (HETE and HPETE) via 5-lipoxygenase. While not strictly a pathway of arachidonic acid metabolism, platelet activating factor (PAF) may also be produced from arachidonic acid.

toxicity leading to fibrosis? The key to this question is that such particles cannot be biodegraded by host systems and that, since the interior of the particles could never be exposed, surface chemistry must be responsible for the constant toxicity. Pandurangi and Seehra[19] have shown that surface silanol groups (SiOH) are important to toxicity linked to hemolysis and fibrosis. Vallayathan et al.[20] have shown that freshly broken silica has surface free radicals that produce greater toxicity than aged, broken silica. In addition, Shi and Dalal[21] demonstrated that Vd and Cr metal ions can be absorbed on mineral dust which can produce free radicals, e.g., OH^-. Mining a variety of minerals produces respirable-sized silica as a by-product which could serve to compound the toxicity of the desired mineral. Some examples of this are lead, iron, and copper mining.[22]

V. MECHANISM OF CALCIUM BINDING TO SILICA

Crystalline silica forms a tetrahedral structure with silicon in the center. These center atoms attach to four oxygen atoms, each of which in turn attach to silicon atoms. The terminal silicon atoms attach to only

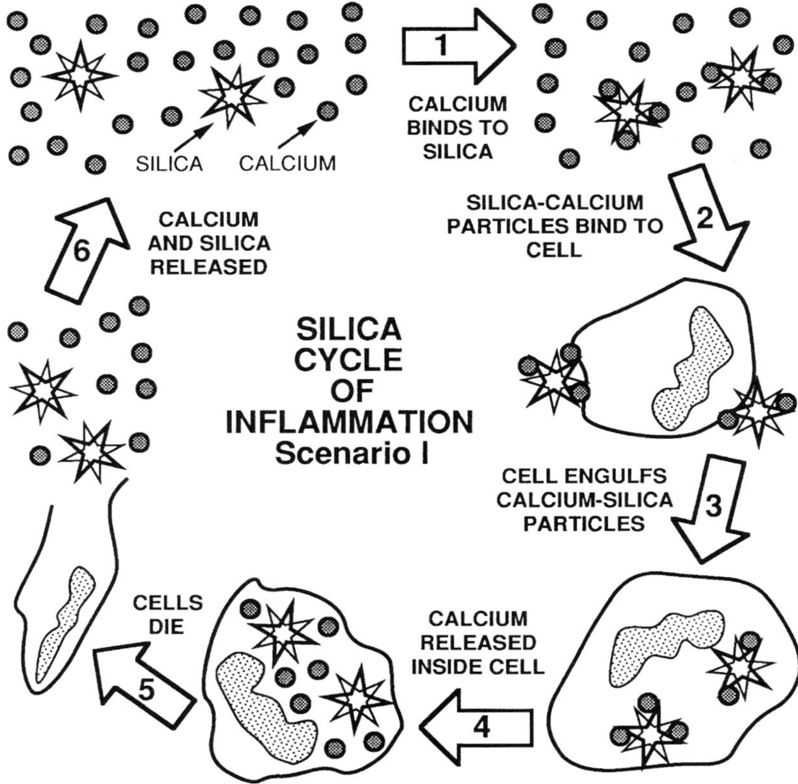

FIGURE 5 A proposed cycle of inflammation caused by silica. In this scenario, extracellular calcium binds to respired silica. The calcium-silica complex is then phagocytized. The calcium is then released inside the phagocyte, and the resulting increase in internal calcium concentration results in the death of the cell. Following death, the cell releases its contents, permitting the cycle to continue.

two oxygen atoms (see Figure 7). When cleavage occurs, SiO^- may be formed which can bind calcium ions as well as other ions. The ability of silica to bind to physiological calcium (10^{-3} *M*) is well known.[9] We have shown that aged, respirable-sized silica binds at least 6 to 10% of calcium at extracellular concentrations,[16] a quantity of Ca^{++} which is toxic if transported into phagocytes. We have seen x-ray evidence as well (see Figure 8). To demonstrate that the surface causes the toxicity, we coated silica with a water-soluble organosilane which binds to silanol groups (see Figure 9). Silica so treated was found to be 60 to 80% less toxic[16] and also bound 60% less radioactive calcium than uncoated silica. These results may indicate that the protection by organosilane coating is due to its ability to inhibit the binding of ionic calcium to the surface of silica or that covering the surface covers toxic groups on the silica. Following inhalation, respirable-sized silica contacts the alveolar liquid, which contains 10^{-3} *M* calcium; thus a ready supply of extracellular, ionic calcium is available in the lungs.

VI. MACROPHAGES AND NEUTROPHILS WITH SILICA PRODUCE PAF

Etherated phospholipids constitute 50% of the phospholipids of neutrophils.[22] Predictably, phagocytosis of silica produces extensive quantities of PAF (see Figure 10). PAF is generated from the activation of PLA_2, which in turn generates lyso-PAF and arachidonate. Lyso-PAF is acetylated to PAF via acetyl coenzyme A (CoA) in the presence of calcium and adenosine 5′-triphosphate (ATP) (see Figure 11). The arachidonate is metabolized via the lipoxygenase pathway as discussed previously. PAF serves to magnify the inflammation present, like the addition of gasoline makes a fire greater. Further, inhaled PAF by itself has been demonstrated to produce fibrosis after inhalation.[23]

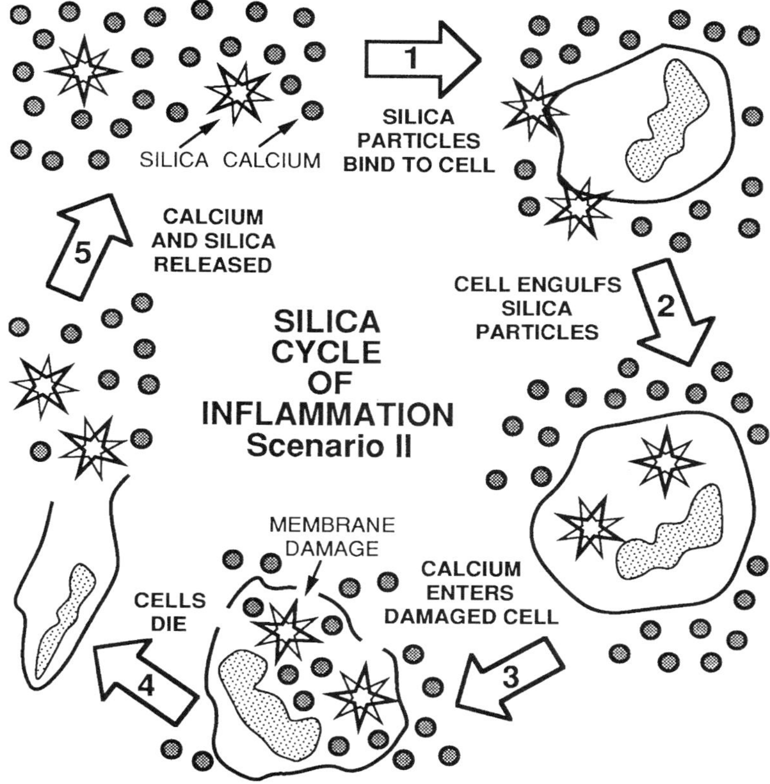

FIGURE 6 A proposed cycle of inflammation caused by silica. Following phagocytosis, the silica inside the phagocyte causes damage to the membrane, allowing calcium to leak in. This results in an increase in internal calcium concentration and the death of the cell. Following death, the cell releases its contents, perpetuating the cycle.

VII. MECHANISMS CAUSING CHRONIC TOXICITY OF SILICA

Regardless of the actual mechanism of the toxicity of silica, it must be cyclical to account for the chronic nature of its damage. Since our data indicate that calcium is involved, we propose the following cycle of toxicity (see Figures 5 and 6). First, silica binds to calcium. The silica with calcium bound to it is engulfed by the phagocytic cell (neutrophils, macrophages, etc.). The silica could release the calcium inside the cell, exert toxicity with calcium bound to it, or cause membrane damage and allow ionic calcium to leak in. Since the silica cannot be digested by cellular mechanisms, the silica particles are released by the cell following their death. The silica particles are then freed to be ingested and perpetuate the cycle (see Figure 12).

The above proposed mechanism bears many similarities to uric acid crystals in gouty inflammation. In gout, indigestible uric acid crystals result in a continuous cycle of inflammation in the affected joint unless the solubility of the uric acid is moderated using drugs inhibiting the formation of uric acid, i.e., allopurinol.

VIII. POSSIBLE METHODS TO DETOXIFY INHALED SILICA

A. SILICA COATING CONVERTS THE LIPOXYGENASE METABOLISM TO CYCLOOXYGENASE METABOLISM

Since it is clear that the surface of silica is responsible for the toxicity, an obvious ploy is to coat the particles before inhalation. The water-soluble organosilane Prosil-28® can be used in either 1/100 or 1/1000 dilutions to coat the silanol groups or OH groups. As discussed above, such a coating dramatically reduces in parallel the toxicity of the silica (see Figures 13 and 16)[21] and the binding of ^{45}Ca to silica (see

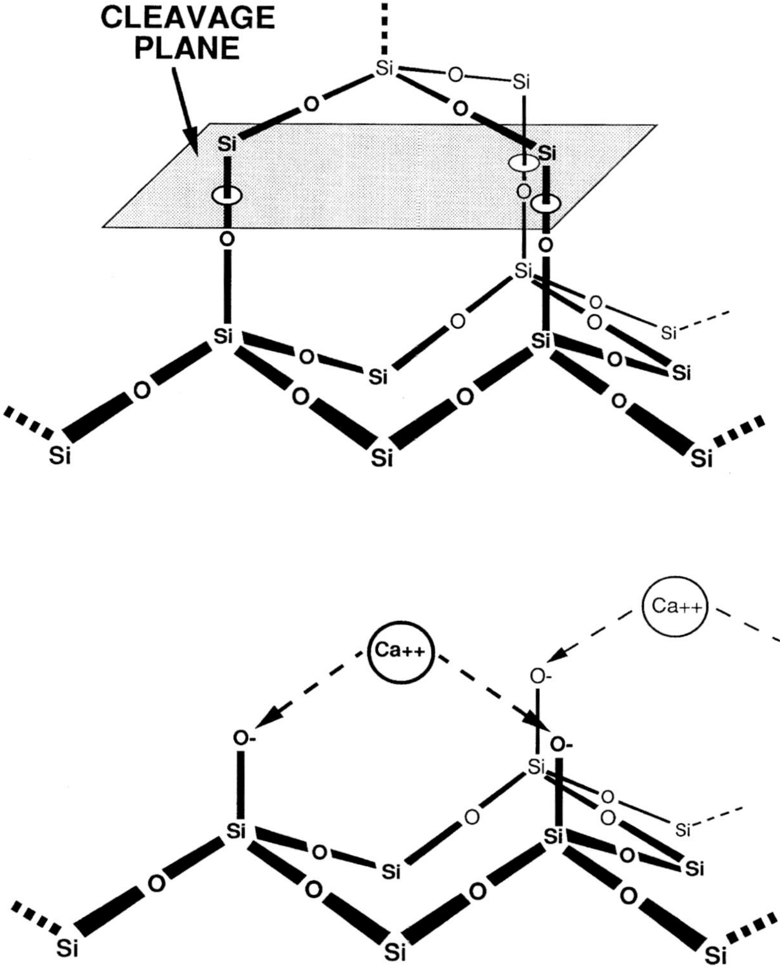

FIGURE 7 The top figure shows the three-dimensional crystalline structure of silica and a likely cleavage plane. A fracture along this plane results in the exposure of negatively charged oxygen groups which could bind ionic calcium (bottom). If calcium binds to broken silica in this manner, it might explain the toxicity of silica.

Figure 14) by 60% or greater. Thus calcium binding and the surface toxicity of silica are apparently linked. Silica coating could be particularly useful in cases when drilling machinery is water cooled or when water sprays are employed. The organosilane could be added to the cooling water or water spray in appropriate concentrations to coat the particles as they are produced. We have shown that coated silica produces much less chemiluminescence (CL) compared to uncoated silica when exposed to neutrophils or macrophages (see Figure 13).[21] This cellular CL is lipoxygenase dependent because direct or indirect lipoxygenase inhibitors decrease the measured CL.[24] Silica coated with polyvinylpyridine-*N*-oxide or aluminum lactate has been shown to produce prostaglandin inflammation rather than LT inflammation as compared to noncoated silica.[25] We have recently shown that organosilane-coated silica produces no more inflammation *in vivo* than low-silica coal dust (see Figure 15). Again, this evidence suggests that nonfibrogenic particles produce cyclooxygenase inflammation rather than the more toxic lipoxygenase products. This may be the reason fibrogenesis is not produced by nonfibrogenic particles.

B. INHIBITION OF THE RISE IN INTRACELLULAR CALCIUM

Since the ingestion of respirable-size silica particles produces calcium-activated increases in PAF and LT, an obvious ploy is to inhibit the increase of intracellular calcium. Even though controlling the internal

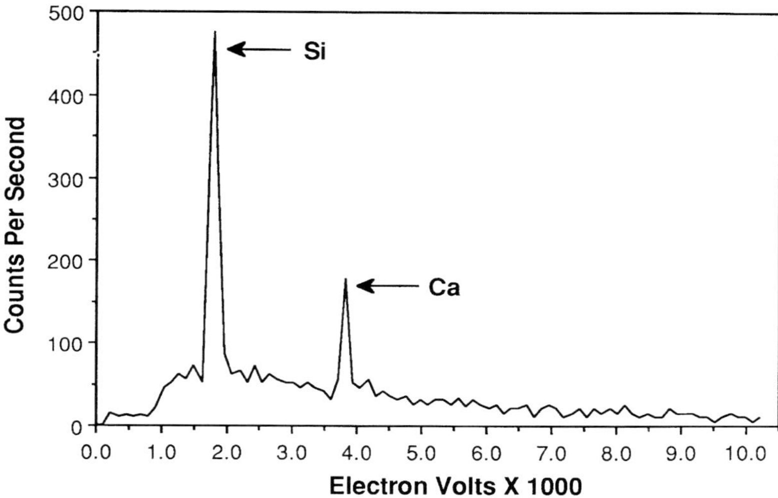

FIGURE 8 X-Ray dispersion analysis from a sample of fumed silica (see Methods for details). Note that the sample contains measurable amounts of both elemental silicon and calcium. Thus calcium is associated with the silica, indicating that calcium binding does occur.

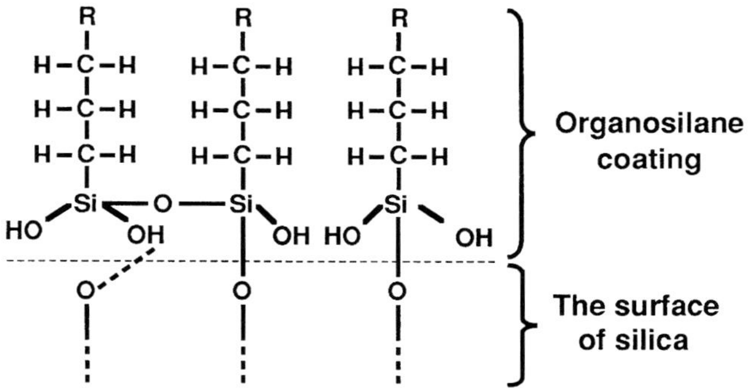

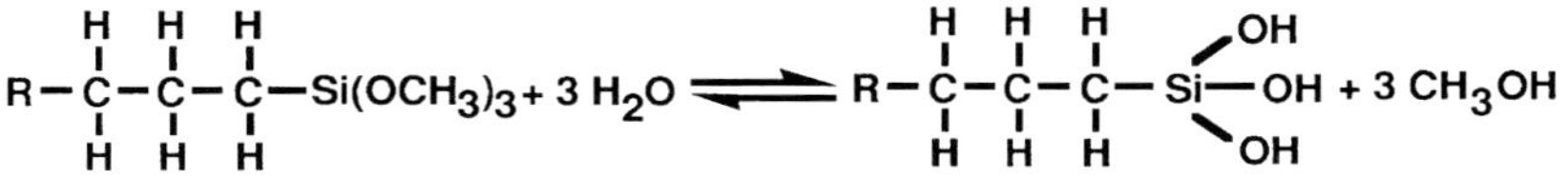

$$R-CH_2-CH_2-CH_2-Si(OCH_3)_3 + 3\,H_2O \rightleftharpoons R-CH_2-CH_2-CH_2-Si(OH)_3 + 3\,CH_3OH$$

Organosilane coating

The surface of silica

FIGURE 9 Formula showing the hydration of organosilane (top). The trisilanol compound so produced binds to the surface of silica (below). While a monolayer is shown, the actual coating may consist of multiple layers.

calcium concentration of the cell could be problematic given the importance of calcium for internal metabolic processes, we tested this approach with phagocytic cells incubated *in vitro* with INDO-1AM (see Figure 16). This highly lipid-soluble substance is transported into the cell where nonspecific esterases metabolically de-esterify INDO-1AM into the active form INDO-1. INDO-1 is a specific chelator of calcium which thus acts only inside cells. The active form binds ionic calcium five orders of magnitude greater than magnesium.[26] We have shown that this treatment can protect against the lethal toxicity of silica, demonstrating that the toxicity is linked to the rise in internal calcium. While the death of the phagocytes is inhibited *in vitro,* this approach may be contraindicated *in vivo* due to the importance of calcium in other cellular processes.

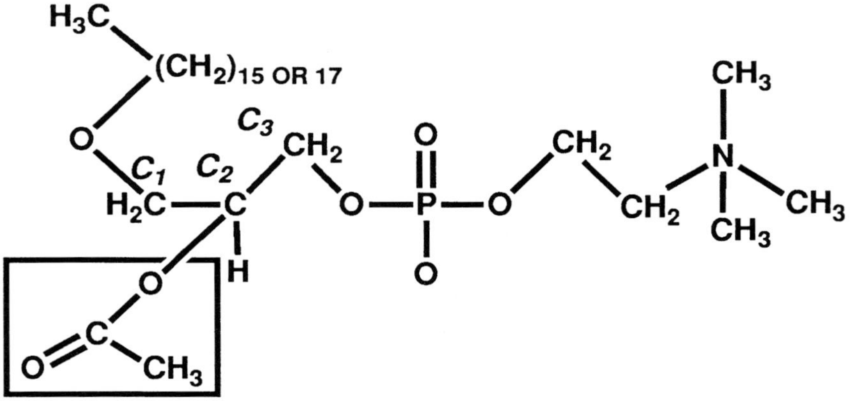

FIGURE 10 Generalized formula for platelet activating factors. The polyhydrocarbon attached to the oxygen at C_1 is usually C_{16} or C_{18}, but C_{20} has also been demonstrated. Note that PAF is acetylated in the C_2 position of the glycerol backbone. The formal name for PAF is 1-O-alkyl-2-acetyl-sn-glyceryl-3-phosphorylcholine. Lyso-PAF is formed by replacing the acetate at the C_2 position (boxed above) with a hydroxyl group.

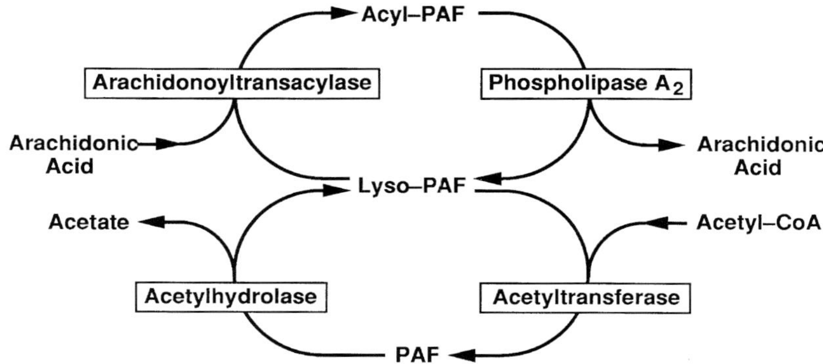

FIGURE 11 Enzymatic pathways for the synthesis and degradation of platelet activating factor from precursors.

C. INHIBITION OF LIPOXYGENASE ACTIVITY OR LEUKOTRIENE RECEPTORS

The inhibition of lipoxygenase would serve to inhibit the formation of the inflammatory mediators found due to silica ingestion. We have used specific lipoxygenase inhibitors to decrease lipoxygenase CL in HL-60 cells, neutrophils, and macrophages. CL from the above cell types was clearly inhibited by A63162 (Abbott), AA-861 (Takeda) antilipoxygenase, tetrandrine, and — the less specific, but more active — nordihydroguaiarectic acid (see Figures 17 and 18). However, tetrandrine did not directly inhibit soybean lipoxygenase activity, suggesting that it acts indirectly, possibly affecting lipoxygenase activation or docking mechanisms within the cell (see Figure 19). Recently, quinolones have been shown to produce indirect inhibition of FLAP-lipoxygenase[27] (tetrandrine is a bisbenzylisoquinoline).

D. INHIBITION OF PAF PRODUCTION OR BINDING

In addition to inhibiting lipoxygenase and calcium activity, inhibition of PAF production or receptor binding activity is clearly possible. Released PAF can activate the metabolic response of neutrophils as measured by luminol-dependent CL. We have shown that 63–072 (Sandoz) and kadsurenone inhibited PAF-dependent luminol CL at a 50% inhibitory concentration (IC_{50}) of 3.2×10^{-7} *M* and 2.78×10^{-6} *M*, respectively.[28] We have shown that rat macrophages and human neutrophils exposed to silica release PAF;[4] drug inhibition of this response could be an important treatment of silicosis. Given that silica can cause fibrosis[29] and that PAF is released when phagocytic cells are exposed to silica, it is not surprising that inhaled PAF can produce fibrosis by itself.[23] Further, tetrandrine inhibits PAF production as well as

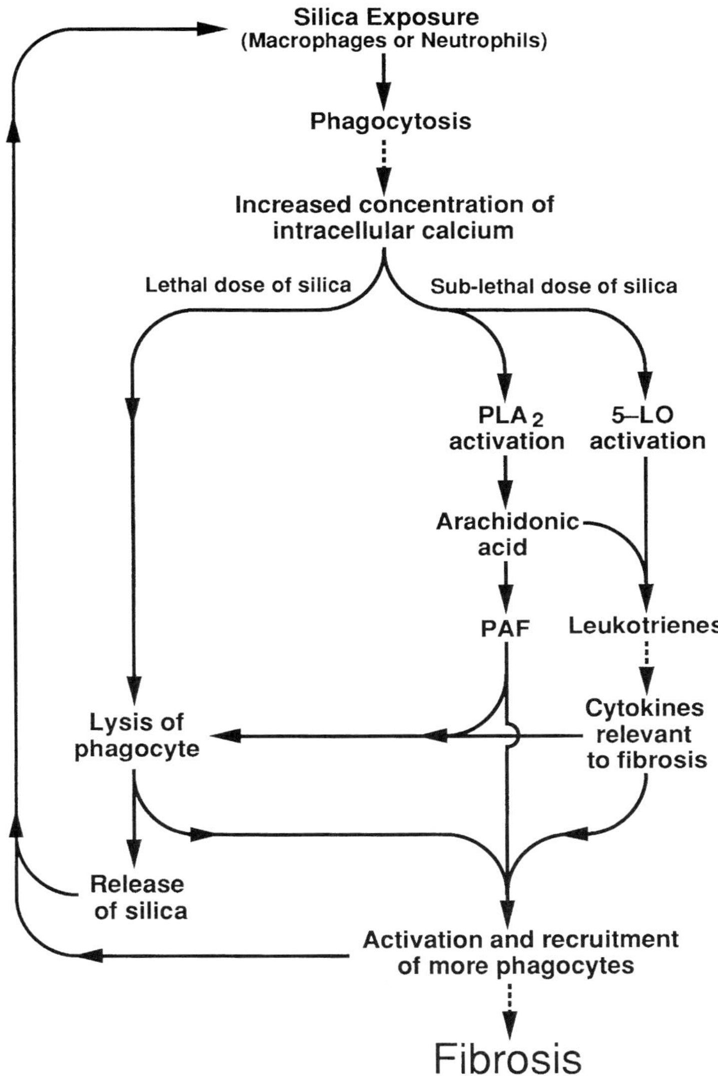

FIGURE 12 Hypothetical cyclical pathway to link inflammation to fibrosis caused by the inflammation of silica.

lipoxygenase activity.[4,24] These two actions of tetrandrine may account for some of its observed antifibrotic effect observed in silica-produced fibrosis.[29]

IX. LINKAGE OF SILICOSIS TO FIBROSIS VIA UNIQUE INFLAMMATION

Silica eventually produces fibrosis in the parenchyma, which results in the thickening of the alveolar wall and thus decreased oxygen exchange. Given this fact, there must be a linkage between the initial, novel inflammatory sequence and fibrosis. Fibrosis clearly arises from fibroblasts inside the alveolar wall, but what triggers the fibroblasts to initiate this unusual action? The growth stimulation of the fibroblast must come from other cell types in the area.

Silica contacts phagocytic cells first, either macrophages or neutrophils in the lung. One of the following happens:

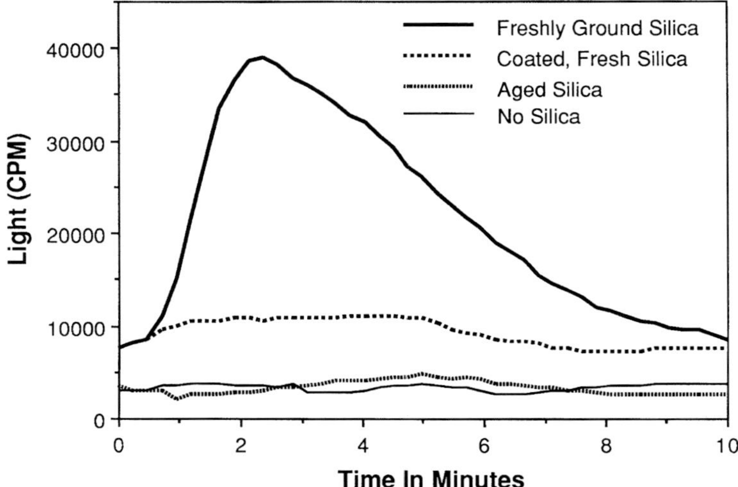

FIGURE 13 Chemiluminescence (lucigenin dependent) from silica-activated rat macrophages. Freshly ground silica, freshly ground silica coated with Prosil 28® organosilane, aged silica, and no silica controls were measured at 37°C for 20 min. Aged silica was prepared in the same manner as fresh silica, but was aged several weeks (see Methods for details). Display of chemiluminescence vs. time is from an assay representative of three separate experiments.

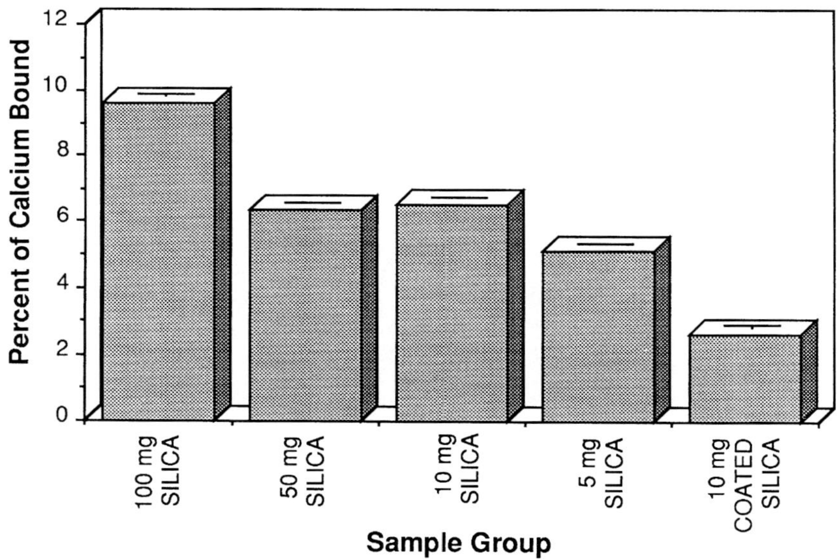

FIGURE 14 The binding of ^{45}Ca to silica (5 µm or less in diameter). 3.3 m*M* $^{45}CaCl_2$ was incubated with various amounts of silica and with coated silica (see Methods for details). Significant amounts of silica were bound by all samples. However, organosilane-coated silica bound approximately one third the amount of ionic calcium as the parallel, uncoated sample.

1. The phagocyte engulfs a sublethal amount of silica and elaborates cytokines such as tumor necrosis factor, interleukin 1, gamma interferon, platelet-derived growth factor, fibroblast growth factor, interleukin 4, PAF, LTB_4, etc.
2. The phagocyte engulfs a lethal amount of silica and elaborates its contents which results in the recruitment of more neutrophils into the area via LTB_4 stimulation of chemotaxsis and the production of more macrophages from monocytes.
3. The phagocyte does not engulf particles but is activated by the stimulants created by the previous interaction of silica and phagocytes as per 1 and 2 above. The activation of the cell results in the production of more cytokines.

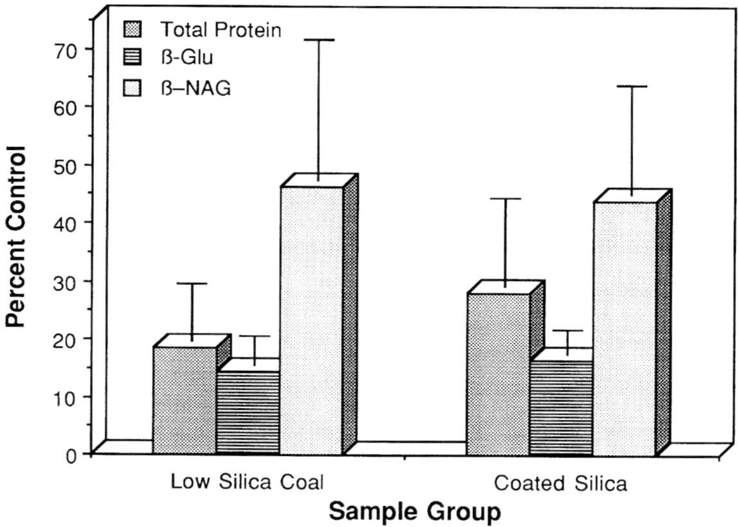

FIGURE 15 Inflammatory indicators from the lungs of rats instilled with either low-silica coal or coated silica as compared to control (rats instilled with untreated silica alone). Total protein, *N*-acetyl glucosaminidase (NAG), and β-glucuronidase (β-GLU) were measured 14 d post instillation (see methods for details). Notice that the response due to coated silica is greatly reduced as compared to control and that this response is similar to that of low-silica coal. Thus, organosilane coating greatly reduces the inflammation.

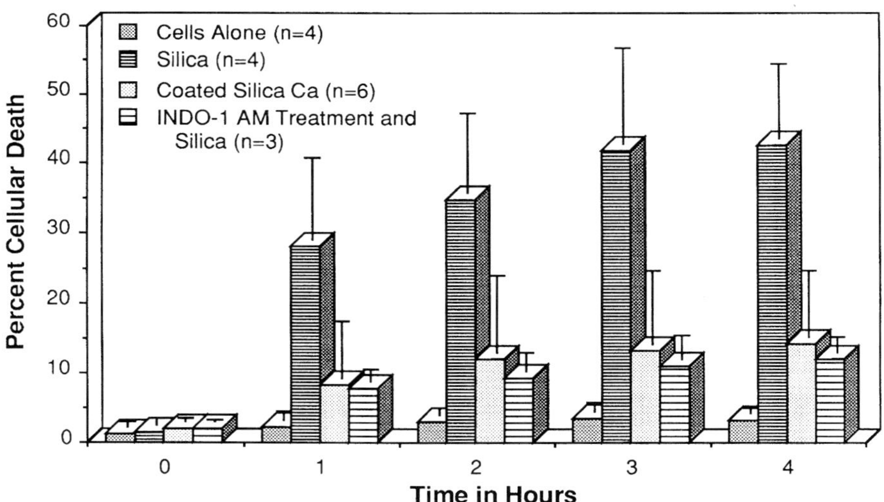

FIGURE 16 Flow cytometry of human neutrophils either unexposed, exposed to silica, or coated silica vs. time at room temperature. The INDO-1AM treatment group was preincubated with INDO-1AM, which penetrates the cells and is de-esterified inside the cell to form an EGTA-like compound which binds intracellular calcium. Note that both organosilane coating and pretreatment with INDO-1AM significantly decrease death as measured propidium iodide assay (see Methods for details). Englen et al.[25] have shown that coating causes a reversion to the prostaglandin pathway from the 5-lipoxygenase pathway.

The cytokines thus produced activate and recruit T and B lymphocytes, fibroblasts, endothelial cells, etc., to play their respective roles in the fibrotic process.

Interdiction in this process is clearly possible. Likewise, the earlier interdiction occurs, the more likely it is to be effective. Therefore the simplest method is to avoid the inhalation of dusts containing respirable-sized silica. If this is not possible or practical, the next most logical method is to coat the silica prior to inhalation, preventing the reactive surface from interacting with the lung.

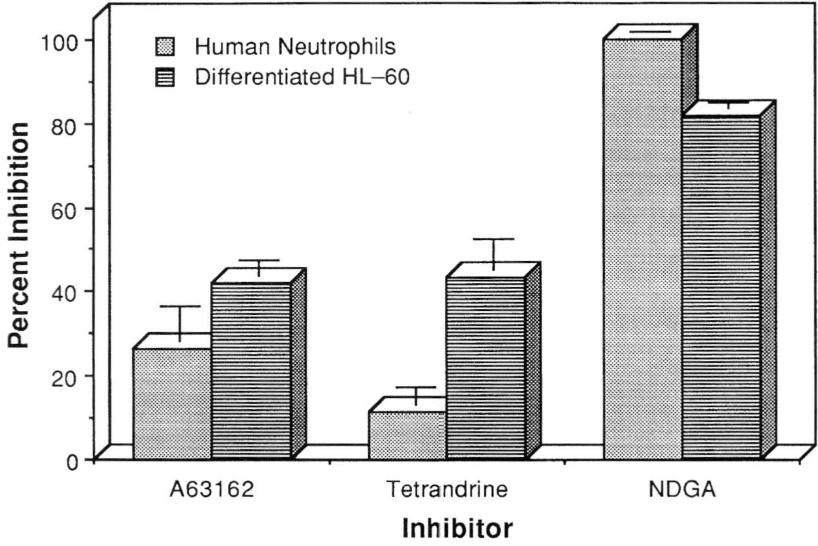

FIGURE 17 Inhibition of luminol-dependent chemiluminescence from 10^6 silica-activated human neutrophils and differentiated human leukemia (HL-60) cells. We used A63162 and nordihydroguaiaretic acid (NDGA) at 2×10^{-5} *M* and tetrandrine at 2×10^{-6} *M*. This shows the direct (A63162 and NDGA) and indirect inhibition (tetrandrine) of 5-lipoxygenase (see Methods for details).

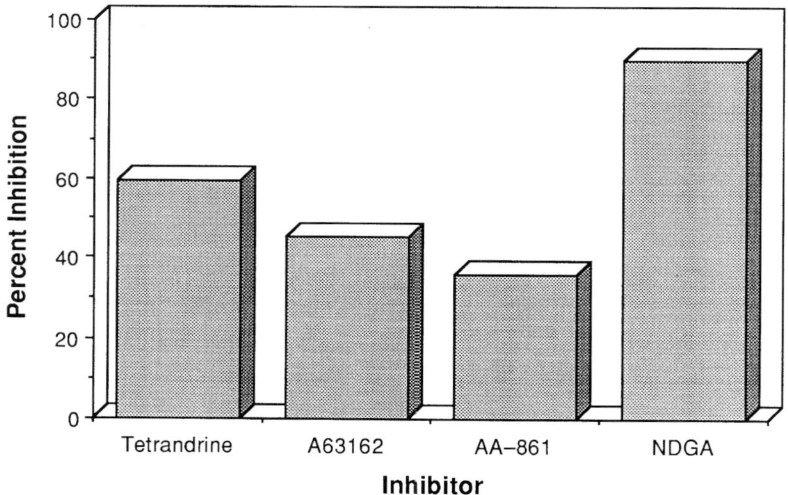

FIGURE 18 Inhibition by various drugs of luminol-dependent chemiluminescence of rat lung macrophages stimulated by silica. The dose of the drugs was 2×10^{-5} *M* except for tetrandrine, which was 2×10^{-6} *M*.

If neither of the above methods are feasible, early interdiction of inflammatory mediators may be possible. Likely candidates are

1. blockade of increased intracellular calcium concentration
2. inhibition of the activation of PLA_2 via PLAP
3. blockade of the release or metabolism of arachidonic acid
4. inhibition of the activation of lipoxygenase via FLAP
5. receptor antagonists of lipoxygenase products

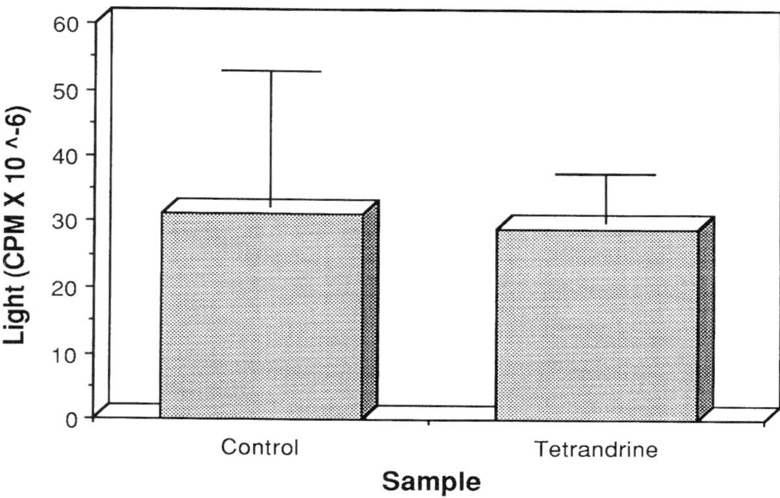

FIGURE 19 The lack of direct inhibition of soybean lipoxygenase by tetrandrine at 2×10^{-6} *M*. This demonstrates that tetrandrine does not inhibit 5-lipoxygenase activity directly.

6. inhibition of cytokine elaboration
7. receptor antagonists of cytokines

As in most disease states, the treatment of silicosis should occur immediately following the inhalation of silica before fibrosis is advanced, preferably before the fibroblast commits to the production of collagen fibers. Therefore, this final approach will be much more effective with early detection. The list above also identifies some possible approaches to early detection.

X. SUMMARY

It was once thought that the inhalation of silica and silica-containing minerals — such as asbestos and coal — would inevitably end in fibrosis. Clearly, the toxicity of silica can be ameliorated by coating the silica prior to inhalation or lessened by a variety of drugs that interdict in the inflammatory process which produces cytokines and thus fibrosis. Much of the elaboration of fibrotic and inflammatory mediators are probably activated by an increase in intracellular calcium. We know that silica increases the elaboration of cytokines important to the fibrotic process, such as interleukin 1,[30] tumor necrosis factor,[31,32] fibroblast growth factor,[33] interleukin 4,[34] interleukin 8,[35] and possibly platelet-derived growth factor.[32] Ultimately, the inhibition of the inflammatory system, calcium, or cytokine action may block the fibrotic process.

XI. METHODS

A. REAGENTS

1. Hepes buffer contains 10 m*M* Hepes, 5 m*M* KCl, 5.5 m*M* glucose, and 145 m*M* NaCl and has a pH of 7.4. Calcium Hepes was prepared as above with the addition of 2 m*M* $CaCl_2$.
2. Dimethyl sulfoxide (DMSO) was obtained from Fisher Scientific Co., Fair Lawn, NJ. A portion was heat sterilized and kept as stock solution that was later used to differentiate the HL-60 cells into neutrophils.
3. A63162 was a gift from Abbott Labs, North Chicago, IL, and was diluted in 1 ml of DMSO and then brought to a final concentration of 1×10^{-4} *M* in Hepes buffer. The drug was stored at –2°C as a stock solution and was prepared each week.

4. NDGA 1,4 bis[3,4 dihydroxyphenyl] 2,3 dimethylbutane was obtained from Sigma Chemical Co., St. Louis, MO. It was diluted to a final concentration of 1×10^{-4} *M* in Hepes buffer without calcium and stored at –2°C as a stock solution.
5. Tetrandrine was a gift from the National Cancer Institute Chemical Carcinogen Reference Standard Repository, Chicago, IL. Tetrandrine was converted to the salt form by the addition of a few drops of 1 N HCl. The solution was titrated with diluted 0.1 N NaOH up to pH 6.8. Next, tetrandrine was diluted in Hepes without calcium up to a final concentration of 1×10^{-4} *M* and pH 7.2. This served as a stock solution and was stored at –2°C.
6. Luminol (5-amino-2,3-dihydro-1,4 phthalazinedione) was obtained from Aldrich Chemical Co., Milwaukee, WI. A stock solution was prepared by dissolving luminol in 1 ml of DMSO, diluting in 99 ml of Hepes buffer without calcium for a final luminol concentration of 5×10^{-5} *M*.
7. Lucigenin (bis-*n*-methylacridinium nitrate) was obtained from Sigma, St. Louis, MO. A stock solution was prepared by dissolving luminol in 1 ml of DMSO, diluting in 99 ml of Hepes buffer without calcium for a final luminol concentration of 2.5×10^{-6} *M*.
8. A23187 was obtained from Sigma, St. Louis, MO, and was diluted in calcium Hepes for a concentration of 1×10^{-5} *M*. This served as a stock solution and was stored at –2°C.
9. AA-861 was supplied by Takeda Chemical Industries, Japan, and was diluted in 1 ml of DMSO and then brought to a final concentration of 1×10^{-4} *M* in Hepes buffer. This served as a stock solution and was stored at –2°C.

B. PREPARATION AND/OR ISOLATION OF CELLS

1. Neutrophils. Neutrophils were isolated from human blood collected via venipuncture in heparinized Vacutainer® tubes. In a 13 × 100-mm Falcon® tube, 3 ml of blood was carefully layered onto 3 ml of Mono-Poly® Resolving Media (Flow Labs, McLean, VA). The tube and its contents were centrifuged at 300 × g for 30 min, at room temperature, in a swinging bucket rotor. The upper band, containing monocytes, platelets, and lymphocytes, was aspirated and discarded. The lower band, containing neutrophils, was collected in a Falcon 50-ml, conical-bottom centrifuge tube containing 47 ml of Hepes buffer. The collected lower band was centrifuged at 250 × g for 5 min and the resulting supernatant discarded. The neutrophil pellet was resuspended in 1 ml of Hepes, counted with a hemocytometer and microscope, and adjusted to a final concentration of 10^7 cells per ml.
2. HL-60 cells. The human promyelocytic HL-60 leukemic cells were provided by Dr. John Durham, Medical Center, West Virginia University (this cell line was originally isolated from a leukemic patient by Robert C. Gallo, National Cancer Institute, Bethesda, MD). The cells were cultured in Corning polystyrene tissue culture flasks. Medium for the cultures was prepared in 100-ml batches by mixing: RPMI-1640 medium without glutamine (Whittaker Bioproducts, Walkersville, MD), 87.5 ml; glutamine (Whittaker Bioproducts, Walkersville, MD), 2 m*M;* fetal bovine serum (Whittaker Bioproducts, Walkersville, MD) heat inactivated (57°C for 30 min), 10 ml; gentamicin sulfate (Whittaker Bioproducts, Walkersville, MD), 5 mg; and amphotericin-B (Gibco Laboratories, Grand Island, NY), 250 μg. The HL-60 cells were grown in Corning® 100 × 20-mm-style polystyrene culture dishes (Corning® Glass Works, Corning, NY) in suspension culture at 37°C in a 100% humidified atmosphere containing 5% CO_2. DMSO (13 μl of sterilized DMSO was added per each ml of medium contained in the dishes) in a final concentration of 1.3% was used to differentiate the HL-60 cells into neutrophil-like cells for 4 d. The culture cells were then removed from the dishes, centrifuged at 500 g for 5 min, and suspended in 1 ml Hepes buffer without calcium, counted with a hemocytometer and microscope and adjusted to a final concentration of 10^7 cells per ml. Morphological assessment of the differentiated cells was performed by Wright-Giemsa staining, and the vitality of the cells was evaluated with the trypan blue exclusion test. The cells so differentiated activate the lipoxygenase mechanism and destroy myeoloperoxidase.[36,37]
3. Rat alveolar macrophages. Alveolar macrophages for CL assays were obtained from male Sprague-Dawley rats approximately 250 to 300 g by bronchoalveolar lavage.[38] Briefly, rats were anesthetized with sodium pentobarbitol (200 mg/kg, i.p.). The trachea was cannulated and the lungs lavaged 10 times with 8-ml aliquots of Hank's balanced salt solution without Ca^{++} or Mg^{++}. Cells were washed twice and suspended in Hepes buffer. The cells were electronically counted and adjusted to a final concentration of 10^7 cells per ml.

C. PREPARATION OF PARTICLE STIMULANTS

1. Silica. Unless otherwise noted, the silica for all samples was 5 μm or less in diameter and was obtained from Dr. Vincent Castranova (ALOSH/NIOSH). In 5 ml of Hepes, 10 mg of silica was suspended for a concentration of 2 mg/ml.
2. Fresh and aged silica. Fresh silica was prepared by grinding crystalline silica for 30 min in a ball grinder equipped with an agate ball (centrifugal ball mill, IEC, Needham, MA). Ground silica was sieved through a 20-μm-mesh filter for 10 min prior to use. Aged silica was prepared in the same manner but was allowed to age in sealed vials at room temperature for two weeks. Prior to use, 10 mg of either aged or fresh silica was suspended in 5 ml of Hepes for a concentration of 2 mg/ml.
3. Organosilane coating of silica. "Coated silica" samples were prepared using the water-soluble organosilane, Prosil 28® (A.H. Thomas, Swedesboro, NJ). Ten ml of a 1% solution of Prosil 28® was added to 10 mg of silica and heated at 100°C for 10 min with constant mixing. The particles were centrifuged at 300 × g for 5 min. The supernatant was aspirated and the particles resuspended in 5 ml of calcium Hepes for a concentration of 2 mg/ml.
4. Coal samples. Bituminous coal particles were obtained from Dr. Hogg, Department of Mineral Sciences, Generic Dust Center, Penn State University. These particles had originally been obtained from a mine in southern West Virginia and had a silica content of 0.2% and a diameter of 7 μm or less. The "coal" suspension was prepared by diluting 10 mg of coal particles in 5 ml of calcium Hepes for a concentration of 2 mg/ml.

D. INDO-1AM TREATMENT

INDO-1AM (Molecular Bioprobes, Eugene, OR) 0.10 m*M* in Hepes (pH = 7.4) was incubated with an equivalent volume of neutrophils for 30 min at room temperature. The cells were then washed in 50 ml of Hank's balanced salt solution, centrifuged to remove the buffer, and resuspended in Hepes buffer (pH = 7.4).

E. CHEMILUMINESCENT ASSAYS

CL was measured using a Berthold® LB 9505-C luminometer. Before each assay the luminometer was adjusted to 37°C, and all determinations were made after the background counts were stabilized. All reactions were carried out in 3-ml round-bottom plastic cuvettes inserted into the counting chamber of the luminometer. Each sample was counted for either 10 or 20 min, and the integrated counts were read from the computer linked to the luminometer. A printed copy of the data was obtained.

Experiments involving neutrophils, macrophages, or HL-60 cells and silica were done as follows: each plastic cuvette contained 100 μl cells (final concentration 1×10^6 cells/ml); 100 μl Hepes with calcium; 10 μl of luminol (final concentration 5×10^{-7} *M*) or lucigenin (final concentration 2.5×10^{-8} *M*). In all the cuvettes except the blank, 100 μl of suspended silica was added as stimulant of the reaction for a total of 0.5 mg per tube. When assayed, A63162, AA-861, tetrandrine, or NDGA were added in an amount of 100 μl each to the cuvettes for a final concentration of 2×10^{-5} *M*, except tetrandrine which was assayed at a final concentration 2×10^{-6} *M*. Hepes without calcium was added to each cuvette to bring the final volume to 500 μl.

F. FLOW CYTOMETRY ASSAY

Neutrophils and particles were mixed together with propidium iodide (Sigma, St. Louis, MO). The final concentration of propidium iodide was 5 μg/ml, the particle stimulants were 0.2 mg/ml, and 10^6 neutrophils were present in a final volume of 1 ml. In the relevant samples, the final concentration of A23187 was 1×10^{-6} *M*. The assay was performed on a FACScan® fluorescence-activated cell analysis unit (Becton-Dickinson, Mt. View, CA) utilizing an air-cooled, laser-producing light at a wavelength of 488 nm with an output of 15.5 mW. At each time point sampled, 10,000 events were measured and saved for subsequent data analysis. The instrument settings were as follows:

Forward scatter: E–1 × 6.00 (linear amplification)
Side scatter: 330v × 1.00 (linear amplification)
Fluorescence 1: green, 630v × log; emission 530 nm ± 15 nm
Fluorescence 2: red, 600v × 8.00; emission 585 nm ± 24 nm

G. ^{45}CA BINDING EXPERIMENTS

$^{45}CaCl_2$ (ICN Radiochemicals, Irvine, CA) used in these experiments had a specific activity of 7.13 mCi/mg Ca. One µCi of ^{45}Ca was incubated with 100-, 50-, 10-, and 5-mg silica samples (5 µm diameter or less) for 30 min at room temperature. The concentration of calcium used was approximately equal to 3.3 m*M* or two to three times greater than the physiological concentration.

After incubation, the silica was washed multiple times with 50 ml of Hepes buffer. Next, the particles were vacuum filtered through a 0.45-µm Millipore® filter. A prefilter (Whatman® GF/C fiberglass filter) was placed on top of the Millipore® filter before aspiration. Moist filters were placed in 10 ml of Instagel® aqueous liquid scintillation fluid. The samples were counted in a Packard Tricarb® liquid scintillation counter 1900 CA set for ^{45}Ca energy equivalent to 256 keV.

H. TETRANDRINE AND SOYBEAN LIPOXYGENASE ASSAY

A 0.2-*M* sodium borate buffer at pH 9.0 was prepared and degassed under vacuum for 45 min. Solutions of 19 m*M* sodium arachidonate in the borate buffer and a solution of 9 mg of luminol (5-amino-2,3-dihydro-1,4 phthalazinedione) in 50 ml of borate buffer were prepared. Lipoxygenase-1 (Sigma Chemical Co., St. Louis, MO) from soybean was used. This solution contained 5.0 mg of the powdered enzyme [170,000 units/mg (Sigma)] dissolved in 10.0 ml of the borate buffer.

The lipoxygenase assay was conducted at 37°C using a Berthold® Luminometer model 9505C-six channel instrument. The assay was established in standard 3-ml, round-bottom plastic cuvettes in a total volume of 500 µl as follows:

1. 350 µl of 0.2 *M* borate buffer, pH 9.0
2. 100 µl drug in borate buffer or buffer (borate) — no drug control
3. 20 µl 10 m*M* sodium arachidonate in deoxygenated borate buffer
4. 20 µl of 10^{-4} *M* luminol
5. 10 µl of soybean lipoxygenase in borate buffer, 5.0 mg enzyme dissolved in 10 ml of borate buffer, enzyme powder is 170,000 units/mg

I. SILICA, COATED SILICA, LOW SILICA COAL INSTILLATION, AND ACELLULAR ASSAYS IN RATS

In 1 ml of 0.9% sterile saline, 20 mg of silica or low-silica coal was suspended. Coated silica was prepared as described above, dried, and 20 mg suspended in 1 ml of 0.9% sterile saline. Prior to instillation, the suspensions were sonicated to assure uniformity. Following anesthesia with sodium brevital (35 mg/kg, i.p.), male Fischer-344 rats of approximately 250 g and 8 to 12 weeks old (Hilltop Lab Animals, PA) were placed on a vertical restraint board and the suspension instilled near the bronchial bifurcation.[1]

After 14 d, bronchoalveolar lavage was performed on all sample groups. The rats were sacrificed using an overdose of pentobarbital followed by exsanguination via the abdominal aorta. The lungs were then lavaged with multiple separate washings with warm, sterile Hank's balanced salt solution, the first lavage fluid kept separate. The volume of fluid put in was 2% of the rat's body weight for the first lavage and then 6 ml for every lavage thereafter. Each time, the buffer was inserted for 30 s, withdrawn, and reinserted for 30 s. The lavages were collected until a total of 80 ml of fluid had been recovered. Lavage fluid was centrifuged for 300 × g at 4°C for 15 min, and the supernatant from the first was collected and immediately assayed for enzymes and total protein as detailed later. The pellets were pooled, counted with a hemocytometer, and viability determined via trypan blue exclusion. Cells were differentiated on slides after staining with eosin and methylene blue.

The supernatant fluid from the first lavage fluid was assayed for *N*-acetyl glucosaminidase (NAG), β-glucuronidase (β-GLU), and total protein. All three levels were determined via colorimetric assays and measured with a Gilford spectrophotometer model 240. NAG was assayed at 400 nm,[39] β-GLU at 400 nm,[40] and total protein at 650 nm.[41]

J. X-RAY DISPERSION ANALYSIS OF FUMED SILICA

Approximately 10 mg of fumed silica (a gift from Mark Hayes, M.D., Ohio College of Podiatric Medicine, Cleveland, OH) was prepared for electron microscopy by mixing it with 10 ml of methanol and then dropping 0.2 ml onto a carbon planchet to air dry. The planchets were mounted onto aluminum stubs and carbon coated on a Polaron® E-6100 evaporator. The samples were then analyzed with an ORTEC energy dispersive system attached to an ETEC® Autoscan scanning electron microscope using an accelerating voltage of 20 kV and an acquisition time of 60 s.

ACKNOWLEDGMENTS

We gratefully acknowledge the support of the Generic Dust Center (grant number 1195142–5423) funded by the U.S. Department of Energy, who have supported the majority of this work. The endorsement of the Generic Dust Center has allowed us to explore a variety of issues related to the inflammatory process and to the toxicity of silica.

In addition, we wish to thank Catherine Nowack for her assistance with flow cytometry, Dianne Schwegler-Berry for her assistance with electron microscopy, Jim Antonini for his assistance with silica instillation into rats and the subsequent measurements, and Dr. Vincent Castranova for his assistance and encouragement throughout much of the work above.

REFERENCES

1. **Lindenschmidt, R. C., Driscoll, K. E., Perkins, M. A., Higg, J. M., Maurer, J. K., and Belfiore, K. A.,** The comparison of a fibrogenic and two nonfibrogenic dusts by bronchoalveolar lavage, *Toxicol. Appl. Pharmacol.,* 102, 268, 1990.
2. **Hepplestone, G.,** Pulmonary toxicology of silica, coal and asbestos, *Environ. Health Perspect.,* 55, 111, 1984.
3. **Kagan, E. and Hartmarn, D. P.,** Elimination of macrophages with silica and asbestos, in *Methods of Enzymology,* Di Sabato, G., Langone, J. J., and Van Vunakis, H., Eds., Academic Press, Orlando, FL, 108, 325, 1984.
4. **Kang, J. H., Van Dyke, K., Pailes, W. H., and Castranova, V.,** Potential role of platelet-activating factor in the development of occupational lung disease: action as an activator or potentiator of pulmonary phagocytes, in *3rd Symposium on Respirable Dust in the Mineral Industries,* Franz, R. L. and Ramani, R. V., Eds., Society for Mining, Metallurgy, and Exploration, Littleton, CO, 1991, 183.
5. **Englen, M. D., Taylor, S. W., Laegreid, W. W., Liggitt, H. D., Silflow, R. M., Breeze, R. C., and Leid, W.,** Stimulation of arachidonic acid metabolism in silica exposed alveolar macrophages, *Exp. Lung Res.,* 15, 511, 1989.
6. **Van Dyke, K., Matamoros, M., Van Dyke, C. J., and Castranova, V.,** Calcium ionophore stimulated chemiluminescence from human granulocytes, *Microchem. J.,* 28, 568, 1983.
7. **Galardi, S. H., Morris, H. R., and DiMarzo, V.,** Novel interactions between second messengers in rat basophilic leukemia (RBL-1) cells, *Biochem. Int.,* 22, 379, 1990.
8. **Lim, W. H. and Stewart, A. G.,** Macrophage activation reduces mobilization of arachidonic acid by guinea pig and rat peritoneal macrophages, *Agents Actions,* 31, 290, 1990.
9. **Fuerstenan, M. C. and Palmer, B. R.,** Anionic floatation of oxides and silicates, in *Floatation (A.M. Gandid Memorial Volume),* Vol. 1, Fuerstenan, A.M., Ed., American Institute of Mining, Metallurgical, and Petroleum Engineers, New York, 1976, 148.
10. **Sigal, E.,** The molecular biology of arachidonic acid metabolism, *Am. Phys. Soc.,* L13, 1991.
11. **Schatz-Munding, M., Hatzelmann, A., and Ulrich, V.,** The involvement of extracellular calcium in the formation of 5 lipoxygenase metabolites by human polymorphonuclear leukocytes, *Eur. J. Biochem.,* 197, 487, 1991.
12. **Yoshihara, Y. and Watanabe, Y.,** Translocation of phospholipase A_2 from cytosol to membranes in rat brain induced by calcium ions, *Biochem. Biophys. Res. Commun.,* 120, 484, 1990.
13. **Bomalaski, J. S., Baker, D. G., Brophy, L., Resurreccion, N. V., Spilberg, I., Muniain, M., and Clark, M. A.,** A phospholipase A_2-activating protein (PLAP) stimulates human neutrophil aggregation and release of lysosomal enzymes, superoxide and eicosanoids, *J. Immunol.,* 142, 3957, 1989.
14. **Rouzer, C. A., Ford-Hutchinson, A. W., Morton, H. E., and Gillard, J. W.,** MK886, a potent and specific leukotrene biosynthesis inhibitor blocks and reverses the membrane association of 5-lipoxygenase in ionophore-challenged leukocytes, *J. Biol. Chem.,* 265, 1436, 1990.
15. **Warheit, D. B., Carakostas, M. C., Kelly, D. P., and Hartsky, M. A.,** Four week inhalation toxicity study with ludox colloidal silica in rats, *Fundam. Appl. Toxicol.,* 16, 590, 1991.
16. **Van Dyke, K., Gutierrez, J., Van Dyke, C., and Nowack, C.,** "Piggy back" mechanism with calcium explains how silica exerts its toxicity to phagocytic cells, *Microchem. J.,* 48, 34, 1993.
17. **Van Rooijen, N.,** High and low Ca^{+2} induced macrophage death, *Cell Calcium,* 12, 38, 1991.

18. **Chen, J., Armstrong, L. C., Liu, S., Garriets, J. E., and Last, J. A.,** Silica increases cytosolic free calcium ion concentration of alveolar macrophages *in vitro, Toxicol. Appl. Pharmacol.,* 111, 211, 1991.
19. **Pandurangi, R. S. and Seehra, M. S.,** Hemolytic ability of different forms of silica and role of the surface silanol species, in *3rd Symposium on Respirable Dust in the Mineral Industries,* Franz, R.L. and Ramani, R.V., Eds., Society for Mining, Metallurgy, and Exploration, Littleton, CO, 1991, 183.
20. **Vallayathan, V., Kang, J. H., Van Dyke, K., Dalal, N. S., and Castranova, A.,** Freshly fractured silica exerts greater toxicity toward lung macrophages than aged dust: organosilane (Prosil 28®) coating markedly reduces dust toxicity to cells, in *3rd Symposium on Respirable Dust in the Mineral Industries,* Franz, R.L. and Ramani, R.V., Eds., Society for Mining, Metallurgy, and Exploration, Littleton, CO, 1991, 117.
21. **Shi, X. and Dalal, N. S.,** Free radical generation by metal ions adsorbed on mineral dust, in *3rd Symposium on Respirable Dust in the Mineral Industries,* Franz, R.L. and Ramani, R.V., Eds., Society for Mining, Metallurgy, and Exploration, Littleton, CO, 1991, 307.
22. **Record, M., Ribbes, G., Terce, F., and Chap, H.,** Subcellular localization of phospholipids and enzymes involved in PAF-acether metabolism, *J. Cell Biochem.,* 40, 353, 1989.
23. **Camussi, G., Pawlowski, I., Tetta, C., Raffirello, C., Algerton, M., Brenjens, J., and Anders, G.,** Acute inflammation induced in the rabbit by local administration of 1-O-octadecyl-2-acetyl-sn-glyceryl-3-phosphorylcholine or of native platelet activating factor, *Am. J. Pathol.,* 122, 78, 1983.
24. **Gutierrez, J., Van Dyke, K., Wu, L., Vallayathan, V., and Castranova, V.,** Inhibition of antilipoxygenase drugs of cellular chemiluminescence in silica activated phagocytic cells, alveolar macrophages, and human leukemia (HL-60) cells, in *3rd Symposium on Respirable Dust in the Mineral Industries,* Franz, R.L. and Ramani, R.V., Eds., Society for Mining, Metallurgy, and Exploration, Littleton, CO, 1991, 171.
25. **Englen, M. D., Taylor, S. W., Laegreid, W. W., Silflow, R. M., and Leid, W.,** Diminished arachidonic acid metabolites release by bovine alveolar macrophages exposed to surface-modified silica, *Am. J. Respir. Cell Mol. Biol.,* 6, 527, 1992.
26. **Tsien, R. Y.,** Fluorescent probes of cell signaling, *Am. Rev. Neurosci.,* 12, 227, 1989.
27. **Charleson, S., Prasit, P., Leger, S., Gillard, J. W., Vickens, P. J., Mancini, J. A., Charleson, P., Guay, J., Ford-Hutchinson, A. W., and Evans, J. F.,** Characterization of a 5-lipoxygenase-activating protein binding assay: correlation of affinity for leukotriene synthesis inhibition, *Mol. Pharmacol.,* 41, 873, 1992.
28. **Van Dyke, K. and Castranova, V.,** Detection of receptor and synthesis antagonists of platelet activating factor in human whole blood and neutrophils using luminol-dependent chemiluminescence, in *New Horizons in Platelet Activating Factor Research,* Winslow, C.M. and Lee, M.L., Eds., John Wiley & Sons, New York, 1987, 181.
29. **Li, Q.-L., Xu, Y.-H., Zhou, Z.-S., Chen, X.-W., Huang, X.-Q., Chen, S.-L., and Zhang, Q.-X.,** The Observation of the treatment effect on 33 cases of silicosis treated with tetrandrine, *J. Clin. Tuberc. Res. Syst. Dis.,* 4, 321, 1981.
30. **Lemaire, I.,** Selective difference in macrophage populations and monokine production in resolving pulmonary granuloma and fibrosis, *Am. J. Pathol.,* 138, 487, 1991.
31. **Mohr, C., Gamsa, D., Graebner, C., Hemenway, D. R., Leslie, K. O., Absher, P. M., and Davis, G. S.,** Systemic macrophage stimulation in rats with silicosis: enhanced release of tumor necrosis factor-alpha from alveolar and peritoneal macrophage, *Am. J. Respir. Cell Mol. Biol.,* 5, 395, 1991.
32. **Piguet, P. F., Collart, M. A., Grau, G. E., Sappino, A. P., and Vassalli, P.,** Requirement of tumor necrosis factor for development of silica-induced pulmonary fibrosis, *Nature,* 344, 245, 1990.
33. **Sjostrand, M., Absher, P. M., Hemenway, D. R., Trombley, L., and Baldor, L. C.,** Comparison of lung alveolar and tissue cells in silica-induced inflammation, *Am. Rev. Respir. Dis.,* 143, 47, 1991.
34. **Terkeltaub, R., Zachariae, C., Santoro, D., Martin, J., Peveri, P., and Matsushima, K.,** Monocyte-derived neutrophil chemotactic factor/interleukin-8 is a potential mediator of crystal-induced inflammation, *Arthritis Rheum.,* 34, 894, 1991.
35. **Gillery, P., Fertin, C., Nicolas, J. F., Chastang, F., Kalis, B., Banchereau, J., and Maquart, F. X.,** Interleukin-4 stimulates collagen gene expression in human fibroblast monolayer cultures: potential role in fibrosis, *FEBS,* 302, 231, 1992.
36. **Kargman, S. and Rouzer, C. A.,** Studies on the regulation, biosynthesis, and activation in differentiated HL60 cells, *J. Biol. Chem.,* 264, 13313, 1989.
37. **Ardekani, A. M. and Van Dyke, K.,** Myeloperoxidase involvement in PMA-induced chemiluminescence in retinoic-acid-differentiated HL-60 cells, *Microchem. J.,* 39, 317, 1989.
38. **Sweeney, T. D., Castranova, V., Bowman, L., and Miles, P. R.,** Factors which effect superoxide anion release from rat alveolar macrophages, *Exp. Lung Res.,* 2, 85, 1981.
39. **Sellinger, O. Z., Beaufay, H., Jacques, P., Doyan, A., and DeDuve, C.,** Tissue fractionation studies, intracellular distribution and properties of β-N-acetyl-glucosaminidase and β-galactosidase in rat liver, *Biochem. J.,* 74, 450, 1960.
40. **Lockard, V. G. and Kennedy, R. E.,** Alterations in rabbit alveolar macrophages as a result of traumatic shock, *Lab. Invest.,* 35, 501, 1976.
41. **Hartree, E. F.,** Determination of protein: a modification of the Lowry method that gives a linear photometric response, *Anal. Biochem.,* 48, 422, 1972.

Section III
Chapter 8

ACUTE SILICOSIS AND THE ACTIVATION OF ALVEOLAR TYPE II CELLS

Gary E. R. Hook and Charles J. Viviano

CONTENTS

I. INTRODUCTION

Lung disease due to the inhalation of silica and silicates occurs in a wide variety of industries. In developing countries where less attention is given to rigid health standards, problems of dust-induced lung disease continue to escalate, and even in the industrialized nations where protection of workers is a high priority subclinical evidence of lung disease is very common.[1–3]

Inhalation of silica dust can give rise to two distinct disease states known, respectively, as acute silicosis and chronic silicosis. Acute silicosis generally occurs in the lungs of humans within a relatively short period of time following exposure to silica, a period ranging from a few months to a few years; whereas chronic silicosis develops over a period of many years and may take as long as 20 years before becoming debilitating. The relationship between acute and chronic silicosis is not clear, although presumably one might lay the foundation for the development of the other. It seems reasonable to suppose that to begin to understand the chronic disease we should begin by understanding the acute condition.

In this review, the hypothesis that acute silicosis begins with the activation of alveolar Type II cells and that activation of Type II cells leads to hypersecretion of pulmonary surfactant and its subsequent accumulation in the alveoli of the lungs will be examined.

0-8493-4709-2/96/$0.00+$.50

II. ACUTE SILICOSIS

Acute silicosis is a sometimes fatal condition that quickly develops in the lungs of humans and animals upon exposure to silica dust. Far less attention has been paid to acute silicosis compared with the chronic disease in spite of the fact that the foundation for the development of the chronic condition is undoubtedly laid during the acute phase. The course taken by the chronic lung disease and hence the long-term survival of the patient may also be determined during this early phase.

Acute silicosis was first described as a distinct entity by Middleton[4] in 1929, who reported that a rapidly fatal illness began 2.5 to 4 years after exposure to silica dust. The symptoms of the disease resembled miliary tuberculosis. Buechner and Ansari[5] in 1969 reported four cases of acute silicosis in which silicotic nodules were uncommon and that the alveoli were filled with granular material that histologically resembled the alveolar accumulations found in the lungs of patients with pulmonary alveolar proteinosis. Heppleston et al.[6–8] reported that the disease induced in rats by inhaled silica resembled very closely the material that accumulated in the lungs of patients with pulmonary alveolar proteinosis. It would appear that an end point similarity had been established between acute silicosis and alveolar proteinosis, although the causative agent(s) in the latter case have not been identified.

Acute silicosis has been called "acute silico-proteinosis"[5] and "silicotic alveolar proteinosis,"[9] although in this review we have chosen to use its original designation of simply "acute silicosis."[4,10,11] The disease in its extreme debilitating form sometimes develops in workers exposed to high concentrations of silica dust, although today its occurrence in the industrialized nations is relatively infrequent. Acute silicosis has been reported in the lungs of workers exposed to silica dust during sandblasting, tunneling, pottery production, and silica flour milling,[5,10,12–15] as well as through the inhalation of domestic scouring powder.[16]

III. INFLAMMATION IN THE LUNGS

The rat is a good model for the study of the human lung disease, because in both the human and the rat the lipidosis characteristic of acute silicosis is established early in the lungs and from that point the eventual development of silicotic nodules can occur. In the early stages following instillation of silica into the lungs of rats its effects appear primarily destructive in nature. Initially there is damage to the Type I epithelium, but this is soon repaired, presumably through the proliferation of Type II cells.[17] Within 24 h there is evidence of Type II cell proliferation and hypertrophy (Figure 1), and by 3 d secreted lamellar bodies are seen to accumulate in the alveoli.[17,18] These changes occur very rapidly following intratracheal injection of silica, but are not seen as rapidly if silica is supplied via the inhalation route. It may take many months to produce significant changes in the phospholipid status of the lungs when silica is supplied via the inhalation route,[19] since development of the condition is dose dependent.[17,19] In the initial stages of acute silicosis there is an intense inflammatory reaction in the lungs with marked increases in the number of alveolar macrophages, neutrophils, and lymphocytes in the alveoli and airways of the lungs.[20–25] It is likely that much of the pulmonary damage induced by silica might be mediated by the release of tissue damaging factors by inflammatory cells.[26,27]

IV. BIOCHEMICAL CHANGES

At the same time as the inflammatory response is progressing, the lung is undergoing several marked changes in its biochemical composition (Table 1). The cellularity of the lungs increases in response to silica as indicated by the increase in its DNA content. This increase in cellularity is primarily associated with the inflammatory reaction and to a lesser extent by hyperplasia of the Type II cell population.[22,28] The water and protein content of the lungs also increases, as does the phospholipid; however, the increase in phospholipid content is markedly greater than the increase in protein or DNA. Clearly, silica has a particularly strong effect on the phospholipid content of the lungs.

This increase in phospholipid content of the lungs is not a generalized effect involving all phospholipid-containing compartments. Most of the increase in pulmonary protein can be accounted for by increases in the protein content of the soluble, mitochondrial, and 600 *g* fractions, but increases in phospholipid are associated with quite different compartments. As shown in Table 2, the phospholipid content of all phospholipid-containing compartments increases in response to silica, but the most marked increase is seen in the two surfactant compartments. These increases in the intra- and extracellular

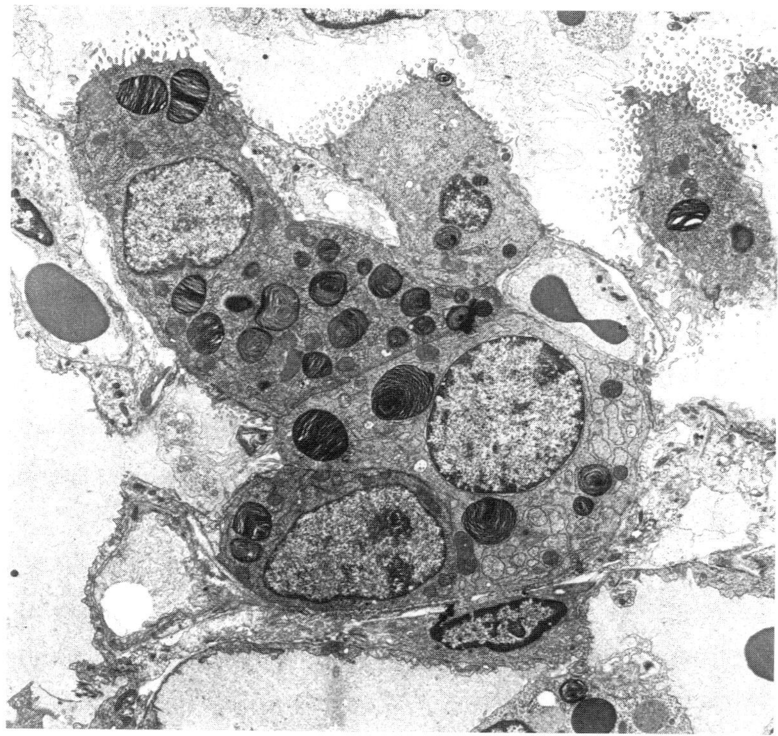

FIGURE 1 Proliferation of alveolar Type II cells in response to intratracheal injection of silica (50 mg) into the lungs of adult (250-g) rats. The rats were killed after 3 d.

TABLE 1
Effect of Silica on the DNA, Protein, Water, and Phospholipid Content of Rat Lungs

	Control	Silica	Increase (Fold)
Lung weight			
Wet weight (g)	1.22 ± 0.14	5.65 ± 0.25	4.6
Dry weight (g)	0.12 ± 0.01	1.05 ± 0.04	8.8
Fluid (g/pair of lungs)	1.13 ± 0.13	4.66 ± 0.31	4.1
DNA			
(mg/pair of lungs)	7.0 ± 0.4	23.9 ± 6.0	3.4
Protein			
(mg/pair of lungs)	239 ± 44	841 ± 148	3.5
Phospholipid			
(mg/pair of lungs)	29.6 ± 4.4	476 ± 129	16.1

Note: Male rats (225–250 g) were injected intratracheally with a single 50-mg dose of silica on day 0 and killed on day 28. Results are mean ±SD (n = 4).

Data from Dethloff et al., *Biochem. J.*, 233, 111–118, 1986.

compartments account for more than 80% of the total increase in pulmonary phospholipid, whereas they account for only about 4% of the protein increase. Quite clearly, the biochemical effects of silica on phospholipid metabolism in the lungs are focused on the surfactant system.

TABLE 2
Silica-Induced Increases in Rat Lung Phospholipid and Protein

	Protein	Phospholipid
	% of total protein increase contained in compartment	% of total phospholipid increase contained in compartment
Unfractionated lung	100	100
600 × g fraction	24.0	0.5
Heavy mitochondrial fraction	21.8	0.7
Light mitochondrial fraction	0.8	2.6
Microsomal fraction	4.6	9.2
Soluble fraction	27.3	1.4
Intracellular surfactant	2.0	59.1
Extracellular surfactant	1.7	24.6

Note: Male rats (225–250 g) were injected intratracheally with 50 mg of silica on day 0 and killed on day 28. Subcellular fractions of the lungs were isolated. Results are mean ± SD (n = 4). In the unfractionated lung the total protein increased from 230 ± 35 to 887 ± 66 mg, and the total phospholipid increased from 24.9 ± 4.6 to 269 ± 21 mg; thus the total protein increase was 657 mg, and the total phospholipid increase was 244 mg. Values of intracellular and extracellular phospholipid and protein are not corrected for recoveries, which in the intracellular pool were approximately 75% and in the extracellular pool were approximately 98%.

Data from Dethloff et al., *Biochem. J.*, 233, 111–118, 1986.

V. PULMONARY SURFACTANT

Pulmonary surfactant is a complex mixture of lipids and proteins that is absolutely essential for the maintenance of normal pulmonary functions such as gas exchange. The alveolar and airway epithelium is covered with a very thin layer of fluid, and surface tension forces at this air/lining layer interface would, in the absence of surfactant, cause the alveoli and distal airways to collapse.[29]

Pulmonary surfactant is made and secreted by alveolar Type II cells. The material is stored in cytoplasmic structures called lamellar bodies. Lamellar bodies are extruded into the alveoli where surfactant phospholipids are released to form the surfactant film. Surfactant inside Type II cells will be referred to as the intracellular pool and surfactant outside those cells as the extracellular pool. The intracellular pool of surfactant consists of primarily lamellar bodies; however, some surfactant probably resides in the endoplasmic reticulum where it is synthesized and possibly in other cytoplasmic structures. The extracellular pool consists of surfactant in the alveoli and distal airways.

Pulmonary surfactant from mammalian lungs consists of approximately 90% lipid and 10% proteins that are synthesized and secreted by alveolar Type II cells.[30] Both lipids and proteins are essential for the correct functioning of surfactant. Surfactant lipid consists of about 90% phospholipids, of which the most important class is phosphatidylcholine, accounting for from 60–80% of the phospholipid present in mammalian surfactants.[29,30]

Phospholipids found in surfactant are no different from phospholipids found in mammalian cells; however, the relative abundance of disaturated phosphatidylcholines in surfactant distinguishes the surfactant system from other membrane systems.[31–33] Phosphatidylcholine and phosphatidylglycerol are unusually high in pulmonary surfactant, and, compared with cellular membranes, the content of phosphatidylethanolamine is unusually low.[32–34] Phosphatidylcholine appears to be especially important in surfactant because dipalmitoylphosphatidylcholine is thought to be the ultimate agent responsible for the lowering of surface tension at the air/extracellular lining interface.[29]

VI. SURFACTANT PROTEINS

Phospholipid is the major component of the surfactant complex, but it is not the only component. About 10% of the surfactant complex consists of protein, of which about half appears to be relatively

TABLE 3
Effect of Silica on Intra- and Extracellular Compartments of Pulmonary Surfactant Phospholipid in the Lungs of Rats

Surfactant phospholipid compartment	Control (mg)	Silica (mg)	Increase (Fold)
Extracellular	1.17 ± 0.04 (3)	25.1 ± 7.1 (5)	22
Intracellular	1.18 ± 0.65 (3)	144 ± 53.8 (5)	123

Note: Male rats (225–250 g) were injected intratracheally with a single 50-mg dose of silica on day 0 and killed on day 28. Recovery of extracellular surfactant phospholipid was 98.4 ± 0.6% and 99.6 ± 0.4% for control and silica-treated rats, respectively. Recovery of intracellular surfactant was 73.7 ± 0.3% and 74.4 ± 4.3% for control and silica-treated rats, respectively. Results are mean ± SD (n) and have not been corrected for recoveries.

Data from Dethloff et al., *Biochem. J.*, 233, 111–118, 1986.

specific for the complex. This specificity has been recognized in four major proteins, designated surfactant proteins A (SP-A), B (SP-B), C (SP-C), and D (SP-D).[35] The relative abundance of these proteins in the complex does not appear to be fixed, because it changes substantially when the complex is secreted by Type II cells. In the lamellar bodies SP-A accounts for only 1% of the total protein, whereas SP-B and SP-C account for 28 and 22%, respectively. However, in the extracellular form of the surfactant complex SP-A accounts for 50% of the protein and SP-B and SP-C account for 8 and 4% of the total protein, respectively.[36]

VII. THE EFFECTS OF SILICA ON THE SURFACTANT SYSTEM

Pulmonary surfactant exists in two major compartments in the lungs. These compartments are the intracellular, or storage, compartment found in the cytoplasm of alveolar Type II cells and the extracellular compartment found in the alveoli and distal airways.[37] Under normal circumstances these two pools exist together in dynamic equilibrium such that the relationship between the two pools is maintained relatively constant; silica severely disturbs this relationship.[38,39] Silica causes expansion of both pools of surfactant phospholipid, but the expansion of the intracellular pool occurs to a degree considerably greater than that of the extracellular pool (Table 3). The composition of surfactant is not affected to any large degree insofar as the major component, phosphatidylcholine, is concerned,[37,40] although among the minor components the greatest change was seen in the phosphatidylinositol component, which increased in both compartments.[37] In addition, Adachi et al.[40] reported a corresponding decrease in the phosphatidylglycerol content of surfactant.

The accumulation of phospholipid in the intracellular and extracellular pools is both time and dose dependent. The expansion rate of the intracellular pool is greater than that of the extracellular pool. In our hands, the effects of silica on rat lungs was to elevate the biosynthetic rate of surfactant phosphatidylcholine 12.6-fold, elevate the secretion rate 7.3-fold, and elevate the clearance rate 5.0-fold.[39] Thus the differential expansion of the two pools is due to imbalances among the rate of biosynthesis of phosphatidylcholine, its secretion, and its clearance from the extracellular pool.[39] Because the imbalance between biosynthesis and secretion is greater than the difference between secretion and clearance, the rate of expansion of the intracellular pool must exceed the expansion rate of the extracellular pool. Heppleston et al.[41] came to a similar conclusion regarding phospholipid biosynthesis in the lungs of silica-treated rats. The differences between the two studies are that Heppleston et al.[41] measured the rate of incorporation of radiolabel into total lung phospholipids, whereas we measured the biosynthesis of surfactant associated with both intra- and extracellular pools as well as the fluxes between the two pools.

VIII. HYPERTROPHIC TYPE II CELLS

The effects of silica on phospholipid metabolism in the lungs appears to be highly focused on the surfactant system, and consequently these effects of silica must be highly concentrated on the alveolar

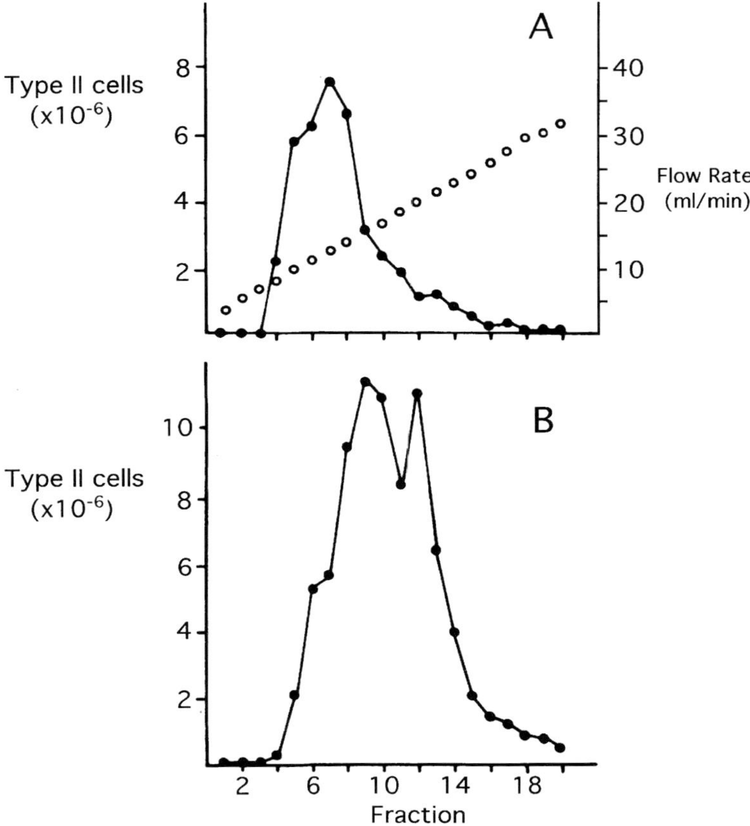

FIGURE 2 Centrifugal elutriation of Type II cells from control (A) and silica-treated (B) rat lungs. (Data from Miller, B. E., and Hook, G. E., *Lab. Invest.,* 58, 565–575, 1988.)

Type II cell. The mechanisms through which silica influences phospholipid metabolism in Type II cells are not known, although some aspects of this phenomenon have recently been clarified.

Microscopic examination of the lungs reveals two major effects of silica on the Type II cell population. First, and most obvious, is the proliferation of Type II cells. Proliferation of Type II cells following silica is most easily demonstrated by using the alkaline phosphatase stain of Miller et al.[28,42] In the alveolar regions of the lungs of rats, Type II cells are the only cells that contain alkaline phosphatase. Neutrophils also stain for alkaline phosphatase but are easily distinguishable from Type II cells by their segmented nuclei and cytoplasmic staining patterns. Not all alveoli show evidence of Type II cell proliferation, but where it does occur it is most marked at the edges of monocyte accumulations. Using morphometric procedures coupled with the alkaline phosphatase stain, we specifically quantitated Type II cells during the course of acute silicosis extending over a period of 28 d and found that the population of Type II cells in the lungs only doubled;[28] however, during this same period the intracellular pool of surfactant phospholipid increased about 20-fold. Consequently, it is clear that the increase in the number of Type II cells cannot account for the increase in the amount of intracellular surfactant phospholipid.[30]

Type II cells may be isolated from the lungs of rats by digesting the lungs using pancreatic elastase. The distribution of these dispersed Type II cells on a flow gradient during centrifugal elutriation is shown in Figure 2. The distribution of Type II cells from the lungs of silica-treated rats is not the same as that found with Type II cells from the lungs of control rats. Many Type II cells are elutriated at significantly higher flow rates than required for the elutriation of control Type II cells. It appears that a new population of Type II cells is present in the lungs of silica-treated rats, a population that is bigger than normal. That is, the Type II cell population from the lungs of silica-treated rats contains many hypertrophic cells.[42–45] The number of hypertrophic Type II cells appears to increase with time (Figure 3) and by 28 d following a single intratracheal injection of silica may account for as much as 65% of the Type II cells. These studies

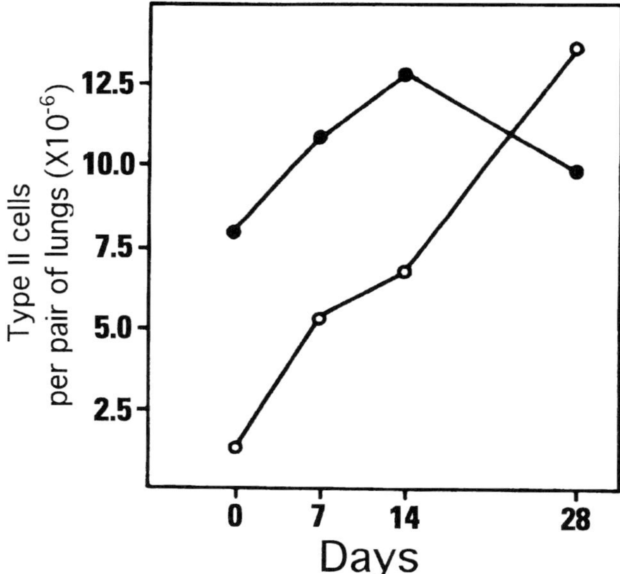

FIGURE 3 Appearance of hypertrophic Type II cells in the lungs of rats following a single 10-mg intratracheal dose of silica (animals were killed after 7 d). Cells were isolated by centrifugal elutriation. Hypertrophic Type II cells from silica-treated rats (open circles). Type II cells from control rats (closed circles). (Data from Miller, B. E., Dethloff, L. A., Gladen, B. C., and Hook, G. E., *Lab. Invest.*, 57, 546–554, 1987.)

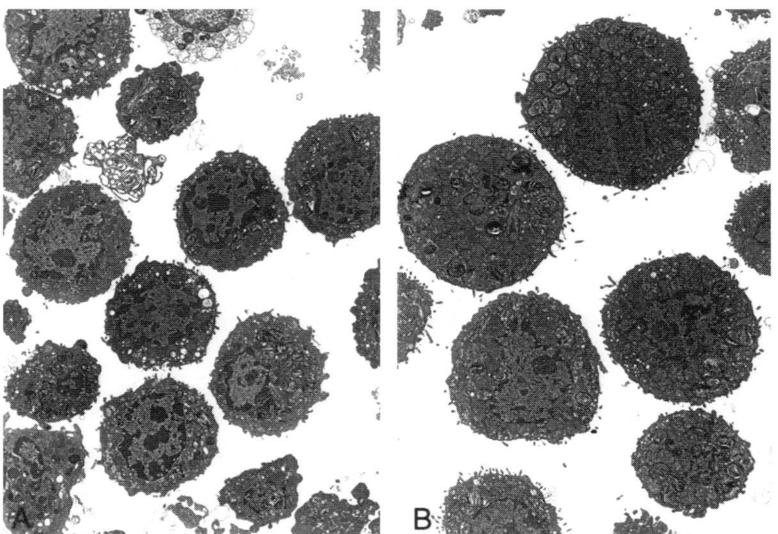

FIGURE 4 Type II cells from the lungs of control rats (A) and hypertrophic Type II cells (B) isolated from the lungs of silica-treated rats (10 mg; 7 d). The cells were isolated by using centrifugal elutriation.

were the first to show that the Type II cell population of the lungs was not uniform during the progression of silica-induced pulmonary inflammation.

From these studies on the development of Type II cell hypertrophy we developed a routine procedure for the isolation of hypertrophic Type II cells from the lungs of silica-treated rats (Figure 4). The basic procedure is similar to that of Dobbs et al.,[46] who used pancreatic elastase to isolate Type II cells from the lungs of rats. As with the Dobbs procedure we also used centrifugal elutriation, but then we used

TABLE 4
Morphometric Analysis of Type II Cells Isolated from the Lungs of Control and Silica-Treated Rats

	Control	Hypertrophic
Cell volume (μ^3)	354 ± 18	523 ± 29[a]
	(311)	(261)
Lamellar body volume (μ^3)	0.32 ± 0.07	0.66 ± 0.10[a]
	(381)	(409)
Lamellar bodies per cell	96 ± 43	131 ± 84[a]
	(41)	(32)

Note: Lungs were digested with trypsin. Cells in the lung digest were separated using centrifugal elutriation into two populations according to their position on a flow gradient. Numbers in parentheses = number of individual profiles measured.

[a] Mean ± SD, $p < 0.05$ (Tukey-Kramer procedure).

Data from Miller et al., *Lab. Invest.*, 55, 153–163, 1986.

differential adherence on IgG-coated plates as described by Dobbs et al.[47] The fundamental difference arises through the use of centrifugal elutriation to separate hypertrophic Type II cells from normal Type II cells. Under the electron microscope hypertrophic Type II cells look like normal Type II cells except for their larger size, increased number of cytoplasmic lamellar bodies, and the presence of dilatations in the endoplasmic reticulum (Table 4).

Type II cells contain surface receptors for SP-A, and it appears likely that these receptors might be involved in the uptake of the protein. Hypertrophic Type II cells from the lungs of rats treated with silica appear to contain many more SP-A receptors than normal, suggesting that if SP-A receptors are involved in the recycling of SP-A then in the hypertrophic Type II cells active recycling of SP-A may be enhanced.[48]

IX. THE CDP-CHOLINE PATHWAY

Hypertrophic Type II cells are biochemically and metabolically different from normal Type II cells. Biochemical analysis shows that hypertrophic Type II cells contain more phospholipid, more protein, more RNA, and more surfactant phospholipid than normal Type II cells (Table 5).[45] The increase in phospholipid arises primarily because of activation of the CDP-choline pathway. This pathway consists of three enzymes, choline kinase, choline phosphate cytidylyltransferase, and choline phosphotransferase and, of these enzymes, cytidylyltransferase is recognized as being rate limiting in normal Type II cells.[49] The specific activities of all of these enzymes except choline kinase are increased in hypertrophic Type II cells (Table 6). On a per cell basis, however, all of the enzyme activities are increased.[50]

Regulation of the CDP-choline pathway by choline phosphate cytidylyltransferase in normal Type II cells is said to involve the distribution of the enzyme between the soluble phase of the cell and the endoplasmic reticulum.[51] Choline phosphate cytidylyltransferase in the soluble phase of the cell is supposed to be inactive insofar as the CDP-choline pathway is concerned.[52] Transfer of the enzyme to the endoplasmic reticulum results in the enzyme now being actively engaged in phospholipid biosynthesis. It is by this means that the CDP-choline pathway is regulated, at least in Type II cells of the normal adult lung. However, this mechanism may not be universally applicable because in the fetal lung Rooney et al.[53,54] have found that stimulation of cytidylyltransferase by dexamethasone in the lungs of fetal animals may be due to activation of the protein and not to increased amounts. In addition, regulation by redistribution of choline phosphate cytidylyltransferase might not be operational in the human lung as

TABLE 5
Biochemical Composition of Type II Cells from the Lungs of Control and Silica-Treated Rats

Parameter (μg/10^6 cells)	Control (n = 8)	Hypertrophic (n = 5)
DNA	5.1 ± 0.3	5.5 ± 0.3
RNA	10.7 ± 1.1	21.1 ± 1.3[a]
Protein	78.6 ± 10.9	114.5 ± 6.6[a]
Phospholipid	20.5 ± 4.1	51.1 ± 3.0[a]

Note: Lungs were digested with trypsin. Cells in the digest were separated by centrifugal elutriation into two populations according to their position on a flow gradient.

[a] Mean ± SEM, $p < 0.05$.

Data from Miller, B. E. and Hook, G. E., *Lab. Invest.*, 58, 565–575, 1988.

TABLE 6
Specific Activities of Enzymes of the CDP-Choline Pathway in Type II Cells from Normal and Silica-Treated Rat Lungs

Enzyme	Control	Hypertrophic
Choline kinase[a]	7.04 ± 0.14	6.03 ± 0.36
Cytidylyltransferase		
Soluble phase	0.92 ± 0.06	0.83 ± 0.10
Particulate phase	2.31 ± 0.27	4.67 ± 0.22[c]
Choline phosphotransferase[b]		
With endogenous 1,2-DAG	0.15 ± 0.02	0.27 ± 0.02[c]
With exogenous 1,2-DAG	5.52 ± 0.23	10.51 ± 2.38[c]

Note: 1,2-DAG = 1,2-diacylglycerols used as substrate in the reaction.

[a] nmol/min/mg protein (soluble phase).
[b] nmol/min/mg protein (particulate phase).
[c] Mean ± SEM (n = 4), $p < 0.05$.
Data from Miller, B. E. and Hook, G. E., *Am. J. Respir. Cell Mol. Biol.*, 1, 127–136, 1989.

indicated by Hunt et al.[55] In addition, some of the observed cytidylyltransferase translocation phenomena might be mediated by cytoskeletal interactions.

In hypertrophic Type II cells from the lungs of silica-treated rats, the activity of the CDP-choline pathway is stimulated by increases in the activities of its constituent enzymes, resulting in increased biosynthesis of phosphatidylcholine.[50] The specific activity of choline kinase activity in the soluble phase of the Type II cell is not increased by silica, but the total amount of activity present in the cell is increased. Choline phosphate cytidylyltransferase activity is increased both in terms of total and specific activity as would be expected if, indeed, this enzyme is rate limiting for the pathway. Perhaps surprisingly, the total and specific activity of choline phosphotransferase is also increased. It seems likely that the increase in choline phosphotransferase activity occurs in order to offset the increase in activity of the choline phosphate cytidylyltransferase because, if this did not occur then, choline phosphotransferase might otherwise become rate limiting. These data suggest that the CDP-choline pathway in alveolar Type II cells, especially under disease conditions, might be regulated not only by the choline phosphate cytidylyltransferase, but that choline phosphotransferase might also be important. Regulation of the pathway might require some kind of coordination between the two enzymes.

Another aspect that must be considered relates to the manner in which choline phosphate cytidylyltransferase is regulated. As mentioned above, it is thought that regulation involves the distribution of the enzyme between the soluble phase of the cell and the endoplasmic reticulum. If choline phosphate cytidylyltransferase is regulated by its transfer between soluble and endoplasmic reticulum, then an increase in choline phosphate cytidylyltransferase activity associated with the endoplasmic reticulum should be accompanied by a corresponding decrease in activity associated with the soluble phase. Although an increase in the total activity of choline phosphate cytidylyltransferase was found in the particulate fraction, no change in the amount of activity associated with the soluble phase was seen.[50] However, it is possible that in the injured lung the increase in activity of choline phosphate cytidylyltransferase might arise from selective activation of the membrane-associated enzyme in a manner similar to that reported by Rooney et al.[53,54] and not through its redistribution.

X. SURFACTANT PROTEINS IN HYPERTROPHIC TYPE II CELLS

SP-A also accumulates in the lungs of silica-treated rats and, as with the phospholipid, appears to be due to the appearance of the hypertrophic Type II cell. Hypertrophic Type II cells contain substantially more SP-A than normal Type II cells. In hypertrophic Type II cells the synthesis of SP-A is enhanced, possibly due to the presence of increased levels of SP-A mRNA.[56] The presence of increased levels of SP-A in hypertrophic Type II cells isolated from the lungs of silica-treated rats has also been reported by Kawada et al.,[57] however, these investigators did not find increased levels of SP-A mRNA and attributed the increased levels of SP-A to some mechanism other than enhanced biosynthesis.

In addition to SP-A, other surfactant proteins also appear to be increased in the lungs of rats treated with silica. SP-D is a collagenous protein somewhat like SP-A that is secreted by Type II cells. The primary translation product is a protein with molecular mass of 39.3 kDa.[59] The surfactant-associated form has a molecular mass of 43 kDa.[59] It is a calcium-dependent, carbohydrate-binding protein[60] with primary sequence homology to SP-A that is secreted by alveolar Type II cells.[61,62] SP-D increases substantially in the lungs of silica-treated rats, and much of the material is found extracellularly in the alveoli.[58]

XI. ALVEOLAR PROTEINOSIS

Acute silicosis closely resembles pulmonary alveolar proteinosis, although in the latter case the causative agent(s) has not been identified. The resemblance between silica-alveolar proteinosis as produced in the lungs of rats by silica and the human disease known as pulmonary alveolar proteinosis was first noted by Heppleston and co-workers.[6–8,63] Silica particles have been reported in the lungs of many patients with pulmonary alveolar proteinosis, although other mineral particulates have also been detected,[64] and it is not possible to identify any particular particle as the causative agent.

The relationship between alveolar proteinosis and acute silicosis was first noticed by Heppleston and co-workers[6–8,41] 20 years ago. In studying the reaction of rat lungs to inhaled silica they were struck by the similarity of appearance between the rat lungs and the lungs of humans with alveolar proteinosis. Ostensibly the lungs of rats developed a periodic acid-Schiff base (PAS) positivity that was like that of the human. Acute silicosis resembles alveolar proteinosis insofar as PAS-positive material accumulates in the alveoli of the lungs.

Pulmonary alveolar proteinosis is a human lung disease in which complex lipid/protein structures accumulate in the alveoli and distal airways of the lungs.[65–67] The disease was first described by Rosen et al.[68] in 1958, and the most characteristic manifestation of this disease was the accumulation of periodic acid-Schiff base positive material in the alveoli of the lungs. Under the electron microscope this material has been shown to consist of a variety of complex structures, the major one of which has been designated tubular myelinlike and multilamellated.[66] These tubular myelinlike multilamellated structures appear to be a complex of phospholipid membranes separated by layers of protein. Digestion of tubular myelinlike multilamellated structures with proteases results in loss of the intermembranous layers without loss of the membranes, indicating that the intervening material is protein in nature. Digestion of tubular myelinlike multilamellated structures with phospholipase c results in loss of the membranes without loss of structural organization in the intervening protein layers.

Tubular myelinlike multilamellated structures are called such because they resemble tubular myelin. Tubular myelin is a structure virtually unique to the lungs. Its functions in the extracellular lining are not entirely clear. Tubular myelin consists of two sets of spaced membranes that intersect at right angles.[69] The membranes are probably phospholipid in nature, and SP-A may be part of the intermembranous material. It is thought that tubular myelin might be the penultimate surfactant complex insofar as the formation of the surface film is concerned. Certainly we have observed tubular myelin structures intermediate between, but continuous with, the surfactant film and secreted lamellar bodies[70,71] suggestive of a close relationship between them. Tubular myelinlike multilamellated structures appear to be abnormal forms of tubular myelin. Structurally these multilamellated structures appear abnormal insofar as tubule formation is often distorted or even absent.[65] In normal tubular myelin, tubules are square in lateral section, whereas in the multilamellated structures from patients, tubules may be polygonal in appearance.[65] Studies from my laboratory have shown that the major protein constituents of the tubular myelinlike multilamellated structures from the lungs of patients[72] have molecular weights in the same range as SP-A. In view of studies by Voss et al.,[73] it is highly likely that the major protein constituent of the multilamellated structures is SP-A. The origin of this protein is the alveolar Type II cell. We have shown previously that biosynthesis and secretion of SP-A is enhanced in the lungs of rats exhibiting silica-induced alveolar proteinosis, and obviously we have to consider the possibility that in human lung alveolar proteinosis similar processes are underway.

SP-A from the alveoli of patients with pulmonary alveolar proteinosis shows a number of differences from that which is found in the lungs of healthy individuals.[73] For example, a large proportion of SP-A from the lungs of patients is irreducibly cross linked. SP-B and SP-C are also different from that found in the lungs of healthy humans. Consequently, the ability of these proteins to function in the pulmonary environment may be severely impaired. The origin of these changes is not known, although it is possible that they might occur in the extracellular environment rather than prior to their secretion by alveolar Type II cells.

Tubular myelinlike multilamellated structures are the major structural entity to accumulate in the lungs of patients, but they are not the only one. Many kinds of structures may be seen in the lungs of patients, including some that probably arise from cell debris.[67] A cytotoxic agent must be responsible for the cell destruction, although the responsible agent has never been identified. However, many kinds of particles have been identified in the lungs of patients with pulmonary alveolar proteinosis, including silica and silicates, but the causative agent remains unknown.[64]

These multilamellated structures appear to be an abnormal form of tubular myelin which is formed as a complex between SP-A and surfactant phospholipids.[72] Similar structures have been seen in the lungs of rats exposed to silica dust, although, in general, the structures are not as extensive as those seen in the lungs of patients.[30] However, it is reasonable to say that alveolar proteinosis induced in the lungs of rats by silica is a model for the human lung disease known as pulmonary alveolar proteinosis.[8] The rat model of acute silico-alveolar proteinosis is also the model for this human disease.

XII. MECHANISMS

The biochemical mechanisms of quartz-induced pneumoconiosis are incompletely understood. Dust overloading is probably required before the acute silicotic response is triggered.[74,75] It is assumed that the initiating event is the interaction of silica with cell or cell membranes,[76] leading to cell damage. It is assumed that the cell damage leads to further cell and tissue injury by the release of lytic enzymes. Ultimately, fibrosis occurs presumably as an overstatement of the repair process. Interaction of Type II cells with silica can occur directly in the alveoli. Indeed, it has been shown that these cells will respond directly to the effects of silica, while other dusts such as titanium dioxide and aluminum-treated silica are without effect.[77] In response to this direct interaction, Type II cells showed evidence of cytotoxicity and initiated repair, replication, and growth.[77] Consistent with this is the report by Panos et al.[78] that Type II cells from the lungs of silica-treated rats are committed to DNA synthesis *in vitro*.[78]

It seems reasonable to suppose that there is a threshold beneath which the alveolar proteinosis-like condition will not develop. Such a threshold has not been established, but is reasonable in view of the fact that not everyone who inhales silica dust develops acute silicosis. On the other hand, very low doses of silica could produce very low levels of alveolar proteinosis, and it is only at the higher doses that the condition becomes debilitating. Accumulation of surfactant in the alveoli might not be noticeable until it begins to interfere with gas exchange. It is likely that this threshold would vary considerably with the individual and that some might have a propensity towards developing the condition more than others. Such a propensity might be related to the "silicosis risk" discussed by Polzik et al.[79] Surfactant appears to play a role in the protection of the lungs by helping to clear particles from the alveoli,[80] although the possibility also exists that the unsaturated phospholipid components of surfactant might play a role in protecting the lungs against free radicals generated either directly from the surfaces of the particles or from activated neutrophils present in the alveoli of the silica-exposed lungs.[81]

REFERENCES

1. **Craighead, J. E. and Vallyathan, N. V.,** Cryptic pulmonary lesions in workers occupationally exposed to dust containing silica, *JAMA,* 244, 1939–1941, 1980.
2. **Green, F. H., Althouse, R., and Weber, K. C.,** Prevalence of silicosis at death in underground coal miners, *Am. J. Ind. Med.,* 16, 605–615, 1989.
3. **Valiante, D. J. and Rosenman, K. D.,** Does silicosis still occur? (see comments.), *JAMA,* 262, 3003–3007, 1989.
4. **Middleton, E. L.,** The present position of silicosis in industry in Britain, *Br. Med. J.,* 2, 485, 1929.
5. **Buechner, H. A. and Ansari, A.,** Acute silico-proteinosis. A new pathologic variant of acute silicosis in sandblasters, characterized by histologic features resembling alveolar proteinosis, *Dis. Chest,* 55, 274–278, 1969.
6. **Heppleston, A. G., Wright, N. A., and Stewart, J. A.,** Experimental alveolar lipo-proteinosis following the inhalation of silica, *J. Pathol.,* 101, 293–307, 1970.
7. **Heppleston, A. G. and Young, A. E.,** Alveolar lipo-proteinosis: an ultrastructural comparison of the experimental and human forms, *J. Pathol.,* 107, 107–117, 1972.
8. **Heppleston, A. G.,** Animal model of human disease. Pulmonary alveolar lipo-proteinosis. Animal model: silica-induced pulmonary alveolar lipo-proteinosis, *Am. J. Pathol.,* 78, 171–174, 1975.
9. Silicosis and Silicate Disease Committee, Diseases associated with exposure to silica and nonfibrous silicate minerals, *Arch. Pathol. Lab. Med.,* 112, 673–720, 1988.
10. **Gardner, L. U.,** Pathology of so-called acute silicosis, *Am. J. Public Health,* 23, 1240–1249, 1933.
11. **MacDonald, G., Piggott, A. P., Gilder, F. W., et al.,** Cases of acute silicosis with a suggested theory of causation, *Lancet,* 846–848, 1930.
12. **Suratt, P. M., Winn, W. C., Jr., Brody, A. R., Bolton, W. K., and Giles, R. D.,** Acute silicosis in tombstone sandblasters, *Am. Rev. Respir. Dis.,* 115, 521–529, 1977.
13. **Banks, D. E., Morring, K. L., Boehlecke, B. A., et al.,** Silicosis in silica flour workers, *Am. Rev. Respir. Dis.,* 124, 445–450, 1981.
14. **Giles, R. D., Sturgill, B. C., Suratt, P. M., and Bolton, W. K.,** Massive proteinuria and acute renal failure in a patient with acute silicoproteinosis, *Am. J. Med.,* 336–342, 1978.
15. **O'Donnell, D. M., Worrell, J. A., and Carroll, F. E.,** Acute silicosis, *Am. J. Roentgenol.,* 158, 1361–1362, 1992.
16. **Dumontet, C., Biron, F., Vitrey, D., Guerin, J. C., Vincent, M., Jarry, O., Meram, D., and Peyramond, D.,** Acute silicosis due to inhalation of a domestic product, *Am. Rev. Respir. Dis.,* 143, 880–882, 1991.
17. **Dethloff, L. A., Gilmore, L. B., Gladen, B. C., George, G., Chhabra, R. S., and Hook, G. E.,** Effects of silica on the composition of the pulmonary extracellular lining, *Toxicol. Appl. Pharmacol.,* 84, 66–83, 1986.
18. **Gross, K. B., White, H. J., and Smiler, K. L.,** Functional and morphologic changes in the lungs after a single intratracheal instillation of silica, *Am. Rev. Respir. Dis.,* 129, 833–839, 1984.
19. **Heppleston, A. G.,** Determinants of pulmonary fibrosis and lipidosis in the silica model, *Br. J. Exp. Pathol.,* 67, 879–888, 1986.
20. **Absher, M. P., Trombley, L., Hemenway, D. R., Mickey, R. M., and Leslie, K. O.,** Biphasic cellular and tissue response of rat lungs after eight-day aerosol exposure to the silicon dioxide cristobalite, *Am. J. Pathol.,* 134, 1243–1251, 1989.
21. **Cantin, A., Dubois, F., and Begin, R.,** Lung exposure to mineral dusts enhances the capacity of lung inflammatory cells to release superoxide, *J. Leukocyte Biol.,* 43, 299–303, 1988.
22. **Dethloff, L. A., Gladen, B. C., Gilmore, L. B., and Hook, G. E.,** Quantitation of cellular and extracellular constituents of the pulmonary lining in rats by using bronchoalveolar lavage. Effects of silica-induced pulmonary inflammation, *Am. Rev. Respir. Dis.,* 136, 899–907, 1987.
23. **Callis, A. H., Sohnle, P. G., Mandel, G. S., Wiessner, J., and Mandel, N. S.,** Kinetics of inflammatory and fibrotic pulmonary changes in a murine model of silicosis, *J. Lab. Clin. Med.,* 105, 547–553, 1985.
24. **Driscoll, K. E., Lindenschmidt, R. C., Maurer, J. K., Higgins, J. M., and Ridder, G.,** Pulmonary response to silica or titanium dioxide: inflammatory cells, alveolar macrophage-derived cytokines, and histopathology, *Am. J. Respir. Cell Mol. Biol.,* 2, 381–390, 1990.

25. **Driscoll, K. E. and Maurer, J. K.,** Cytokine and growth factor release by alveolar macrophages — potential biomarkers of pulmonary toxicity, *Toxicol. Pathol.*, 19, 398–405, 1991.
26. **Dalal, N. S., Shi, X. L., and Vallyathan, V.,** ESR spin trapping and cytotoxicity investigations of freshly fractured quartz: mechanism of acute silicosis, *Free Radical Res. Commun.*, 9, 259–266, 1990.
27. **Dalal, N. S., Shi, X., and Vallyathan, V.,** Oxygenated radical formation by fresh quartz dust in a cell-free aqueous medium and its inhibition by scavengers, in *Effects of Mineral Dusts on Cells,* Mossman, B.T. and Begin, R.O., Eds., Springer-Verlag, Berlin, NATO ASI Series Vol. H30, 1989.
28. **Miller, B. E., Chapin, R. E., Pinkerton, K. E., Gilmore, L. B., Maronpot, R. R., and Hook, G. E.,** Quantitation of silica-induced type II cell hyperplasia by using alkaline phosphatase histochemistry in glycol methacrylate embedded lung, *Exp. Lung Res.*, 12, 135–148, 1987.
29. **Clements, J. A.,** Functions of the alveolar lining, *Am. Rev. Respir. Dis.*, 115, 67–71, 1977.
30. **Hook, G. E. R.,** Alveolar proteinosis and phospholipidoses of the lungs, *Toxicol. Pathol.*, 19, 482–513, 1991.
31. **Rooney, S. A. and Gobran, L. I.,** Alveolar lavage and lavaged lung tissue phosphatidylcholine composition during fetal rabbit development, *Lipids,* 12, 1050–1054, 1977.
32. **Rooney, S. A., Nardone, L. L., Shapiro, D. L., Motoyama, E. K., Gobran, L., and Zaehringer, N.,** The phospholipids of rabbit type II alveolar epithelial cells: comparison with lung lavage, lung tissue, alveolar macrophages, and a human alveolar tumor cell line, *Lipids,* 12, 438–442, 1977.
33. **Rooney, S. A., Page-Roberts, B. A., and Motoyama, E. K.,** Role of lamellar inclusions in surfactant production: studies on phospholipid composition and biosynthesis in rat and rabbit lung subcellular fractions, *J. Lipid Res.*, 16, 418–425, 1975.
34. **Rooney, S. A., Canavan, P. M., and Motoyama, E. K.,** The identification of phosphatidylglycerol in the rat, rabbit, monkey and human lung, *Biochim. Biophys. Acta,* 360, 56–67, 1974.
35. **Possmayer, F.,** A proposed nomenclature for pulmonary surfactant-associated proteins, *Am. Rev. Respir. Dis.*, 138, 990–998, 1988.
36. **Oosterlaken-Dijksterhuis, M. A., van Eijk, M., van Buel, B. L., van Golde, L. M., and Haagsman, H. P.,** Surfactant protein composition of lamellar bodies isolated from rat lung, *Biochem. J.*, 274, 115–119, 1991.
37. **Dethloff, L. A., Gilmore, L. B., Brody, A. R., and Hook, G. E.,** Induction of intra- and extra-cellular phospholipids in the lungs of rats exposed to silica, *Biochem. J.*, 233, 111–118, 1986.
38. **Dethloff, L. A., Gilmore, L. B., and Hook, G. E.,** The relationship between intra- and extra-cellular surfactant phospholipids in the lungs of rabbits and the effects of silica-induced lung injury, *Biochem. J.*, 239, 59–67, 1986.
39. **Dethloff, L. A., Gladen, B. C., Gilmore, L. B., and Hook, G. E.,** Kinetics of pulmonary surfactant phosphatidylcholine metabolism in the lungs of silica-treated rats, *Toxicol. Appl. Pharmacol.*, 98, 1–11, 1989.
40. **Adachi, H., Hayashi, H., Sato, H., Dempo, K., and Akino, T.,** Characterization of phospholipids accumulated in pulmonary-surfactant compartments of rats intratracheally exposed to silica, *Biochem. J.*, 262, 781–786, 1989.
41. **Heppleston, A. G., Fletcher, K., and Wyatt, I.,** Changes in the composition of lung lipids and the "turnover" of dipalmitoyl lecithin in experimental alveolar lipo-proteinosis induced by inhaled quartz, *Br. J. Exp. Pathol.*, 55, 384–395, 1974.
42. **Miller, B. E. and Hook, G. E.,** Hypertrophy and hyperplasia of alveolar type II cells in response to silica and other pulmonary toxicants, *Environ. Health Perspect.*, 85, 15–23, 1990.
43. **Miller, B. E., Dethloff, L. A., Gladen, B. C., and Hook, G. E.,** Progression of type II cell hypertrophy and hyperplasia during silica-induced pulmonary inflammation, *Lab. Invest.*, 57, 546–554, 1987.
44. **Miller, B. E., Dethloff, L. A., and Hook, G. E.,** Silica-induced hypertrophy of type II cells in the lungs of rats, *Lab. Invest.*, 55, 153–163, 1986.
45. **Miller, B. E. and Hook, G. E.,** Isolation and characterization of hypertrophic type II cells from the lungs of silica-treated rats, *Lab. Invest.*, 58, 565–575, 1988.
46. **Dobbs, L. G., Geppert, E. F., Williams, M. C., Greenleaf, R. D., and Mason, R. J.,** Metabolic properties and ultrastructure of alveolar type II cells isolated with elastase, *Biochim. Biophys. Acta,* 618, 510–523, 1980.
47. **Dobbs, L. G., Gonzalez, R., and Williams, M. C.,** An improved method for isolating type II cells in high yield and purity, *Am. Rev. Respir. Dis.*, 134, 141–145, 1986.
48. **Suwabe, A., Panos, R. J., and Voelker, D. R.,** Alveolar type II cells isolated after silica-induced lung injury in rats have increased surfactant protein A (SP-A) receptor activity, *Am. J. Respir. Cell Mol. Biol.*, 4, 264–272, 1991.
49. **Post, M., Batenburg, J. J., Schuurmans, E. A., and Van Golde, L. M.,** The rate-limiting step in the biosynthesis of phosphatidylcholine by alveolar type II cells from adult rat lung, *Biochim. Biophys. Acta,* 712, 390–394, 1982.
50. **Miller, B. E. and Hook, G. E.,** Regulation of phosphatidylcholine biosynthesis in activated alveolar type II cells, *Am. J. Respir. Cell Mol. Biol.*, 1, 127–136, 1989.
51. **Vance, D. E.,** Boehringer Mannheim Award Lecture. Phosphatidylcholine metabolism: masochistic enzymology, metabolic regulation, and lipoprotein assembly, *Biochem. Cell Biol.*, 68, 1151–1165, 1990.
52. **Feldman, D. A., Rounsifer, M. E., Charles, L., and Weinhold, P. A.,** CTP: phosphocholine cytidylyltransferase in rat lung: relationship between cytosolic and membrane forms, *Biochim. Biophys. Acta,* 1045, 49–57, 1990.

53. **Rooney, S. A., Dynia, D. W., Smart, D. A., Chu, A. J., Ingleson, L. D., Wilson, C. M., and Gross, I.,** Glucocorticoid stimulation of choline-phosphate cytidylyltransferase activity in fetal rat lung: receptor-response relationships, *Biochim. Biophys. Acta,* 888, 208–216, 1986.
54. **Rooney, S. A., Smart, D. A., Weinhold, P. A., and Feldman, D. A.,** Dexamethasone increases the activity but not the amount of choline-phosphate cytidylyltransferase in fetal rat lung, *Biochim. Biophys. Acta,* 1044, 385–389, 1990.
55. **Hunt, A. N., Normand, C. S., and Postle, A. D.,** CTP: cholinephosphate cytidylyltransferase in human and rat lung: association in vitro with cytoskeletal actin, *Biochim. Biophys. Acta,* 1043, 19–26, 1990.
56. **Miller, B. E., Bakewell, W. E., Katyal, S. L., Singh, G., and Hook, G. E.,** Induction of surfactant protein (SP-A) biosynthesis and SP-A mRNA in activated type II cells during acute silicosis in rats, *Am. J. Respir. Cell Mol. Biol.,* 3, 217–226, 1990.
57. **Kawada, H., Horiuchi, T., Shannon, J. M., Kuroki, Y., Voelker, D. R., and Mason, R. J.,** Alveolar type II cells, surfactant protein A (SP-A), and the phospholipid components of surfactant in acute silicosis in the rat, *Am. Rev. Respir. Dis.,* 140, 460–470, 1989.
58. **Crouch, E., Persson, A., Chang, D., and Parghi, D.,** Surfactant protein D. Increased accumulation in silica-induced pulmonary lipoproteinosis, *Am. J. Pathol.,* 139, 765–776, 1991.
59. **Crouch, E., Rust, K., Persson, A., Mariencheck, W., Moxley, M., and Longmore, W.,** Primary translation products of pulmonary surfactant protein D, *Am. J. Physiol.,* 260, L247–253, 1991.
60. **Persson, A., Chang, D., Rust, K., Moxley, M., Longmore, W., and Crouch, E.,** Purification and biochemical characterization of CP4 (SP-D), a collagenous surfactant-associated protein, *Biochemistry,* 28, 6361–6367, 1989.
61. **Persson, A., Chang, D., and Crouch, E.,** Surfactant protein D is a divalent cation-dependent carbohydrate-binding protein, *J. Biol. Chem.,* 265, 5755–5760, 1990.
62. **Persson, A., Rust, K., Chang, D., Moxley, M., Longmore, W., and Crouch, E.,** CP4: a pneumocyte-derived collagenous surfactant-associated protein. Evidence for heterogeneity of collagenous surfactant proteins, *Biochemistry,* 27, 8576–8584, 1988.
63. **Heppleston, A. G.,** Atypical reaction to inhaled silica, *Nature,* 213, 199, 1967.
64. **Abraham, J. L. and McEuen, D. D.,** Inorganic particulates associated with pulmonary alveolar proteinosis: SEM and X-ray microanalysis results, *Appl. Pathol.,* 4, 138–146, 1986.
65. **Hook, G. E., Gilmore, L. B., and Talley, F. A.,** Multilamelled structures from the lungs of patients with pulmonary alveolar proteinosis, *Lab. Invest.,* 50, 711–725, 1984.
66. **Gilmore, L. B., Talley, F. A., and Hook, G. E.,** Classification and morphometric quantitation of insoluble materials from the lungs of patients with alveolar proteinosis, *Am. J. Pathol.,* 133, 252–264, 1988.
67. **Hook, G. E., Bell, D. Y., Gilmore, L. B., Nadeau, D., Reasor, M. J., and Talley, F. A.,** Composition of bronchoalveolar lavage effluents from patients with pulmonary alveolar proteinosis, *Lab. Invest.,* 39, 342–357, 1978.
68. **Rosen, S. H., Castleman, B., and Liebow, A. A.,** Pulmonary alveolar proteinosis, *N. Engl. J. Med.,* 258, 1123–1142, 1958.
69. **Weibel, E. R., Kistler, G. S., and Tondury, G.,** A stereologic electron microscope study of "tubular myelin figures" in alveolar fluids of rat lungs, *Z. Zellforsch. Mikrosk. Anat.,* 69, 418–427, 1966.
70. **Hook, G. E. R., Spalding, J. W., Ortner, M. J., Tombropoulos, E. G., and Chignell, C. F.,** Investigation of phospholipids of the pulmonary extracellular lining by electron paramagnetic resonance: the effects of phosphatidylglycerol and unsaturated phosphatidylcholines on the fluidity of dipalmitoylphosphatidylcholine, *Biochem. J.,* 223, 533–542, 1984.
71. **Williams, M. C.,** Conversion of lamellar body membranes into tubular myelin in alveoli of fetal rat lungs, *J. Cell Biol.,* 72, 260–277, 1977.
72. **Hook, G. E., Gilmore, L. B., and Talley, F. A.,** Dissolution and reassembly of tubular myelin-like multilamellated structures from the lungs of patients with pulmonary alveolar proteinosis, *Lab. Invest.,* 55, 194–208, 1986.
73. **Voss, T., Schafer, K. P., Nielsen, P. F., Schafer, A., Maier, C., Hannappel, E., Maassen, J., Landis, B., Klemm, K., and Przybylski, M.,** Primary structure differences of human surfactant-associated proteins isolated from normal and proteinosis lung, *Biochim. Biophys. Acta,* 1138, 261–267, 1992.
74. **Bolton, R. E., Vincent, J. H., Jones, A. D., Addison, J., and Beckett, S. T.,** An overload hypothesis for pulmonary clearance of IUCC amosite fibers inhaled by rats, *Br. J. Ind. Med.,* 40, 1983.
75. **Morrow, P. E.,** Dust overloading of the lungs: update and appraisal, *Toxicol. Appl. Pharmacol.,* 113, 1–12, 1992.
76. **Allison, A. C., Harington, J. S., and Birbeck, M.,** An examination of the cytotoxic effects of silica on macrophages, *J. Exp. Med.,* 124, 141–154, 1966.
77. **Lesur, O., Cantin, A. M., Tanswell, A. K., Melloni, B., Beaulieu, J. F., and Begin, R.,** Silica exposure induces cytotoxicity and proliferative activity of type-II pneumocytes, *Exp. Lung Res.,* 18, 173–190, 1992.
78. **Panos, R. J., Suwabe, A., Leslie, C. C., and Mason, R. J.,** Hypertrophic alveolar type II cells from silica-treated rats are committed to DNA synthesis *in vitro, Am. J. Respir. Cell Mol. Biol.,* 51–59, 1990.
79. **Polzik, E. V., Katsnelson, B. A., Kochneva, M. Y. U., and Kasantsev, V. S.,** The principles of predicting the individual risk of silicosis and silicotuberculosis, *Med. Lav.,* 81, 87–95, 1990.
80. **Curti, P. C. and Genghini, M.,** Role of surfactant in alveolar defence against inhaled particles, *Respiration,* 55 (Suppl. 1), 60–67, 1989.
81. **Hook, G. E. R.,** Does pulmonary surfactant aid in defense of the lungs? *Environ. Health Perspect.,* 101, 98, 1994.

Section III
Chapter 9

FIBROGENIC FACTORS: IDENTITY AND MODE OF RELEASE

Leslie Couch and Peter B. Bitterman

CONTENTS

I. INTRODUCTION

Silica remains an important cause of pneumoconiosis worldwide despite improvements in environmental standards and industrial hygiene procedures. Our understanding of the molecular and cellular pathogenesis of silicosis has increased greatly during the past decade. This has brought health care professionals closer to the point where standards can be set based on this understanding, and workers at risk of disease can be identified prior to the development of physiological derangements. In this review we will highlight recent advances that have further elucidated the pathogenesis of pulmonary fibrosis, the principle manifestation of silica-induced pneumoconiosis. We will examine data specifically developed from studies of silica-induced pulmonary fibrosis but also will use information derived from other causes of pulmonary fibrosis that are pertinent to our understanding of the process.

The discussion will begin with a brief overview of fibroblast biology and develop some important principles governing the interaction between fibroblasts and two key elements of the provisional matrix, fibrin and fibronectin. The development of acute inflammation in response to silica and the mechanisms of macrophage activation will be considered by Drs. Driscoll and Castranova in Section III, Chapters 4 and 5. In this chapter we will focus on selected macrophage-derived peptide ligands that illustrate general principles of regulation of the fibrotic process. We will also consider key ligands involved in autocrine regulation of fibroblast function. Our discussion will conclude by considering the role of the epithelium and epithelial-derived products in modulating fibroblast function.

II. GENERAL FIBROBLAST BIOLOGY

The interstitial cells in the lung are located in the interlobular septa, the bronchial and vascular adventitia, and the alveolar wall between the epithelium and the capillary endothelium. These cells are similar to the fibroblasts located elsewhere in that they have abundant rough endoplasmic reticulum, ribosomes, and golgi apparatus. However, some interstitial cells possess bundles of intracellular filaments and are termed myofibroblasts. When activated by appropriate signals in the context of alveolar injury,

0-8493-4709-2/96/$0.00+$.50

these myofibroblasts migrate into the alveolar airspace where they proliferate and synthesize connective tissue. The activation of myofibroblasts is initiated and controlled by an interaction among regulatory signals provided by the extracellular matrix, inflammatory cells, alveolar epithelial cells, endothelial cells, and fibroblasts. As fibroblasts are stimulated to migrate, they move from the physiological matrix in the interstitium onto a provisional matrix within the alveolar airspace.[1]

The physiological matrix is composed of a variety of proteins and carbohydrates. Membrane receptors for these moieties regulate cell-cell and cell-matrix interactions. Several membrane receptor superfamilies have been characterized. Each receptor type has ligand specificity. The integrins comprise one such superfamily. These heterodimeric transmembrane glycoproteins serve as receptors for several matrix components, including fibrin and fibronectin, which are involved in cell migration, attachment, and proliferation. Integrins consist of a common β subunit noncovalently associated with a distinct α subunit. The β subunit defines one of four integrin subfamilies (β1, β2, β3, βD). Integrins with the same β subunit and different α subunits bind different ligands, suggesting the α subunit dictates ligand specificity. Antibodies to the β1 integrin family block cell migration and cytodifferentiation. Ligand binding to integrins causes enhanced cell attachment and spreading on ligand-coated surfaces. In the lung, the $\alpha_5\beta_1$ fibronectin receptor is required for fibronectin matrix assembly by the fibroblast.[2–4]

Fibroblasts express cell surface receptors for a number of peptide ligands modulating migration, proliferation, and connection tissue deposition. Among these are platelet-derived growth factor (PDGF) receptors which belong to a family of receptor proteins characterized by an extracellular domain composed of five immunoglobulin-like repeats, similar patterns of cysteine distribution, a hydrophobic membrane sparing domain, and intracellular tyrosine kinase activity. The functional PDGF receptor exists as a heterodimer or homodimer of two subunits, α and β. Each differs in its binding specificity for the three major dimeric isoforms of PDGF (AA, BB, and AB). The expression of PDGF receptor is tightly controlled, reflecting its role in growth and development. The α and β receptors appear to be independently regulated with pro-inflammatory proteins, such as transforming growth factor-β (TGF-β), able to regulate cell-specific expression of PDGF receptor subunits. The response repertoire varies for a given type of fibroblast to a specific PDGF ligand, since receptor composition varies between fibroblast types. Some fibroblasts and smooth muscle cells have mainly β receptors, while others have equal amounts of α and β receptors. Of note, PDGF-AA binds mainly to type α receptors, PDGF-AB to a heterodimeric receptor, with PDGF-BB binding predominantly to β type receptors. The interaction of the receptor with PDGF ligand causes induction of receptor tyrosine kinase activity, leading to autophosphorylation. This in turn increases phospholipase A2 and alters intracellular ions by mobilizing Ca^{2+} and stimulating the Na/H exchanger. This results in the expression of a new set of growth regulatory genes, including the immediate early genes fos and jun, as well as the cyclins. In addition to autophosphorylation of the receptor on tyrosine residues, phosphate is also found bound to serine residues. This suggests the receptor may be regulated by two types of kinases, autophosphorylation on tyrosine residues and phosphorylation on serine residues.[5–8]

Receptors for the fibroblast growth factor (FGF) family of growth factors (both basic and acidic) have been identified on the fibroblast cell surface. The FGF-related ligands appear to bind to the same receptor. These receptors may belong to the same family as PDGF receptors exhibiting internal tyrosine kinase domains. Interaction of aFGF, bFGF, or kFGF with its receptor results in receptor autophosphorylation on tyrosine residues. The details of FGF receptor regulation remain to be elucidated. Some studies suggest that regulation may be through glycosylation of the receptor, which may be essential for receptor stability.[9,10]

Two insulin-like growth factor (IGF) receptors have been identified on the fibroblast surface, type 1 and type 2. The type 1 receptor appears to be situated on basolateral aspects of the cell. Type 1 receptors are more prevalent in proliferating cells and are composed of four subunits, two α and two β chains. Signal transduction occurs in a manner similar to PDGF and FGF via tyrosine kinase activity and autophosphorylation.[11–13]

The TGF-β receptor is composed of serine/thronine kinases, termed receptors I and II. The receptors are characterized by a small extracellular domain, a single transmembrane domain, and a cytoplasmic protein containing the kinase activity. Ligand binds directly to receptor II, which is constitutively active. The ligand receptor II complex binds to receptor I. Phosphorylation of receptor I by receptor II permits receptor I to begin the process of signal transduction. There are a number of Type I isoforms; the nature of the Type I receptor appears to dictate the nature of the biological response upon ligand binding.[13a]

III. PROVISIONAL MATRIX

Deposition of provisional matrix composed mainly of fibrin and fibronectin is prominent in many acute and chronic inflammatory reactions in the lung. In idiopathic pulmonary fibrosis, fibrin is present in the interstitium and along the alveolar surface. Immediately following acute lung injury, fibrin and fibronectin are present along the alveolar ducts and in the alveolar airspaces. Observations by Pratt[14] and Spencer[15] suggest that these areas of fibrin deposition subsequently evolve into fibrotic areas with the lung parenchyma. These data are supported by *in vitro* studies which demonstrate that fibrin and fibronectin are important matrix molecules for fibroblast and epithelial adherence and proliferation.

Fibronectin is a potent haptoattractant and growth factor for lung fibroblasts. It is a 440,000-Da glycoprotein that is synthesized by alveolar macrophages as well as fibroblasts. It provides one mechanism for fibroblast attachment to the connective tissue matrix via the $\alpha_2\beta_1$ integrins.[16] Also, it can act as a growth factor inducing mesenchymal cells to enter the cell cycle G1. Immunohistochemical studies indicate that virtually all alveolar macrophages stain positively for intracellular fibronectin and its synthesis is a property of alveolar macrophages obtained from the terminal respiratory tract of normal individuals.[17,18] Rom and associates[19] have shown increased release of fibronectin from alveolar macrophages isolated from those workers exposed to mineral dusts, including asbestos, silica, and coal, who had functional evidence of lung disease. Also, an increased amount of fibronectin has been identified in the epithelial lining fluid of the lower respiratory tract under these circumstances. Immunohistochemical staining of pneumoconiotic lesions from patients exposed to coal, silica, or asbestos demonstrates large amounts of fibronectin.[19–21] Taken together, these data implicate fibronectin as one of the major matrix elements regulating fibroblast function in occupational dust exposure.

In normal lung, there is little procoagulant activity found at the air-lung interface and a corresponding high level of fibrinolytic activity consistent with the absence of extravascular fibrin deposition. The normal alveolar compartment contains factor VII, tissue factor, and factor V but lacks factor X, prothrombin, and fibrinogen. Also, plasminogen and plasminogen activator inhibitor 1 are very low or absent. When the lung is injured, these factors of the coagulation and fibrinolytic cascade traverse into the alveolar compartment and are also locally elaborated by alveolar macrophages and epithelial cells. This has been demonstrated in cells obtained from patients with idiopathic pulmonary fibrosis and sarcoidosis, patients with acute lung injury, and marmosets with bleomycin-induced lung injury. The increased procoagulant factors are due mainly to increased tissue factor associated with factor VII, despite increases in antithrombin III and extrinsic pathway inhibitors. In patients with acute lung injury, bronchoalveolar lavage fluid has been shown to impair fibrinolytic activity, effectively inhibiting both plasmin and plasminogen activator. Under these circumstances, plasminogen activator inhibitor 1 has been variably detected, and levels of plasminogen activator inhibitor 2 are low or undetectable. The net effect is the presence of polymerized fibrin at the air-lung interface which provides a provisional matrix onto which myofibroblasts can adhere and proliferate. Persistent fibrin deposits are seen in areas of pulmonary scarring, supporting a role for fibrin as a nidus for pulmonary fibrosis.[22–25]

IV. PEPTIDE LIGANDS

Among the proteins expressed locally and systemically after injury are Interleukin 1 (IL-1) and tumor necrosis factor-α (TNF-α). These moieties have pleiotropic effects on fibroblast function and differentiated state and can initiate the molecular processes involved in dust-induced pulmonary fibrosis.

IL-1 is produced by several cell types but is particularly important as an alveolar macrophage mediator. Two forms exist, IL-1α, the major membrane form, and IL-1β, the secreted form. IL-1 stimulates the proliferation and activation of the T helper lymphocyte population, which in turn stimulates the monocyte/macrophage population and other cells to secrete growth factors. Schmidt et al.[26] showed that IL-1 regulates the growth of dermal fibroblasts and that monocytes stimulated with silica release IL-1. This in turn induces proliferation of fibroblasts, primarily through autocrine stimulation of PDGF.[26–30] A number of other biological effects relevant to the pathogenesis of pneumoconiosis have been attributed to IL-1. IL-1 increases collagen and collagenase production by fibroblasts as well as a number of extracellular matrix-associated proteins. IL-1 regulates the plasminogen activator profile of a number of cell types.[27] Immunohistochemistry of patients with sarcoidosis reveals intracytoplasmic IL-1 in macrophages and epithelioid cells surrounding granulomas.[28–30] Some animal models suggest IL-1 may be involved in modulating the production of granulomas, although direct evidence in silicotic lesions is lacking.

TNF is able to regulate mesenchymal cell population size by regulating programmed death and proliferation. Comprised of two or more identical 17-kDa disulfide subunits, TNF-α is primarily synthesized and excreted by activated mononuclear phagocytes, including the alveolar macrophage.[31] It regulates fibroblast proliferation and growth by induction of IL-6.[32] In alveolar macrophages from patients with sarcoidosis there is upregulation of TNF-α.[33] Piguet and co-workers[34] demonstrated alveolar macrophage-derived TNF as a mediator of pulmonary fibrosis in silica-exposed mice.[3] The use of neutralizing anti-TNF antibodies in this model prevented increased collagen accumulation in the lungs.[34] Gosset et al.[35] showed coal dust exposure of alveolar macrophage-induced mRNA expression and secretion of both TNF and IL-6. These studies demonstrated that upregulation of TNF is due to cellular activation by coal dust rather than demise of the cell. Silica was found to have similar effects.[36]

Growth factors provide the defined cell cycle-specific signals regulating cell proliferation. They act in a paracrine or autocrine fashion by binding to specific cell surface receptors. Growth factors may act singly or together to stimulate proliferation of a given population of cells. Each growth factor is active for specific target cells and tissues, often signaling both directed migration and proliferation as well as preserving cell viability. In fibroproliferative lung disorders such as sarcoidosis, idiopathic pulmonary fibrosis, pneumoconiosis, and acute lung injury, a set of trophic signals for mesenchymal cells in the fluid lining the air-lung interface has been identified. Among these are PDGF-related peptides, fibronectin, TGF-β, FGF, and IGF.

The family of genes designated proto-oncogenes are now recognized to play an important role in the regulation of cell proliferation. The growth factor-receptor interaction leads to rapid expression of immediate early proto-oncogenes such as c-fos, c-myc, and c-jun. The products of c-myc and c-fos are nuclear proteins which may regulate transcription or, together with other nuclear moieties, act as a transcriptional activation complex. Some proto-oncogenes are structurally and functionally homologous to growth factors such as c-sis for PDGF B chain or growth factor receptors such as erb B for epidermal growth factor. These data support a close relationship between oncogenes, growth factors, and the regulation of fibroblast growth.

PDGF was discovered in 1974 as a material released from platelets that is a major source of fibroblast growth-promoting activity in whole blood serum. It promotes the growth of many cells which are serum dependent. There are two genes, designated A and B, which encode the PDGF peptides. Each contains seven exons and spans approximately 22 to 24 kilobases (kb) in length. There is a 60% homology in amino acid sequence and similarity in exon size and number between the two chains. The A chain gene is located on the short arm of chromosome 7, coding for three mRNA species: 1.9, 2.3, and 2.8 kb. The B chain gene is located on the long arm of chromosome 22, producing mRNA in the range of 3.4 to 4.2 kb. Regulation of gene expression involves both transcriptional and post-transcriptional events.[37]

The PDGF protein is bioactive in the picomolar to nanomolar range for target cells that possess the appropriate high-affinity cell surface receptors. It can direct both migration and proliferation of mesenchymal cells.[38,39] The active protein usually is a disulfide-linked homo- or heterodimer of two peptides designated A and B (AA, AB, and BB). It is cationic in aqueous solution and demonstrates high-affinity binding to stromal glycosaminoglycans such as heparan sulfate as well as anionic glycoproteins in plasma. α2 Macroglobulin may serve a physiologic role as a PDGF binding moiety. Alveolar macrophages release α2 macroglobulin which, through its binding and release of PDGF, may modulate the biologic response to PDGF-related peptides. Target cell responsiveness is either enhanced or inhibited to the PDGF-α2 macroglobulin complex, depending on whether the PDGF is bound to a receptor recognized or unrecognized α2 macroglobulin.[40]

Using immunological tools, the molecular mass of PDGF-related peptides are being identified and quantified in integumentory wounds as well as the lungs of patients with pulmonary fibrosis and acute lung injury. One form has a molecular mass corresponding to platelet-derived PDGF-AB (29 kDa). However, a number of PDGF-related peptides with molecule masses ranging from 14 to 67 kDa have been identified from active fibrotic processes *in vivo*. Of note, platelets, mononuclear phagocytes, endothelial cells, and mesenchymal cells release PDGF-related peptides with molecular masses ranging from 14 to 67 kDa. The precise amino acid sequence of the bioactive peptides *in vivo* and their respective cellular sources remain to be elucidated. This information will be important to establish a role for these ligands in both physiological and pathological circumstances.[41–45]

Pathologically, abnormal expression and secretion of PDGF and PDGF-related peptides are felt to have a role in cancer, pulmonary fibrosis, and atherosclerosis. Vignaud and associates[43] demonstrated that interstitial macrophages of idiopathic pulmonary fibrosis patients exhibited a level of B chain expression that was three-fold higher than control subjects. Using *in situ* hybridization, positive macrophages were noted in areas of fibrosis as well as in anatomically normal areas of lung, suggesting that PDGF may be involved in all phases of the fibrotic process. Brown and associates[46] have shown that supernatants of human alveolar macrophages stimulated with silica contain growth factor activity for human lung fibroblasts. These investigators suggested that silica may be a particularly potent fibrogenic agent *in vivo* by allowing macrophages to release growth factors for fibroblasts without triggering the release of prostaglandin E2, an inhibitor of fibroblast proliferation. Rom and co-workers[19] examined alveolar macrophages from patients with occupational disease related to inorganic dust exposure (asbestosis, silicosis, and coal worker's pneumoconiosis) who had physiological evidence of interstitial disease. These alveolar macrophages were found to release increased amounts of PDGF-related peptides compared to normal macrophages.

TGFβ includes a family of closely related molecules TGF-β1, TGF-β2, TGF-β3, and TGF-β4. It also includes more distantly related molecules such as Mullerian-inhibiting substance, inhibins, and actins. Biologically active TGF-β1 is composed of two identical 12.5-kDa monomers linked by cysteine-cysteine disulfide bonds. Generally it is found to be secreted in latent form and activated either by changes in pH or enzymatically, for example, by plasmin. It modulates proliferation of mesenchymal cells and inhibits proliferation of epithelial and endothelial cells. Within the lung, the ability of TGF-β to control production of extracellular matrix is a bioactivity of significance for the evolution of fibrosis. TGF-β1 increases fibroblast synthesis of collagen types I, III, and V and glycosaminoglycans. It also prevents degradation of matrix by inducing protease inhibitors and inhibiting the production of proteases targeting extracellular matrix.

TGF-β has been shown to increase the number of cell surface receptors for fibronectin and collagen by activating genes encoding these receptors. TGF-β has been demonstrated in primary human skin fibroblast culture to delay entry of cells into S phase, yet increase net DNA synthesis.[47–50] Soma and Grotendorst[51] demonstrated the effect to be dependent upon the autocrine production of PDGF-related peptides. In particular, antibodies to PDGF A chain blocked the DNA synthesis-inducing activity of TGF-β. Evidence suggests this may occur *in vivo,* since intradermal injection of TGF-β in rat skin upregulates the expression of the PDGF A chain gene. While TGF-β stimulates autocrine production of PDGF-related peptides, this is probably not enough to sustain new tissue growth without additional growth factors in the microenvironment.

IGF-I stimulates proliferation of various types of cells, including fibroblasts. It is a nonglycosolated single chain polypeptide composed of 70 amino acids, with a molecular mass of 7.6 kDa. The IGF-I gene has at least five exons and four introns that code for at least two mRNA transcripts formed by alternative splicing. Tissue forms of IGF-I have been identified with higher molecular masses. Human fibroblast cultures produce IGF-I with a molecular mass of 21.5 kDa. The IGF-I receptor is composed of two α chains that bind the ligand and two β chains that span the cellular membrane. The receptor has tyrosine kinase activity and is capable of undergoing autophosphorylation. Alveolar macrophage-derived growth factor (AMDGF) was described as a polypeptide with progression type growth factor activity. It is released by alveolar macrophages in the idiopathic fibrotic lung diseases as well as in some pneumoconioses but not by normal alveolar macrophages. AMDGF is a member of the IGF-I family, with the mRNA transcripts of exons I-III of the IGF-I gene being complementary to the macrophage-derived IGF-I mRNA. AMDGF and molecules of the IGF-I family are recognized by polyclonal and monoclonal anti-IGF-I antibodies. The macrophage form of IGF-I will displace rIGF-I from its receptor and exhibit tyrosine kinase activity similar to rIGF-I. The IGF-I signal has an unknown pathway to the nucleus but can rapidly induce the immediate early proliferation-related genes such as c-fos.[52–55]

V. EPITHELIAL-FIBROBLAST INTERACTION

Epithelial-fibroblast interactions have long been regarded as playing an integral role in lung repair and the development of a thickened remodeled interstitium. Despite this, a limited amount of information about this complex interplay is available. Recent research in lung development has shown that when surfactant synthesis begins, there is disruption of epithelial basement membrane and an increased

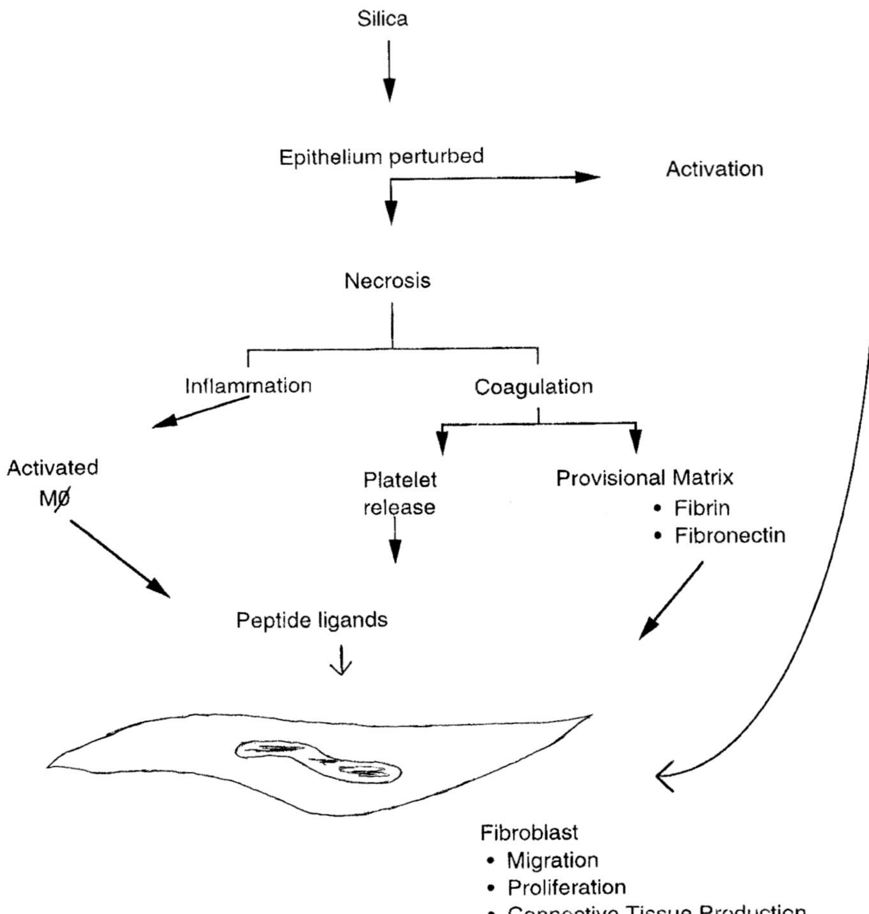

FIGURE 1 Silica interacts with the epithelium to result in functional activation or necrosis. Activated epithelium can either directly modulate fibroblast function, or augment pro-inflammatory pathways. Necrotic epithelium stimulates inflammatory pathways leading to macrophage (MØ) activation with release of acute response proteins like IL-1 and TNF, as well as the sustained release of profibrotic peptide ligands. Coagulation results in platelet release of profibrotic ligands as well as formation of a provisional matrix acting as a nidus for subsequent fibrosis.

cell-cell contact between alveolar fibroblasts and cuboidal epithelial cells. Patterns of cellular renewal after injury appear to follow the patterns established in lung development. Epithelial injury in organ culture studies is associated with fibroblast proliferation.[56,57] Adamson et al.[58] showed that with prolonged and severe epithelial injury induced by bleomycin and BHT there is an associated increase in fibroblast growth. These findings suggest that failure to maintain or restore normal epithelium in a timely manner results in fibroblast activation with proliferation and increased collagen formation. Type I cells do not appear to have epithelial-interstitial cell contacts, as the basement membranes of these cells are continuous and possess a smooth basal surface.

VI. CONCLUSION

The proposed pathogenesis of silica-induced fibrosis is via two pathways (see Figure 1). Silica activates the alveolar macrophages to release trophic factors, which in turn activate lung fibroblasts to migrate, proliferate, and produce connective tissue. Silica also damages the epithelium, causing activation of epithelial cells and fibroblasts. The necrosis created by epithelial disruption leads to influx of procoagulant factors, thus allowing provisional matrix to be deposited in the airspace in concert with an inflammatory response. Under the direction of solid phase signals from provisional matrix and soluble signals from growth factors, fibroblasts migrate into the airspace where they proliferate and deposit connective tissue matrix. The extent of the original injury, the preservation of structure, and the intensity of dust exposure all influence the development of fibrosis and determine if obliteration of normal architecture will ensue or if there will be normal repair.

REFERENCES

1. **Goldstein, R. and Fine, A.,** Fibrotic reaction in the lung: the activation of the lung fibroblast, *Exp. Lung Res.,* 11, 245–261, 1986.
2. **McDonald, J.,** Receptors for extracellular matrix components, *Am. J. Physiol.,* 257, L331–L337, 1989.
3. **McDonald, J.,** Extracellular matrix assembly, *Annu. Rev. Cell Biol.,* 4, 183–207, 1988.
4. **Schwartz, M. H., Lechene, C., and Ingbar, D. E.,** Activation of a cytoplasmic signal by integrin $\alpha5\beta1$, *J. Cell Biol.,* 111, 263a, 1990.
5. **Ross, R., Rains, E., and Bowen-Pope, D.,** The biology of platelet derived growth factor, *Cell,* 46, 155–169, 1986.
6. **Heldin, C., Backstrom, G., Ostman, A., Hammacher, A., Ronnstrand, L., Rubin, K., Nister, M., and Westermark, B.,** Binding of different dimeric forms of PDGF to human fibroblasts: evidence for two separate receptor types, *EMBO J.,* 7, 1387–93, 1988.
7. **Hart, C. E., Forstrom, J. W., and Kelly, J. D.,** Two classes of PDGF receptor recognize different isoforms of PDGF, *Science,* 240, 1529–1534, 1988.
8. **Heldin, C. H., Betsholtz, C., Johnsson, A., Nister, M., Ek, B., Ronnstrand, L., Wasteson, A., and Westermark, B.,** Platelet-derived growth factor: mechanism of action and relation to oncogenes, *J. Cell. Sci. Suppl.,* 3, 65–76, 1985.
9. **Gospodarowicz, D., Ferrara, N., Schweigerer, L., and Newfeld, G.,** Structural characterization and biological functions of fibroblast growth factor, *Endocr. Rev.,* 8, 95–114, 1987.
10. **Rifkin, D. B. and Moscatelli, D.,** Recent developments in the cell biology of basic fibroblast growth factor, *J. Cell Biol.,* 109, 1–6, 1989.
11. **Clemmons, D. R., Van Wyk, J. J., and Pledger, W. J.,** Sequential addition of platelet factor and plasma to BALB/c3T3 fibroblast cultures stimulates somatomedin C binding early in cell cycle, *Proc. Natl. Acad. Sci. U.S.A.,* 77, 6664–6668, 1980.
12. **Nissley, S. P. and Rechler, M. M.,** Somatomedin/insulin-like growth factor tissue receptors, *Clin. Endocrinol. Metab.,* 13, 43–67, 1984.
13. **Ong, J., Yamashita, S., and Melmed, S.,** Insulin-like growth factor I induces c-fos messenger ribonucleic acid in L6 rat skeletal muscle cells, *Endocrinology,* 120, 353–357, 1987.

13a. **Wrana, J. L., Sttisano, L., Wierer, R., Ventura, F., and Massague, J.,** Mechanism of activation of the TGF b receptor, *Nature,* 370, 241–247, 1994.

14. **Pratt, P.,** *The Lung: Structure, Function and Disease,* Williams & Wilkins, Baltimore, 1978, 45–7.
15. **Spencer, H.,** *Pathology of the Lung,* 3rd ed., W. B. Saunders, Philadelphia, 1977, 234–40.
16. **Clark, R., Lanigan, J., DellaPelle, P., Manseau, E., Dvarak, H., and Cloven, R.,** Fibronectin and fibrin provide a provisional matrix for epidermal cell migration during wound reepithelialization, *J. Invest. Dermatol.,* 79, 264–269, 1982.
17. **Adachi, K., Yamauchi, K., Bernaudin, J., Fouret, P., Ferrans, V., and Crystal, R.,** Evaluation of fibronectin gene expression by *in situ* hybridization, *Am. J. Pathol.,* 133, 193–203, 1988.
18. **Yamauchi, K., Martinet, Y., and Crystal, R.,** Modulation of fibronectin gene expression in human mononuclear phagocytes, *J. Clin. Invest.,* 80, 1720–1727, 1987.
19. **Rom, W., Bitterman, P., Rennard, S., Cantin, A., and Crystal, R.,** Characterization of the lower respiratory tract inflammation of nonsmoking individuals with interstitial lung disease associated with chronic inhalation of inorganic dusts, *Am. Rev. Respir. Dis.,* 136, 1429–1434, 1987.
20. **Rom, W.,** Relationship of inflammatory cell cytokines to disease severity in individuals with occupational inorganic dust exposure, *Am. J. Ind. Med.,* 19, 15–27, 1991.
21. **Davis, G.,** Pathogenesis of silicosis: current concepts and hypotheses, *Lung,* 164, 139–154, 1986.
22. **Chapman, H., Stahl, M., Allen, C., Yee, R., and Fair, D.,** Regulation of the procoagulant activity within the bronchoalveolar compartment of normal human lung, *Am. Rev. Respir. Dis.,* 137, 1417–1425, 1988.

23. **Idell, S., James, K., Levin, E., Schwartz, B., Manchanda, N., Maunder, R., Martin, T., McLarty, J., and Fair, D.,** Local abnormalities in coagulation and fibrinolytic pathways predispose to alveolar fibrin deposition in the adult respiratory distress syndrome, *J. Clin. Invest.,* 84, 695–705, 1989.
24. **Idell, S., Koenig, K., Fair, D., Martin, T., McLarty, J., and Maunder, R.,** Serial abnormalities of fibrin turnover in evolving adult respiratory distress syndrome, *Am. J. Physiol.,* 261, 240–248, 1991.
25. **Chapman, H., Allen, C., and Stone, O.,** Abnormalities in pathways of alveolar fibrin turnover among patients with interstitial lung disease, *Am. Rev. Respir. Dis.,* 133, 437–443, 1986.
26. **Schmidt, J., Oliver, C., Lepe-Zuniga, J., Green, I., and Gery, I.,** Silica-stimulated monocytes release fibroblast proliferation factors identical to interleukin 1, *J. Clin. Invest.,* 73, 1462–1472, 1987.
27. **Michel, J. and Quertermous, T.,** Modulation of mRNA levels for urinary and tissue type plasminogen activator and plasminogen activator inhibitors 1 and 2 in human fibroblasts by interleukin I, *J. Immunol.,* 143, 890–895, 1989.
28. **Wewers, M. D., Saltini, C., and Sellers, S.,** Evaluation of alveolar macrophages in normals and individuals with active pulmonary sarcoidosis for the spontaneous expression of the interleukin I Beta gene, *Cell Immunol.,* 107, 479–488, 1987.
29. **Chilosi, M, Menestrina, F., and Capelli, P.,** Immunohistochemical analysis of sarcoid granulomas. Evaluation of Ki67+ and interleukin 1+ cells, *Am. J. Pathol.,* 131, 191–198, 1988.
30. **Postlethwaite, A. E., Lachman, L. B., Mainardi, C. L., and Kang, A. H.,** Interleukin 1 stimulation of collagenase production by cultured fibroblasts, *J. Exp. Med.,* 157, 801–806, 1983.
31. **Aggarwal, B. B., Kohr, W. J., Hass, P. E., et al.,** Human tumor necrosis factor: production, purification and characterization, *J. Biol. Chem.,* 260, 2345–54, 1985.
32. **Martinet, Y., Yamauchi, K., and Crystal, R.,** Differential expression of the tumor necrosis factor/cachectin gene by blood and lung mononuclear phagocytes, *Am. Rev. Respir. Dis.,* 138, 659–665, 1988.
33. **Bachwich, P. R., Lynch, J. P., III, Larrick, J., et al.,** Tumor necrosis factor production by human sarcoid alveolar macrophages, *Am. J. Pathol.,* 125, 421–425, 1986.
34. **Piguet, P. F., Collart, M. A., Grau, G. E., Sappino, A. P., and Vassalli, P.,** Requirement of tumor necrosis factor for development of silica-induced pulmonary fibrosis, *Nature,* 344, 245–247, 1990.
35. **Gosset, P., Lassalle, P., Vanhee, D., Wallaert, B., Aerts, C., Noisin, C., and Tonnel, A.,** Production of tumor necrosis factor α and interleukin 6 by human alveolar macrophages exposed *in vivo* to coal mine dust, *Am. J. Respir. Cell Mol. Biol.,* 5, 431–436, 1991.
36. **Borm, P., Pakmen, J., Engelen, J., and Buurman, W.,** Spontaneous and stimulated release of tumor necrosis factor-alpha (TNF) from blood monocytes of miners with coal worker's pneumoconiosis, *Am. Rev. Respir. Dis.,* 138, 1589–1594, 1988.
37. **Ross, R., Rains, E., and Bowen-Pope, D.,** The biology of platelet-derived growth factor, *Cell,* 46, 155–169, 1986.
38. **Bitterman, P., Wewers, M. D., Rennard, S., Adelberg, S., and Crystal, R.,** Modulation of alveolar macrophage-driven fibroblast proliferation by alternative macrophage mediators, *J. Clin. Invest.,* 177, 700–708, 1986.
39. **Clark, R., Folkvord, J., Hart, C., Murray, M., and McPherson, J.,** Platelet isoforms of platelet-derived growth factor stimulate fibroblasts to contract collagen matrices, *J. Clin. Invest.,* 84, 1036–1040, 1989.
40. **Bonner, J., Badgett, A., Osornio-Vargas, A., Hoffman, M., and Brody, A.,** PDGF-stimulated fibroblast proliferation is enhanced synergistically by receptor-recognized a2 macroglobin, *J. Cell Physiol.,* 145, 1–8, 1990.
41. **Martiner, Y., Rom, W., Grotendorst, G., Martin, G., and Crystal, R.,** Exaggerated spontaneous release of platelet-derived growth factor by alveolar macrophages from patients with idiopathic pulmonary fibrosis, *N. Engl. J. Med.,* 317, 202–209, 1987.
42. **Mornex, J., Martinet, Y., Yamauchi, K., Bitterman, P., Grotendorst, G., Chytil-Wein, A., Martin, G., and Crystal, R.,** Spontaneous expression of the c-sis gene and release of a platelet-derived growth factor-like molecule by human alveolar macrophages, *J. Clin. Invest.,* 78, 61–66, 1986.
43. **Vignaud, J. M., Allan, M., Martinet, N., Pech, M., Plenat, F., and Martinet, Y.,** Presence of platelet-derived growth factor in normal and fibrotic lung is specifically associated with interstitial macrophages while both interstitial macrophages and alveolar epithelial cells express the c-sis proto-oncogene, *Am. J. Respir. Cell Mol. Biol.,* 5, 531–538, 1991.
44. **Synder, L. S., Hertz, M. I., Peterson, M. S., et al.,** Acute lung injury: pathogenesis of intraalveolar fibrosis, *J. Clin. Invest.,* 88, 663–673, 1991.
45. **Marinelli, W., Polunovsky, V., Harmon, K., and Bitterman, P.,** Role of platelet-derived growth factor in pulmonary fibrosis, *Am. J. Respir. Cell Mol. Biol.,* 5, 503–504, 1991.
46. **Brown, G. P., Monick, M., and Hunninghake, G. W.,** Fibroblast proliferation induced by silica-exposed human alveolar macrophages, *Am. Rev. Respir. Dis.,* 138, 85–89, 1988.
47. **Pelton, R. W. and Moses, H. L.,** The B type transforming growth factors: mediators of cell regulation in the lung, *Am. Rev. Respir. Dis.,* 142, S31–S35, 1990.
48. **Raghow, R., Postlethwaite, A., Keski-Oja, J., Moses, H., and Kang, A.,** Transforming growth factor β increases steady state levels of type 1 procollagen and fibronectin messenger RNAs posttranscriptionally in cultured human dermal fibroblasts, *J. Clin. Invest.,* 79, 1285–1288, 1987.

49. **Dubaybo, B. and Thet, L.,** Effect of transforming growth factor beta on synthesis of glycosaminoglycans by human lung fibroblasts, *Exp. Lung Res.*, 16, 389–403, 1990.
50. **Khalil, N., Bereznay, O., Sporn, M., and Greenberg, A.,** Macrophage production of transforming growth factor β and fibroblast collagen synthesis in chronic pulmonary inflammation, *J. Exp. Med.*, 170, 727–737, 1989.
51. **Soma, Y. and Grotendorst, G.,** TGF-β stimulates primary human skin fibroblast DNA synthesis via an autocrine production of PDGF-related peptides, *J. Cell. Physiol.*, 140, 246–253, 1989.
52. **Nissley, S. P. and Rechler, M. M.,** Insulin-like growth factors: biosynthesis, receptors and carrier proteins, in *Hormonal Proteins and Peptides*, Li, C. H., Ed., Academic Press, New York, 127–203, 1984.
53. **Clemmons, D. R. and Shaw, D. S.,** Purification and biological properties of fibroblast somatomedin, *J. Biol. Chem.*, 261, 10293–10298, 1986.
54. **Rom, W., Basset, P., Fells, G., Nukiwa, T., Trapnell, B., and Crystal, R.,** Alveolar macrophages release an insulin-like growth factor 1 type molecule, *J. Clin. Invest.*, 82, 1685–1693, 1988.
55. **Ong, J., Yamashita, S., and Melmed, S.,** Insulin-like growth factor I induces c-fos messenger ribonucleic acid in L6 rat skeletal muscle cells, *Endocrinology*, 120, 353–357, 1987.
56. **Adamson, I. Y. R., and Bowden, D. H.,** The type 2 cell as progenitor of alveolar epithelial regeneration: a cytodynamic study in mice after exposure to oxygen, *Lab. Invest.*, 30, 35–42, 1974.
57. **Witschi, H.,** Role of the epithelium in lung repair, *Chest (Suppl.)*, 99, 3, 22S–25S, 1991.
58. **Adamson, I. Y. R., Hedgecock, C., Bowden, D. H.,** Epithelial cell-fibroblast interactions in lung injury and repair, *Am. J. Pathol.*, 137, 385–392, 1990.

Section III
Chapter 10

IMMUNOLOGICAL ASPECTS OF SILICOSIS

Rashi Iyer and Andrij Holian

CONTENTS

I. INTRODUCTION

Silicosis is a chronic progressive lung disease associated with macrophage-dominated granulomatous inflammation caused by the inhalation of silica dust.[1] Histopathological studies of silicotic lungs in experimental animals are characterized by macrophage aggregates, followed by a significant increase in the lymphocyte population, along with alveolar type II cell hyperplasia.[2] Bronchoalveolar lavage (BAL) analysis of silica-treated mice show an increase in macrophages, as well as lymphocytes, in the lavage fluid.[3,4] Furthermore, macrophages from silicotic patients[5] and silica-treated macrophages *in vitro*[6,7] release fibrogenic factors. Therefore, most current observations indicate that pulmonary macrophages play a key role in the development of silicosis. However, the exact mechanism by which macrophages are activated and mediate further inflammatory responses resulting in fibrosis is not clear.

This chapter attempts to describe potential roles of the immune system in the development of silicosis and the several loci where the immune system could be involved with the ultimate effect of collagen deposition. The information obtained to date about the effect of silica on the immune system and the mechanisms that might play a major role in the immunopathogenesis of silica, starting with the major role player, the macrophage, will be discussed. This will be followed by the proposed roles of lymphocytes in lung fibrosis, as well as the possible correlation of silicosis with autoimmunity. Based on the information collected and evaluation of the available data, a number of hypotheses and possible explanations

0-8493-4709-2/96/$0.00+$.50

will be put forward in an effort to describe the involvement of the immune system in silicosis. Finally, suggestions for future lines of research that will help to further elucidate the sequence of events occurring in the course of silicosis will be presented.

II. SILICA AND THE MACROPHAGE

A. SILICA STIMULATION OF MACROPHAGES

Certain particulates, such as silica, can induce pulmonary inflammation and have the ability to stimulate alveolar macrophages to produce a variety of fibrogenic factors *in vitro*.[6,7] Based on these and related observations, macrophages have been implicated as a major role player in silica-induced fibrosis. However, the mechanisms involved in the development of pulmonary fibrosis probably include a repertoire of immune cells and fibroblasts interacting with one another at various levels. In this context, macrophages will be considered the focus of the immune system having a wide array of immunological functions and capable of interacting with T cells, B cells,[8] and fibroblasts.[9]

Initial events after inhalation of silica include the movement of macrophages towards the particulates followed by phagocytosis of the particulates.[6,7,10] These events are accompanied by release of growth factors and cytokines, such as tumor necrosis factor-α (TNF-α)[11] and interleukin 1 (IL-1),[12] that have growth-promoting activity on fibroblasts and stimulate increased collagen deposition.[13] A variety of other cytokines have also been shown to influence fibroblasts *in vitro,* such as platelet-derived growth factor,[14] IL-2,[15] transforming growth factor-β (TGF-β),[16] and macrophage-derived growth factor (MDGF).[17] Therefore, a complex network of cytokines has been implicated in the induction of lung fibrosis. For the most part, these cytokines are derived from pulmonary macrophages,[18] as well as from activated T lymphocytes.[19] Of the many cytokines that are involved, IL-1 and TNF-α have been shown to play an important, if not central, role in the development of fibrosis.[20] For example, it is well established that silica stimulates the production of IL-1 by monocytes.[21] and macrophages,[22,23] and IL-1 in turn increases the secretion of TNF-α by macrophages.[24] In addition, IL-1 has been shown to play a crucial role in lymphocyte proliferation,[25] generation of immunoglobulin (Ig)-secreting cells,[26] and is also a potent chemoattractant for T lymphocytes in the blood.[27]

TNF-α, which functions as a fibroblast growth factor,[9] is also released from macrophages on exposure to silica.[11] However, it may work synergistically with IL-1 to inhibit fibroblast proliferation.[28] Therefore, the relative contributions of each of these cytokines to the development of fibrosis is not understood. Clearly, these and many other cytokines and prostanoids are involved in the overall balance of factors in determining the regulation of fibroblast proliferation and collagen deposition involved in fibrosis. This is a complex and rapidly evolving area of research that is beyond the scope of this review. However, the pleiotropic cytokines TNF-α and IL-1 appear to be important in fibrogenesis and are therefore good markers of macrophage activation and are probably good surrogates for the factors that are released by macrophages in fibrogenesis. Furthermore, other immune cells regulate the ability of macrophages to produce these cytokines. For example, an *in vitro* study using a bleomycin-induced fibrotic model showed that T lymphocytes are required for an increase of pulmonary TNF-α mRNA levels.[29] This suggested that T cells probably secreted a cytokine(s) that stimulated the proliferation of macrophages, resulting in enhanced secretion of TNF-α by these cells.

B. UNIQUE BIOACTIVITY OF SILICA

It is important to note that particulate-stimulated migration and phagocytic activity of macrophages seem to occur regardless of the fibrogenic potential of the particulate.[30,31] For example, it has been demonstrated that macrophages release growth factors in response to both fibrogenic and nonfibrogenic stimuli.[32,33] Although a similar macrophage response is observed with silica and nonfibrogenic titanium dioxide,[30] including an influx of polymorphonuclear neutrophils (PMN),[32–35] the ultimate factors or mechanisms responsible for the differential host response resulting in fibrosis or no fibrosis to a particulate are not clear. It may be that the magnitude and profile of secretory factors released by macrophages are in part responsible for the fibrotic response unique to silica (and probably asbestos). If that is so, it is possible that there may be one or several mechanisms involved in regulating the secretion of growth factors by macrophages. Due to the marked increase of lymphocytes observed in the lungs of silica-treated mice[4,36] and patients with silicosis,[37] it is probable that these lymphocytes regulate the release of growth factors by macrophages via the lymphokines secreted by these lymphocytes.

III. SILICA AND THE IMMUNE SYSTEM

As discussed above, there is a growing appreciation of the role of the immune system in the development of lung fibrosis. As described earlier, several studies have demonstrated the rapid influx of lymphocytes to sites of silicotic lesions within the lung.[38–41] Therefore, it is possible that IL-1 released from silica-treated macrophages may result not only in the proliferation of resident lymphocytes[42] but also recruitment of circulating lymphocytes to the affected/diseased site.[42] It is likely, therefore, that the silica-macrophage interaction triggers a cascade of inflammatory and fibrotic events involved in a cell-mediated/humoral immune response.

While macrophages can regulate lymphocyte recruitment, proliferation, and activation, the secretory activity of pulmonary macrophages may be regulated in turn by lymphocytes.[43] It has also been proposed that T cells directly or indirectly can influence macrophage infiltration into the lung after exposure to silica.[44] In silicotic animals, lymphokines released by activated lymphocytes have been shown to stimulate the secretion of mitogenic factors by macrophages.[45] Furthermore, it has been shown that T lymphocytes isolated from the lung tissue of animals administered intratracheal silica are able to stimulate naive macrophages to secrete MDGF.[43] This process is facilitated by cell-to-cell contact between lymphocytes and macrophages,[45] implying that the lymphokines might be expressed on the surface of activated lymphocytes or secreted at sites of cell-to-cell contact.

Another component of the lung immune system that has been of recent interest is the bronchus-associated lymphoid tissue (BALT). The BALT is composed of isolated lymphoid aggregates mostly present near bifurcations within the large bronchi where particles tend to deposit. However, since little is known about the identity and presence of cells required for the generation of an immune response in BALT,[46] it is difficult to draw any conclusions about the potential involvement of these lymphoid tissues in the development of silicosis. Furthermore, the presence of this organ in humans is not yet firmly established. Therefore, for the purpose of this review we acknowledge that BALT may be involved, but it is not needed for the model that we are presenting.

A. POTENTIAL MECHANISMS INVOLVED IN THE IMMUNE RESPONSE TO SILICA

The mechanistic aspects of the immune response to a given particulate may well depend on the respiratory tract deposition of the particulate and the immune cells encountered. Several hypotheses, described below and each diagrammed in Figure 1, can be constructed to account for the immunologic correlates of lung fibrosis resulting from silica exposure.

First, a particulate may stimulate a nonspecific polyclonal response. Nonspecific polyclonal responses are generally ascribed to an "adjuvant" effect.[47] The role of silica as an adjuvant is well known[47,48] and might be responsible for enhancing a nonspecific immune response to an antigen.[49] The antigen for a particulate-activated macrophage could be a host protein that has adsorbed onto the particulate.[50–52] This silica-protein interaction may result in denaturation of the protein molecule, thus exposing novel proteolytic sites on the host protein. Phagocytosis of the particulate could then lead to activation of an antigen-presenting cell, such as a macrophage, and the subsequent presentation of this host antigen to immune cells, resulting in an autoimmune response.

A second mechanism whereby a particulate could generate an immune response is by interacting directly with a T cell. For example, it has been demonstrated that cross linking of T cell receptors is sufficient to cause release of lymphokines by T cells that can then stimulate B cells in a polyclonal fashion.[53,54] Thus, it may be possible for a large polyvalent particulate, such as silica, with a repeating unit structure to cross link T cell receptors, thereby stimulating B cells.

Another possible mechanism whereby a particulate can generate an immune response would be for it to interact directly with B cells, resulting in their activation. For example, many antigens can activate B cells without any T cell intervention by effectively cross linking cell-surface antigen receptors (cytophilic Ig) on resting B cells.[55] This could also be a possible mechanism involved in the production of autoantibodies in silicotic patients.[9]

The extent to which any or all of these above mechanisms contribute to inducing silicosis has not been described. Furthermore, with the evolving realization of the overlap of functional properties among the immune cells it has become increasingly difficult to determine whether the cell-mediated or humoral response is the dominant immune response in silicosis.

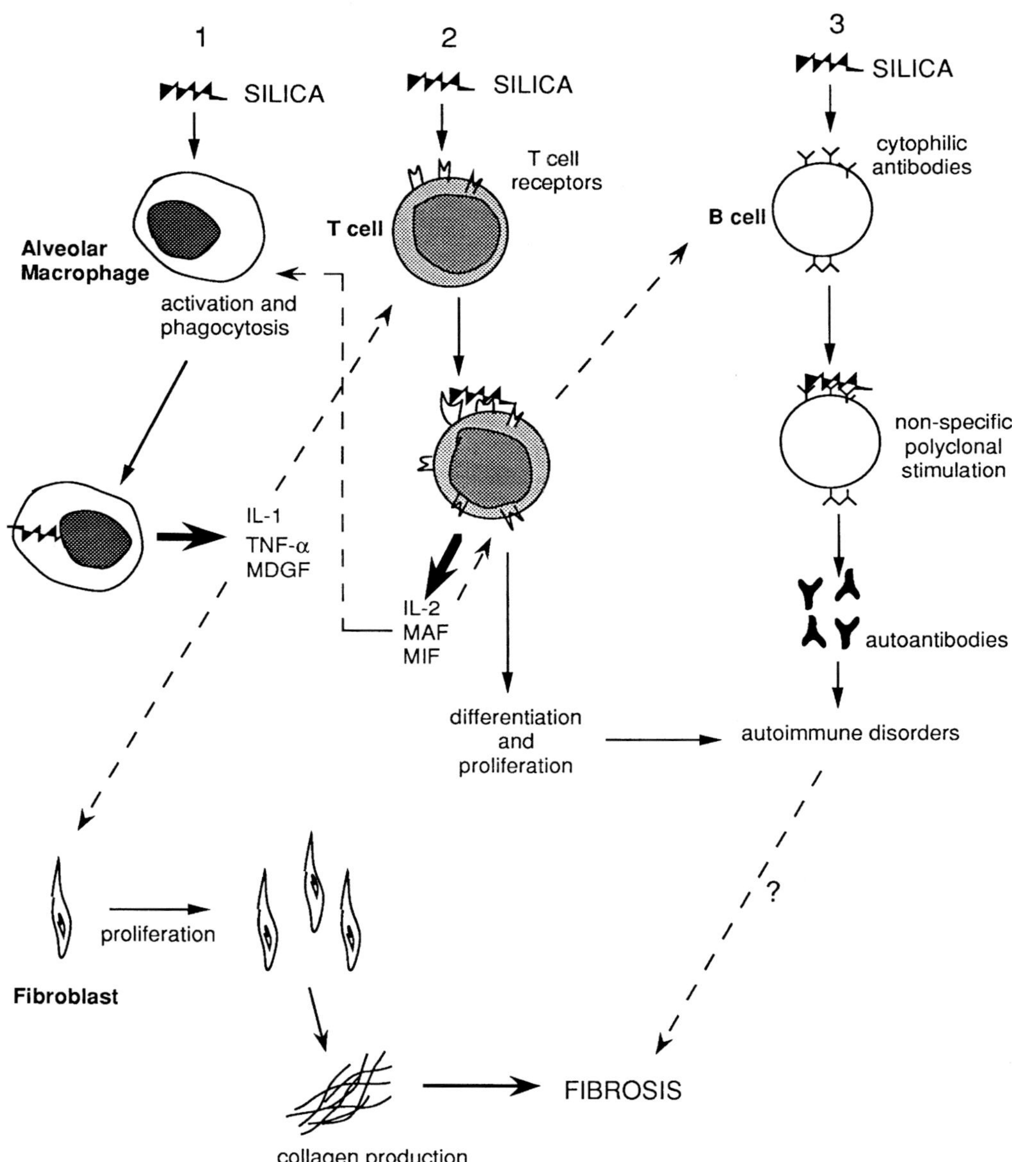

FIGURE 1 Schematic diagram of potential interactions between silica and major cells of the immune system, namely macrophages, T cells, and B cells. 1. Silica-macrophage interaction. 2. Direct interaction of silica with a T cell: cross linking of T cell receptors. 3. Direct interaction of silica with a B cell: cross linking of cytophilic Igs. Bold arrows indicate secretion of cytokines and dashed arrows indicate their target cells.

B. LYMPHOCYTE POPULATIONS IN SILICOSIS

Silica has been shown to have profound regulatory effects on the function of mononuclear cells obtained from healthy individuals and thus on lymphocyte activation and proliferation.[56] Both enhancement[47,57] and suppression[58] of immune responses have been observed *in vivo* after exposure to silica. A possible explanation for this may be the ratio or relative number of macrophages to lymphocytes present at the site of silica deposition. For example, it has been shown that at low levels of monocytes/macrophages, the net effect of exposure to silica was found to be immunosuppressive.[56] In contrast, in cultures with a high macrophages-to-lymphocyte ratio, an enhancement of the immune response was observed.[56] Thiele and Lipsky proposed that the immune response enhancement was due to macrophage lysis by silica, thus inhibiting the immune suppression mediated by macrophages. In contrast, in conditions of a decreased ratio of macrophages to lymphocytes, decreased antigen presentation by macrophages may be responsible for the suppression of the immune system. If this occurs *in vivo,* it might in part explain a variety of abnormal immune phenomena observed in some patients with silicosis.

Several studies have been done to quantitate and define lymphocyte populations in animal models exposed to silica.[4,44,56] Quantitation of immune cells in animals and humans exposed to silica have demonstrated a predominance of T helper cells in the BAL fluid throughout the immune response, as compared to T suppressor cells.[4,57] Immunohistologic assessment of lymphocyte populations in silica-induced pulmonary inflammation in mice have reported a significant influx of Thy-1+ T cells early in the course of fibrosis.[36] In addition, antibodies to CD4+ and CD8+ demonstrated increased levels of both CD4+ and CD8+ T cells in silica-treated mice.[36] These T lymphocytes may be involved in the recruitment and proliferation of B lymphocytes[55] and may serve to explain the influx of B cells into the lungs in murine models. Although this concomitant increase in B cells has been observed, it lags behind the T cell increase.[4] This variance observed in the level of lymphocytes may be due to either differences in proliferation within the two lymphocyte populations or rate of migration to the site of injury. Furthermore, lymphocyte responses are also dependent on the particular cytokines secreted by the activated macrophages as well as the subset of lymphocytes that initially respond to the stimuli.

C. SUBPOPULATIONS OF T LYMPHOCYTES

Considerable evidence has accumulated confirming the existence of two well-defined T cell subsets, namely, Th1 and Th2.[59,60] Th1 cells on activation release cytokines such as IL-2 and IFN-γ (Interferon), whereas the Th2 cells predominantly secrete IL-4, IL-5, IL-6, and IL-10.[60,61] Therefore, Th1 cells could be considered immunostimulatory and Th2 immunosuppressive by virtue of the cytokines secreted by them.[62] It has been shown that IFN-γ inhibits the proliferation of Th2 cells but not Th1 cells,[63,64] while IL-10 (produced by Th2 cells) inhibits the synthesis of cytokines by Th1 cells but not Th2 cells.[60] Immunostimulatory cytokines such as IL-2 are responsible for the autocrine growth of T cells,[65] whereas IL-10 has been shown to stimulate the proliferation of antibody-secreting B cells.[60] In addition, Th2 cells have been demonstrated to be more efficacious in recruiting B cell help and are associated with high antibody levels.[66,67] Therefore, the specific subset of T cells recruited during the initial phase of an immune response would be an important factor in the course of an immune response to an antigen in the lungs. The regulation of immune effector functions may thus consist of the regulation of different T cell subsets by the activated macrophages and cytokines released by both cell types.

Importantly, Th2 cells have been shown to be present in lungs by using glycolipid markers.[68] Also, BAL cells from atopic asthmatic patients showed a predominance of cells expressing mRNA for IL-2, IL-3, IL-4, IL-5, and granulocyte macrophage colony stimulating factor (GM-CSF).[69] Furthermore, isolated T cells from these patients expressed elevated levels of mRNA for IL-4 and IL-5. This pattern of mRNA expression is compatible with predominant activation of Th2 cells.[69]

Therefore, if Th1 cells were the chief responders to the silica-activated macrophages, they would initiate activation of cytolytic CD8+ T cells and generate basically a cell-mediated immune response as diagrammed in Figure 2. In contrast, if Th2 cells were initially recruited, the cytokines released by these cells such as IL-4, IL-5, IL-6, and IL-10 would ultimately stimulate the proliferation and differentiation of antibody-producing B lymphocytes. IL-10 would also suppress the ability of Th1 cells to induce a cell-mediated immune response. As described earlier, it has been shown that T cells are required for the proliferation of macrophages and secretion of TNF-α.[29] However, it is not yet clear whether a particular subset of T cells is responsible for this expansion of macrophages. It could be speculated, thus, that development of fibrosis might be dependent not only on activation of macrophages and the subsequent recruitment of lymphocytes but also on the specific populations of lymphocytes that proliferate in response to the stimuli. Also, the release of MDGF may be regulated by mediators secreted by lymphocytes, further emphasizing the important role of the specific lymphocyte populations that proliferate in response to silica in any given individual.

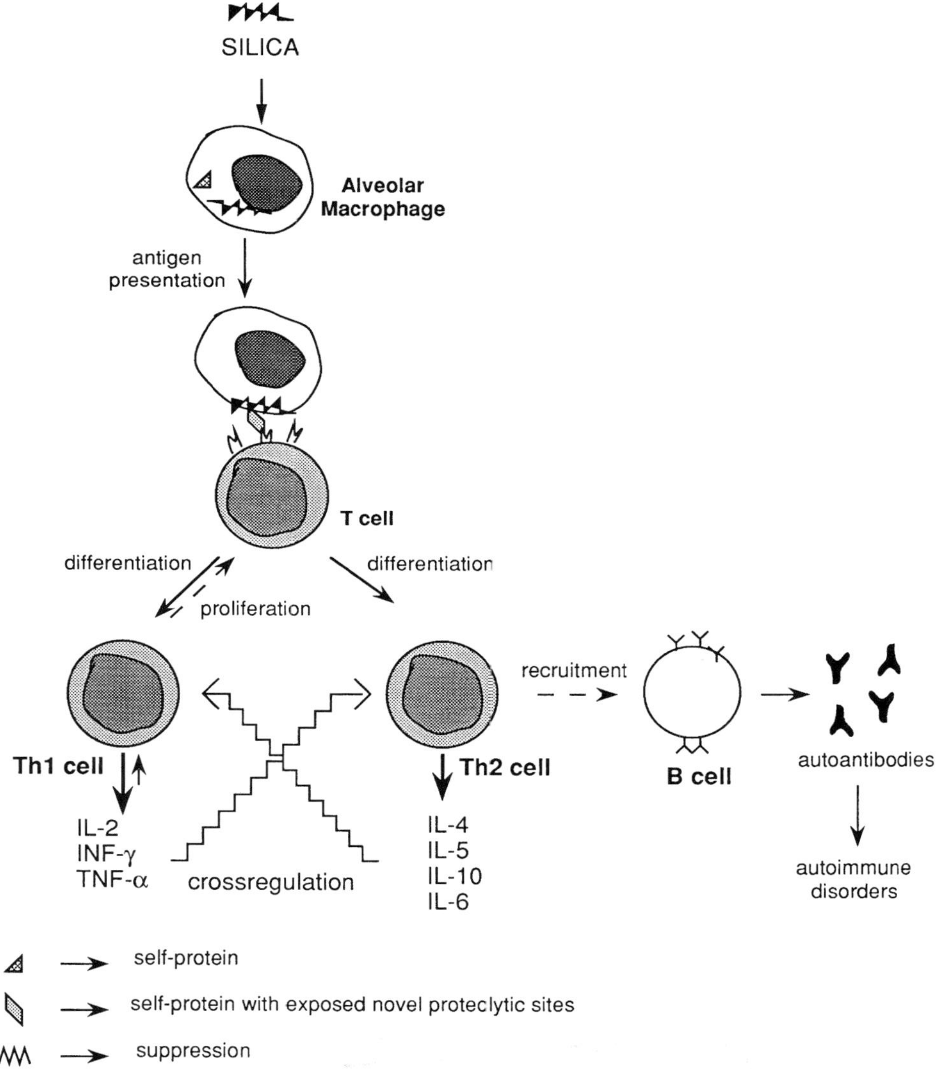

FIGURE 2 Schematic diagram of the T cell subtypes Th1 and Th2 and their proposed role in the development of silicosis and associated autoimmune disorders. Silica-macrophage interaction results in the enhanced presentation of antigen to T cells. This is followed by the selective differentiation and proliferation of Th1 or Th2 cells, resulting in either a cell-mediated or humoral immune response, respectively. Bold arrows indicate secretion of cytokines and dashed arrows indicate their target cells.

IV. ROLE OF SILICA IN AUTOIMMUNITY

A. ASSOCIATION OF SILICA WITH AUTOIMMUNITY

Habeeb, as early as 1945, hypothesized a role for autoimmunity in the development of silicosis based primarily on the eosinophilia, often associated with silicosis.[70] Over the next few years, autoimmune phenomena gained increasing attention as possible etiologies for many conditions, including systemic lupus erythematosus (SLE), rheumatoid arthritis, and scleroderma. Patients with pulmonary diseases including pneumoconiosis showed a significantly higher level of antibodies to the insoluble antigens as compared to normal. Furthermore, one of these antigens appeared to be a collagen-like compound.[71]

Early investigations also demonstrated increased antinuclear antibodies (ANA) in patients with silicosis,[72,73] while others found an association between connective tissue diseases such as rheumatoid arthritis and scleroderma.[74] Furthermore, the presence of ANA was demonstrated to be associated with abnormal chest X-rays and pulmonary function studies.[72,73]

Although silicosis has been associated with autoimmune diseases, such as SLE, RF, and dermatomyositis,[75,76] perhaps the greatest number of studies have been published documenting the association between silicosis and scleroderma.[74–82] Anti-Scl 70, thought to be specific for scleroderma, was found in 47% of patients with silicosis-associated systemic sclerosis in a study by Rustin et al.[77] This is comparable to levels found in scleroderma not associated with silica exposure (34–77%).

Elevated anticollagen antibody levels have also been detected in sera of silicotic patients at an early stage of the disease.[83] Furthermore, levels of anticollagen antibodies tended to be higher in patients positive for ANA and RF; however, this was not statistically significant. Finally, levels of procollagen III peptide, a marker for fibrotic changes in other organs, was also elevated early. While levels of procollagen III peptide were previously found to be elevated in silicotic patients,[82,84] this was the first study documenting elevated levels of anticollagen antibodies.

B. POTENTIAL MECHANISMS OF AUTOIMMUNITY IN SILICOSIS

Thus far we have presented evidence to support a role of the immune system in the pathogenesis of silicosis. As mentioned earlier, an increasing incidence of autoimmune diseases in silicotic patients have been reported. However, the interplay of events involved between development of silicosis and autoimmunity are not well defined. As described above, a number of studies have demonstrated a high incidence of antinuclear antibodies in humans occupationally exposed to silica dust.[72,73] In addition, Ig and Ig-secreting cells are present in and around silicotic nodules.[85] Immunological studies of patients with silicosis have shown elevation of serum polyclonal gamma-globulin, especially IgG.[86–89] These results support B cell hyperactivity in silicosis. Furthermore, increased levels of IgG and IgA have also been reported in BAL in experimental and human silicosis.[90] The existence of IgM, IgA, and IgG antibodies in several autoimmune disorders and the presence of immune complexes of IgG, IgA, and IgM in silicotic patients emphasizes the importance of the potential relationship between silicosis and autoimmunity.[91,92] Interestingly, generation of the IgA class of antibodies is more dependent on T helper cells, in agreement with the observed increase in T helper cells seen in animals exposed to silica.[44]

Other evidence that supports the association of autoimmunity with silicosis is a perturbation in the complement system. It is interesting to note that even partial complement dysfunction can predispose patients to the development of autoimmune disorders.[93] Consistent with this observation, elevated C4 levels were measured in silicotic patients also known to have autoimmune disorders.[91]

Finally, since human leukocyte antigen (HLA) antigens are linked with immune response capability and might indicate a genetic susceptibility to silicosis, a study of HLA levels was done in 49 silicotic patients.[94] The prevalence of HLA antigen, specifically B44 and A9, was significantly elevated in these patients. Other studies have shown excesses of AW19 and B12 and other histocompatibility antigens.[95] Whether these findings reflect a genetic predisposition to silicosis is yet unknown but reflects an important area of potential research.

In summary, the incidence and significance of antibodies against various nuclear antigens and immune complexes in the pathology of lung fibrosis is unknown. However, a couple of mechanisms have been proposed whereby exposure to silica could result in autoimmune disorders.

First, expression of Ia antigen on alveolar macrophages has been shown to increase during pulmonary fibrosis.[96] Cells which are activated by silica show an increased expression of major histocompatibility complex (MHC) class II antigen.[97] Since the efficiency of presentation varies with the level of expression of Ia antigen,[98] activated alveolar macrophages may present antigen more efficiently to resident lymphocytes, and this might in turn increase the magnitude or duration of the immune response in lungs. It is possible that adsorption of a self-protein on a particulate could change the conformation of the protein such that it is now recognized by the immune cells as a foreign protein.[51] Phagocytosis of this protein-particulate complex may then lead to more efficient presentation of an essentially self-protein as an immunogenic molecule due to the increased expression of MHC by these cells. This self-antigen may then be recognized by a T cell in a MHC-restricted fashion which subsequently stimulates a B cell response.

Therefore, antibodies generated against this altered host protein may then recognize normal host proteins leading to an autoimmune response.

Second, the occurrence of hypergammaglobulinemia, rheumatoid factor (RF), antinuclear factors, and immune complexes are indicative of a nonspecific polyclonal stimulation of the humoral immune system.[99,100] Particulates such as silica have been shown to interact directly with T cells/B cells, resulting in a nonspecific polyclonal immune response. This is possible in silicosis, since silica has often been implicated to function as an adjuvant.[47,49] This might explain the presence of immune complexes observed in silicotic patients.

V. ROLE OF STRESS PROTEINS IN SILICOSIS

A. STRESS RESPONSE

The stress response, more commonly known as heat shock response, is a rapid and reversible response of cells to various types of stress, such as bacterial and viral infection, ischemia, transition metals, drugs, and various environmental insults.[101,102] It is characterized by the increased synthesis of a highly conserved family of proteins, frequently referred to as heat shock or stress proteins and the concomitant inhibition of normal protein synthesis.[103,104] The stress protein family share remarkable structural homology between species, exhibiting a 50% homology in the hsp70 gene between *Escherichia coli* and human.[105]

Stress proteins were first discovered when cells were exposed to elevated but nonlethal temperatures.[104] The increased synthesis of stress proteins appears to afford cells some degree of protection against subsequent exposure to lethal temperatures.[106] The major effect of heat shock is the unfolding or the improper folding of cellular proteins. Therefore, it has been suggested that it is the improperly folded polypeptide that actually initiates the induction of the heat shock response. As has been described in a number of recent reviews,[105–108] stress proteins appear to have many other important functions in unstressed cells as well. A few of the several functions suggested for stress proteins include chaperoning,[107] prevention of denaturation, and renaturation of proteins.[108]

The relevance of stress proteins in this discussion stems from the increasing interest regarding a potential role of stress proteins in immune regulation.[109,110] Stress proteins can elicit a potent immunological response and have been shown to be immunogenic.[111,112] Although there are varying opinions about the involvement of stress proteins in the immune response, their prevalence in a number of autoimmune disorders is consistent with their potential role in autoimmunity.[113,114] Studies have reported the presence of antibodies to self-stress proteins in autoimmune disorders such as SLE[115] and RF.[114,116] In addition, the presence of antibodies to stress protein, particularly hsp 65, in the human immune response to mycobacterial infections is believed to be significant.[114] Many pathogenic organisms are put under stress when they first invade the host, resulting in the synthesis of stress proteins by these organisms.[104] However, what may be significant in potentiating an autoimmune phenomena is that host cells, such as macrophages, involved in the initial elimination of these organisms also undergo stress, switching on the synthesis of host or self-stress proteins. Therefore, considering the sequence homology within stress proteins across species, it is quite possible that T cells and Ig specific for stress proteins synthesized by the pathogenic organisms will now start killing and/or activating host cells expressing homologous self-stress proteins, resulting in an autoimmune phenomena.[104]

B. IMMUNE RESPONSE, STRESS PROTEINS, AND SILICOSIS

T lymphocytes which recognize autologous proteins have been isolated from a number of patients suffering from autoimmune diseases.[113] The $\gamma\delta$ T cells have been shown to be predominant among the T cell clones that recognize stress proteins.[117] The $\gamma\delta$ T cells are a subclass of T cells with a receptor composed of γ and δ chains. These T cell receptors were found to recognize various antigens from the mycobacterium family.[109] It has also been established that at least one subset of $\gamma\delta$ T cells recognize conserved peptide sequences on stress proteins, including autologous stress proteins.[118] $\gamma\delta$ T cells have been shown to proliferate in the presence of activated $\alpha\beta$ T cells.[119] It may also be relevant that there are comparatively high levels of $\gamma\delta$ T cells in the neonatal phase that is followed by a gradual decrease of this T cell subset in the adult, leading to the general concept that $\gamma\delta$ T cells respond to some highly conserved epitopes on stress proteins across species. Therefore, these cells may be specialized to remove autologous stressed cells as well as infected cells, perhaps as a first line of defense against viral or bacterial invasion.[120]

Taken together, these observations and the association of silicosis with autoimmune diseases generate the following line of reasoning. Since stress proteins have been shown to be present in a number of autoimmune disorders[113,114] and in mycobacterial infections,[114] and these very same diseases have been associated with silicosis, it may then logically follow that stress proteins are the common factor in stimulating an abnormal immune response observed in these varied conditions.

Based on the above, phagocytosis of silica by macrophages may result in the chronic induction, processing, and significant cell surface expression of stress proteins by macrophages due to the persistence of silica in the lung. At the same time, release of IL-1 by silica-activated macrophages can result in an initial influx of $\alpha\beta$ and $\gamma\delta$ T cells. Release of IL-2 and IL-4 by the $\alpha\beta$ T cells can stimulate the expansion of autoreactive $\gamma\delta$ T cells capable of recognizing the self-stress protein,[121] thus initiating an autoimmune response as illustrated in Figure 3. Therefore, the initial subset of T cells recruited and cytokines released in response to silica would play a crucial role.

As described earlier, cell-to-cell contact between macrophages and lymphocytes is required to activate lymphocytes in silicosis.[45] This activation may be mediated by lymphokines or some other protein expressed on the cell surface. Therefore, there is a possibility that stress proteins expressed by macrophages on exposure to silica may in fact be the molecule recognized by T cells resulting in the T cell response observed in silicosis.

As stated earlier, silicosis predisposes humans to mycobacterial infections.[122] It appears that the chronic presence of silica in the lung leads to a suppression of cell-mediated immunity.[123] The predominant immunoregulatory function of alveolar macrophages is to suppress the T cell response to antigenic and mitogenic stimuli.[124,125] It has been shown that cell contact between macrophages and T cells is required for the suppression of the immune response.[126] It remains to be determined whether this suppressive factor, present on macrophages or lymphocytes, is a stress protein expressed on the cell surface. Therefore, the expression of stress proteins on activated macrophages in silicotic patients may result in the suppression of a cell-mediated response while the humoral response may be unaffected. These events could render the individual more susceptible to mycobacterial infection.

In summary, local accumulation of self-stress proteins on prolonged insult with silica may provide a stimulus for proliferation of autoreactive lymphocytes. This may be a possible mechanism whereby particulates such as silica induce an autoimmune response sometimes associated with fibrosis.

VI. SUMMARY AND HYPOTHESIS

The initial events following inhalation of silica involve its phagocytosis, followed by macrophage activation and release of various growth factors and cytokines. These factors can stimulate the chemotactic migration of the T and B cells towards the activated macrophages. Lymphokines released by these immune cells would initiate a sequence of events involving the various components of the immune system. Furthermore, the pattern of cytokines released by subpopulations of lymphocytes, particularly Th1 and Th2 cells, could provide an explanation for individual susceptibility for the development of silicosis following silica exposure.

Although in silicosis the proposed role of the stress response is unproven, it could provide a plausible mechanism for a number of observations related to silicosis. Furthermore, the stress response has recently been observed in other fibrotic models,[127] suggesting that stress proteins could have a role in silicosis. It is our hypothesis that stress proteins play a well-defined and central role in the development of silica-induced lung fibrosis and the autoimmune disorders often associated with silicosis. There are several possible mechanisms by which stress proteins could induce an autoimmune disorder and enhance the secretion of growth factors by macrophages. The following possible mechanisms are proposed.

1. Silica-macrophage interaction could result in the increased synthesis of stress proteins by the stressed macrophage, resulting in the expression of these stress proteins on the cell surface. This could then result in the activation of autoreactive T cells specific for self-stress proteins precipitating an immune response.

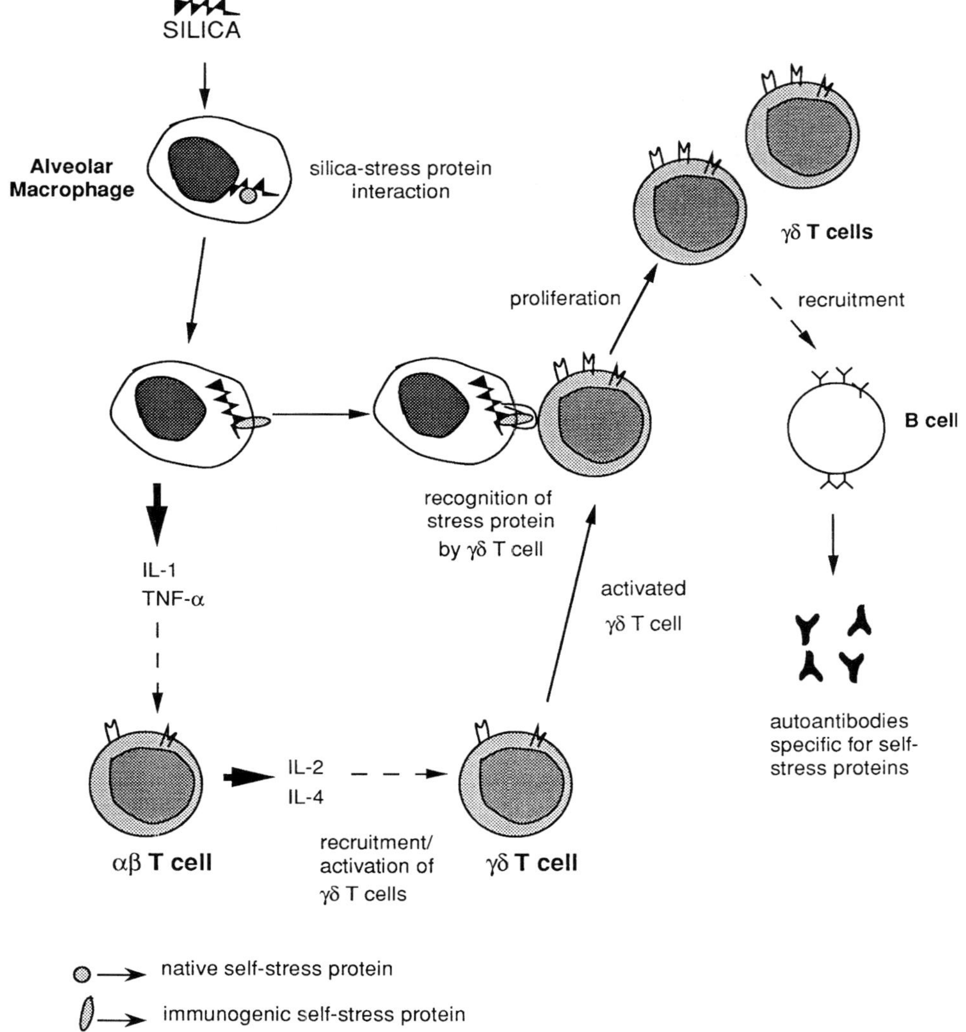

FIGURE 3 Schematic diagram of the potential role of the stress response in silicosis. Phagocytosis of silica is followed by the interaction of silica with the stress protein, macrophage activation, and stress protein presentation on the cell surface. Activated macrophages release chemotactic factors, resulting in the influx and activation of $\alpha\beta$ and $\gamma\delta$ T cells and the recognition of stress proteins by these cells. Activated $\gamma\delta$ T cells may then further recruit Ig-secreting B cells specific for self-stress proteins. Bold arrows indicate secretion of cytokines and dashed arrows indicate their target cells.

2. Silica may interact with the self-stress proteins in such a manner so as to expose some novel antigenic sites on the stress proteins, thus rendering them immunogenic. This altered self-protein may then be recognized by an autoreactive T cell.
3. Alternatively, silica may influence endogenous stress proteins, increasing the concentration of these proteins on the cell surface, thereby altering the fine balance between tolerance and immunity.

Any or all of the above mechanisms could be instrumental in stimulating immune cells and inducing the production of cytokines. This stimulation could further trigger a cascade of other pathways and in turn affect events responsible for fibroblast proliferation and collagen secretion, resulting in fibrosis. Obviously, these hypotheses remain to be tested and their significance in silicosis determined.

REFERENCES

1. **Davis, G. S.,** Pathogenesis of silicosis: current concepts and hypotheses, *Lung*, 164, 1339, 1986.
2. **Spencer, H .,** Pathology of the lung, 3rd ed., W. B. Saunders, Philadelphia, 1977, 379.
3. **Davis, G. S., Hemenway, D. R., Evans, J. N., Lapenas, D. J., and Brody, A. R.,** Alveolar macrophages stimulation and population changes in silica-exposed rats, *Chest*, 80, 8, 1981.
4. **Struhar, D., Harbeck, R. J., and Mason, R. J.,** Lymphocyte populations in lung tissue, BAL, and peripheral blood in rats at various times during the development of silicosis, *Am. Rev. Respir. Dis.*, 139, 28, 1989.
5. **Flint, A.,** Pathologic features of interstitial lung disease, in *Interstitial Lung Disease*, Schwarz, N. M. I. and King, T. E., Eds., B. C. Decker, Philadelphia, 1988, 45.
6. **Schmidt, J. A., Oliver, C. N., Lepe-Zuniga, J. L., Green, I., and Gery, I.,** Silica stimulated monocytes release fibroblast proliferation factors identical to interleukin-1. A potential role for interleukin-1 in the pathogenesis of silicosis, *J. Clin. Invest.*, 73, 1462, 1984.
7. **Martin, T. R., Altman, L. C., Albert, R. K., and Henderson, W. R.,** Leukotriene B_4 production by the human alveolar macrophages: a potential mechanism for amplifying inflammation in the lung, *Am. Rev. Respir. Dis.*, 129, 106, 1984.
8. **Thiele, D. L. and Lipsky, P. E.,** The accessory function of phagocytic cells in human T cells and B cell responses, *J. Immunol.*, 129, 1033, 1982.
9. **Scheule, R. K., and Holian, A.,** Immunologic aspects of pneumoconiosis, *Exp. Lung Res.*, 17, 661, 1991.
10. **Benson, S. C., Belton, J. C., and Scheve, L. G.,** Regulation of lung fibroblasts proliferation and collagen synthesis by alveolar macrophage in experimental silicosis. I. Effect of macrophage conditioned medium from silica instilled in rats, *J. Environ. Pathol. Toxicol. Oncol.*, 7, 87, 1986.
11. **Davis, G. S., Leslie, K., Scwarz, J. E., Pfeiffer, L. M., Eubanks, L. H., and Hemenway, D. R.,** Altered patterns of lymphocyte accumulation in silicosis in cytokine-sufficient and cytokine-deficient mice, *Chest*, 103, 121S, 1993.
12. **Schmidt, J. A., Oliver, C. N., Lepe-Zuniga, J. L., Green, I., and Gery, I.,** Silica-stimulated monocytes release fibroblast proliferation factors identical to interleukin 1, *J. Clin. Invest.*, 73, 1462, 1984.
13. **Sugarman, B. J., Aggarwal, B. B., Figari, I. S., and Palladino, M. A.,** Recombinant human tumor necrosis factor a: effects on proliferation of normal and transformed cells *in vitro*, *Science (Washington D.C.)*, 230, 943, 1985.
14. **Ross, R., Raines, E. W., and Bowen-Pope, D. F.,** The biology of platelet derived growth factor, *Cell*, 46, 155, 1986.
15. **Schmidt, J. A., Mizel, S. B., Cohen, D., and Green, I.,** Interleukin 1 a potential regulator of fibroblast proliferation, *J. Immunol.*, 128, 2177, 1982.
16. **Roberts, A. B., Sporn, M. B., Assoian, R. K., Smith, J. M., Roche, N. S., Wakefield, L. M., Heine, U. I., Liotta, L. A., Falanga, V., Kehrl, J. H., and Fauci, A. S.,** Transforming growth factor type-beta: rapid induction of fibrosis and angiogenesis *in vivo* and stimulation of collagen formation *in vitro*, *Proc. Natl. Acad. Sci. U.S.A.*, 83, 4167, 1986.
17. **Rom, W. N., Travis, W. D., and Brody, A. R.,** Cellular and molecular basis of asbestos related disease, *Am. Rev. Respir. Dis.*, 143, 408, 1991.
18. **Martinet, Y., Rom, W. N., Grotendorst, G. R., Martin, G. R., and Crystal, R. G.,** Exaggerated spontaneous release of PDGF by alveolar macrophages from patients with idiopathic pulmonary fibrosis, *N. Engl. J. Med.*, 317, 202, 1987.
19. **O'Gara, A., Umland, S., De France, T., and Christiansen, J.,** B cell factors are pleitropic, *Immunol. Today*, 9, 45, 1988.
20. **Piguet, P. F., Collart, M. A., Grau, G. E., Sappino, A. P., and Vassalli, P.,** Requirement of tumor necrosis factor for the development of silica-induced pulmonary fibrosis, *Nature*, 344, 245, 1990.
21. **Schmidt, J. A., Oliver, C. N., Green, I., and Gery, I.,** Silica stimulated macrophages release a fibroblast proliferation factor identical to interleukin 1, *Fed. Proc., Fed. Am. Soc. Exp. Biol.*, 41, 438, 1982.
22. **Stuhar, D., Harbeck, R. J., and Mason, R. J.,** Lymphocyte populations in lung tissue, bronchoalveolar lavage fluid, and peripheral blood in rats at various times during the development of silicosis, *Am. Rev. Respir. Dis.*, 139, 28, 1989.
23. **Oghiso, Y. and Kubota, Y.,** Enhanced interleukin-1 production by alveolar macrophages and increase in 1a-positive lung cells in silica exposed rats, *Microbiol. Immunol.*, 30, 1189, 1986.
24. **Roitt, I., Brostoff, J., and Male, D.,** *Immunology*, 2nd ed., Gower Medical Publishers, New York, 1989.
25. **Falkoff, R. J., Butler, J. L., Dinarello, C. A., and Fauci, A. S.,** Direct effects of a monoclonal B-cell differentiation factor and of purified interleukin-1 on B-cell differentiation, *J. Immunol.*, 133, 692, 1984.
26. **Hunninghake, G. W., Glazier, A. J., Monick, M. M., and Dinarello, C. A.,** IL-1 is a chemotactic factor for human T-lymphocytes, *Am. Rev. Respir. Dis.*, 135, 66, 1987.
27. **Unanue, E. R.,** The regulatory role of macrophages in antigenic stimulation. Part two: Symbiotic relationship between lymphocytes and macrophages, *Adv. Immunol.*, 31, 1, 1981.
28. **Elias, J. A., Gustilo, K., and Freundlich, B.,** Human alveolar macrophage and blood monocyte inhibition of fibroblast proliferation: evidence for synergy between interleukin-1 and tumor necrosis factor, *Am. Rev. Respir. Dis.*, 138, 1595, 1988.
29. **Piguet, P. F., Collart, M. A., Grau, G. E., Kapanci, Y., and Vassalli, P.,** Tumor necrosis factor/cachectin plays a key role in bleomycin-induced pneumopathy and fibrosis, *J. Exp. Med.*, 170, 655, 1989.

30. **Lindenschmidt, R. C., Driscoll, K. E., Perkins, M. A., Higgins, J. M., Maurer, J. K., and Belfiore, K. A.,** The comparison of a fibrogenic and two nonfibrogenic dusts by bronchoalveolar lavage, *Toxicol. Appl. Pharmacol.,* 102, 268, 1990.
31. **Chang, L. Y., Overby, L. H., Brody, A. R., and Crapo, J. D.,** Progressive lung cell reactions and extracellular matrix production after a brief exposure to asbestos, *Am. J. Pathol.,* 131, 156, 1988.
32. **Morgan, A., Moores, S., Holmes, A., Evans, J. C., Evans, N. H., and Black, A.,** The effect of quartz administered by intratracheal instillation on the rat lung. I. The cellular response, *Environ. Res.,* 22, 1, 1980.
33. **Sykes, S. E., Morgan, A., Moores, S. R., Holmes, A., and Davison, W.,** Dose-dependent effects in the subacute response of the rat lung to quartz, *Exp. Lung Res.,* 5, 227, 1983.
34. **Miller, K. and Kagan, E.,** The *in vitro* effects of quartz on alveolar macrophage membrane topography and on the characteristics of the intrapulmonary cell population, *J. Reticuloendothel. Soc.,* 21, 307, 1977.
35. **Davis, G. S., Hemenway, D. R., Evans, J. N., Lapenas, D. J., and Brody, A. R.,** Alveolar macrophage stimulation and population changes in silica exposed rats, *Chest,* 80, 8S, 1981.
36. **Kumar, R. K.,** Quantitative immunohistologic assessment of lymphocyte populations in the pulmonary inflammatory response to intratracheal silica, *Am. J. Pathol.,* 135, 605, 1989.
37. **Newman, L., Storey, E., and Kreiss, K.,** Immunologic evaluation of occupational lung disease, in *State of the Art Reviews: Occupational Pulmonary Diseases,* Vol. 2, Rosenstock, L., Ed., Hanley and Belfus, Philadelphia, 1987, 345.
38. **Allison, A. C., Harington, J. S., and Birbeck, M.,** An examination of the cytotoxic effects of silica on macrophages, *J. Exp. Med.,* 124, 141, 1966.
39. **Christman, J. W., Emerson, R. J., Graham, W. G. B., and Davis, G. S.,** Mineral dust and cell recovery from BAL of healthy Vermont granite workers, *Am. Rev. Respir. Dis.,* 132, 393, 1985.
40. **Schuyler, M., Gauner, H. R., Stankus, R. P., Kaimal, V., Hoffman, E., and Salvaggio, J.,** Bronchoalveolar lavage in silicosis, *Lung,* 57, 95, 1980.
41. **Callis, A. H., Sohnle, P. G., Mandel, G. S., Weissner, J., and Mandel, N. S.,** Kinetics of inflammatory and fibrotic pulmonary changes in murine model of silicosis, *J. Lab. Clin. Med.,* 105, 547, 1985.
42. **Schmidt, J. A., Oliver, C. N., Lepe-Zuniga, J. L., Green, I., and Gery, K.,** Silica stimulated monocytes release fibroblast proliferation factors identical to interleukin 1 in the pathogenesis of silicosis, *J. Clin. Invest.,* 73, 1462, 1984.
43. **Kovacs, E. J. and Kelley, J.,** Lymphokine regulation of macrophage derived growth factor secretion following pulmonary injury, *Am. Rev. Respir. Dis.,* 129, 833, 1985.
44. **Hubbard, A. K.,** Role of T-lymphocytes in silica-induced pulmonary inflammation, *Lab. Invest.,* 61, 46, 1989.
45. **Wei, L., Kumar, R. K., O'Grady, R., and Velan, G.,** Role of lymphocytes in silicosis: regulation of secretion of macrophage-derived mitogenic activity for fibroblasts, *Int. J. Exp. Pathol.,* 73, 793, 1992.
46. **Daniele, R. P.,** *Immunology and Immunologic Diseases of the Lung,* Blackwell Scientific, Oxford, 1991.
47. **Pernis, B. and Paroetto, F.,** Adjuvant effect of silica on antibody production, *Proc. Soc. Exp. Biol. Med.,* 110, 390, 1962.
48. **Haustein, U. F., Ziegler, V., and Herrmann, K.,** Chemically induced scleroderma, *Hautarzt,* 43(8), 469, 1992.
49. **Brozena, S. J., Fenske, N. A., and Cruse, C. W.,** Human adjuvant disease following augmentation mammoplasty, *JAMA,* 260, 236, 1988.
50. **Scheule, R. K. and Holian, A.,** IgG specifically enhances chrysotile asbestos-stimulated superoxide anion production by the alveolar macrophage, *Am. J. Respir. Cell Mol. Biol.,* 1, 313, 1989.
51. **Scheule, R. K. and Holian, A.,** Modification of asbestos bioactivity for the alveolar macrophage by selective protein adsorption, *Am. J. Respir. Cell Mol. Biol.,* 2, 441, 1990.
52. **Soderquist, M. E. and Walton, A. G.,** Structural changes in proteins adsorbed on polymer surfaces, *J. Colloid Interface Sci.,* 75, 385, 1980.
53. **Perkins, R. C., Scheule, R. K., and Holian, A.,** *In vitro* bioactivity of asbestos for the human alveolar macrophage and its modification by IgG, *Am. J. Respir. Cell Mol. Biol.,* 4, 532, 1991.
54. **DeFranco, A. L., Ashwell, J. D., Schwartz, R. H., and Paul, W. E.,** Polyclonal stimulation of resting B lymphocytes by antigen specific T lymphocytes, *J. Exp. Med.,* 159, 861, 1984.
55. **Hirohata, S., Jelinek, D. F., and Lipsky, P. E.,** T cell-dependent activation of B cell proliferation and differentiation by immobilized monoclonal antibodies to CD3, *J. Immunol.,* 140, 3736, 1988.
56. **Moseley, P. L., Monick, M., and Hunninghake, G. W.,** Divergent effects of silica on lymphocyte proliferation and Ig production, *Am. Physiol. Soc.,* 350, 1988.
57. **Mancino, D., and Bevilaciqua, N.,** Persistent and boosterable IgE production in mice infected with low doses of ovalbumin and silica, *Int. Arch. Allergy Appl. Immunol.,* 57, 155, 1978.
58. **Levy, N. H. and Wheelock, E. F.,** Effects of intravenous silica on immune functions and nonimmune functions of the immune host, *J. Immunol.,* 115, 41, 1975.
59. **Parronchi, P., Macchia, D., Piccinni, M. P., Biswas, P., Simonelli, C., Maggi, E., Ricci, M., Ansari, A. A., and Romagnani, S.,** Allergen and bacterial antigen specific T cell clones established from atopic donors show a different profile of cytokines production, *Proc. Natl. Acad. Sci. U.S.A.,* 88, 4538, 1991.
60. **Romagnani, S.,** Human Th1 and Th2 subsets: regulation of differentiation and role in protection and immunopathology, *Int. Arch. Allergy Immunol.,* 98, 279, 1992.

61. **Mosmann, T. R., Cherwinski, H., Bond, M. W., Giedlin, M. A., and Coffman, R. L.,** Two types of murine helper T cell clone. I. Definition according to profiles of lymphokine activities and secreted proteins, *J. Immunol.*, 136, 2348, 1986.
62. **Mosmann, T. R. and Moore, K. W.,** The role of IL-10 in crossregulation of TH1 and TH2 responses, *Immunol. Today*, 12(3), A49, 1991.
63. **Gajesski, T. F., Joyce, J., and Fitch, F. W.,** Anti proliferative effect of IFN-γ in immune regulation. III. Differential selection of Th1 and Th2 murine helper T lymphocyte clones using recombinant IL-2 and recombinant IFN-γ, *J. Immunol.*, 140, 4245, 1988.
64. **Parronchi, P., De Carli, M., Manetti, R., Simonelli, C., Piccinni, M. P., Macchia, D., Maggi, E., Del Prete, G. F., and Romagnani, S.,** Il-4 and IFN-γ exert opposite regulatory effects on the development of cytolytic potential by TH1 or Th2 human T cell clones, *J. Immunol.*, 180, 63, 1992.
65. **Kroemer, G., Toribio, M. L., and Martinez, C.,** Interleukin-2: counteracting pleiotropy by compartmentalization, *New Biol.*, 3(3), 219, 1991.
66. **Kim, J., Woods, A., Becker-Dunn, E., and Bottomly, K.,** Distinct functional phenotypes of cloned Ia restricted helper T cells, *J. Exp. Med.*, 162, 188, 1985.
67. **Killar, L., MacDonald, G., West, J., Woods, A., and Bottomly, K.,** Cloned Ia-restricted T cells that do not produce IL-4/B cell stimulatory factors 1 fail to help antigen specific B cells, *J. Immunol.*, 138, 1674, 1987.
68. **Ebel, F., Schmitt, E., Peter-Katalinic, J., Kniep, B., and Muhlradt, P. F.,** Gangliosides: differentiation markers for murine T helper lymphocyte subpopulations TH1 and TH2, *Biochemistry*, 31(48), 12190, 1992.
69. **Robinson, D. S., Hamid, Q., Ying, S., Tsicopoulos, A., Barkans, J., Bentley, A. M., Corrigan, C., Durham, S. R., and Kay, A. B.,** Predominant TH2-like bronchoalveolar T-lymphocyte population in atopic asthma, *N. Engl. J. Med.*, 326(5), 298, 1992.
70. **Burrell, R. G.,** Autoantibodies in pulmonary disease, *Am. Rev. Respir. Dis.*, 87, 389, 1963.
71. **Burrell, R. G., Wallace, J. P., and Andrews, C. E.,** Lung antibodies in patients with pulmonary disease, *Am. Rev. Respir. Dis.*, 89, 697, 1963.
72. **Jones, R. N., Turner-Warick, M., Ziskind, M., and Weill, H.,** High prevalence of antinuclear antibodies in sandblasters' silicosis, *Am. Rev. Respir. Dis.*, 113, 393, 1976.
73. **Kang, K. Y., Yagura, T., and Yamamura, Y.,** Antinuclear factor in pneumoconiosis, *N. Engl. J. Med.*, 288, 164, 1973.
74. **Rodnan, G. P., Benedek, T. B., Medsger, T. A., Jr., and Cammarata, R. J.,** The association of progressive systemic sclerosis with coal miners pneumoconiosis and other forms of silicosis, *Ann. Intern. Med.*, 66, 323, 1967.
75. **Matsuoka, Y., Tomita, M., Yoshino, I., and Hosoda, Y.,** Relationship between autoimmune diseases and pneumoconiosis, *Jpn. J. Ind. Health*, 34(5), 421, 1992.
76. **Koeger, A. C., Alcaix, D., Rozenberg, S., and Bourgeois, P.,** Occupational exposure to silicone and dermatopolymyositis. 3 cases, *Ann. Med. Int.*, 142(6), 409, 1991.
77. **Rustin, M. H. A., Bull, H. A., Ziegler, V., Mehlhorn, J., Haustein, U.-F., Maddison, P. J., James, J., and Dowd, P. M.,** Silica-associated systemics sclerosis is clinically, serologically and immunologically indistinguishable from idiopathic systemic sclerosis, *Br. J. Dermatol.*, 123, 725, 1990.
78. **Herrmann, K., Schulze, E., Heckmann, M., Schubert, K., Meurer, M., Ziegler, V., Haustein, U. F., Mehlhorn, J., and Krieg, T. H.,** Type III collagen aminopropeptide and laminin PI levels in serum of patients with silicosis-associated and idiopathic systemic scleroderma, *Br. J. Dermatol.*, 123, 1, 1990.
79. **Yanez Diaz, S., Moran, M., Unamuno, P., and Armijo, M.,** Silica and trichloroethylene-induced progressive systemic sclerosis, *Dermatology*, 184(2), 98, 1992.
80. **Mehlhorn, J., Ziegler, V., Keyn, J., and Vetter, J.,** Quartz crystals in the skin as a cause of progressive systemic scleroderma, *Z. Gesamte Inn. Med. Ihre Grenzgeb.*, 45(6), 149, 1990.
81. **Mehlhorn, J., Herrmann, K., Taubig, H., Dohler, B., Ziegler, V., and Vietze, K.,** Early detection of scleroderma in quartz dust exposed workers and workers with silicosis by determining serum beta-galactosidase activity, *Z. Gesamte Hyg. Ihre Grenzgeb.*, 36(1), 48, 1990.
82. **Haustein, U. F., Ziegler, V., Herrmann, K., Mehlhorn, J., and Schmidt, C.,** Silica-induced scleroderma, *J. Am. Acad. Dermatol.*, 22(3), 444, 1990.
83. **Nagaoka, T., Tabata, M., Kobayashi, K., and Okada, A.,** Studies on production of anticollagen antibodies in silicosis, *Environ. Res.*, 60, 12, 1993.
84. **Schulze, E., Herrmann, K., Haustein, U. F., Mehlhorn, J., and Bohme, H. J.,** N-procollagen (III) peptide and lysosomal beta-galactosidase in progressive scleroderma and silicosis, 176(11), 687–93, 1990.
85. **Vigliani, E. C. and Pernis, B.,** An immunological approach to silicosis, *J. Occup. Med.*, 1, 319, 1959.
86. **Deshazo, R. D.,** Current concepts about the pathogenesis of silicosis and asbestosis, *J. Allergy Clin. Immunol.*, 70, 41, 1982.
87. **Jones, R. N., Turner, W. M., Ziskind, M., and Weill, H.,** High prevalence of antinuclear antibodies in sandblaster's silicosis, *Am. Rev. Respir. Dis.*, 113, 393, 1976.
88. **Doll, N. J., Hughes, J., Weill, H., and Salvagio, J. E.,** Autoantibodies in silicosis, *J. Allergy Clin. Immunol.*, 65, 170, 1980.

89. **Doll, N. J., Stankus, R. P., Hughes, J., Weill, H., Gupta, R. C., Rodriguez, M., Jones, R. N., Alsaugh, M. A., and Salvagio, J. E.,** Immune complexes and autoantibodies in silicosis, *Clin. Immunol.*, 68(4), 281, 1981.
90. **Doll, N. J., Stankus, R. P., and Salvagio, J. E.,** Hypersensitivity lung disease, in Simmons, P. H., Ed., *Current Pulmonology,* 13, 61, 1981.
91. **Nigam, S. K., Saiyed, H. N., Malaviya, R., Suthar, A. M., Desai, U. M., Venkaiah, K., Sharma, Y. K., and Kashyap, S. K.,** Role of circulating immune complexes in the immunopathogenesis of silicosis, *Toxicol. Lett.*, 51(3), 315, 1990.
92. **Calhoun, W. J., Christman, J. W., Ershler, W. B., Graham, W. G., and Davis, G. S.,** Raised immunoglobulin concentrations in BAL fluid of healthy granite workers, *Thorax,* 41, 266, 1986.
93. **Schifferli, J. A., Na, Y. C., and Peters, D. K.,** The role of complement and its receptor in the elimination of immune complexes, *N. Engl. J. Med.*, 315, 488, 1986.
94. **Kreiss, K., Danilovs, J. A., and Newman, L. S.,** Histocompatibility antigens in a population based silicosis series, *Br. J. Ind. Med.*, 46, 364, 1989.
95. **Koskinen, H., Tiilikanen, A., and Nordman, H.,** Increased prevalence of HLA-Aw19 and of the phenogroup Aw19, B18 in advanced silicosis, *Chest,* 83, 848, 1983.
96. **Kaltreider, H. B., Byrd, P. K., and Curtis, J. L.,** Expression of Ia by murine alveolar macrophages is upregulated during the evolution of a specific pulmonary immune response, *Am. Rev. Respir. Dis.*, 137, 1411, 1988.
97. **Struhar, D. and Harbeck, R. J.,** Anti-Ia antibodies inhibit the spontaneous secretion of IL-1 from silicotic rat alveolar macrophages, *Immunol. Lett.*, 23, 31, 1989/1990.
98. **Unanue, E. R.,** Antigen-presenting function of macrophage, *Immunol. Rev.*, 2, 395, 1984.
99. **Miller, S. D. and Zarkower, A.,** Silica-induced alterations of murine lymphocyte immunocompetence and suppression of B lymphocyte immunocompetence: a possible mechanism, *J. Reticuloendothel. Soc.*, 19, 47, 1976.
100. **Youinou, P., Ferec, C., and Cledes, J.,** Immunological effect of silica dust analysed by monoclonal antibodies, *J. Clin. Immunol.*, 16, 207, 1985.
101. **Nover, L.,** *Heat Shock Response of Eucaryotic Cells,* Springer-Verlag, Berlin, 1984.
102. **Schlesinger, M. J., Tissieres, A., and Ashburner, M., Eds.,** *Heat Shock Proteins: from Bacteria to Man,* Cold Spring Harbor Laboratory, Cold Spring Harbor, NY, 1982.
103. **Lindquist, S. and Craig, E. A.,** The heat shock proteins, *Annu. Rev. Genet.*, 22, 163, 1988.
104. **Tissieres, A., Mitchell, H. K., and Tracy, U.,** Protein synthesis in salivary glands of drosiphila melanogaster: relation to chromosome puffs, *J. Mol. Biol.*, 84, 389, 1974.
105. **Schlesinger, M. J.,** Heat shock proteins, *J. Biol. Chem.*, 265(21), 12111, 1990.
106. **Wakui, H., Itoh, H., Tsahima, Y., Kobayashi, R., Nakamoto, Y., and Miura, A. B.,** Specific antibodies against the stress inducible 72-kDa protein, a member of the heat shock protein hsp70, in healthy human subjects, *Int. J. Biochem.*, 23, 975, 1991.
107. **Ellis, R. J.,** Molecular chaperones: the plant connection, *Science,* 250, 954, 1990.
108. **Beckmann, R. P., Mizzen, L. A., and Welch, W. J.,** Interaction of hsp 70 with newly synthesized proteins: implications for protein folding and assembly, *Science,* 248, 850, 1990.
109. **Haregewoin, A., Soman, G., Hom, R. C., and Finberg, R. W.,** Human gamma delta T cells respond to mycobacterial heat shock proteins, *Nature,* 340, 309, 1989.
110. **Janeway, C. A., Jones, B., and Hayday, A.,** Specificity and function of T cells bearing the gamma delta receptors, *Immunol. Today,* 9, 73, 1990.
111. **Chirgwin, J. M., Przblyla, A. E., MacDonald, R. J., and Rutter, W. J.,** Isolation of biologically active ribonucleic acid from sources enriched in ribonuclease, *Biochemistry,* 18, 5294, 1979.
112. **Lindquist, S.,** The heat shock response, *Am. Rev. Biochem.*, 55, 1151, 1986.
113. **Lamb, J. R., Bal, V., Mendez-Samperio, P., Mehlert, A., So, A., Rothbard, J., Jindal, S., Young, R. A., and Young, D. B.,** Stress proteins may provide a link between the immune response to infection and autoimmunity, 1(2), 191, 1989.
114. **Danielli, M. G., Markovitz, D., Gabrielli, A., Corvetta, A., Giorgi, P. L., van Derzee, R., Van Embden, J. D. A., Danieli, G., and Cohen, I. R.,** Juvenile rheumatoid arthritis patients manifest immune reactivity to the mycobacterial 65-kDa hsp, to its 180–188 peptide, and to a partially homologous peptide of the proteoglycan link protein, *Clin. Immunol. Immunopathol.*, 64(2), 121, 1992.
115. **al Bayati, Z. A. and Stohs, S. H.,** The possible role of phospholipase A2 in hepatic microsomal lipid peroxidation induced by 2,3,7,8-tetrachlorodibenzo-p-dioxin in rats, *Arch. Environ. Contam. Toxicol.*, 20, 361, 1991.
116. **Alexandrova, M. and Farkas, P.,** Stress induced changes of glucocorticoid receptor in rat liver, *J. Steroid Biochem.*, 42, 493, 1992.
117. **Janis, E. M., Kaufmann, S. H. E., Schwartz, R. H., and Pardoll, D. M.,** Activation of γδ T cells in the primary immune response to *Mycobacterium tuberculosis, Science,* 244, 713, 1989.
118. **Ferrick, D. A. and Gemmell-Hori, L.,** Potential development role for self-reactive T cells bearing γδ T cell receptors for heat shock proteins: Hsp and gamma delta T cells, *Chem. Immunol.*, 53, 1, 1992.
119. **Modlin, R. L., Pirmez, C., Hofman, F. M., Torigian, V., Uyemura, K., Rea, T. H., Bloom, B. R., and Brenner, M. B.,** Human lymphocytes bearing antigen specific gamma-delta T-cell receptors accumulate in human infectious disease lesions, *Nature,* 338, 544, 1989.

120. **Kaufmann, S. H. E. and Kabelitz, D.,** Gamma-delta T lymphocytes and heat shock proteins, *Curr. Top. Microbial. Immunol.,* 167, 191, 1991.
121. **Barcena, A., Toribio, M. L., Pezzi, L., and Martinez, C.,** A role for interleukin 4 in the differentiation of mature T cell receptor gamma/delta + cells from human intrathymic T cell precursors, *J. Exp. Med.,* 172, 439, 1990.
122. **Baetjer, A. M. and Vintinner, F. J.,** The effect of silica and feldspar dusts on susceptibility to lobar pneumonia, *J. Invest. Hyg. Toxicol.,* 26, 101, 1944.
123. **Watanabe, S., Shirakaami, A., Takeichi, T., Ohara, T., and Saito, S.,** Alterations in lymphocyte subsets and serum Ig levels in patients with silicosis, *J. Clin. Lab. Immunol.,* 23, 45, 1987.
124. **Yeager, H., Sweeney, J. A., Herscowitz, H. B., Barsoum, I. S., and Kagan, E.,** Modulation of mitogen-induced proliferation of autologous peripheral blood lymphocytes by human alveolar macrophages, *Infect. Immun.,* 38, 260, 1982.
125. **Rich, E. A., Tweardy, D. J., Fujiwara, H., and Ellner, J. J.,** Spectrum of immunoregulatory functions and properties of human alveolar macrophages, *Am. Rev. Respir. Dis.,* 136, 258, 1987.
126. **Schauble, T. L., Boom, W. H., Finegan, C. K., and Rich, E. A.,** Characterization of suppressor function of human alveolar macrophages for T lymphocyte responses to phytohemagglutinin: cellular selectivity, reversibility, and early events in T cell activation, *Am. J. Respir. Cell Mol. Biol.,* 8, 89, 1993.
127. **Pope, L. M., Sally, J. Y., and York, J.,** Bleomycin induces the hsp 70 heat shock promoter in cultured cells, *Am. J. Respir. Cell Mol. Biol.,* 1, 89, 1989.

Section IV
Surface Modification and Disease Prevention Modalities

Section IV
Chapter 1

PULMONARY SURFACTANT ADSORPTION AND THE EXPRESSION OF SILICA TOXICITY

Michael J. Keane and William E. Wallace

CONTENTS

I. INTRODUCTION

In the alveolar regions of the lung, the interface between the epithelial cells and the air within alveoli consists of an aqueous dispersion of materials collectively designated pulmonary surfactant. Particles of silica or any other material that are inhaled into this region do not directly contact cells or tissue; the first contact will be with the hypophase that forms the tissue/air interface. Thus, interaction with the surfactant must precede any physical or chemical surface interaction with lung cells.

II. SURFACTANT PROPERTIES AND FUNCTION

The primary physiological functions of pulmonary surfactant are (a) the reduction of the surface tension of water in the hypophase to levels that eliminate collapse of alveoli under normal inhalation and exhalation, (b) an increase in lung compliance to lessen work of inspiration, (c) the prevention of edema by limiting influx of fluids, and (d) limitation of protein permeability into the alveolar spaces.[1] Additionally, pulmonary surfactant has protective roles, which include (a) hydrolytic enzymes to degrade microbes and foreign particles, (b) antifree-radical effects from catalase activity and unsaturated lipids in surfactant molecules, and (c) the surfactant film limits water evaporation.[1] While these protective effects are generally beneficial, reactions of free radicals with surfactant components such as unsaturated lipids

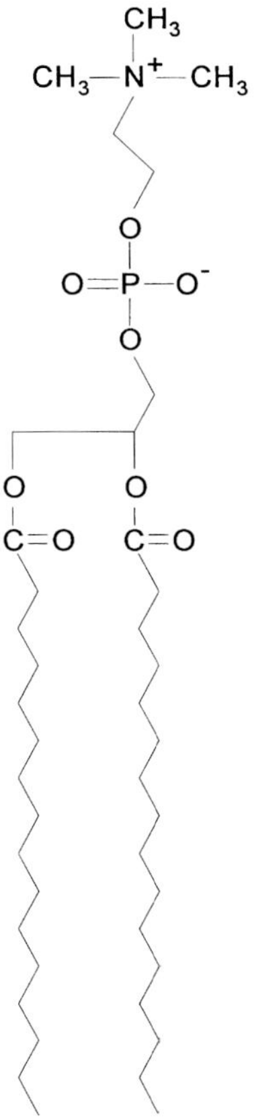

FIGURE 1 Dipalmitoyl phosphatidyl choline (DPPC) molecule.

may generate species that are toxic in the lung and elsewhere; free radical and related effects are discussed in Section II, Chapter 3.

Pulmonary surfactant has been extensively studied in the past several decades and is known to contain numerous components, primarily lipids (mostly phospholipids), carbohydrates, and proteins.[2,3] The phospholipid fraction is composed primarily of phosphatidyl cholines, principally dipalmitoyl phosphatidyl choline (DPPC), which is often 70–80% of that fraction.[4] Pulmonary surfactant composition studies have been reviewed recently.[5,6]

The protein fraction consists of many components, and surfactant proteins A, B, C, and D (SP-A, SP-B, SP-C, and SP-D) are important components of surfactant.[6,7] Other proteins such as albumin and immunoglobulins are also present.[7]

The DPPC is the surfactant component that is the major contributor to surface tension reduction,[8] but surfactant proteins are also considered to be important in configuring DPPC to provide minimum surface tension conditions.[9] For instance, SP-A and SP-B, along with calcium ions, are important in assembling DPPC in arrangements that provide optimal surface tension reduction.[7] Overall, the surface tension is reduced from about 71 dyn/cm to as low as 1 dyn/cm.[1]

Phospholipid molecules, especially phosphatidyl cholines, are so distinctive in their structure that some discussion is in order here. Referring to Figure 1, it can be seen that the molecule can be divided into several domains: an esterified glycerol/fatty acid domain, a highly polar phosphate ester region, and a highly polar choline region. The fatty acids are generally 16 carbons or more in length, and this end of the molecule is always very hydrophobic and lipophilic. The phosphate ester region has a unit negative charge shared between the two oxygen atoms not involved in ester linkages. The choline region of the molecule has a unit positive charge distributed throughout the trimethylammonium moiety. The charge on this group is not exchangeable with H^+ or other ions or groups in aqueous solution. As might be

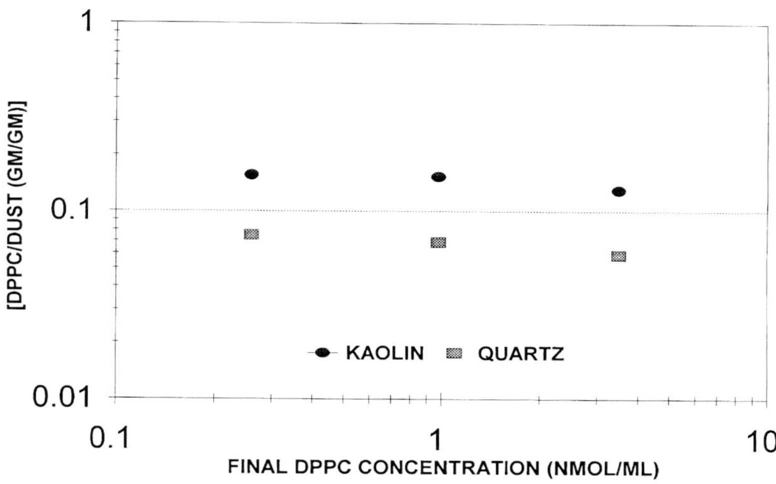

FIGURE 2 Adsorption isotherms for DPPC on quartz and kaolin at 37°C.

expected, these three domains all interact with appropriate basic, acidic, or hydrophobic regions of other molecules in very specific ways, forming very ordered structures. Other phospholipids, e.g., phosphatidyl ethanolamines, have similar molecular structure and have surfactant properties, but none are present in surfactant at comparable concentration to DPPC or other phosphatidyl cholines.

III. QUARTZ/SILICA SURFACE CHEMISTRY

As detailed in Section II, Chapter 2, quartz and other forms of silica have important surface chemistries. Most importantly, in most situations involving interactions with physiological systems, quartz and amorphous silicas exhibit significant numbers of surface silanol (SiOH) groups that manifest a moderate surface acidity in aqueous environments at typical pH values found *in vivo.* Measured and estimated values of pK_a range down to 6.5, which is comparable to carbonic acid or HOCl.[10]

Silica has been extensively studied, especially in regard to surface charge (ζ potential) and the point of zero charge (PZC) which is a function of pH. The PZC is about two for silica, which is highly acidic; at most physiological conditions, silica particles will be highly charged.[10] A typical surface concentration of silanols on silica materials is five SiOH per nm^2.[10] Thus silica is highly likely to interact with any materials that carry positive charges in solution at pH levels centered about neutral; a typical industrial application for removal of silica from minerals involves amine complexation/flotation.[11] This is not the case with all silicate minerals; while most have silica tetrahedra in their structure and carry a net negative charge in solution, they may carry surface groups that are amphoteric in character; thus the mineral surfaces can exhibit both acid and basic behavior, depending on pH and other factors, such as composition of solution. An example would be the aluminosilicate mineral kaolinite, or kaolin clay. Layers of silica tetrahedra alternate with layers of aluminol octahedra, and the aluminol groups are an important feature of the kaolin surface. The aluminol groups can react with either acidic or basic groups, depending on pH.

IV. INTERACTION OF SILICA AND OTHER MINERAL DUSTS WITH SURFACTANT COMPONENTS

Inhaled mineral particles/surfactant interactions include surface adsorption of phospholipids and possibly other surfactant components on the particles. Additionally, silica and other dusts may induce the secretion of excess surfactant;[13] this has been recently reviewed by Heppleston.[14] The adsorption of the DPPC component of pulmonary surfactant with both quartz and kaolin has been studied by Wallace et al.;[15] adsorption isotherms at 37°C are shown in Figure 2. The data shown are for a kaolin material less than 5 μm particle size and 13 m^2/g specific surface area, and a quartz sample of <5 μm particle size and

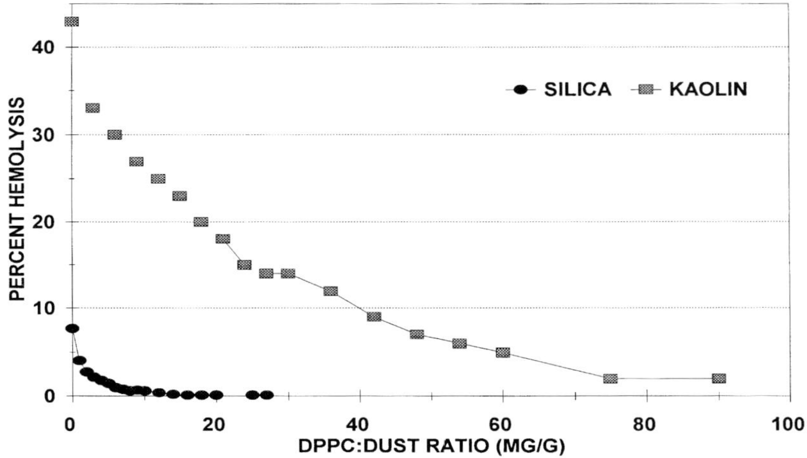

FIGURE 3 Hemolysis vs. DPPC: dust ratio for silica (quartz) and kaolin.

4 m^2/g area. Wallace et al.[12] have estimated the possibility of surfactant depletion in the lung by mineral dust adsorption, but dust loadings would need to be extremely high for this to be possible. Using literature values for the dimensions of the DPPC molecule and measured values of specific surface area, it is evident that a number of layers of DPPC are adsorbed to the mineral surfaces in these isotherm studies. Additional studies indicate that even after extensive rinsing, several layers of DPPC persist on the mineral dust surfaces.[15] Limited evidence from Fourier transform infrared spectroscopy (FTIR) studies indicate a strong trimethylammonium interaction with both quartz and kaolin surfaces.[16] Typical values of retained DPPC are 150 mg/g before and 80 mg/g after rinsing for kaolin, and 60–70 mg/g before and 15–20 mg/g after rinsing for quartz. Typically, 24-mg samples are sedimented, the supernatant discarded, and resuspended in 5 ml of fresh medium. Even after several such rinsing cycles, those amounts remain.[15]

V. SURFACTANT MODIFICATION OF THE INTERACTION OF MINERAL DUST WITH BIOLOGICAL SYSTEMS

As detailed in Section III, there are a number of current theories on the initial events involved in silicosis but no *in vitro* assays that are unequivocally predictive of silicosis induction *in vivo*. A simple assay involving plasma membrane lysis in erythrocytes by mineral dusts has been used for many types of dusts encountered in the workplace.[17,18]

While this hemolysis assay is sensitive and has a dose-related linear response for quartz, it is also about equally as sensitive for other dusts that are not generally considered to be fibrogenic, such as kaolin, when normalized for specific surface area.[15] The situation is similar with assays based on release of lysosomal enzymes such as β-glucuronidase and β-*N*-acetylglucosaminidase; the assays respond well to quartz but equally as well to other dusts not generally considered fibrogenic. Thus, many dusts are capable of generating false positives in both these membranolytic assays.

When mineral dusts such as quartz or kaolin are treated with DPPC[15] or lung lavage fluid[19] the toxicity in membranolytic assays is almost entirely eliminated. Typically, dusts are incubated with phospholipid dispersions or bronchial washings for periods of up to several hours with gentle agitation, then exposed to appropriate cell suspensions in membranolytic assays. Typical responses in these assays generally fall to levels close to the negative controls.[15,19] The effect is generally dose related for low surfactant loadings (below the isotherm amounts for dusts of a given specific surface area).[16] Figure 3 shows membranolytic strength vs. DPPC (dust ratio in milligrams DPPC per gram of dust for quartz and kaolin).

The elimination of membranolysis by coating mineral with genuine or simulated surfactant indicates that there are clearly other events involved in fibrotic disease initiation *in vivo*. The false positives of the assays for nonfibrogenic dusts are now false negative results for quartz, a fibrogenic dust. Obviously, quartz particles that are inhaled by individuals who have competent pulmonary surfactant systems are still subject to silicosis, so either the prophylactic effects of surfactants are temporary, or there may be quartz functional groups or other attributes that are completely distinct from those involved in membranolytic effects. It is possible, however, that the retention strength or removal rate of surfactant materials are important factors in distinguishing fibrogenic and nonfibrogenic dusts. In any case, membranolytic assays are not good indicators of fibrogenic potentials of mineral dusts.

The pulmonary macrophage is considered to have a central role in silicosis, as detailed in Section III of this book; this would be a probable location of surfactant removal from particles *in vivo*. Epithelial cells as well as interstitial cells may well also be involved, but those cell types have not been as well studied, especially in *in vitro* studies. After phagocytosis and fusion of the phagosome with lysosomes to form phagolysosomes in pulmonary macrophages, any material will be subjected to a variety of enzymes at low pH, typically 4–5. These enzymes include phospholipase A_2 (PLA_2), which hydrolyzes phosphatidyl cholines to lyso-PC and free fatty acids, as well as proteases and other enzymes. The situation within epithelial and interstitial cells may be different with regards to both enzyme types, amounts, and pH dependence.

Other materials can also adsorb to mineral surfaces; proteins, in particular, have been studied in *in vitro* experiments. Allison[20] has shown adsorption and removal of dye-labeled proteins on quartz.

VI. REMOVAL OF SIMULATED SURFACTANT IN CELL-FREE STUDIES

The removal of adsorbed phospholipids has been studied by Wallace et al.[15] in cell-free experiments. Respirable quartz (Min-U-Sil® <5 μm [U.S. Silica, Berkeley Springs, WV]) and kaolin (<5 μm) were used to contrast quartz, a known fibrogenic and cytotoxic material, with kaolin, a cytotoxic but less fibrogenic dust. Cell-free studies used a commercially available PLA_2 isolated from porcine pancreas; this enzyme is a neutral pH optimum enzyme, and studies were done at neutral pH. Briefly, dusts were coated in DPPC dispersions in excess of isotherm amounts for 60 min at 37°C, rinsed twice with buffer, and subjected to varying amounts of PLA_2 in neutral Ca^{2+}-supplemented buffer for times ranging from 2–72 h. Samples were then rinsed twice in buffer supplemented with EDTA and divided into two portions. One portion from each treatment was dried, and all lipids were extracted and DPPC separated from lyso-PC and other products by thin-layer chromatography (TLC). Both DPPC and the hydrolysis product lyso-PC were quantitated by isolation of bands and phosphate analysis. The hemolysis assay using sheep erythrocytes was used to measure the membranolytic strength of dusts in the other portion of each sample. Selected results from the studies are shown in Figures 4 and 5. Rapid removal of about half of the adsorbed DPPC at 2 h is evident for both dusts, as shown in Figure 4. The results for longer times, ranging up to 144 h, indicate a much more rapid loss of DPPC and its hydrolysis products (lyso-PC and palmitic acid) from quartz than from kaolin. The empirical data have been modeled for first-order coupled kinetics, and this treatment confirms a much higher removal rate for quartz when the results are normalized for differing specific surface areas of the two dusts.

VII. REMOVAL OF SURFACTANT FROM MINERAL PARTICLES *IN VITRO* BY A MACROPHAGE-LIKE CELL LINE

Removal of DPPC from quartz and kaolin particles by cells in culture has been studied by Hill[21,22] using a macrophage-like rat cell line, $P388D_1$. Dusts were treated with DPPC as above, with the addition of ^{14}C-labeled DPPC, with the labels at the fatty acid carbonyl carbons at both the 1- and 2- positions (DuPont, Boston, MA). Cells were cultured in RPMI 1640 with serum and antibiotics in six-well plates, at cell densities of $2 \times 10^5/cm^2$. DPPC-treated dusts were added at levels of 100, 400, 800, and 1600 μg per million cells for quartz and 25, 50, 100, 400, and 1600 μg per million cells for kaolin. Cells and dusts were incubated at 37°C in 5% CO_2 for periods up to 9 d. After incubation, cells were harvested with Triton® X-100 and total lipids were extracted with 2:1 v/v $CHCl_3$:CH_3OH. Disaturated phospholipids were isolated using the method of Mason et al.;[23] recovered disaturated phospholipids were determined by liquid scintillation counting. Results were normalized to the controls, which were dusts not exposed to cells. In order to determine whether fatty acids hydrolyzed from DPPC might be reincorporated into disaturated phospholipids, ^{14}C palmitic acid was added to similar cultures of cells for periods from 1 to 9 d; no significant label was found in the recovered phospholipids. Viability of cells exposed to quartz

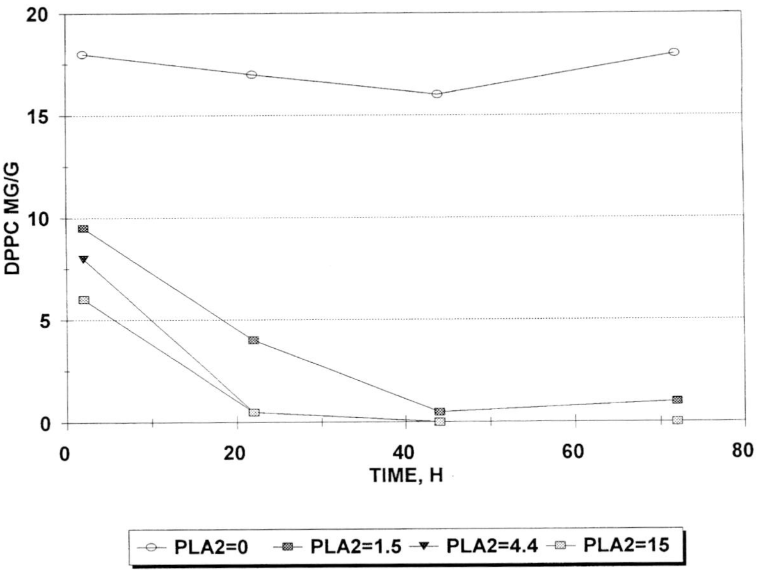

FIGURE 4 DPPC remaining on quartz vs. time following phospholipase A_2 hydrolysis *in vitro*.

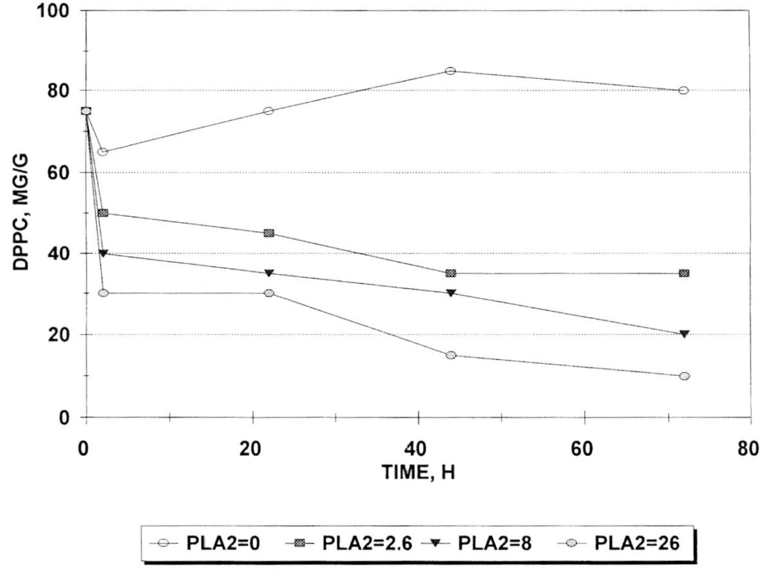

FIGURE 5 DPPC remaining on kaolin vs. time following phospholipase A_2 hydrolysis *in vitro*.

and kaolin was determined by trypan blue exclusion for all samples; viability was near 100% for low loadings of both dusts at day 1 but fell strongly for the 800- and 1600-μg loadings.

The removal rates are shown in Figures 6 and 7; controls at each time point are treated dusts incubated but not exposed to cells. The removal of DPPC from both dusts is evident from the initial time, but the rate slows considerably between days 6 and 9 and stays in the vicinity of 20% for both dusts at day 9.

Since the hypothesis of this study postulated lysosomal hydrolysis of dust-adsorbed lipids, studies of lysosomal inhibition by drugs were also included in the study. Chlorphentermine, imipramine, and

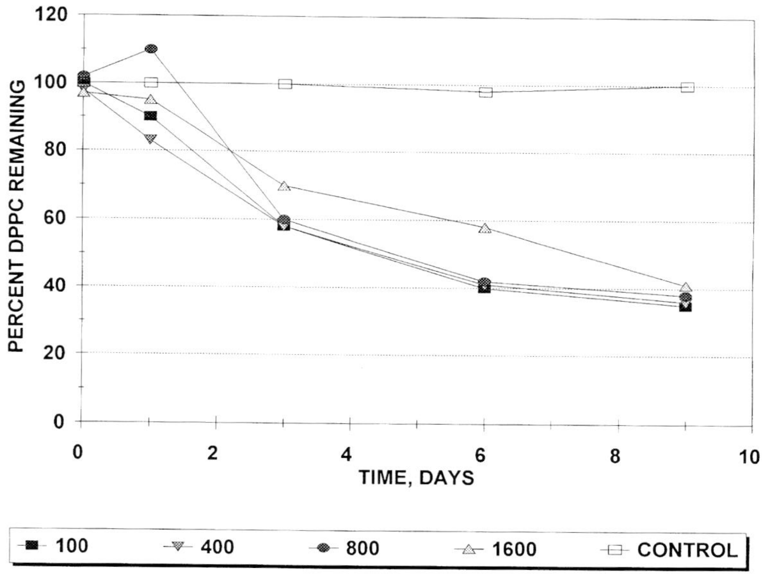

FIGURE 6 DPPC remaining on quartz vs. time following incubation with P388D$_1$ cells.

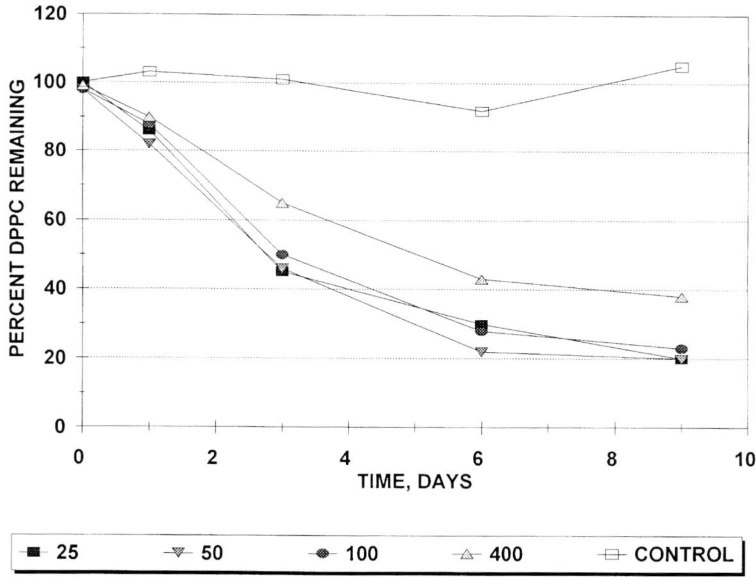

FIGURE 7 DPPC remaining on kaolin vs. time following incubation with P388D$_1$ cells.

chloroquine, at nontoxic concentrations, were added to the medium with quartz-challenged cells. After 3-d incubation, lipids were extracted, assayed, and compared to parallel samples without the drugs. Results show that all except imipramine at the low concentration significantly lower the DPPC removal rate from quartz. This demonstrates clearly that digestion of adsorbed lipids from dusts must be at least partially lysosomal in nature.

The study also examined the extracellular phospholipase activity of the P388D$_1$ cell line, since conditioned medium seemed to degrade dust-adsorbed DPPC, while there was no degradation of DPPC

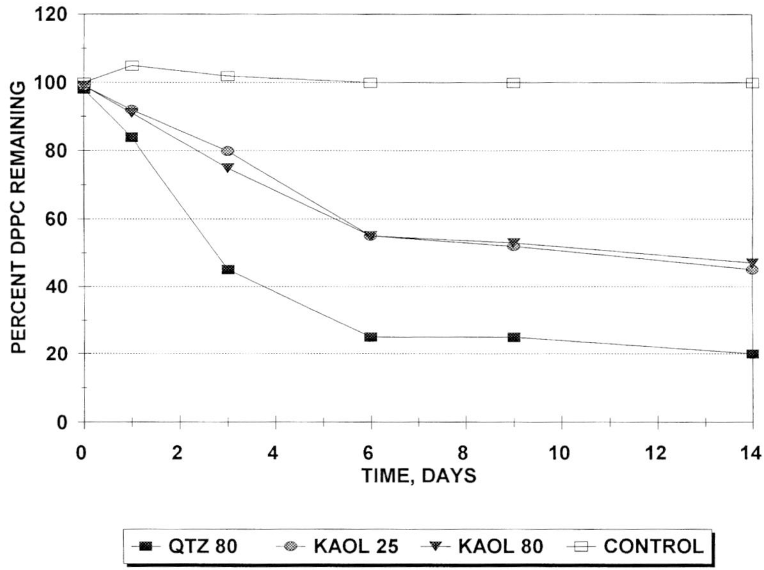

FIGURE 8 DPPC remaining on quartz and kaolin vs. time following incubation with conditioned medium from P388D$_1$ cells.

in plain medium. The conditioned medium was prepared by incubating cells in the presence of DPPC-treated quartz for 3 d at 37°C. Figure 8 shows the removal of DPPC for times up to 14 d. To demonstrate that this effect was enzymatic in nature, several methods of protein denaturation were applied to the conditioned medium; heating for 30 min at 56°C was effective in eliminating hydrolysis of DPPC from quartz by the conditioned medium.

The results from the P388D$_1$ cells in this study were not conclusive in establishing whether there might be a rate difference of DPPC removal from quartz and kaolin.

VIII. REMOVAL RATE STUDIES OF FLUORESCENT-LABELED SURFACTANT FROM MINERAL PARTICLES *IN VITRO*

A study by Das[24] of removal of fluorescent-labeled surfactant from mineral surfaces *in vitro* in rat primary alveolar macrophages examined particles within individual cells. Dioleoyl phosphatidyl choline (DOPC) was supplemented with 10% dipyrrometheneboron difluoride (BODIPY®) fluorescent label (Molecular Probes, Eugene, OR). Quartz and kaolin dusts were incubated overnight with the DOPC mixture and added to cultures of cells at a loading of 50 µg per million cells. Cells were incubated up to 7 d at 37°C in minimal essential medium with 10% calf serum and antibiotics; culture medium was changed every 72 h. Excitation of 488 nm was focused on the cells, and a 10-µm aperture was used to limit the viewing area to particles or particle clusters within cells. Emitted light passing a 510-nm filter was measured by a photomultiplier. Measurements were made at 0, 6, 24, 48, 72, 120, 144, and 168 h; 20 cells containing dust particles were measured at each time point. Fluorescence intensity minus background fluorescence was normalized to the time zero values. Results are illustrated in Figure 9; the estimated rates for quartz and kaolin appear to be equal for the time points up to 7 d. Even at 7 d, not all DOPC has been removed from either dust; more than 10% of the initial amount remains. This study has not unequivocally answered the question of quartz and kaolin surface restoration within cells because of this residual amount remaining, but the rates for both quartz and kaolin are very similar for times ranging to 7 d.

In order to assure that the fluorescent label was an unequivocal indicator of adsorbed DOPC, cell-free experiments using porcine PLA$_2$ followed by TLC separation and phosphate determination were done; results indicated a good correspondence between fluorescence values and DOPC as measured by the phosphate assay.

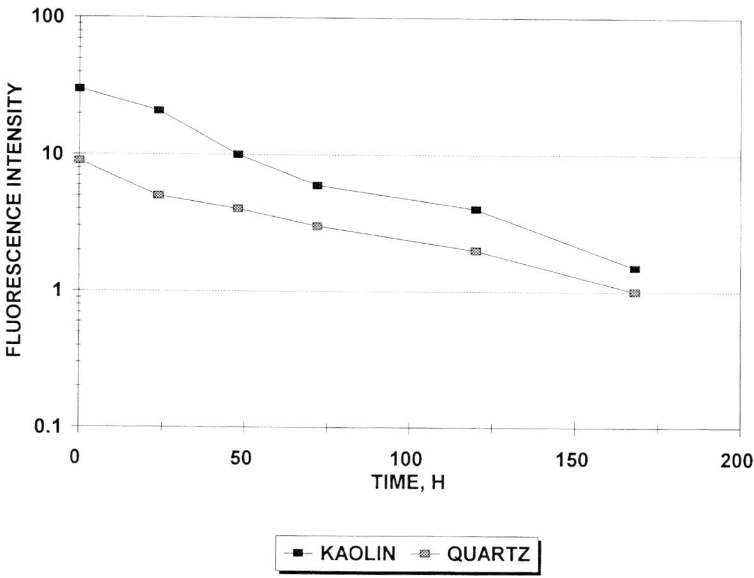

FIGURE 9 Fluorescence intensity of BODIPY-labeled DOPC on quartz and kaolin vs. time in rat primary alveolar macrophages.

A. DUAL FLUORESCENT LABEL STUDIES

In vitro studies of internalized mineral particles within primary cells have been studied by Das[23] using light microscopy with multiple fluorescent dyes. Primary alveolar macrophages from rats were exposed to rhodamine B isothiocyanate-dextran (RITC-dextran), followed by exposure to quartz and kaolin particles that had been coated with DPPC phospholipids containing 10% BODIPY®-fluorescent-labeled lipids.

Results indicate that RITC-dextran is taken up promptly (6–24 h) and lysosomes are clearly visible as small red spots. At 48–72 h, intact spots were seen as randomly distributed throughout the cytoplasm; nuclei were clear of spots. After 120–168 h, the red fluorescence was spread throughout all of the cytoplasm, suggesting lysis of the lysosomal vesicles.

Phospholipid-treated quartz and kaolin particles within cells were observed as well-defined green spots when properly excited approximately 24 h after phagocytosis. The green fluorescence spread considerably by 48–120 h and was pale and uniform throughout the cytoplasm after 144 h, suggesting loss of considerable label in contact with mineral particles.

The use of two-color overlay images permits visualization of both the BODIPY® green fluorescence and the red RITC-dextran fluorescence. The presence of greenish-yellow spots is evidence for lysosome-phagosome fusion at 24 h after challenge. Between 72 and 120 h, mixing of the green and red fluorescent regions was revealed by the spreading of a uniform yellow color throughout the cytoplasm. After 144 h, all fluorescence was weak and diffuse, suggesting degradation and redistribution of both labels, consistent with the evidence from the RITC-dextran-only study.

While these studies indicate loss and redistribution of phospholipids adsorbed on minerals within macrophages within several days, the techniques are not sufficient to resolve whether the mineral surfaces are completely cleared of adsorbed phospholipids or their hydrolysis products within the course of these studies.

IX. CONCLUSIONS

Pulmonary surfactant, a complex mixture of lipids, proteins, and other components, is the surface of initial contact of inhaled silica particles in the alveolar region of the lung and thus may be important in the development of fibrosis. *In vitro* studies have established that there is a strong adsorption of DPPC, a dominant component of pulmonary surfactant, on respirable quartz and other mineral dusts. Treatment of mineral dusts with authentic or simulated pulmonary surfactant in *in vitro* studies shows complete elimination of membranolytic damage in several similar short-term assays.

Noting the lysosomal environment typical of macrophages and other cells, it is reasonable to assume hydrolysis of adsorbed phospholipids and other materials adsorbed on mineral particles such as silica. Evidence from cell-free studies of adsorbed phospholipids on dusts hydrolyzed by porcine PLA_2 indicate that there is a substantial difference in the kinetics of DPPC removal from quartz and kaolin at neutral pH. This could be an important factor in disease initiation if removal rates for quartz are greater than clearance rates from the lung.

In vitro studies with a macrophage-like cell line, $P388D_1$, indicate comparable rates of DPPC removal from both quartz and kaolin, but significant amounts of DPPC remain after 9 d; much of the enzyme activity was shown to be extracellular in nature, which limits the use of this cell line to determine rate differences for quartz and kaolin.

Studies using rat primary alveolar macrophages tracked a fluorescent-labeled phospholipid adsorbed on quartz and kaolin dusts. Again, similar hydrolysis rates were shown for quartz and kaolin, but neither dust was cleared even at 7 d. Cell viability was also very low at that time; the primary macrophages were not hardy enough to answer the question of rate differences.

Overall, the goal of determining rates of surfactant removal from mineral particles within cells has been elusive. While there is little question that surfactant and its components have important interactions with inhaled mineral particles such as quartz, the complete role has not been established. Future studies, especially *in vivo* procedures, should elucidate the role of pulmonary surfactant in the initiation and development of silicosis.

REFERENCES

1. **Bourbon, J. R.,** Pulmonary surfactant — an overview, in *Pulmonary Surfactant: Biochemical, Functional, Regulatory, and Clinical Concepts,* Bourbon, J., Ed., CRC Press, Boca Raton, FL, 1991, chap. 1.
2. **King, R. J. and Clements, J. A.,** Surface active materials from dog lung. I. Method of isolation, *Am. J. Physiol.,* 223, 707–726, 1972.
3. **King, R. J., Klass, D. J., Gikas, E. G., and Clements, J. A.,** Isolation of apoproteins from canine surface active material, *Am. J. Physiol.,* 224, 788, 1973.
4. **Gilfillan, A. M., Chu, A. J., Smart, D. A., and Rooney, S. A.,** Single plate separation of lung phospholipids including disaturated phosphatidyl choline, *J. Lipid Res.,* 24, 1651, 1983.
5. **Haagsman, H. P. and van Golde, L. M. G.,** Lung surfactant and pulmonary toxicology, *Lung,* 163, 275, 1985.
6. **Rooney, S. A.,** The surfactant system and pulmonary toxicology, *Am. Rev. Respir. Dis.,* 131, 439, 1985.
7. **Whitsett, J. A. and Weaver, T. E.,** Structure, function, and regulation of pulmonary surfactant proteins, in *Pulmonary Surfactant: Biochemical, Functional, Regulatory, and Clinical Concepts,* Bourbon, J., Ed., CRC Press, Boca Raton, FL, 1991, chap. 4.
8. **Notter, R. H. and Finkelstein, J. N.,** Pulmonary surfactant: an interdisciplinary approach, *J. Appl. Physiol.,* 57, 1613, 1984.
9. **Schurch, S., Goerke, L., and Clements, J. A.,** Direct determination of surface tension in the lung, *Proc. Nat. Acad. Sci. U.S.A.,* 73, 4698, 1976.
10. **Iler, R. K.,** *The Chemistry of Silica,* Wiley-Interscience, New York, 1979, chap. 6.
11. **Fuerstenau, M. C., Ed.,** *Flotation,* American Institute of Mining, Metallurgy, and Petroleum Engineers, New York, 1976.
12. **Wallace, W. E., Headley, L. C., and Weber, K. C.,** Dipalmitoyl lecithin surfactant adsorption by kaolin dust *in vitro, J. Colloid Interface Sci.,* 51, 535, 1975.
13. **Miller, B. E. and Hook, G. E.,** Hypertrophy and hyperplasia of alveolar type II cells in response to silica and other pulmonary toxicants, *Environ. Health Perspect.,* 85, 15, 1990.
14. **Heppleston, A. G.,** Current status review: the role of surfactant in the pulmonary reaction to mineral particles, *Int. J. Exp. Pathol.,* 72, 599, 1991.
15. **Wallace, W. E., Keane, M. J., Mike, P. S., Hill, C. A., Vallyathan, V., and Regad, E. D.,** Contrasting respirable quartz and kaolin retention of lecithin surfactant and expression of membranolytic activity following phospholipase A_2 digestion, *J. Toxicol. Environ. Health,* 37, 391, 1992.

16. **Keane, M. J., Wallace, W. E., Seerha, M., Hill, C., Vallyathan, V., Raghootama, P., and Mike, P.,** Respirable particle surface interactions with the lecithin component of pulmonary surfactant, *Proc. VII Int. Pneumoconiosis Conf.,* U.S. Department of Health and Human Services (NIOSH), Publication 90–108 Part 1, 231, 1990.
17. **Harington, J., Miller, K., and McNab, G.,** Hemolysis by asbestos, *Environ. Res.,* 4, 95, 1971.
18. **Vallyathan, V., Schwegler, D., Reasor, M., Stettler, L., and Green, F. H. Y.,** Comparative *in vitro* cytotoxicity and relative pathogenicity of mineral dusts, *Ann. Occul. Hyg.,* 32, 279, 1988.
19. **Emerson, R. J. and Davis, G. S.,** Effect of alveolar lining material-coated silica on rat alveolar macrophages, *Environ. Health Perspect.,* 51, 81, 1983.
20. **Allison, A. C.,** Lysosomes and the toxicity of particulate pollutants, *Arch. Intern. Med.,* 128, 131, 1971.
21. **Hill, C. A.,** Response of macrophages to surfactant coated quartz and kaolin, Ph.D. dissertation, West Virginia University, Morgantown, WV, 1990.
22. **Hill, C. A., Wallace, W. E., Keane, M. J., and Mike, P. S.,** The enzymatic removal of a surfactant coating from quartz and kaolin by P388D1 cells, *Cell Biol. Tox.,* 11, 119, 1995.
23. **Mason, R. J., Nellenbogen, J., and Clements, J. A.,** Isolation of disaturated phosphatidyl choline with osmium tetroxide, *J. Lipid Res.,* 17, 281, 1976.
24. **Das, A. R.,** Visualization of Particle-Macrophage Interactions During Phagocytosis *In Vitro,* Ph.D. dissertation, West Virginia University, Morgantown, WV, 1993.

Section IV
Chapter 2

SUPPRESSION OF SILICA-INDUCED TOXICITY WITH ORGANOSILANE SURFACE COATING

Vincent Castranova, Knox Van Dyke, Lixin Wu, Nar S. Dalal, and Val Vallaythan

CONTENTS

I. STATEMENT OF PROBLEM

Occupational exposure to crystalline silica can result in the development of pulmonary fibrosis. Chronic silicosis can develop over a period of 20–40 years and may progress from simple silicosis to progressive massive fibrosis.[1,2] In simple silicosis, few symptoms are noted and pulmonary function is relatively normal. However, there is radiographic evidence of small rounded opacities in the upper lobes of the lungs. These lesions represent silicotic nodules which consist of collagen arranged in a spiral pattern. As the disease progresses, these opacities become larger and more numerous, and restrictive lung disease may become discernible in pulmonary function tests. On the other hand, acute silicosis can develop rapidly (1–3 years) following inhalation of relatively high levels of silica dust. This acute disease is associated with dyspnea, fatigue, cough, and weight loss and is characterized histologically by alveolar proteinosis and diffuse, rather than nodular, fibrosis.[3]

Cellular injury and tissue damage are believed to be important steps in the development of silicosis.[4] Surface properties of particles play critical roles in the expression of cytotoxicity. Several theories have been advanced to explain the unique cytotoxicity of crystalline silica.

The first theory is that the surface of silica becomes hydrated in the presence of water to form silanol groups (–SiOH). These –SiOH groups are hydrogen donors.[5] In contrast, most biological macromolecules contain lone-pair electrons on oxygen or nitrogen which serve as hydrogen acceptors.[6,7] Therefore, the formation of hydrogen bonds would result in strong interaction between silica and biological membranes. Such interaction would result in loss of membrane integrity, lysosomal enzyme leakage, tissue injury, and lung scarring.[8] Nash et al.[5] suggested that the ability of polyvinylpyridine-*N*-oxide (PVPNO) to suppress the cytotoxicity and fibrogenicity of silica is due to its capacity to serve as a hydrogen acceptor. Indeed, PVPNO by virtue of its terminal oxygens can form strong hydrogen bonds with silanol groups on the surface of crystalline silica, thus preventing interaction with and damage to pneumocyte membranes.

A second theory is that the surface of silica particles is negatively charged. This negative surface charge is demonstrable by the electrophoretic mobility of silica in physiological buffers.[9] Nolan et al.[8] reported that at pH = 7.0 the ratio of –SiOH to $–SiO^-$ groups on the crystalline surface of silica is 30:1. It is proposed that this negative surface charge is a significant contributor to the cytotoxicity of silica.[10]

As predicted, the cytotoxicity of silica is suppressed by the addition of trace metal cations such as Zn^{2+}, Fe^{3+}, or Al^{3+}. Of these metals, Al^{3+} is the most potent inhibitor of silica-induced hemolysis, i.e., decreasing hemolysis by 98% at $AlCl_3$ levels which reduce the zeta potential of silica to 0 mV, while $ZnCl_2$ is least potent.[8] Nolan et al.[8] have also reported that treatment of silica with $AlCl_3$ does not affect the binding of PVPNO, suggesting that Al^{3+} binds specifically to $-SiO^-$ groups while PVPNO binds to –SiOH surface sites. They suggest that the inhibitory action of PVPNO is not due to elimination of the hydrogen binding potential of silica but rather occurs because the PVPNO coating of the particulate surface would be several hundred Angstroms thick, and this coating would make the surface $-SiO^-$ groups inaccessible to pneumocyte membranes.

A third theory addressing the unique cytotoxicity of freshly crushed silica involves the generation of radicals on fresh cleavage planes. Langer[11] reported that crushing crystalline silica increases its cytotoxicity. Indeed, compared to aged silica, freshly ground silica causes greater peroxidation of membrane lipids, is more hemolytic, and elevates the leakage of lactate dehydrogenase from alveolar macrophages.[12] Dalal et al.[13] have demonstrated that crushing crystalline silica under ambient atmosphere breaks Si–O bonds and results in the generation of $\dot{S}i$ and $Si\text{–}\dot{O}$ radicals on the fresh cleavage planes. In aqueous solution, these surface radical sites can react with water to form hydroxyl radicals ($\dot{O}H$).[12–15] The presence of such radicals could explain the increased incidence of acute silicosis in workers, such as sandblasters, rock drillers, and silica mill operators, who are exposed to freshly sheared dust.

II. CHEMISTRY OF ORGANOSILANE COATING AGENTS

From the discussion above, it is clear that surface properties play an important role in the cytotoxicity of silica. Therefore, it has been proposed that application of an organosilane material to the surface of silica particles would decrease their ability to cause lung disease.[16,17] A class of silane coupling agents proposed as protective coatings has the following chemical formula:

$$R'\text{–Si–}(R^3)_3$$

where R' = a lower alkyl, (R^2)-lower alkyl, (lower alkyl) amine, or [(R^2)-lower alkyl] amine group
R^2 = a phenyl, carboxy, amino, amido, mercapto, (amino) lower alkyl, [(amino) lower alkyl] amine, (lower alkylene) carbonyl, or (epoxy) lower alkyl group
R^3 = a hydroxyl or lower alkoxy group

The chemical groups listed are defined as follows:

lower alkyl = alkyl radicals having one to eight carbon atoms
lower alkylene = alkylene radicals having two to eight carbon atoms
(amino) lower alkyl = lower alkyl radical substituted by an amino moiety
[(amino) lower alkyl] amine = [(NH_2)-lower alkyl]-NH-
(lower alkyl) amine = (lower alkyl)-NH-
[(R^2)-lower alkyl] amine = [(R^2)-lower alkyl]-NH-
(epoxy) lower alkyl = lower alkyl radical connected to two adjacent carbon atoms
(lower alkylene) carbonyl = (lower alkylene)-CO-

Common to this class of silane coupling agents is that the R^3 groups are hydroxy or lower alkoxy groups. The lower alkoxy groups are hydrolyzable and form silanol groups as follows:

$$R' - Si - (\text{lower alkoyl})_3 + 3H_2O \longrightarrow R' - Si - (OH)_3 + 3[(OH)\text{lower alkyl}]$$

These silanol groups can interact with the surface of the silica crystal forming Si–O or hydrogen bonds to surface oxygens. In addition, adjacent organosilane molecules could form hydrogen bond cross links, thus coating the silica particle with a film of relatively inert material. Such a reaction is shown in Figure 1.

Prosil 28® is an example of this class of organosilane material. This water-soluble material is produced by PCR Incorporated (Gainesville, FL) and is commonly used to silicanize laboratory glassware, thus preventing cell adhesion. It forms a relatively long-lasting coating on glassware and has proven to be

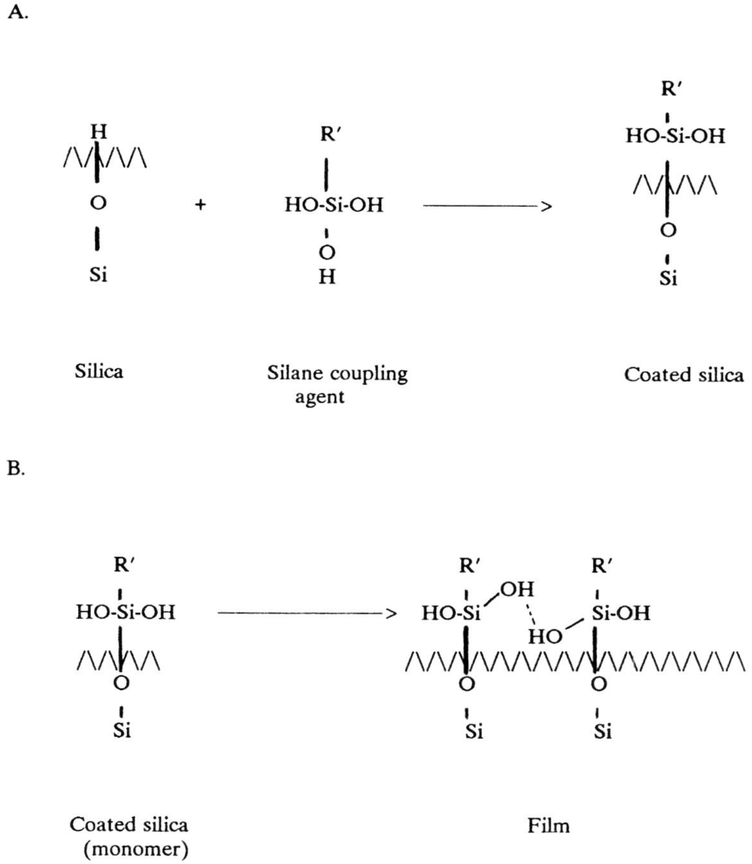

A.

B.

FIGURE 1 Chemical interaction of silane-coupling agents with the surface of crystalline silica.

nontoxic and nonmutagenic to cells in culture.[18] This chapter presents data indicating that Prosil 28® can be used to coat crystalline silica particles and is effective in reducing the cytotoxicity of α-quartz.

III. METHODOLOGY OF COATING APPLICATION

Prosil 28® concentrate is diluted 100:1 (vol:vol) with distilled water and added to silica (2 mg/ml). This suspension is heated at 100°C for 10 min. The suspension is then cooled, centrifuged at 1800 × g for 10 min, and the supernate removed. The coated silica is then washed three times by alternate addition, centrifugation, and aspiration of a buffered solution (145 m*M* NaCl, 5 m*M* KCl, 1 m*M* $CaCl_2$, 10 m*M* HEPES, and 5.5 m*M* glucose; pH = 7.4).

IV. SUPPRESSION OF THE CYTOTOXIC ACTIVITY OF SILICA: *IN VITRO* STUDIES

Coating of silica with Prosil 28® is effective in decreasing the *in vitro* cytotoxicity of this dust.[17] As shown in Figure 2, the lytic potency of silica is significantly suppressed after organosilane coating; i.e., silica-induced hemolysis is decreased by 78% after treatment of the dust with Prosil 28®. Similarly, organosilane coating also reduces silica-induced membrane damage of alveolar macrophages. Data shown in Figure 3 indicate that *in vitro* exposure to uncoated silica decreases membrane integrity of these phagocytes in a time-dependent fashion; i.e., cellular viability is decreased by 17% after a 1-h exposure to silica and by 60% after 5 h. However, coated silica is much less toxic. Indeed, Prosil 28® treatment significantly reduces the cytotoxicity of silica by as much as 73% (5 h silica exposure).

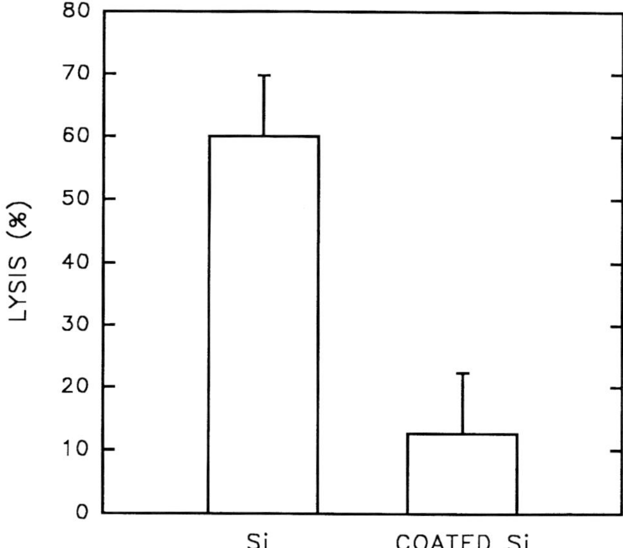

FIGURE 2 Suppression of the hemolytic activity of silica with Prosil 28®. Sheep red blood cells (2% suspension) were exposed to uncoated (Si) or coated silica (10 mg/ml) for 1 h at 37°C and hemoglobin release monitored spectrophotometrically at 540 nm. Data are means ± SE of three experiments.

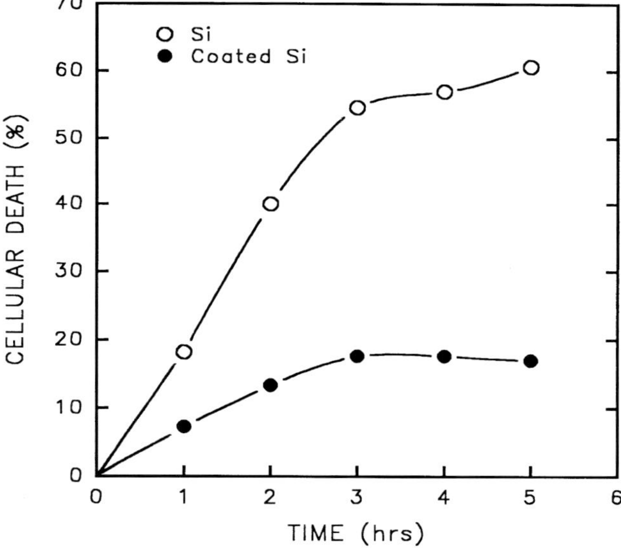

FIGURE 3 Protective effect of Prosil 28® in alveolar macrophages. Alveolar macrophages were obtained by bronchoalveolar lavage of rat lungs. These phagocytes (10^6 cells) were exposed to uncoated (Si) or coated silica (5 mg/ml) for 1–5 h at 37°C. Cell death was determined by monitoring the uptake of a propidium probe using the fluorescence detector of a FAC Scan Flow Cytometer. Propidium uptake indicates loss of membrane integrity. Data are from a single representative experiment.

In addition to preventing the cytotoxic effects of silica, organosilane coating also effectively decreases the ability of silica particles to activate oxidant production by alveolar macrophages. Figure 4 indicates that *in vitro* exposure of alveolar macrophages to uncoated silica results in significant generation of chemiluminescence; i.e., oxidant release is increased by 735%. Coating silica with Prosil 28® signifi-

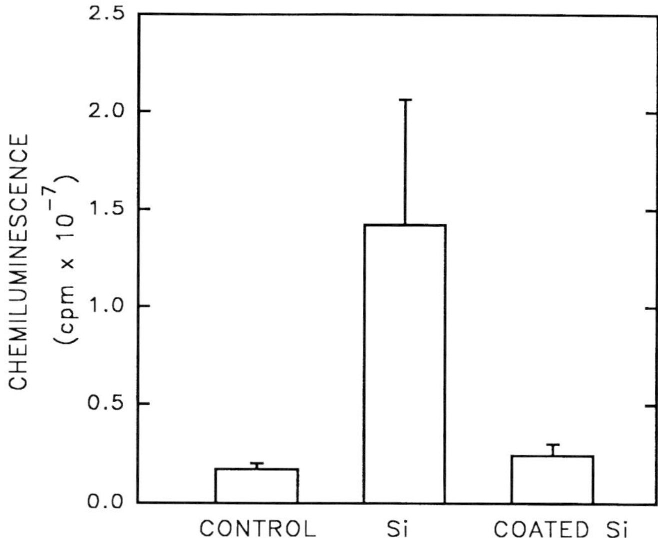

FIGURE 4 Inhibitory effect of a Prosil 28® coating on the ability of silica to activate alveolar macrophages. Rat alveolar macrophages (10^6 cells) were exposed to uncoated (Si) or coated silica (0.5 mg/ml) at 37°C. Activation of oxidant generation was determined by monitoring chemiluminescence in the presence of luminol (2.5×10^{-8} *M*) using a luminometer. Data are means ± SE of three experiments.

cantly reduces this stimulatory potency by 83%. These data suggest that an organosilane coating not only decreases cellular damage caused directly by silica but also decreases oxidant injury due to reactive products secreted from silica-activated phagocytes.

V. SUPPRESSION OF THE CYTOTOXIC ACTIVITY OF SILICA: *IN VIVO* STUDIES

Preliminary data also suggest that coating silica with organosilane materials may reduce the *in vivo* toxicity of α-quartz.[19] Intratracheal instillation of untreated silica results in a decline in the viability of cells harvested by bronchoalveolar lavage, an increase in lavagable acellular protein, elevation of acellular levels of β-glucuronidase, and infiltration of granulocytes into the airspaces. Although more data are needed, results obtained thus far suggest that Prosil 28® treatment of silica tends to decrease these dust-dependent pulmonary reactions. Figure 5 shows that Prosil 28®-coated silica causes slightly less (8%) cell damage to pulmonary phagocytes *in vivo,* measured as the viability of cells lavaged from silica-exposed rats. Another suggestion of less lung damage with coated silica is given in Figure 6. The data indicate that coating decreases protein leakage into the airspaces by 16% compared to native silica. Coated silica is significantly less potent in causing lysosomal enzyme release *in vivo* (Figure 7). This 63% decrease in β-glucuronidase levels in lavage fluid suggests that intratracheally instilled coated silica causes less damage to pulmonary macrophages. Coated silica is also significantly less inflammatory *in vivo;* i.e., silica-induced infiltration of granulocytes into the airspaces is decreased by 35% in rats instilled with Prosil 28®-treated silica compared to untreated silica (Figure 8).

Wiessner et al.[22] have also reported protective effects with chemically coated quartz. The organosilane coatings used in their study were trimethylchlorosilane and 3-aminopropyltriethoxysilane (Figure 9). Although chemically different from Prosil 28®, these compounds can also form Si–O bonds with silanol groups on the silica surface. Comparison of their results from mice six weeks after intratracheal instillation of uncoated or coated silica indicate that coating significantly decreased the *in vivo* toxicity of silica. That is, coated silica was significantly less inflammatory and fibrotic, determined by measuring lung weight and hydroxyproline content, respectively.

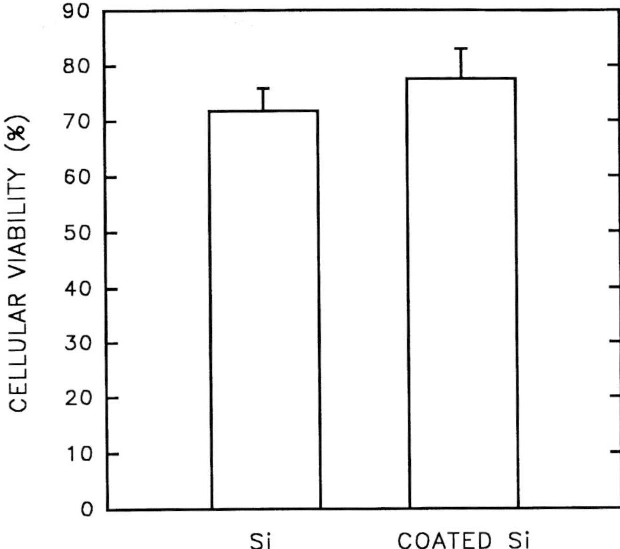

FIGURE 5 Viability of lavaged cells after silica exposure. Rats were exposed to silica by intratracheal instillation of 20 mg of uncoated (Si) or Prosil 28®-coated α-quartz. Cells were obtained by bronchoalveolar lavage 1 d postexposure and viability determined by trypan blue dye exclusion. Data are means ± SE of three experiments.

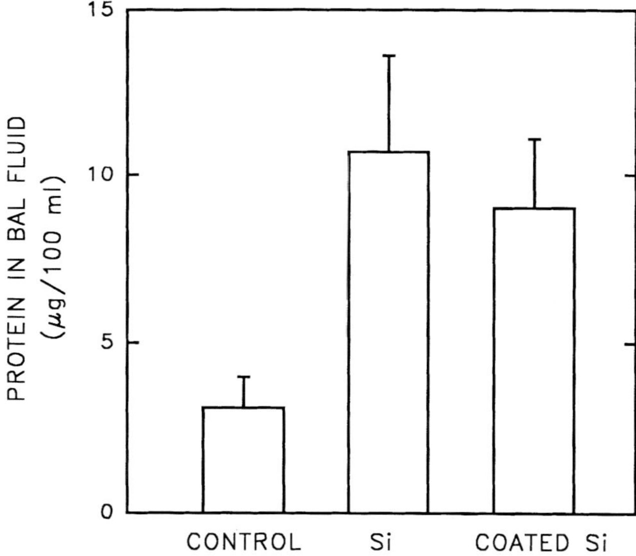

FIGURE 6 Protein leakage after silica exposure. Rats were exposed to silica by intratracheal instillation of 20 mg of uncoated (Si) or Prosil 28®-coated α-quartz. Acellular protein in the bronchoalveolar lavage fluid was measured 1 d postexposure by the method of Lowry et al.[20] Data are means ± SE of three experiments.

VI. PROPOSED PRACTICAL APPLICATION

Organosilane materials such as Prosil 28® are effective in coating silica particles, masking reactive surface sites on this dust, and reducing its toxicity *in vitro. In vivo* data, while preliminary, are supportive of a suppression of cytotoxicity. To pursue this hypothesis, future research should test if it is possible to

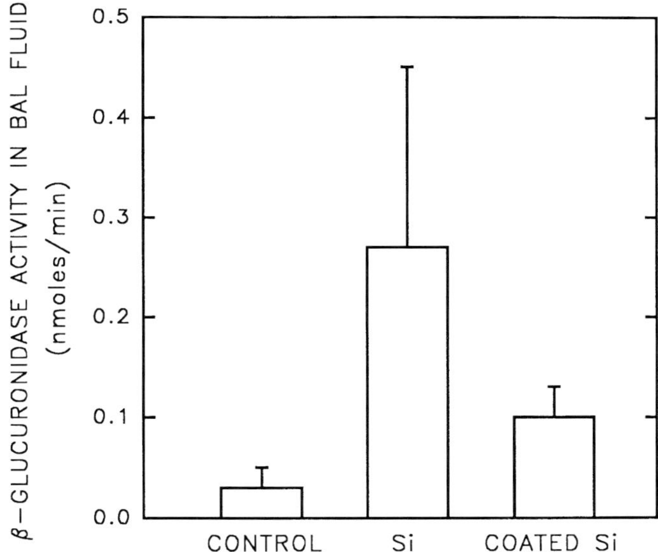

FIGURE 7 Lysosomal enzyme release due to silica exposure. Rats were exposed to silica by intratracheal instillation of 20 mg of uncoated (Si) or Prosil 28®-coated α-quartz. Acellular levels of β-glucuronidase in bronchoalveolar lavage fluid were measured 1 d postexposure by the method of Fishman et al.[21] Data are means ± SE of three experiments.

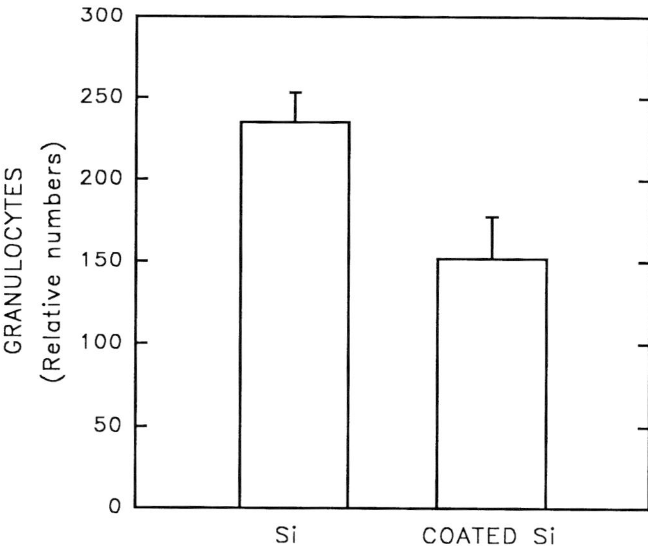

FIGURE 8 Granulocyte influx in silica-exposed lungs. Rats were exposed to silica by intratracheal instillation of 20 mg of uncoated (Si) or Prosil 28®-coated α-quartz. Granulocytes harvested by bronchoalveolar lavage were counted microscopically 1 d postexposure. Data are means ± SE of three experiments.

incorporate organosilane coating agents into water sprays of drill bits or rock grinders, thus coating silica particles as they are generated, and to determine if such treatment would decrease the pathogenic potential of silica dust. In addition, a full evaluation of the potential toxicity of organosilane materials must be conducted in animal models before its commercial use as a coating agent can be considered.

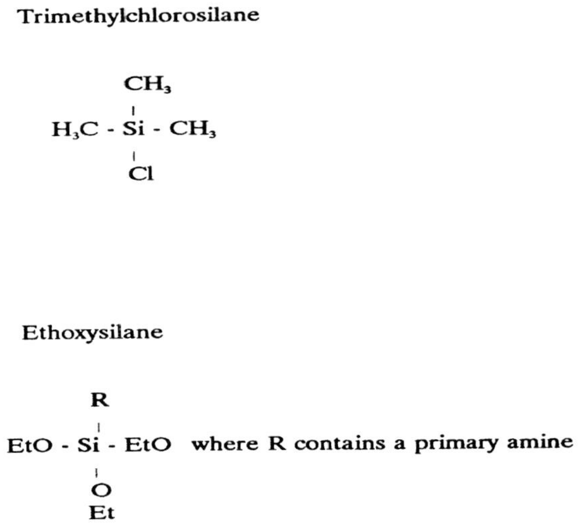

Trimethylchlorosilane

$$H_3C - \underset{\underset{Cl}{|}}{\overset{\overset{CH_3}{|}}{Si}} - CH_3$$

Ethoxysilane

$$EtO - \underset{\underset{\underset{Et}{O}}{|}}{\overset{\overset{R}{|}}{Si}} - EtO$$ **where R contains a primary amine**

FIGURE 9 Chemical formula of organosilane coating materials used by Wiessner et al.[22]

REFERENCES

1. **Ziskind, M., Jones, R. N., and Weill, H.,** Silicosis, *Am. Rev. Respir. Dis.,* 113, 643–65, 1976.
2. **Parkes, W. R.,** *Occupational Lung Disorders,* 2nd ed., Butterworths, Boston, 1982.
3. **Banks, D. E.,** Acute silicosis, in *Occupational Respiratory Diseases,* Merchant, J. A., Boehlecke, B. A., Taylor, G., and Pickett-Harner, M., Eds., DHHS (NIOSH) Publ. No. 86–102, U.S. Government Printing Office, Washington, D.C., 1986, 239–241.
4. **Davis, G. S.,** The pathogenesis of silicosis, *Chest,* 89, 166–169, 1986.
5. **Nash, T., Allison, A. C., and Harington, J. S.,** Physico-chemical properties of silica in relation to its toxicity, *Nature (London),* 210, 259–261, 1966.
6. **Allison, A. C.,** Silicon compounds in biologic systems, *Proc. R. Soc. London Ser. B,* 171, 19–30, 1968.
7. **Stöber, W. and Brieger, H.,** On the theory of silicosis, *Arch. Environ. Health,* 16, 706–708, 1968.
8. **Nolan, R. P., Langer, A. M., Harington, J. S., Oster, G., and Selikoff, I. J.,** Quartz hemolysis as related to its surface functionalities, *Environ. Res.,* 26, 503–520, 1981.
9. **Mehrishi, J. N., and Seamen, G. V. F.,** Temperature dependence of the electrophoretic mobility of cells and quartz particles, *Biochim. Biophys. Acta,* 112, 154–159, 1966.
10. **Stalder, K. and Stöber, W.,** Hemolytic activity of suspension of different silica modification and inert dust, *Nature (London),* 206, 874–875, 1965.
11. **Langer, A. M.,** Crystal faces and cleavage planes in quartz as templates in biological processes, *Q. Rev. Biophys.,* 11, 543–575, 1978.
12. **Vallyathan, V., Shi, X., Dalal, N. S., Irr, W., and Castranova, V.,** Generation of free radicals from freshly fractured silica dust: potential role in acute silica-induced lung injury, *Am. Rev. Respir. Dis.,* 138, 1213–1219, 1988.
13. **Dalal, N. S., Suryan, M. M., Jafari, B., Vallyathan, V., and Green, F. H. Y.,** EPR detection of reactive free radicals in coal and quartz dusts and its implication to pneumoconiosis and silicosis, in *Proc. 1st Int. Symp. on Respirable Dusts in the Mineral Industry,* Ramani, R. V. and Frantz, R., Eds., 1986 24–29, 1986.
14. **Shi, X., Dalal, N. S., and Vallyathan, V.,** ESR evidence for hydroxyl radical generation in aqueous suspension of quartz particles and its possible significance to lipid peroxidation in silicosis, *J. Toxicol. Environ. Health,* 25, 237–245, 1988.
15. **Dalal, N. S., Shi, X., and Vallyathan, V.,** The role of free radicals in the mechanisms of hemolysis and lipid peroxidation by silica: comparative ESR and cytotoxicity studies, *J. Toxicol. Environ. Health,* 29, 307–316, 1990.
16. **Vallyathan, V., Castranova, V., Dalal, N. S., and Van Dyke, K.,** Prevention of the acute cytotoxicity associated with silica containing minerals, U.S. Patent No. 5096733, 1992.
17. **Vallyathan, V., Kang, J. H., Van Dyke, K., Dalal, N. S., and Castranova, V.,** Response of alveolar macrophages to *in vitro* exposure to freshly fractured vs aged silica dust: the ability of Prosil 28, an organosilane material, to coat silica and reduce its biological reactivity, *J. Toxicol. Environ. Health,* 33, 303–315, 1991.
18. PCR Incorporated, Gainesville, FL (personal communications).

19. **Wu, L.,** Intervention of Silica Toxicity Using Inhibition of Lipoxygenase, Thesis, West Virginia University, Morgantown, WV, 1993.
20. **Lowry, O. H., Rosebrough, N. J., Farr, A. L., and Randall, R. J.,** Protein measurement with the folin phenol reagent, *J. Biol. Chem.,* 193, 265–275, 1951.
21. **Fishman, W. H., Kato, K., Anstiss, C. L., and Green, S.,** Human serum β-glucuronidase: its measurement and some of its properties, *Clin. Chim. Acta,* 15, 435–447, 1967.
22. **Wiessner, J. H., Mandel, N. S., Sohnle, P. G., Hasegana, A., and Mandel, G. S.,** The effect of chemical modification of quartz surfaces on particle-induced pulmonary inflammation and fibrosis in the mouse, *Am. Rev. Respir. Dis.,* 141, 111–116, 1990.

Section IV
Chapter 3

SUPPRESSION OF THE CYTOTOXICITY AND FIBROGENICITY OF SILICA WITH PVPNO

Vincent Castranova

CONTENTS

I. INTRODUCTION

The unique cytotoxic potency of crystalline silica has been attributed, in part, to the presence of silanol groups (–SiOH) on the particulate surface.[1] Silanol groups are formed by the hydration of the silica surface in the presence of water. The –SiOH groups are hydrogen donors and can form hydrogen bonds with a wide variety of biological macromolecules which contain hydrogen acceptors, such as oxygen or nitrogen groups with lone-pair electrons.[2,3] Such hydrogen bonding between silica particles and biological membranes has been cited to explain the silica-induced loss of membrane integrity and the resulting leakage of lysosomal enzymes, tissue injury, and lung scarring.[4] The following sequence of events has been proposed to explain the pathogenesis of silica:[5,6]

1. Initially inhaled silica dust is phagocytized by alveolar macrophages.
2. Lysosomes fuse with phagocytic vesicles containing silica.
3. Hydrogen binding between silica particles and the phagolysosome disrupts the vesicle membrane.
4. Released lysosomal enzymes kill the macrophages and cause damage to surrounding lung tissue.
5. Fibrogenic factors are released from alveolar macrophages.
6. Lung scarring results and progresses to fibrosis with continued exposure.

Schlipköter and collaborators[10] postulated that it should be possible to mask these surface –SiOH groups with hydrogen acceptor molecules and that this coated silica would no longer interact strongly with biological membranes. Compounds with such properties include polymers of 2-vinylpyridine-*N*-oxide. The monomeric structure of polyvinylpyridine-*N*-oxide (PVPNO) is given in Figure 1. The O^- group of this compound is a hydrogen acceptor which may interact strongly with –SiOH groups on the surface of α-quartz. The PVPNO polymer, with a chemical formula of $(C_7H_7NO)_n$, might thus coat the surface of silica, theoretically rendering it nontoxic (Figure 2).

PVPNO polymers with molecular weights ranging from 30,000 to 200,000 kDa have been shown to decrease the cytotoxicity of silica.[7] The most thoroughly tested formulation is Bay 3504, P-204 which is produced by Bayer (Germany). This chapter will review data supporting the effectiveness of PVPNO in decreasing the cytotoxicity of silica *in vitro* and its fibrogenicity *in vivo*.

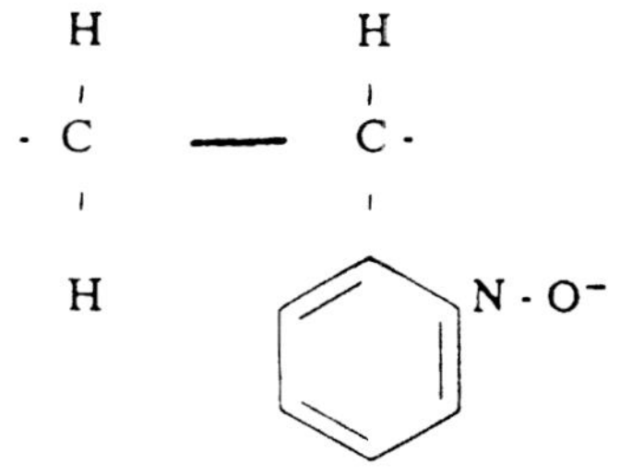

FIGURE 1 Monomeric structure of PVPNO.

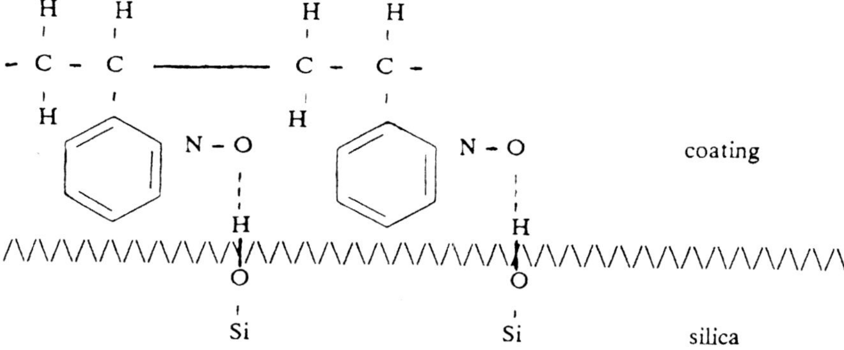

FIGURE 2 A PVPNO coating on silica.

II. SUPPRESSION OF THE CYTOTOXIC ACTIVITY OF SILICA: *IN VITRO* STUDIES

Schlipköter and Brockhaus[8] were the first to report that treating silica with PVPNO significantly depresses its hemolytic potency. The ability of PVPNO to decrease silica-induced lysis of red blood cells has been verified.[4,9] Indeed, as little as 0.7% (w/w) PVPNO is capable of reducing silica-induced hemolysis by 85%. The amount of PVPNO required to detoxify silica is directly proportional to the surface area of the α-quartz particles. This is consistent with the hypothesis that PVPNO acts by forming a protective monolayer on the silica surface. Similarly, treating silica with PVPNO also decreases its ability to lyse L cells in culture.[10]

The ability of silica to damage macrophages and cause enzyme release is thought to play an important role in the development of silicosis.[5] Schlipköter and Beck[11] have shown that PVPNO reduces the toxicity of silica toward macrophages. Such suppression of silica-induced macrophage damage is reported with both crystalline and amorphous silica after PVPNO treatment.[12,13] Indeed, exposure of mouse peritoneal macrophages to silica results in a 44-fold increase in leakage of β-glucuronidase and a 50-fold increase in phosphatase leak 24 h after exposure in culture. Treatment of silica or cells with PVPNO decreases cell death and lysosomal enzyme release by approximately 86%. Microscopic observation of these peritoneal macrophages indicates that PVPNO does not alter the rate of phagocytosis of the silica particles but rather prevents lysis of the phagosomes containing the engulfed silica.[14]

Silica is also a potent stimulator of oxidant production by phagocytic cells. This excess oxidant load is thought to contribute to silica-induced lung damage. Klockars et al.[15] have shown that *in vitro* silica exposure results in the generation of chemiluminescence from polymorphonuclear leukocytes. The induction of chemiluminescence is rapid, peaking 15 min after silica exposure. Treating silica with PVPNO completely inhibits this oxidant production. Half-maximal inhibition occurs with 0.08% PVPNO (w/w of silica), while maximal inhibition occurs at 1% PVPNO. Evidence suggests that the ability of PVPNO to inhibit silica-induced chemiluminescence is due specifically to interaction with the silica particles rather than a nonspecific antioxidant or membrane stabilizing effect, since PVPNO does not affect asbestos-induced chemiluminescence generated by polymorphonuclear leukocytes (PMN).

TABLE 1
***In Vitro* Effects of PVPNO on the Cytotoxicity of Silica**

Protective action	Ref.
↓ Hemolysis	4,8,9
↓ Cytotoxicity toward cultured cells	10
↓ Damage to peritoneal macrophages	11,12–14
↓ Damage to alveolar macrophages	16
↓ Chemiluminescence by PMN	15
↓ Lipoxygenase in alveolar macrophages	16
↑ Cyclooxygenase in alveolar macrophages	16

Englen et al.[16] have reported that silica is highly inflammatory; i.e., it stimulates alveolar macrophage production of inflammatory mediators such as leukotriene B_4 and 5-HETE. These lipoxygenase products cause infiltration of phagocytes into the lung and increase oxidant-induced lung injury. Treating silica with PVPNO not only decreases the cytotoxicity of silica toward macrophages by 70%, but also completely blocks activation of the lipoxygenase pathway of arachidonic acid metabolism while increasing cyclooxygenase products, such as thromboxane and prostaglandin E_2. It is of interest that prostaglandins released from alveolar macrophages have an inhibitory effect on fibroblast proliferation.[17] This suggests another mechanism by which PVPNO may protect the lung from fibrosis.

In conclusion, PVPNO seems to interact with silica to reduce its cytotoxicity. The protective effects of PVPNO treatment are summarized in Table 1. Data suggest that PVPNO may bind strongly to silanol groups on the surface of α-quartz and that this hypothetical coating is not degraded by lysosomal enzyme activity.

III. SUPPRESSION OF THE FIBROGENICITY OF SILICA: ANIMAL MODELS

Schlipköter and colleagues[8,10,18,19] were the first to report that PVPNO administered either by subcutaneous or intravenous injection decreases the pulmonary fibrotic response of rats to intratracheally instilled silica. PVPNO treatment also decreases peritoneal fibrosis resulting from silica injected into the abdominal cavity.[8,20] Along with a decrease in fibrosis, PVPNO treatment increases the clearance of silica and decreases damage to mitochondrial and lysosomal membranes.[21,22]

The antifibrotic action of PVPNO is evidenced by decreases in the following silica-induced parameters: (1) increased lung weight, (2) elevated collagen content, and (3) nodular proliferation.[7,23,24] For example, eight months after an intratracheal exposure to silica, rats treated with PVPNO exhibit 65% lower lung weight, 86% less collagen, and significantly less severe lung pathology changes than silica-exposed rats without PVPNO therapy.[24] PVPNO exhibits significant antifibrotic effects, i.e., lower lung weight, lower lung collagen, and lower pathologic scores for fibrosis, even when administered three weeks prior to or as long as four months after intratracheal exposure to silica.[7]

PVPNO therapy also diminishes a number of other responses to intratracheally instilled silica in rats. PVPNO decreases silica-induced immunological changes, such as increased compliment C_3, elevated circulating immune complexes, and increased susceptibility to histoplasmosis infection.[12,25] Lastly, PVPNO significantly blocks the rise in serum angiotensin-I-converting enzyme in silica-exposed rats.[26]

PVPNO is also effective in protecting animals against the adverse effects of silica administered via inhalation. Subcutaneous injections of PVPNO for six months significantly decreased the fibrotic, lipidotic, and granulomatous reactions of rats to inhalation of silica (20 mg/m^3, 5 d/week, 18 h/d).[27] In addition, PVPNO given by inhalation was also effective in decreasing silica-induced elevations in pulmonary hydroxyproline and phospholipid levels, as well as histological changes.[28] However, Goldstein and Randall[29] suggested the fibrosis would progress after cessation of PVPNO therapy.

A number of animal studies reported no major side effects resulting from PVPNO treatment.[8,10,18,19] However, Cheng et al.[30] reported that chronic subcutaneous administration of PVPNO was associated with abnormal liver morphology and impairment of hepatic function. Furthermore, evidence exists that PVPNO caused cancerous tumor formation at the injection site.[31] Li and Yao[32] have suggested that

TABLE 2
Effects of PVPNO Treatment of Animals on the Pulmonary Responses to Silica

Protective action	Ref.
↓ Lung weight gain	7,23,24
↓ Lipidosis	27,28
↓ Excess collagen content	7,24,29
↓ Excess hydroxyproline levels	23
↑ Clearance of silica	21
↓ Abnormal immune reactions	25
↓ Excess susceptibility to infection	12
↓ Angiotension-I-converting enzyme levels	26
↓ Pathologic score for fibrosis	7,8,10,18–21,23,24,27,29

cytotoxicity may be reduced and excretion increased when PVPNO polymers with molecular weights below 50,000 kDa are used.

In conclusion, PVPNO administration to animals is effective in diminishing adverse pulmonary reactions to silica. The protective effects of PVPNO are summarized in Table 2. PVPNO can be effectively administered subcutaneously, intravenously, or by inhalation. Protective effects are noted when PVPNO is administered prior to, during, or months after silica exposure. However, there is evidence that the protective action of PVPNO is compromised as the period between silica exposure and subsequent PVPNO treatment becomes greater and protection may dissipate with time following discontinuation of the PVPNO therapy. Furthermore, questions have been raised as to adverse effects of PVPNO, such as cirrhosis and tumors.

IV. CLINICAL STUDIES WITH PVPNO

A number of clinical studies have suggested that PVPNO may exert a positive therapeutic action in workers with various degrees of silicosis. Schlipköter and colleagues[33] reported that PVPNO given intravenously reduced reported symptoms in miners and stone cutters. Similarly, complaints of cough, shortness of breath, and chest pain decreased in miners, tunnelers, and foundry workers treated with aerosols of PVPNO.[34] Furthermore, pulmonary function tests improved in 74% of these treated patients. In a large clinical trial in China, PVPNO therapy for 1 to 2 years reduced reports of chest pain (↓ 63%), cough (↓ 58%), shortness of breath (↓ 60%), and anorexia (↓ 61%).[35] In addition, a decrease in frequency of upper respiratory infections was reported. However, in this study pulmonary function did not improve. Unfortunately, a problem common to these studies is that they were not blinded and did not have the proper control groups. Therefore, the reported subjective improvements are subject to a placebo effect.

Zhao et al.[36] were the first to report effects of PVPNO on the radiographic progression of silicosis. Several studies (evaluating chest X-rays as improved, stationary, or progressed in silicotic patients after a 1 to 2 year course of PVPNO administered either intramuscularly or by inhalation) found that between 45 and 78% of the treated patients were classified as stationary.[7,24,35] In contrast, the majority of untreated silicotic patients in these studies exhibited progression of radiographic abnormality over this time. Two problems in these studies are that treatment and control groups may not have been matched properly for severity of disease and that the quality of the radiographs and readers was not strictly controlled. In addition, it must be noted that discontinuation of PVPNO administration leads to renewed progression of silicosis monitored by chest radiographs.[35,36]

Adverse side effects of PVPNO therapy have not been reported in any of the above studies.[33,34] No significant changes in blood enzyme levels have been reported,[28] and no increase in tumors or cancer have been found in these human trials.[28,37]

V. SUMMARY

In summary, PVPNO has been shown *in vitro* to decrease the cytotoxic effects of silica. This action is thought to be due to the ability of PVPNO to strongly bind to surface silanol groups on α-quartz.

Treatment of animals with PVPNO appears to prevent the onset or progression of silicosis. Reports suggest that PVPNO is effective when administered subcutaneously, intramuscularly, intravenously, or by inhalation. However, fibrosis progresses upon cessation of treatment. Clinical trials, while promising, have generally not been sufficiently controlled. Finally, the report that PVPNO was associated with tumors and hepatic damage is a serious concern.

REFERENCES

1. **Nash, T., Allison, A. C., and Harington, J. S.,** Physio-chemical properties of silica in relation to its toxicity, *Nature (London),* 210, 259–261, 1966.
2. **Allison, A. C.,** Silica compounds in biologic systems, *Proc. R. Soc. London, Ser. B,* 171, 19–30, 1968.
3. **Stöber, W. and Brieger, H.,** On the theory of silicosis, *Arch. Environ. Health,* 16, 706–708, 1968.
4. **Nolan, R. P., Langer, A. M., Harington, J. S., Oster, G., and Selikoff, I. J.,** Quartz hemolysis as related to its surface functionalities, *Environ. Res.,* 26, 503–520, 1981.
5. **Heppleston, A. G.,** Silicotic fibrogenesis: a concept of pulmonary fibrosis, *Ann. Occup. Hyg.,* 26, 449–462, 1982.
6. **Heppleston, A. G. and Styles, J. A.,** Activity of a macrophage factor in collagen formation by silica, *Nature (London),* 214, 521–522, 1967.
7. **Lu, S., and Ding, M. B.,** Recent advances in the treatment of selected pneumoconiosis: a report from China, in *Control of Pneumoconiosis (Prevention, Early Diagnosis, and Treatment),* World Health Organization/OCH/90.1, Annex 4, 1990, 1–21.
8. **Schlipköter, H. W., and Brockhaus, A.,** Die hemmung der experimentellen silikase durch subcutane verabreichung von poly vinyl pyridin-N-oxide, *Klin. Wochenschr.,* 39, 1182, 1189, 1961.
9. **Stalder, K., and Stöber, W.,** Hemolytic activity of suspensions of different silica modifications and inert dust, *Nature (London),* 207, 874–875, 1965.
10. **Schlipköter, H. W., Dolgner, R., and Brockhaus, A.,** The treatment of experimental silicosis, *Ger. Med. Monthly,* 8, 509–516, 1963.
11. **Schlipköter, H. W., and Beck, E. G.,** Observations on the relationship between quartz cytotoxicity and fibrogenicity while testing the biological activity of synthetic polymers, *Med. Lav.,* 56, 458–493, 1965.
12. **Von Behren, L. A., Chaudhary, S., Rabinovich, S., Shu, M. D., and Tewari, R. P.,** Protective effect of poly-2-vinyl pyridine-N-oxide on susceptibility of silica-treated mice to experimental histoplasmosis, *Infect. Immun.,* 42, 818–823, 1983.
13. **Davies, R., Griffiths, D. M., Johnson, N. F., Preece, A. W., and Livingston, D. C.,** The cytotoxicity of kaolin towards macrophages *in vitro, Br. J. Exp. Pathol.,* 65, 453–466, 1984.
14. **Allison, A. C., Harington, J. S., and Birbeck, M.,** An examination of the cytotoxic effects of silica on macrophages, *J. Exp. Med.,* 124, 141–154, 1966.
15. **Klockars, M., Hedenborg, M., and Vanhala, E.,** Effect of two particle surface-modifying agents, polyvinylpyridine-N-oxide and carboxymethyl cellulose, on the quartz and asbestos mineral fiber-induced production of reactive oxygen metabolites by human polymorphonuclear leukocytes, *Arch. Environ. Health,* 45, 8–14, 1990.
16. **Englen, M. D., Taylor, S. M., Laegreid, W. W., Silflow, R. M., and Leid, R. W.,** Diminished arachidonic acid metabolite release by bovine alveolar macrophages exposed to surface-modified silica, *Am. J. Respir. Cell Biol.,* 6, 527–534, 1992.
17. **Reist, R. H.,** Cytokine and Pharmacological Regulation of Lung Fibroblast Proliferation, Dissertation, West Virginia University, Morgantown, WV, 1992.
18. **Schlipköter, H. W., and Brockhaus, A.,** The action of polyvinylpyridine on experimental silicosis, *Dtsch. Med. Wochenschr.,* 85, 920–923, 1960.
19. **Schlipköter, H. W.,** Neue therapeutische möglichkeiten bei staublungenerkran kungen, *Zentralbl. Arbeitsmed. Arbeitsschutz,* 16, 221–226, 1966.
20. **Schlipköter, H. W.,** Silicosis-inhibiting substances, *Med. Lav.,* 54, 405–412, 1963.
21. **Golodnikov, Y. N.,** Experimental silicosis induced by extra-pure crystalline silicon dust and the effect of polyvinyl-pyridine-N-oxide on its evolution, *Gig. Tr. Prof. Zabol.,* 12, 21–26, 1978.
22. **Shnaydman, I. M.,** Possible methods of affecting the sclerosis mechanisms in experimental silicosis, *Byull. Eksp. Biol. Med.,* 75, 27–30, 1973.
23. **Idel, H.,** Therapeutic effects of polyvinylpyridine-N-oxide and tetrandrine in experimental silicosis, *Inst. Nat. Sante Rech. Med.,* 155, 471–477, 1987.
24. **Hu, T. and Li, Q.,** Studies of therapeutic effects of drugs on silicosis, in *Proc. Int. Symp. on Pneumoconioses* Li, Y., Yao, P., Schlipköter, H. W., Idel, H., and Rosenbruch, M., Eds., Stefan W. Albers Verlag, Düsseldorf, 1990, 269–272.

25. **Idel, H.,** Silicosis and immunomodulation effects of antisilicotic treatment, in *Proc. Int. Symp. on Pneumoconioses,* Li, Y., Yao, P., Schlipköter, H. W., Idel, H., and Rosenbruch, M., Eds., Stefan W. Albers Verlag, Düsseldorf, 1990, 273–275.
26. **Lin, J.,** Studies on serum angiotensin-I-converting enzyme activity of experimental silicosis in rats, *Chung Hua Yu Fang I Hsuch Tsa Chih,* 24, 274–276, 1990.
27. **Heppleston, A. G.,** Determinants of pulmonary fibrosis and lipidosis in the silica models, *Br. J. Exp. Pathol.,* 67, 879–888, 1986.
28. **Sklensky, B.,** Polyvinylpyridine-N-oxide and treatment of silicosis in steel casting cleaners, in *Proc. Int. Symp. on Pneumoconioses,* Li, Y., Yao, P., Schlipköter, H. W., Idel, H., and Rosenbruch, M., Eds., Stefan W. Albers Verlag, Düsseldorf, 1990, 292–295.
29. **Goldstein, B. and Randall, R. E. G.,** The prophylactic use of polyvinylpyridine-N-oxide (PVPNO) in baboons exposed to quartz dust, *Environ. Res.,* 42, 469–481, 1987.
30. **Cheng, Y. H., Han, S. I., and Zhang, Z. L.,** Studies of the therapeutic effect of Kexiping on silicosis, in *Proc. Ther. Effect of Kexiping on Silicosis,* CAPM Press, Institute of Occupational Medicine, Beijing, China, 1970, 40–45.
31. **Schmadl, D.,** Prufung von polyvinylpyridine-N-oxide auf die carcinogene wirkung bei ratten und mausen, *Arzneim. Forsch.,* 19, 1313–1314, 1969.
32. **Li, Y. R. and Yao, P. P.,** Studies of the absorption, distribution, and excretion of PVNO-^{14}C, in *Proc. Ther. Effect of Kexiping on Silicosis,* CAPM Press, Institute of Occupational Medicine, Beijing, China, 1970, 143–156.
33. **Prügger, F., Mallner, B., and Schlipköter, H. W.,** Polyvinylpyridine-N-oxide (Bay 3504, p-204, PVNO) in the treatment of human silicosis, *Wien. Klin. Wochenschr.,* 96, 848–853, 1984.
34. **Burilkov, T.,** Inhalatory treatment of silicosis with PVNO, in *Proc Int. Symp. on Pneumoconioses,* Li, Y., Yao, P., Schlipköter, H. W., Idel, H., and Rosenbruch, M., Eds., Stefan W. Albers Verlag, Düsseldorf, 1990, 251–255.
35. **Lu, Y. R. and Lu, S. X.,** Therapeutic effect of PVNO in clinical silicosis, from Institute of Health, China National Center for Preventive Medicine, Beijing, China (personal communication).
36. **Zhao, J. D., Liu, J. D., and Li, G. Z.,** Long term follow-up observations of the therapeutic effect of PVNO on human silicosis, *Zentralbl. Bakteriol. Mikrobiol. Hyg.,* 178, 259–262, 1983.
37. **Schlipköter, H. W.,** The aetiology and pathogenesis of silicosis and its causal prophylaxis and treatment, *Natur Ingenieur Gesellschaftswissenschaften,* 197, 39–105, 1970.

Section IV
Chapter 4

MODULATION OF QUARTZ TOXICITY BY ALUMINUM

Geraldine M. Brown and Kenneth Donaldson

CONTENTS

I. MECHANISMS OF QUARTZ TOXICITY

The biological activity of silica, the most common form of which is α-quartz, is related to interactions between the surface of quartz particles and cells,[1] leading to cell damage[2] or cell activation.[3] Although the precise mechanisms are not yet fully elucidated, these quartz/cell interactions are believed to contribute, in the long term, to the tissue derangements which result from chronic inhalation of quartz in its pure form or in mixed dusts, both in man and in experimental animal models. Substances such as aluminum which can bind to the quartz particles and so reduce the reactivity of the quartz surface are therefore of potential importance in limiting quartz toxicity. This has implications for both hazard assessment of mixed dusts containing quartz and aluminum and for therapeutic intervention following silica inhalation.

II. MODIFICATION OF THE QUARTZ SURFACE BY ALUMINUM

Modification of the quartz surface by reaction with aluminum was first indicated in the study of Denny et al.,[4] who observed reduction in the solubility of quartz in the presence of metallic aluminum powder. Reduced solubility of quartz was also shown by Dale and Kings[5] using aluminum chloride solution and, indirectly, by Ulmer,[6] who demonstrated markedly enhanced particle agglomeration following the addition of aluminum to a suspension of quartz. Other indicators of quartz surface activity which have been modified by treatment with aluminum are electron diffraction[7] and zeta potential.[8]

The foregoing studies provided circumstantial evidence that quartz particles could be coated with aluminum. The first actual demonstration of aluminum on the quartz surface was that of Bremner,[9] who

0-8493-4709-2/96/$0.00+$.50

stained the aluminum with aurintricarboxylate. The use of X-ray photoelectron spectrophotoscopy also demonstrated that aluminum strongly bonded to the quartz surface by means of an oxygen bridge[10] and, more recently, Wallace et al.[11] demonstrated an aluminosilicate coating on the surface of quartz particles using energy dispersive X-ray analysis.

III. REDUCTION OF QUARTZ BIOACTIVITY BY ALUMINUM

A. FIBROTIC RESPONSE

The first evidence that aluminum could reduce the toxicity of quartz particles was provided in work by Denny et al.[12] who demonstrated that concomitant inhalation of quartz and aluminum powder resulted in reduced lung fibrosis in rabbits. These results were questioned when experiments by Belt and King[13] failed to show a protective effect of aluminum on quartz toxicity in experiments where the dust was administered by intratracheal injection. However, the same authors did subsequently demonstrate an ameliorative effect of aluminum powder on quartz toxicity[14,15] using a more physiological exposure regimen where rats were exposed to aerosols of the two minerals. Between 1950 and the late 1960s further experimental studies were carried out in America and Europe investigating interactions between quartz and diverse forms of aluminum such as metallic aluminum, aluminum hydroxide, aluminum chloride, and aluminum chlorhydroxyallantoinate (reviewed in Reference 16). These studies demonstrated conclusively that the development of quartz-induced lung damage, measured as the number and severity of fibrotic lesions, altered lung weight or increased amounts of collagen per lung, in rats, guinea pigs, and rabbits, could be reduced and in some cases eliminated entirely by simultaneous treatment with aluminum.

B. BRONCHOALVEOLAR INFLAMMATORY RESPONSE

Evaluation of the mechanisms involved in the modulation of quartz toxicity by aluminum have been facilitated in recent years by the introduction of bronchoalveolar lavage as a research tool. This has enabled quantification of the inflammatory response in the airspaces of lungs exposed to quartz and so has permitted more detailed analysis of how aluminum acts to reduce quartz toxicity. The first work investigating the bronchoalveolar response to aluminum-coated quartz was reported by Begin et al.[17] using a soluble form of aluminum, aluminum lactate. Native quartz and aluminum-coated quartz were administered to sheep by intratracheal injection, and the lung response was assessed over a period of 60 d. The coated quartz elicited a markedly reduced influx of inflammatory leukocytes into the bronchoalveolar space; biochemical markers of inflammation in the lavage fluid, which increased in response to untreated quartz, were also less in the sheep treated with aluminum-coated quartz. The protective effect of aluminum in the sheep model persisted for up to 10 months and was associated with increased clearance of quartz from the lung.[18] Further studies in sheep[19,20] and in rats[21] demonstrated that the inflammatory response to quartz in the lung could be ameliorated even when the aluminum was administered substantially later than the quartz and the inflammatory response was well established. It was notable that there was no suppressive effect of aluminum on the lung response to a bacterial challenge.[21] Thus the suppressive effect of late administration of aluminum on the quartz alveolitis was deemed to be due to interaction of aluminum with quartz particles either following uptake of aluminum into the phagolysosome of live macrophages containing quartz particles or extracellularly when quartz was released by dead macrophages.

C. *IN VITRO* BIOACTIVITY

The mechanisms whereby the pathogenicity of quartz is ameliorated by aluminum have been addressed in a number of studies which investigated specific aspects of quartz bioactivity. In one study, inhibition of the cytochrome C-oxidase system of lung homogenates by silicic acid was suppressed by aluminum chloride.[22] Nolan et al.[8] demonstrated a link between particle surface charge and bioactivity by the observation that change in zeta potential was correlated with a reduced interaction with red blood cells (RBC). There was a concomitant reduction in hemolysis of the RBC, possibly due to the binding of aluminum to ionized silanol groups on the quartz surface which are thought to be involved in the interaction between quartz particles and components of cell membranes.[8]

Specific effects of aluminum on quartz:cell membrane interactions were recently demonstrated by Cao et al.[23] who showed that membrane dehydration in rabbit erythrocytes exposed to quartz was reduced by coating the quartz with aluminum; this was associated with a reduction in the quartz-mediated membrane fluidity and permeability of guinea pig macrophages by aluminum-coated quartz. Further studies by Cao et al.[24] demonstrated conformational changes, measured by Raman spectroscopy, in membrane phospholipids of liposomes exposed to quartz, which were blocked by coating the quartz with aluminum. Thus, the protective effect of aluminum is likely to be related to its ability to reduce the interaction between quartz particles and lipid components of the cell membrane. This may account for the reduced phagocytosis by rat macrophages of aluminum-coated, compared with native quartz particles.[6] It does not, however, explain the increased pulmonary clearance of aluminum-coated quartz reported by Begin et al.[18] and others.[16]

Two key aspects of quartz bioactivity relevant to the development of silicotic lung disease, cytotoxicity, and cell activation have also been investigated *in vitro* and shown to be modified by aluminum. The cytotoxic effect of quartz on guinea pig macrophages was reduced.[23,25] This was related, in rat macrophages, to the concentration of aluminum on the quartz surface as measured by electron spectroscopy for chemical analysis (ESCA) and by Auger spectroscopy.[26] The suppressive effects of aluminum on quartz-mediated lung inflammation and fibrosis may be related to changes in the type of inflammatory mediator secreted by macrophages following phagocytosis of native and aluminum-coated quartz. Englen et al.[27] demonstrated a shift in the type of arachidonic acid product secreted by bovine macrophages exposed *in vitro* to DQ12 quartz. Native quartz caused release of lipoxygenase products, while aluminum-coated quartz caused release of cyclooxygenase products. Effects of aluminum-coating of quartz on the secretion of other inflammatory mediators by macrophages have not yet been assessed.

IV. ASSESSMENT OF QUARTZ TOXICITY IN MIXED DUSTS CONTAINING QUARTZ

The interest in effects of aluminum on the toxicity of quartz in mixed dusts was initiated, in part, by the demonstration that aluminum could be leached from rock dusts and could subsequently coat quartz particles, thus reducing their solubility.[9] On the basis of these findings he postulated that the toxicity of quartz in mixed dusts, such as coal mine dusts containing aluminum-bearing minerals, might be less than predicted for quartz alone due to coating of the quartz by aluminum.

Epidemiological studies of coal miners in Britain substantiate the notion that the harmfulness of a mixed dust containing quartz is not simply related to the quartz content of the dust. While important colliery-related differences between exposure to respirable dust and prevalence of pneumoconiosis have been demonstrated,[28] these are not always related to differences in the quartz content of the coal mine dust. Walton et al.[28] speculated that the presence of other mineral components of the respirable dust cloud (possibly aluminum-bearing clays) could perhaps lessen the impact of the toxic effects of the quartz. In some instances, however, the quartz content of a coal mine dust has had a strong bearing on the harmfulness of that dust.[29,30] These studies suggest that when the quartz content of a mixed dust is sufficiently high (above around 10%), then its toxicity is no longer masked by other minerals in the dust.

A number of experimental studies have demonstrated that coal mine dust and its components could indeed reduce the pathogenic effects of quartz.[31,32] The work of Martin et al.,[33] however, suggested that the protective effect of aluminum may be transient and that, unless there is continual replacement of the aluminum, the fibrotic effect of the quartz will eventually be expressed. Martin's work is in contradiction with that of Begin et al.[18] and Policard et al.,[16] who reported increased quartz clearance from the lung and hence, presumably, reduced quartz toxicity in the presence of aluminum.

V. ALUMINOTHERAPY IN HUMAN SUBJECTS

The use of aluminum inhalation in humans for the treatment of established silicosis was implemented in Canada very soon after the initial reports of success in animal studies. Improved lung function was subsequently reported in patients treated with metallic aluminum[34–36] and hydrated alumina.[37] However, these studies, for the most part, did not control for a possible placebo effect by using mock dust inhalation, and later work showed that improvements in both subjective and objective lung function were similar in silicotics and pneumoconiotics subdivided randomly into treatment and placebo groups.[38] Between the years 1945 and 1979, aluminum powder inhalation was used as prophylaxis against silicosis in the gold mining industry of Ontario.[39] The effect of this treatment resulted in a decrease in the incidence of new cases exhibiting the first radiological signs of silicosis following implementation of aluminum therapy in 1944/45. The summary indicated that there were no ill effects due to aluminum inhalation and that not a single case of silicosis was found where exposure to silica and aluminum treatment was concurrent. Nevertheless, the report concluded that aluminum therapy was not a substitute for sound dust control and that reducing dust levels in mines was a preferable method of disease reduction. Despite this, aluminum therapy continued to be used and later studies again indicated that aluminum treatment could be beneficial in prophylaxis or in the treatment of early lesions of pneumoconiosis,[40] although it did not affect established lesions.[41]

VI. HARMFUL EFFECTS OF ALUMINUM

The benefits of using aluminum therapy in the prophylaxis of silicosis or mixed dust pneumoconiosis must be balanced with the health risks associated with aluminum exposure. Experimental studies have demonstrated toxic effects of aluminum powder in the lungs of rats[15,42] and hamsters.[43] The major limitation of these studies was that the dusts were administered, at high doses, by intratracheal instillation. However, pulmonary aluminosis was also described in humans exposed to aluminum pyrotechnic flake,[44] finely powdered aluminum,[45,46] and, possibly, aluminum fibers.[47]

In addition to lung toxicity, aluminum powder affects cognitive test performance,[48] and there are now fears that aluminum exposure may contribute to the development of Alzheimer's disease.[49]

VII. SUMMARY

From *in vitro* work with quartz and isolated cells, it appears that the well-documented protective effect of aluminum may be mediated by its ability to bind to the surface of quartz particles, probably by interaction with ionized silanol groups on the quartz surface. This in turn attenuates the interaction between quartz particles and components of the cell membrane, thus ameliorating the cytotoxic and/or stimulatory effects of the quartz and therefore preventing the inflammatory and, ultimately, the fibrotic response in the lung. *In vivo* experiments have confirmed the decreased pathogenicity of aluminum-treated quartz. In addition, it has been demonstrated that late treatment with aluminum lactate can reduce the evidence of toxicity to a previous quartz exposure.

This implies that there might be a potential for therapeutic intervention in situations where quartz exposure has been substantial and no alternative therapy exists. However, the risk of neurotoxic effects of aluminum should still preclude the use of prophylactic aluminotherapy except in cases such as acute progressive silicosis with its otherwise bleak prognosis. The controversy over the duration of the protective effect of aluminum suggests that, in such cases, prolonged treatment with aluminum postexposure might be necessary to prevent recurrence of quartz toxicity. Thus the use of aluminum treatment, with its attendant risks, should never replace the imperative of reducing quartz exposure in the workplace.

The presence of aluminum-bearing clays in mixed dusts containing quartz may have a bearing on the predicted toxicity of that dust and should therefore be considered in setting limits for occupational exposure levels. However, the long-term protective effect of aluminum on silicosis is not known, thus complicating hazard assessment in the workplace. In addition, in certain situations the quartz content of a mixed dust, if sufficiently high, can contribute substantially to the harmfulness of that dust, despite the presence of aluminum-bearing minerals.

REFERENCES

1. **Weissner, J. H., Mandel, N. S., Sohnle, P. G., Hasegawa, A., and Mandel, G. S.,** The effect of chemical modification of quartz surfaces on particulate-induced pulmonary inflammation and fibrosis in the mouse, *Am. Rev. Respir. Dis.,* 141, 111–116, 1990.
2. **Donaldson, K. and Brown, G. M.,** Assessment of mineral dust cytotoxicity towards rat alveolar macrophages using a ^{51}Cr release assay, *Fund. Appl. Toxicol.,* 10, 365–366, 1988.

3. **Kusaka, Y., Brown, G. M., and Donaldson, K.,** Alveolitis caused by exposure to coal mine dusts: production of interleukin-1 and immunomodulation by bronchoalveolar leukocytes, *Environ. Res.,* 53, 76–89, 1990.
4. **Denny, J. J., Robson, W. D., and Irwin, D. A.,** The prevention of silicosis by metallic aluminum: first paper, *Can. Med. Assoc. J.,* 37, 1–8, 1937.
5. **Dale, J. C. and King, E. J.,** Adsorption of dyes, amino acids, proteins and metal hydroxides on quartz, *Indust. Hyg. Occup. Med.,* 55, 83–88, 1952.
6. **Ulmer, W. T.,** Prophylaxis of silicosis by aluminum — preliminary report on experimental investigations, *Ind. Med. Surg.,* 33, 52–56, 1964.
7. **Le Bouffant, L., Daniel-Moussard, H., Martin, J. C., Letort, M., and Policard, A.,** Etude du mecanisme de l'action inhibitrice des charbons vis-a-vis des effets fibrogenes du quartz, *C.R. Acad. Sci. Paris,* 267, 1879–1882, 1968.
8. **Nolan, R. P., Langer, A. M., Harrington, J. S., Oster, G., and Selikoff, I. J.,** Quartz hemolysis as related to its surface functionalities, *Environ. Res.,* 26, 503–520, 1981.
9. **Bremner, F.,** Antidotal rocks and silicosis, *Can. Min. J.,* 60, 589–595, 1939.
10. **Czernichowski, M., Erre, R., and Van Damme, H.,** Etude de la liason quartz-aluminum par spectroscopie ESCA in silicosis and mixed-dusts pneumoconiosis, Le Bouffant, L., Eds., *Colloque Inserm,* 155, 289–294, 1987.
11. **Wallace, W. E., Harrison, J., Keane, M. J., Bolsaitis, P., Eppelsheimer, D., Poston, J., and Page, S. J.,** Clay occlusion of respirable quartz particles detected by low voltage scanning electron microscopy-X-ray analysis, *Ann. Occup. Hyg.,* 34, 195–204, 1990.
12. **Denny, J. J., Robson, W. D., and Irwin, D. A.,** The prevention of silicosis by metallic aluminum: second paper, *Ind. Med.,* 8, 133–146, 1939.
13. **Belt, T. and King, E. J.,** Failure of aluminum to prevent experimental silicosis, *J. Pathol.,* 55, 69–73, 1943.
14. **King, E. J., Wright, B. M., Ray, S. C., and Harrison, C. V.,** Effect of aluminum on the silicosis-producing action of inhaled quartz, *Br. J. Ind. Med.,* 7, 27–36, 1950.
15. **King, E. J., Harrison, C. V., and Mohanty, G. P.,** The effect of aluminum and of aluminum containing 5 percent of quartz in the lungs of rats, 75, 429–434, 1958.
16. **Policard, A., Letort, M., Charbonnier, J., Daniel-Moussard, H., Martin, J. C., and Le Bouffant, L.,** Recherches experimentales concernant l'inhibition de l'action cytotoxique du quartz au moyen de substances minerales, notamment de composes de l'aluminum, *Beitr. Silikose-Forsch.,* 23, 3–57, 1971.
17. **Begin, R., Masse, S., Rola-Pleszynski, M., Martel, M., Desmarais, Y., Geoffroy, M., Le Bouffant, L., Daniel, H., and Martin, J.,** Aluminum lactate treatment alters the lung biological activity of quartz, *Exp. Lung Res.,* 10, 385–399, 1986.
18. **Begin, R., Masse, S., Sebastien, P., Martel, M., Bosse, J., Dubois, F., Geoffroy, M., and Labbe, J.,** Sustained efficacy of aluminum to reduce quartz toxicity in the lung, *Exp. Lung Res.,* 13, 205–222, 1987.
19. **Begin, R., Masse, S., Sebastien, P., Martel, M., Geoffroy, M., and Labbe, J.,** Late aluminum therapy reduces the cellular activities of simple silicosis in the sheep model, *J. Leuk. Biol.,* 41, 400–406, 1987.
20. **Dubois, F., Begin, R., Cantin, A., Masse, S., Martel, M., Bilodeau, G., Dufresne, A., Perreault, G., and Sebastien, P.,** Aluminum inhalation reduces silicosis in a sheep model, *Am. Rev. Respir. Dis.,* 137, 1172–1179, 1988.
21. **Brown, G. M., Donaldson, K., and Brown, D. M.,** Bronchoalveolar leukocyte responses in experimental silicosis: modulation by a soluble aluminum compound, *Toxicol. Appl. Pharmacol.,* 101, 95–105, 1989.
22. **Engelbrecht, F. M. and Jordan, M. E.,** The influence of silica and aluminum on the cytochrome c-oxidase activity of rat lung homogenate, *S. Afr. Med. J.,* 46, 769–771, 1972.
23. **Cao, C. J., Liu, S. J., and Lin, K. C.,** The injurious effect of quartz on cell membranes and the preventive effect of aluminum citrate against quartz, in Proc. VIIth Int. Pneumoconiosis Conference, Part II. Pittsburgh, DHHS (NIOSHH) Publ. No. 90–108, II, 947–953, 1990.
24. **Cao, C. J., Liu, S. J., and Lin, K. C.,** Raman spectroscopic studies on the mechanisms of membrane damage induced by quartz and the protective effect of aluminum citrate, in Proc. VIIth Int. Pneumoconiosis Conference, Part II. Pittsburgh, DHHS (NIOSHH) Publ. No. 90–108, II, 1181–1185, 1990.
25. **Marks, J., Mason, M. A., and Nagelschmidt, G.,** A study of dust toxicity using a quantitative tissue culture technique, *Br. J. Ind. Med.,* 13, 187–191, 1956.
26. **Kreigseis, W., Scharmann, A., and Serafin, J.,** Investigations of surface properties of silica dusts with regard to their cytotoxicity, *Ann. Occup. Hyg.,* 31, 417–427, 1987.
27. **Englen, M. D., Taylor, S. M., Laegreid, W. W., Silflow, R. M., and Leid, R. W.,** Diminished arachadonic acid release by bovine alveolar macrophages exposed to surface-modified silica, *Am. J. Respir. Cell Mol. Biol.,* 6, 527–534, 1992.
28. **Walton, W. H., Dodgson, J., Hadden, G. G., and Jacobsen, M.,** The effect of quartz and other non-coal dusts in coalworker's pneumoconiosis. 1. Epidemiological studies, in *Inhaled Particles,* IV, Walton, W. H., Ed., Pergamon Press, Oxford, 1977, 669–690.
29. **Seaton, A., Dick, J. A., Dodgson, J., and Jacobsen, M.,** Quartz and pneumoconiosis in coal miners, *Lancet,* ii, 1272–1275, 1981.
30. **Hurley, J. F., Burns, J., Copeland, L., Dodgson, J., and Jacobsen, M.,** Coalworker's simple pneumoconiosis and exposure to dust at ten British coal mines, *Br. J. Ind. Med.,* 39, 120–127, 1982.

31. **Le Bouffant, L., Daniel, H., and Martin, J. C.,** Quartz as a Causative Factor in Pneumoconiotic Lesions in Coal miners, Luxembourg, Commission of the European Communities, ECSC Industrial Health and Medicine Series No. 19, 1977.
32. **Le Bouffant, L., Daniel, H., Martin, J. C., and Bruyere, S.,** Effect of impurities and associated minerals on quartz toxicity, *Ann. Occup. Hyg.,* 26, 625–634, 1982.
33. **Martin, J. C., Daniel, H., and Le Bouffant, L.,** Short and long-term experimental study of the toxicity of coal mine dust and some of its constituents, in *Inhaled Particles IV,* Walton, W. H., Ed., Pergamon Press, Oxford, 1977, 361–371.
34. **Crombie, D. W., Blaisdell, J. L., and MacPherson, G.,** The treatment of silicosis by aluminum powder, *Can. Med. Assoc. J.,* 50, 318–324, 1944.
35. **Hannon, J. G. W.,** Aluminum therapy in the United States, *Trans. Can. Inst. Min. Metal.,* 47, 180, 1944.
36. **Johns, D. R. and Petronella, S. J.,** Aluminum Therapy for Silicosis, *Monthly Bull. Indiana State Board of Health,* 43, 203, 1945.
37. **Bamberger, P. J.,** Aluminum therapy in silicosis, *Ind. Med.,* 14, 477, 1945.
38. **Berry, J. W.,** Aluminum therapy in advanced silicosis, *Am. Rev. Tuberc.,* 57, 557–573, 1948.
39. **Gent, M., Grey, C. C., and Hewitt, D.,** Report of the Task Force on Aluminum Inhalation Therapy to the Ontario Ministry of Labour, Toronto, Ministry of Labour, 1980.
40. **Baffie, A. S., Delesvaux, C. R., and Riffat, D. J.,** Essai therapeutique d'aerosols d'un sel d'aluminum sur les lesions pneumoconiotiques du mineur de charbon, *Rev. Fr. Mal. Respir.,* 9, 61–62, 1981.
41. **Prevost, J.-M. and Deflandre, J.,** Etude clinique de l'action des sels solubles d'aluminum en aerosols sur la pneumoconiose du houilleur basin du nord pas-de-callais in silicosis and mixed-dusts pneumoconiosis, *Colloq. Inserm,* 155, 493–502, 1987.
42. **White, L. R., Steinegger, A. F., and Schlatter, C.,** Pulmonary response following intratracheal instillation of potroom dust from an aluminum reduction plant into rat lung, *Environ. Res.,* 42, 534–545, 1987.
43. **Renne, R. A., Eldridge, S. R., Lewis, T. R., and Stevens, D. L.,** Fibrogenic potential of intratracheally instilled quartz, ferric oxide, fibrous glass and hydrated alumina in hamsters, *Toxicol. Pathol.,* 13, 306–314, 1985.
44. **Goralewski, G.,** Die Aluminumlunge-Eine Neue Gewerbeerkrankung, *Arch. Gewerbepathol. Gewerbehyg.,* 8, 501–531, 1947.
45. **Mitchell, J., Manning, G. B., Molyneux, M.,and Lane, R. E.,** Pulmonary fibrosis in workers exposed to finely powdered aluminum, *Br. J. Ind. Med.,* 18, 10–20, 1961.
46. **McLaughlin, A. I. G., Kazantzis, G., King, E., Teare, D., Porter, R. J., and Owen, R.,** Pulmonary fibrosis and encephalopathy associated with the inhalation of aluminum dust, *Br. J. Ind. Med.,* 19, 253–263, 1962.
47. **Gilks, B. and Churg, A.,** Aluminum-induced pulmonary fibrosis: do fibres play a role? *Am. Rev. Respir. Dis.,* 136, 176–179, 1987.
48. **Rifat, S. L., Eastwood, M. R., McLachlan, D. R., and Corey, P. N.,** Effect of exposure of miners to aluminum powder, *Lancet,* 336, 1162–1165, 1990.
49. **Raphals, P.,** Study of miners heightens aluminum fears, *New Sci.,* 127, 17, 1990.

Section IV
Chapter 5

BISBENZYLISOQUINOLINE ALKALOIDS: ANIMAL STUDIES

Vincent Castranova, Joseph K. H. Ma, and Jane Y. C. Ma

CONTENTS

I. INTRODUCTION

Hanfangchi is a medicinal extract from the root of the Chinese herb, *Stephania tetrandra S. moore.* It has been used in China as a traditional folk medicine for the treatment of rheumatoid arthritis. Hanfangchi has also been used for the treatment of angina and hypertension.[1] Its efficacy as a cardiovascular agent stems from its properties as a Ca^{2+} antagonist; i.e., it binds to the Ca^{2+} entry blocker receptor complex and allosterically inhibits ligand binding at other stimulatory receptor sites in the complex.[2,3] Hanfangchi also exhibits antitumor properties.[4]

Chen and Chen[5] identified tetrandrine as the pharmacologically active ingredient in hanfangchi. The structure of tetrandrine has since been characterized and the drug synthesized.[6] Tetrandrine is a bisbenzylisoquinoline alkaloid with an empirical formula of $C_{38}H_{42}O_6N_2$. Its molecular weight is 622.73.

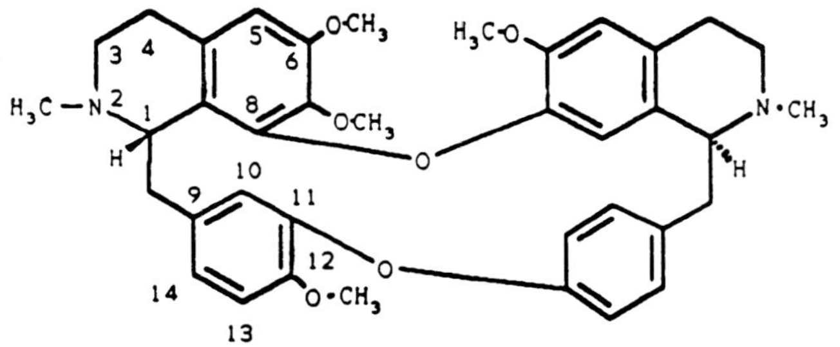

TETRANDRINE

FIGURE 1 Chemical structure of tetrandrine.

It is characterized by methoxy groups at C_7 and C_{12}, uncharged nitrogens at N_2 and N_2', and two 17-carbon ring members connected by a double oxygen bridge between C_8–C_7' and C_{11}–C_{12}'. The chemical structure of tetrandrine is given in Figure 1.

Recently, tetrandrine has been used in China as an antifibrotic drug. Clinical trials suggest that administration of tetrandrine to patients with silicosis results in substantial improvement of symptoms, increases in diffusion capacity, and decreases in the size of shadows on lung X-rays.[7] The purpose of the present chapter is to present current animal and cellular data concerning the biological activities of tetrandrine as they relate to the antifibrotic properties of this drug.

II. PROPOSED MECHANISTIC PATHWAYS IN THE PATHOGENESIS OF SILICOSIS: MODULATION BY TETRANDRINE

Silicosis is an interstitial lung disease which is the consequence of silica-induced damage to lung cells and the resulting lung scarring associated with induction of the fibrotic process. Several mechanisms have been proposed to characterize this cycle of damage and fibrosis:

1. Direct cytotoxicity — direct cellular damage resulting from the interaction of crystalline silica with cell membranes
2. Activation of the respiratory burst in alveolar macrophages — silica-induced stimulation of the production of reactive oxygen species by macrophages resulting in lipid peroxidation and oxidant injury to the lung parenchyma
3. Pulmonary inflammation — silica-induced release of factors from alveolar macrophages which are chemoattractants and/or activators of leukocytes causing further lung damage
4. Activation of fibrogenesis — silica-induced release of fibrogenic factors from alveolar macrophages resulting in proliferation and collagen synthesis by fibroblasts

The effects of tetrandrine on these pathways of fibrosis are detailed.

A. EFFECT OF TETRANDRINE ON THE DIRECT CYTOTOXICITY OF SILICA

Crystalline silica exhibits direct cytotoxicity. Silica can interact with plasma membranes to induce lipid peroxidation of these structures, which results in cell damage and loss of membrane integrity.[8] Even in the absence of cell death, silica has been shown to increase the permeability of monolayers of alveolar type II epithelial cells, suggesting leakage of tight junctions.[9]

The direct toxicity of silica on alveolar macrophages is demonstrated in Figure 2. A 30-min *in vitro* exposure of these phagocytes to 5 mg/ml silica at 37°C results in a 30% decrease in cellular viability. Treatment of these cells with 65 μM tetrandrine fails to protect them from silica-induced damage. Similar results are seen when viability is monitored as lactate dehydrogenase release from alveolar macrophages. Silica decreases viability by 73%, while silica-exposed cells treated with tetrandrine exhibit a 71% decline in viability.[10] Therefore, the antifibrotic action of tetrandrine is not due to a decrease in the direct cytotoxicity of silica.

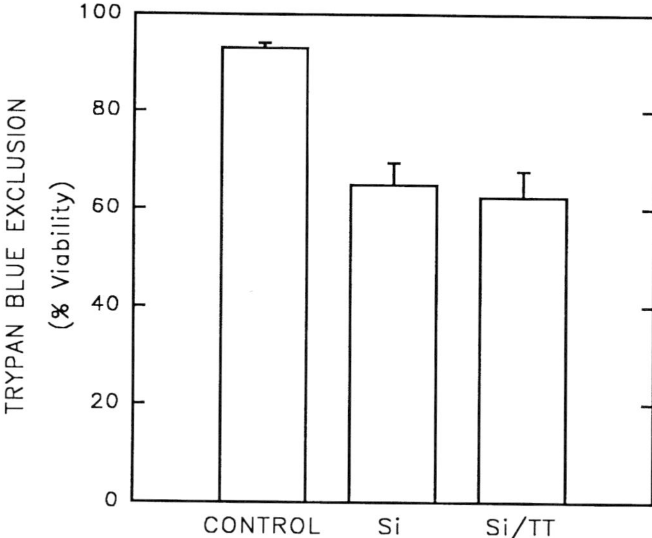

FIGURE 2 Effect of *in vitro* exposure of alveolar macrophages to crystalline silica on cellular viability. Viability was measured as the ability of cells to exclude trypan blue dye. Si indicates exposure of 8×10^5 cells to 5 mg/ml silica for 30 min at 37°C. Si/TT cells were treated with 65 μM tetrandrine 10 min prior to and during the silica exposure. Data are means ± SE of four experiments.

B. INHIBITION OF SILICA-INDUCED ACTIVATION OF ALVEOLAR MACROPHAGES: RELEASE OF OXIDANT SPECIES

Hypersecretion of reactive forms of oxygen by alveolar macrophages can overwhelm the natural protective mechanisms of the lung and result in destruction of the lung parenchyma.[11] These reactive oxygen species include superoxide anion, hydrogen peroxide, and hydroxyl radical.

1. *In Vitro* Studies

Exposure of alveolar macrophages to crystalline silica causes an increase in respiratory burst activity which is effectively inhibited by *in vitro* treatment with tetrandrine.[12] Figure 3 shows that 75 μM tetrandrine decreases the silica-induced increase in oxygen consumption of alveolar macrophages by 95%. The ID_{50} value for this inhibition is 29 μM tetrandrine. Tetrandrine also inhibits silica-induced release of hydrogen peroxide from alveolar macrophages (Figure 4). A maximal inhibition of 87% is observed at 27 μM tetrandrine with an ID_{50} value of 13 μM. Similar inhibition of silica-induced chemiluminescence also is noted (Figure 5). Preincubation of macrophages for 5 min with 40 μM tetrandrine decreases chemiluminescence generated by alveolar macrophages in response to silica exposure by 64%. This inhibition of silica-induced activation of alveolar macrophages by tetrandrine is not explained by a decrease in cellular viability in the presence of tetrandrine. Indeed, *in vitro* treatment of alveolar macrophages with 96 μM tetrandrine for 20 min at 37°C has no adverse effect on either membrane integrity (Figure 6) or resting oxygen consumption (Figure 7). Therefore, tetrandrine may express antifibrotic activity by decreasing oxidant release from silica-exposed alveolar macrophages, thus minimizing oxidant-induced lung damage.

2. *In Vivo* Studies

Inhalation of silica primes alveolar macrophages to release greater amounts of reactive oxygen species upon *in vitro* stimulation. This activation is inhibited *in vivo* by oral administration of tetrandrine. Oral administration of tetrandrine (33 μg/g body wt/d from 4 d prior to exposure until day of sacrifice) decreases zymosan-stimulated oxygen consumption (Figure 8) and hydrogen peroxide release (Figure 9) from alveolar macrophages harvested 1 or 4 d after a single inhalation of 110 mg/m^3 of silica for 6 h.

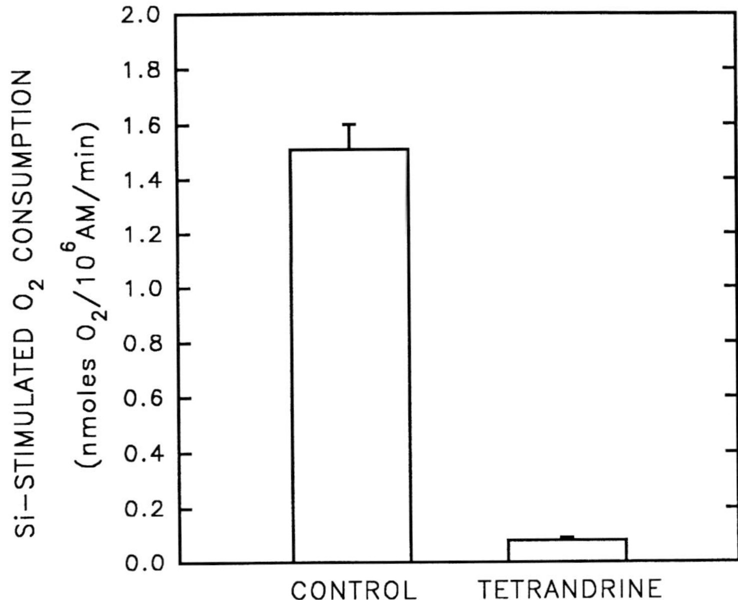

FIGURE 3 Inhibition of silica-stimulated oxygen consumption by tetrandrine. Alveolar macrophages were exposed at 37°C to 1.7 mg/ml silica in the absence (control) or presence of 75 μM tetrandrine. Data are means ± SE of four experiments expressed as the silica minus resting level.

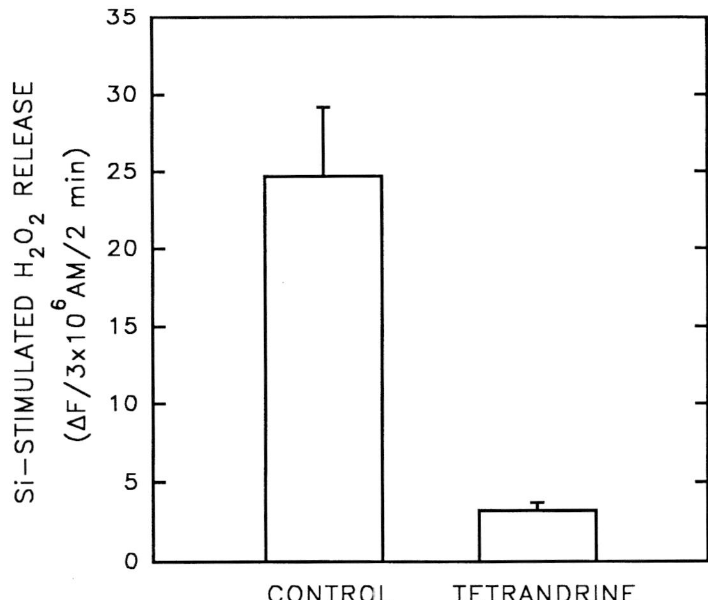

FIGURE 4 Inhibition of silica-stimulated hydrogen peroxide release by tetrandrine. Alveolar macrophages were exposed at 37°C to 1 mg/ml silica in the absence (control) or presence of 27 μM tetrandrine. Data are means ± SE of four experiments expressed as the silica minus resting level.

Zymosan-stimulated oxygen consumption is inhibited by 57 and 43% at 1 and 4 d postexposure, respectively. Similarly, zymosan-induced hydrogen peroxide release is inhibited by 26 and 43% at 1 and 4 d postexposure, respectively. *In vivo* treatment with tetrandrine also inhibits cell spreading of alveolar macrophages *in vitro*. As shown in Figure 10, macrophages from silica-exposed rats exhibit 62% greater

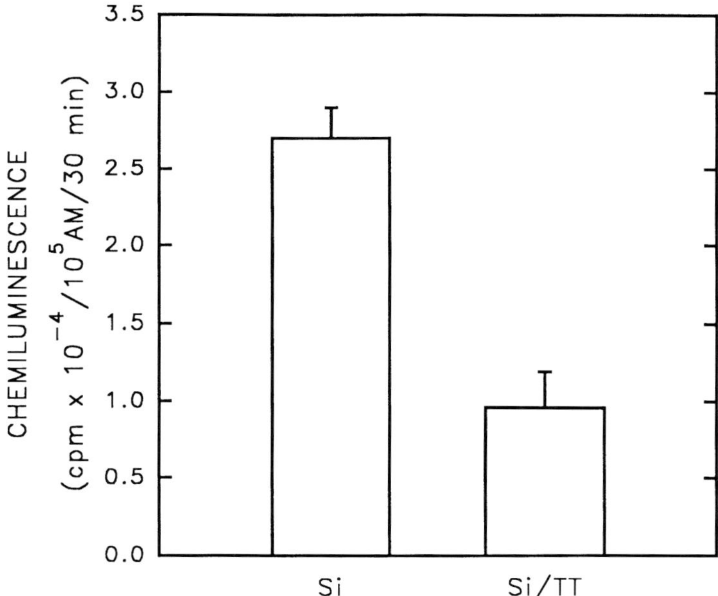

FIGURE 5 Inhibition of silica-stimulated chemiluminescence by tetrandrine. Alveolar macrophages were exposed at 37°C to 0.5 mg/ml silica in the absence or presence of 40 μ*M* tetrandrine. Data are means ± SE of seven experiments expressed as the silica minus resting level.

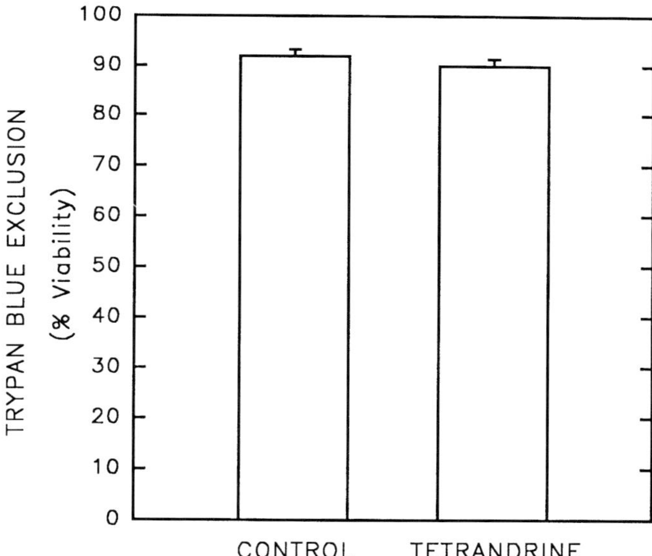

FIGURE 6 Effect of tetrandrine on membrane integrity of alveolar macrophages. Macrophages (8×10^5) were incubated at 37°C in the absence (control) or presence of 96 μ*M* tetrandrine for 20 min and viability monitored by measuring the exclusion of trypan blue dye microscopically. Data are means ± SE of four experiments.

spreading than air controls. Treatment of silica-exposed rats with tetrandrine causes a 74% depression of this surface activity. This inhibitory action of tetrandrine is not due to effects on cellular viability. Indeed, oral administration of tetrandrine for 8 d does not alter membrane integrity (Figure 11) or resting oxygen consumption (Figure 12) of alveolar macrophages. Therefore, as described with *in vitro* studies, *in vivo* treatment with tetrandrine is effective in inhibiting silica-induced priming of alveolar macrophages.

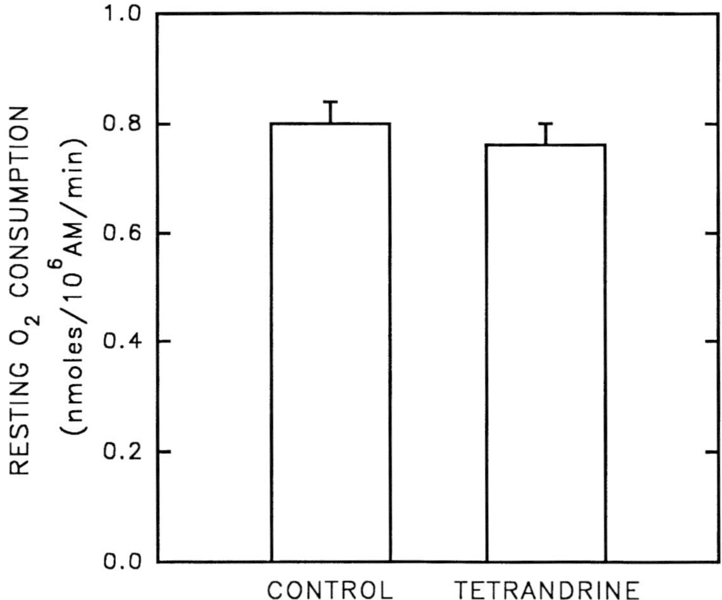

FIGURE 7 Effect of tetrandrine on resting oxygen consumption of alveolar macrophages. Cells were studied at 37°C in the absence (control) or presence of 96 μ*M* tetrandrine. Data are means ± SE of four experiments.

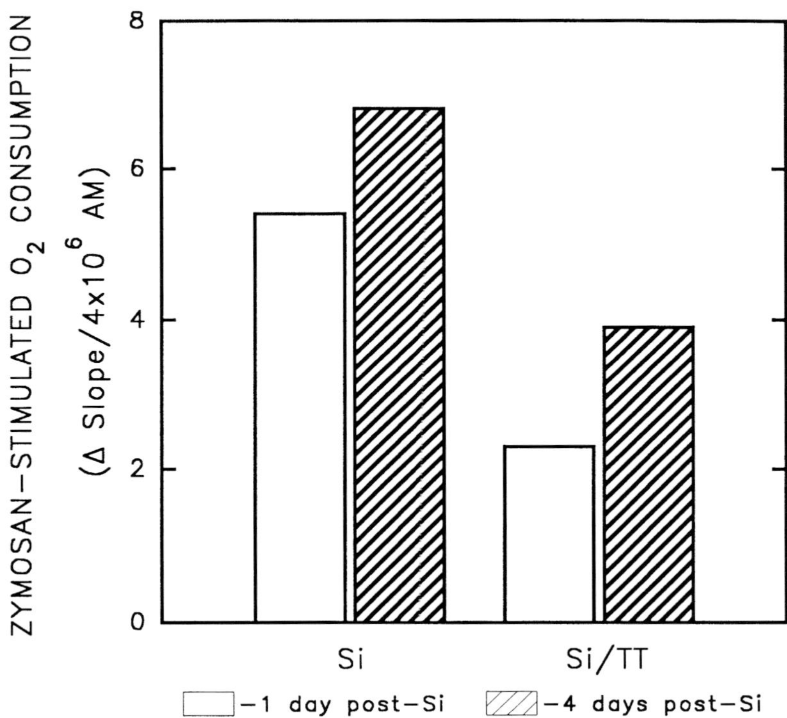

FIGURE 8 Effect of *in vivo* treatment with tetrandrine on the responsiveness of alveolar macrophages after inhalation of silica. Rats received 33 μg/g body wt of tetrandrine daily from 4 d prior to silica inhalation until the day of sacrifice. Exposure was by inhalation of 110 mg/m^3 of silica for 6 h. Zymosan-stimulated oxygen consumption (zymosan minus resting level) was measured 1 or 4 d postexposure. Values are means of three experiments.

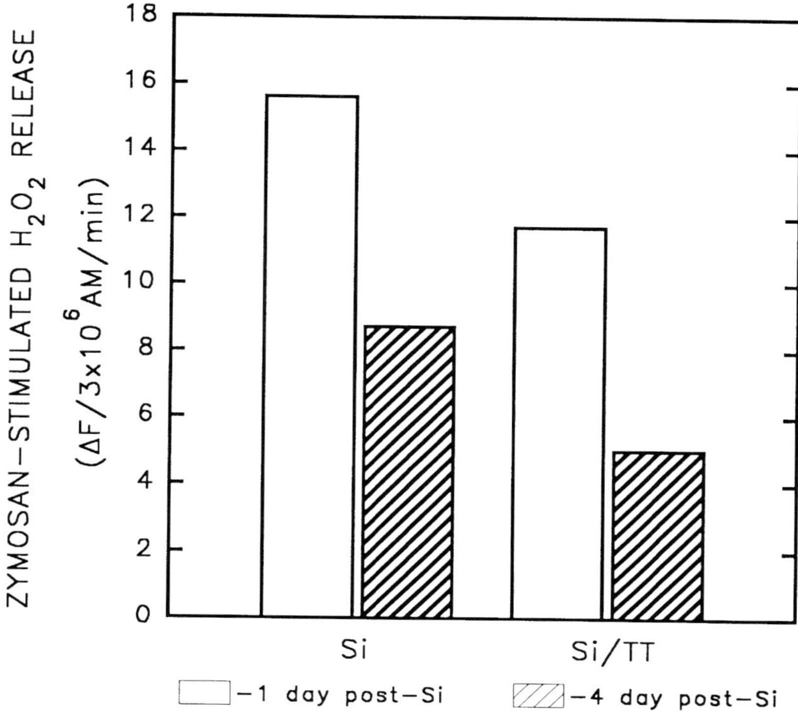

FIGURE 9 Effect of *in vivo* treatment with tetrandrine on the responsiveness of alveolar macrophages after inhalation of silica. Rats received 33 μg/g body wt of tetrandrine daily from 4 d prior to silica inhalation until the day of sacrifice. Exposure was by inhalation of 110 mg/m^3 of silica for 6 h. Zymosan-stimulated hydrogen peroxide release (zymosan minus resting level) was measured 1 or 4 d postexposure. Values are means of three experiments.

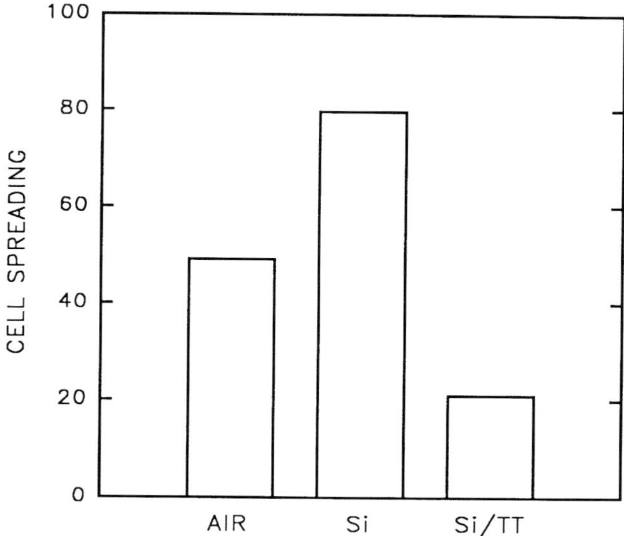

FIGURE 10 Effect of *in vivo* treatment with tetrandrine on cellular spreading of alveolar macrophages after inhalation of silica. Rats received 33 μg/g body wt of tetrandrine daily for 4 d prior to silica inhalation until the day of sacrifice. Exposure was by inhalation of 110 mg/m^3 of silica for 6 h. Cell spreading was measured 4 d postexposure. Values are means of three experiments.

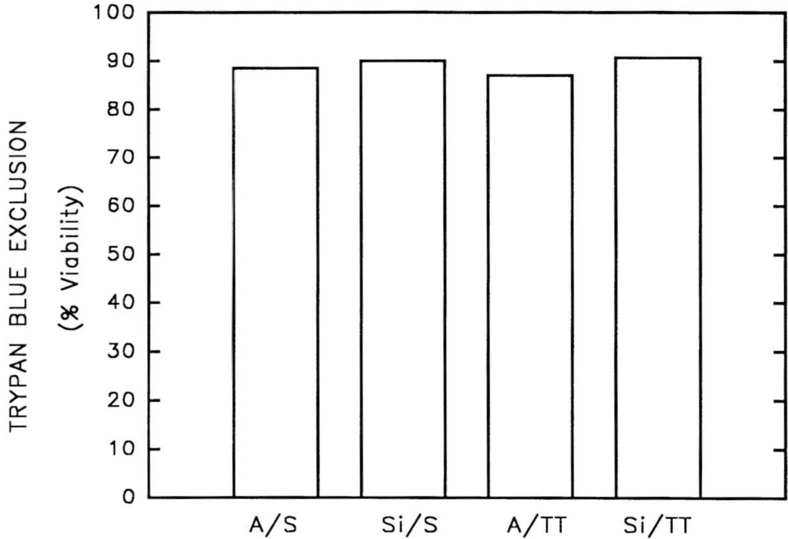

FIGURE 11 Effect of *in vivo* treatment with tetrandrine on membrane integrity of alveolar macrophages. A/S = air inhalation/oral saline (daily for 8 d). Si/S = silica inhalation (110 mg/m³ for 6 h)/oral saline (daily for 8 d). A/TT = air inhalation/oral tetrandrine (33 μg/g body wt daily for 8 d). Si/TT = silica inhalation (110 mg/m³ for 6 h)/oral tetrandrine (33 μg/g body wt daily for 8 d). Data are means of three experiments.

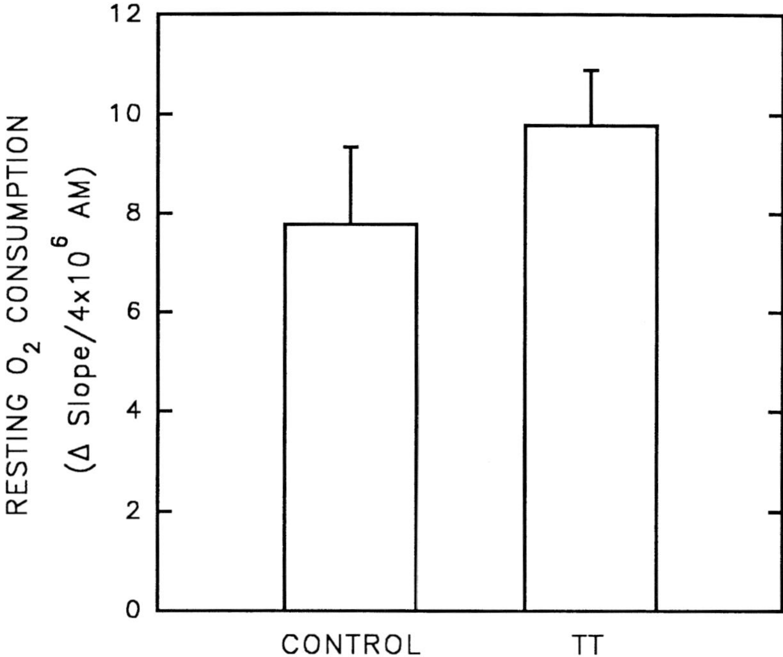

FIGURE 12 Effect of *in vivo* treatment with tetrandrine on resting oxygen consumption of alveolar macrophages. Rats were treated orally with saline (control) or tetrandrine (33 μg/g body wt) daily for 8 d before macrophages were harvested. Data are means ± SE of three experiments.

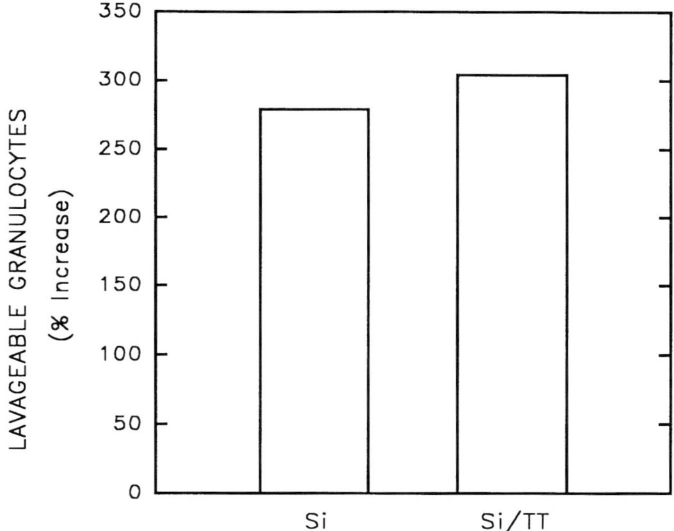

FIGURE 13 Effect of *in vivo* treatment with tetrandrine on silica-induced infiltration of granulocytes into the lung. Rats were treated orally with saline or tetrandrine (33 μg/g body wt) daily for 4 d prior to inhalation exposure to 110 mg/m[3] silica for 6 h. Bronchoalveolar lavage was conducted 1 d postexposure. Data are given as percent increase above the unexposed levels. Values are means of three experiments.

C. INHIBITION OF PULMONARY INFLAMMATION

Pulmonary inflammation occurs in two stages, i.e., infiltration of leukocytes into the airways and activation of these leukocytes. The result is enhanced oxidant-induced lung damage which may lead to lung scarring. Tetrandrine is a potent inhibitor of both of these inflammatory processes.

1. Modulation of Silica-Induced Release of Chemotactic Factors from Alveolar Macrophages

Alveolar macrophages, upon exposure to silica, produce a number of factors which are chemoattractants for leukocytes. Among these factors are platelet activating factor (PAF), platelet-derived growth factor (PDGF), leukotriene B_4, and prostaglandins.[13–15] Teh et al.[16] have reported that tetrandrine is a potent inhibitor of prostaglandin and leukotriene synthesis *in vitro*. This inhibition appears to be mediated by the ability of tetrandrine to block phospholipase A_2.[17] In addition, tetrandrine also decreases the ability of leukocytes to respond *in vitro* to chemotactic agents; i.e., 16 μ*M* tetrandrine decreases the ability of neutrophils to adhere, move randomly, and chemotax by 44, 42, and 25%, respectively.[18,19] In contrast to this *in vitro* depression of chemotactic activity, *in vivo* treatment with tetrandrine does not decrease silica-induced infiltration of granulocytes into the airways (Figure 13). Therefore, whether inhibition of chemotaxis is a major mechanism to explain the antifibrotic potency of tetrandrine remains unresolved.

2. Modulation of the Activity of Polymorphonuclear Leukocytes

Alveolar macrophages exposed to silica produce a number of mediators which activate a respiratory burst in neutrophils. These stimulants of neutrophil oxidant production include tumor necrosis factor (TNF), PAF, and interleukin 1 (IL-1).[13,20,21] *In vitro* treatment of alveolar macrophages with tetrandrine decreases silica-induced IL-1 release from these phagocytes by 63% (Figure 14). The ID_{50} for this inhibition is 17 μ*M* tetrandrine.

Tetrandrine also depresses the responsiveness of neutrophils to known stimulants. Figure 15 demonstrates the inhibitory effect of tetrandrine on the ability of neutrophils to generate chemiluminescence upon stimulation with PAF. Neutrophils are affected by very low concentrations of tetrandrine. Inhibition is complete at 8 μ*M* tetrandrine with an ID_{50} of 1.4 μ*M*. Similar inhibition is seen with n-formyl methionyl lencyl phenylalanine (FMLP)-induced chemiluminescence. Tetrandrine (16 μ*M*) also inhibits FMLP-

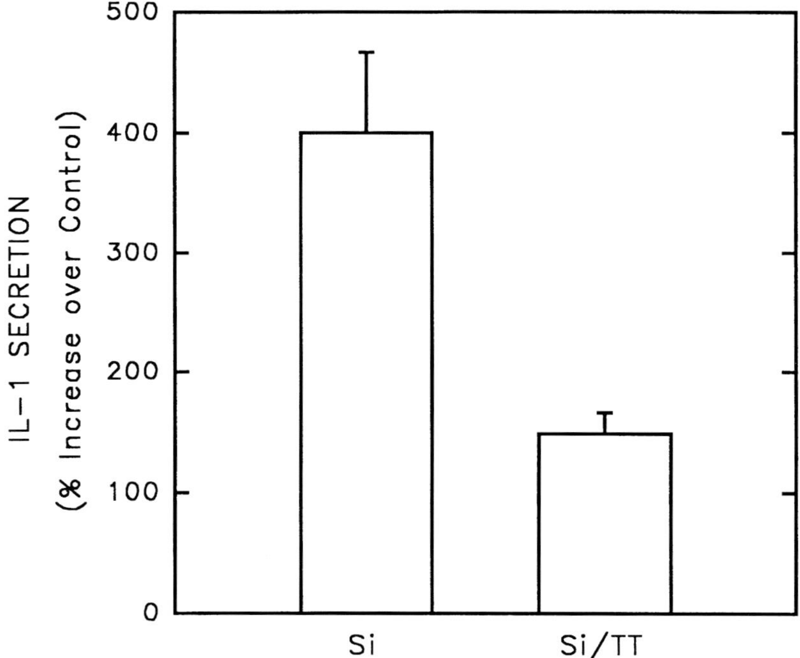

FIGURE 14 Effect of *in vitro* treatment with tetrandrine on silica-induced IL-1 release from alveolar macrophages. Macrophages were treated in culture with 20 μ*M* tetrandrine and exposed to 50 μg/ml silica. After a 20-h culture period, the IL-1 level of the supernate was determined by monitoring its ability to stimulate thymocyte proliferation. Data are means ± SE of three experiments.

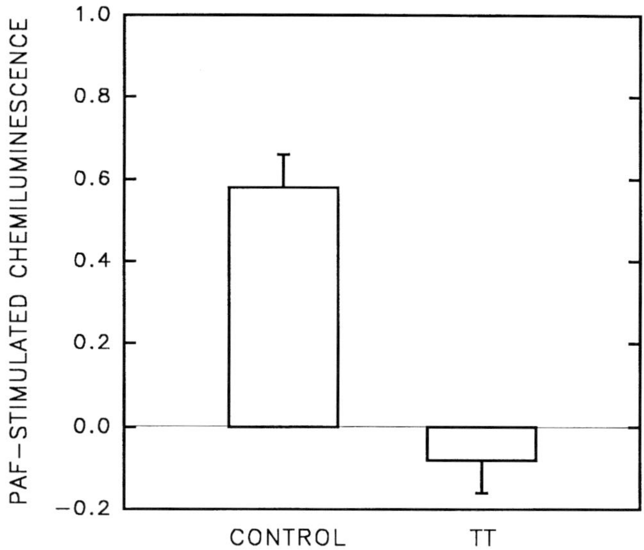

FIGURE 15 Inhibition of neutrophil-generated chemiluminescence after treatment with tetrandrine. Neutrophils were treated with 8μ*M* tetrandrine at 37°C for 10 min prior to stimulation with 10^{-9} *M* PAF. Data are means ± SE of three experiments.

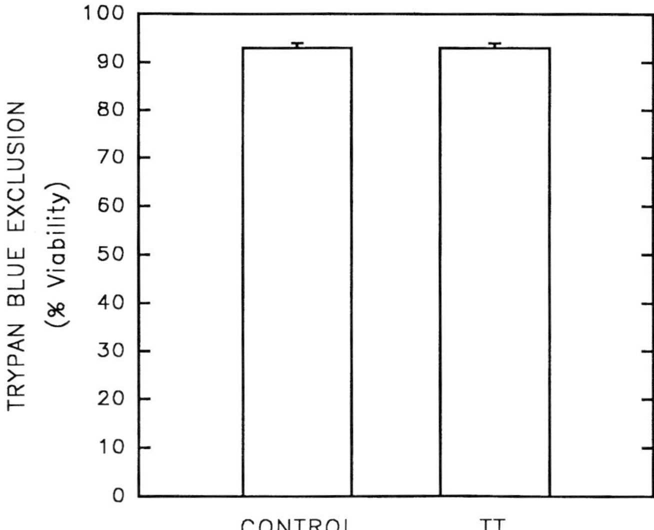

FIGURE 16 Effect of tetrandrine on the cellular viability of neutrophils. Neutrophils were treated with 10 μ*M* tetrandrine for 30 min at 37°C. Viability was determined by measuring the exclusion of trypan blue dye. Data are means ± SE of three experiments.

induced hexose-monophosphate shunt activity, superoxide anion release, hydrogen peroxide secretion, and lysosomal enzyme release from neutrophils.[19,22] These inhibitory effects on neutrophil activation are not due to decreases in cellular viability, since treatment of these phagocytes with 10 μ*M* tetrandrine for 30 min at 37°C has no adverse effect on membrane integrity (Figure 16).

3. Modulation of the Activity of Lymphocytes

Tetrandrine also demonstrates immunosuppressive properties. It decreases the ability of lymphocytes to proliferate in response to mitogens such as concanavalin A, inhibits the production of immunoglobulin by B cells, and suppresses killing by natural killer cells.[23]

D. INHIBITION OF FIBROGENESIS

Silica-induced fibrosis includes the following steps: (1) silica-induced release of fibrogenic factors from alveolar macrophages, (2) proliferation of fibroblasts, and (3) increased production of collagen by pulmonary fibroblasts. Data obtained thus far suggest that tetrandrine is capable of modulating all three of these fibrogenic pathways.

1. Inhibition of the Release of Alveolar Macrophage-Derived Fibrogenic Factors

IL-1 has been reported to exhibit stimulatory activity toward fibroblast growth and collagen synthesis.[24,25] As shown in Figure 14, tetrandrine inhibits the production of IL-1 by silica-exposed alveolar macrophages. Furthermore, Cai et al.[26] reported that media from alveolar macrophages exposed to silica induces the production of hydroxyproline (a collagen substrate) by pulmonary fibroblasts and that treatment of alveolar macrophages with tetrandrine inhibits the production of this fibrogenic mediator.

2. Inhibition of Fibroblast Proliferation

Tetrandrine also exhibits a direct inhibitory action on pulmonary fibroblast; i.e., tetrandrine decreases the responsiveness of fibroblasts to proliferative agents. Figure 17 shows that fibroblast proliferation in response to human serum is decreased by 90% after treatment with 10 μ*M* tetrandrine. Likewise, fibroblast growth in response to plasma plus PDGF, fibroblast growth factor or TNF is also inhibited by tetrandrine. This inhibitory action of tetrandrine persists even after competence has been attained, suggesting modification of a progression step. Furthermore, this inhibition is not due to a reduction in

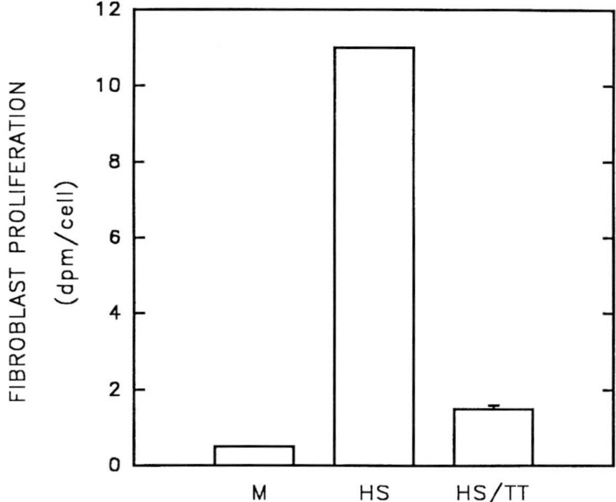

FIGURE 17 Inhibition of fibroblast proliferation by tetrandrine. Fibroblasts were treated with 10 μ*M* tetrandrine for 6 h at 37°C and proliferation in response to 10% human serum determined by measuring the incorporation of tritiated thymidine into DNA over 32 h in culture. M indicates the media negative control; HS is the positive control with human serum; and HS/TT is human serum plus tetrandrine. Data are means of three experiments.

fibroblast viability, since treatment of fibroblast cultures with tetrandrine does not compromise membrane integrity measured by trypan blue exclusion.

3. Inhibition of Fibrosis *In Vivo*

Oral administration of tetrandrine to rats exposed to silica by intratracheal instillation results in significant decreases (up to 52%) in lung collagen.[27–29] Tetrandrine also decreases lung weight gain associated with silica.[29] These actions of tetrandrine result in a significant depression of silica-induced fibrosis; i.e., while nodules are normally apparent microscopically four weeks after instillation of 50 mg silica, tetrandrine-treated silica-exposed rats exhibit only small macules.[30]

III. MECHANISMS INVOLVED IN THE INHIBITORY ACTIONS OF TETRANDRINE

In summary, the antifibrotic activity of tetrandrine may be mediated by decreasing oxidant release from alveolar macrophages, suppressing pulmonary inflammation involving activated leukocytes, and inhibiting fibroblast activity. The net result would be less oxidant-induced damage and less fibrosis. The possible mechanisms by which these inhibitory activities of tetrandrine are expressed are described.

A. RECEPTORS

Several lines of investigation suggest that the inhibitory action of tetrandrine is not mediated at the site of stimulant-receptor interaction. Castranova et al.[31] have shown that membrane depolarization of alveolar macrophages in response to PAF, i.e., an initial response to PAF receptor occupancy, is unaffected by treatment with tetrandrine. Similarly, the binding of concanavalin A or monoclonal reagents to lymphocytes is not altered by tetrandrine.[23] Lastly, since tetrandrine blocks the response of macrophages, neutrophils, lymphocytes, and fibroblasts to a number of chemically unrelated stimulants, it seems unlikely that blockade of agonist-receptor binding is involved in the inhibitory actions of tetrandrine.

B. CALCIUM MOBILIZATION

Silica causes an increase in free cytoplasmic calcium in alveolar macrophages (Figure 18). Similarly, growth factors such as 1% human serum mobilize internal calcium in lung fibroblasts, causing a transient rise in cytoplasmic calcium, which precedes proliferation.[32] In both cell systems, tetrandrine blocks this

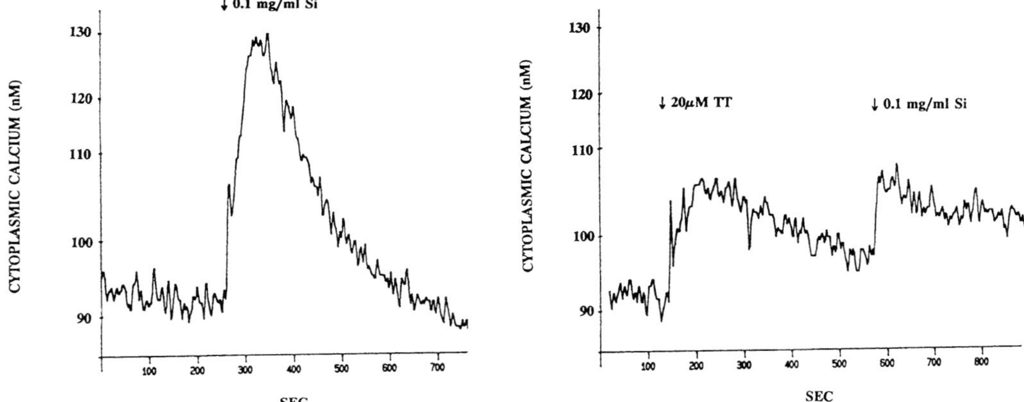

FIGURE 18 Inhibition of silica-induced calcium mobilization in alveolar macrophages by tetrandrine. Alveolar macrophages (5×10^6 cells/ml) were loaded with 2 μ*M* indo-1-acetoxy-methyl ester for 30 min at 22°C, washed, and resuspended in HEPES-buffered solution containing 0.2 m*M* EDTA at 2×10^6 cells/ml. Fluorescence was monitored at an excitation of 350 nm and emission wavelengths of 400 and 450 nm. Cytoplasmic calcium ($[Ca^{2+}]_i$) was determined as follows:

$$[Ca^{2+}]_i = Kd \quad [S_{f2}/S_{b2}] \quad (R - R_{min})/R_{max} - R$$

where Kd = 250, R = the experimental ratio of fluorescence at 400 to 450 nm, R_{max} = the fluorescence ratio when dye is saturated with Ca^{2+}, R_{min} = the fluorescence ratio when no Ca^{2+} is bound to the dye, and S_{f2}/S_{b2} = the ratio of fluorescence at 450 nm for free and bound forms of the dye. Silica and tetrandrine were added as indicated by the arrows.

stimulant-induced calcium mobilization. The inhibitory action of tetrandrine with alveolar macrophages is shown in Figure 18. This inhibition of the stimulant-induced rise in cytoplasmic calcium may be mediated in part by inhibition of agonist-stimulated calcium influx. Indeed, tetrandrine has been shown to be a calcium entry blocker in cardiac muscle.[2,3] This action involves binding of tetrandrine to a Ca^{2+} entry blocker receptor site which allosterically affects the receptor complex to decrease ligand binding to its stimulatory receptor site.

C. SECOND MESSENGERS

Hashizume et al.[17] reported that in platelets tetrandrine suppresses agonist-induced activation of phospholipase C, which is involved in the production of secondary messengers such as inositol triphosphate and diacylglycerol. These results are supported by the finding of Seow et al.[23] that tetrandrine decreases the production of inositol monophosphate in concanavalin A-stimulated lymphocytes. A decrease in inositol metabolism may be responsible for the decrease in calcium mobilization observed with tetrandrine treatment.

D. CYTOSKELETAL COMPONENTS

Our laboratory has extensively investigated factors affecting tetrandrine-membrane interaction.[33–35] Our data indicate that tetrandrine binds strongly and irreversibly to alveolar macrophages while tubocurarine, an inactive analog (characterized by hydroxyl substitutions at C_7 and C_{12}, positively charged ammonium nitrogens at positions N_2 and N_2', and a 20-bond-length oxygen-bridged ring between C_8–C_{12}' and C_{13}–C_7'), binds weakly to these phagocytes. Binding of tetrandrine to pulmonary fibroblasts also appears to be irreversible.[32] Tetrandrine does not bind to sonicated cell membranes, indicating that its binding is not simply hydrophobic interaction with membrane lipids. In contrast, binding is inhibited by microtubule modifiers (vinblastine or taxol) and microfilament agents (cytochalasin B). The suggestion that the cytoskeleton plays a role in the inhibitory action of tetrandrine is supported by data from Liu et al.[36] and Chen et al.,[37] which indicate that tetrandrine binds strongly to isolated microtubules.

E. ANTIOXIDANT PROPERTIES

Some data suggest that tetrandrine may act as a direct antioxidant. Seow et al.[19] have reported that tetrandrine is a scavenger for superoxide anion, decreasing the generation of superoxide in a cell-free

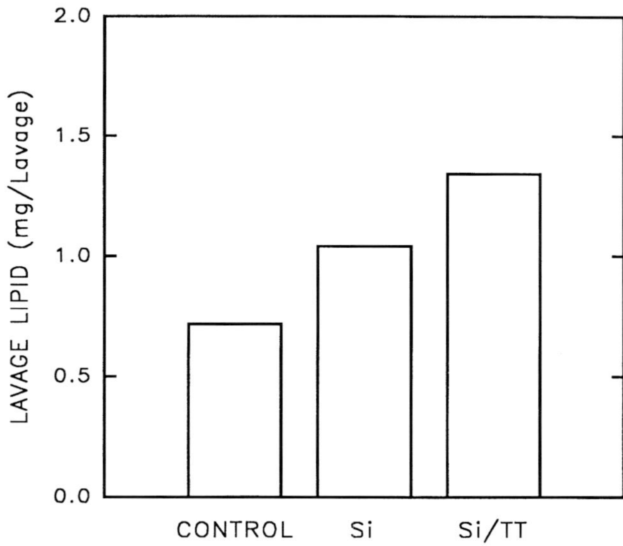

FIGURE 19 Lavagable lipid from silica-exposed, tetrandrine-treated rats. Rats were treated orally with saline or tetrandrine (33 μg/g body wt) daily for 4 d prior to inhalation exposure to 110 mg/m^3 silica for 6 h. Bronchoalveolar lavage was conducted 1 d postexposure. Data are means of three experiments.

hypoxanthine-xanthine oxidase system by 33%. Similarly, Shiraishi et al.[38] have reported that tetrandrine inhibits lipid peroxidation of biological membranes. In contrast, our laboratory has found that tetrandrine is not a strong antioxidant. It has no effect on H_2O_2-induced chemiluminescence or the fluorometric detection of H_2O in a cell-free system. Furthermore, tetrandrine does not inhibit the resting rate of oxygen metabolism or the resting production of superoxide or hydrogen peroxide by alveolar macrophages.[31]

F. LIPIDOSIS

Pulmonary surfactant or its primary constituent, dipalmitoyl lecithin, has been shown to suppress the cytotoxicity of silica.[39,40] It is possible that the antifibrotic action of tetrandrine may be mediated in part by the induction of pulmonary lipidosis. Indeed, oral treatment with tetrandrine increases the lipidotic response of rats to inhalation of silica by 29% (Figure 19). This increased lipid accumulates within alveolar macrophages (Figure 20) and results in a 23% increase in the size of these phagocytes (Figure 21). Note that ingested silica is associated with lipid in tetrandrine-treated macrophages (Figure 20).

IV. SUMMARY

In conclusion, tetrandrine has been shown to exhibit significant antifibrotic activity in animal models of silicosis. This antifibrotic activity is associated with the ability of tetrandrine to inhibit silica-induced secretion of cytokines and reactive species from pulmonary phagocytes. Such inhibition has been demonstrated both *in vitro* and *in vivo* with alveolar macrophages and neutrophils in response to a variety of particulate or soluble stimulants. In addition, tetrandrine directly inhibits the ability of pulmonary fibroblasts to proliferate in response to growth factors.

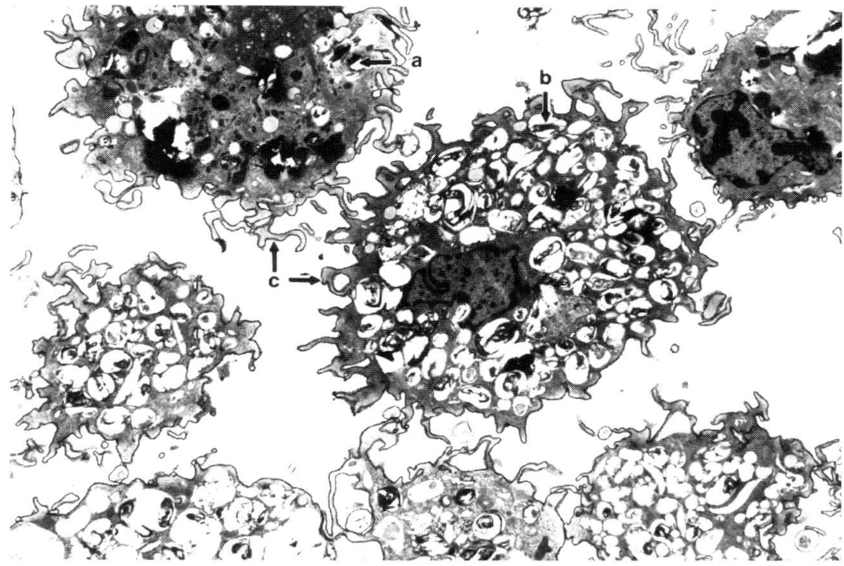

FIGURE 20 Transmission electron micrograph of alveolar macrophages obtained from silica-exposed, tetrandrine-treated rats. Rats were treated orally with tetrandrine (33 µg/g body wt) daily 4 d prior to and 4 d after inhalation of silica (110 mg/m^3 for 6 h). Key: (a) silica inclusions, (b) lipid inclusions, and (c) darkly stained plasma membrane.

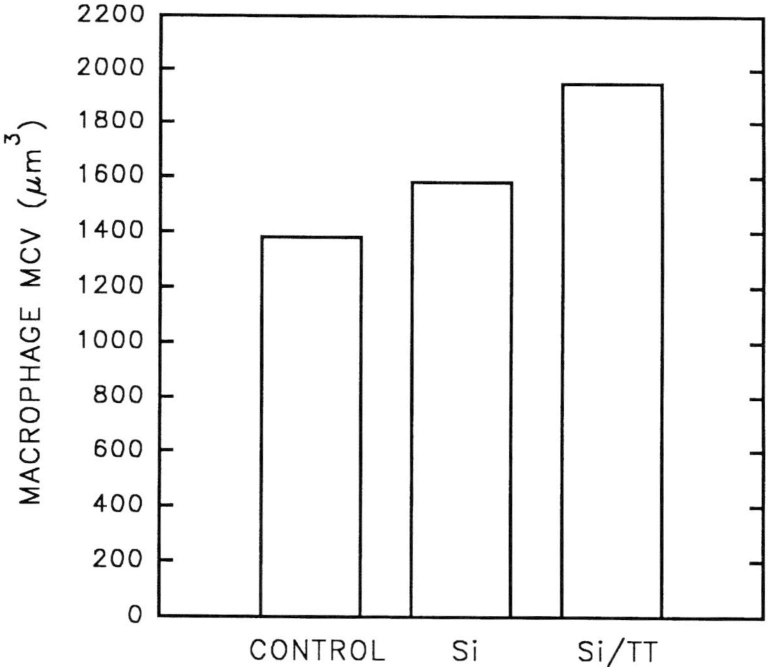

FIGURE 21 Effect of silica inhalation and tetrandrine treatment of the cellular volume of alveolar macrophages. Rats were treated orally with saline or tetrandrine (33 µg/g body wt) daily for 4 d prior to inhalation exposure to 110 mg/m^3 silica for 6 h. Bronchoalveolar lavage was conducted 1 d postexposure. Data are means of three experiments.

REFERENCES

1. **Zeng, F. D., Shaw, D. H., Jr., and Ogilvie, R. I.,** Kinetic disposition and hemodynamic effects of tetrandrine in anesthetized dogs, *J. Cardiovasc. Pharmacol.*, 7, 1034–1039, 1985.
2. **Fang, D. C. and Jiang, M. X.,** Studies on tetrandrine calcium antagonistic action, *Chin. Med. J.*, 99, 638–642, 1986.
3. **King, V. F., Garcia, M. L., Himmel, D., Reuben, J. P., Lam, Y. T., Pan, J., Han, G., and Kaczorowski, G. J.,** Interaction of tetrandrine with slowly inactivating calcium channels: characterization of calcium channel modulation by an alkaloid of Chinese medicinal herb origin, *J. Biol. Chem.*, 263, 2238–2245, 1988.
4. **Kupchan, S. M. and Atland, H. W.,** Requirements for tumor-inhibitory activity among benzylisoquinoline alkaloids and related synthetic compounds, *J. Med. Chem.*, 16, 913–917, 1973.
5. **Chen, K. K. and Chen, A. L.,** The alkaloids of Han-Fang-Chi, *J. Biol. Chem.*, 109, 681–685, 1935.
6. **Inubushi, Y., Masaki, Y., Matsumoto, S., and Takani, F.,** Studies on the alkaloids of Menispermaceous plants. CCXLIX. Total synthesis of optically active natural isotetrandrine, phaeanthine and tetrandrine, *J. Chem. Soc.*, 11, 1547–1556, 1969.
7. **Li, Q., Xu, Y., Zhou, Z., Chen, X., Huang, X., Chen, S., and Zhan, C.,** The therapeutic effect of tetrandrine on silicosis, *Chin. J. Tuberc. Respir. Dis.*, 4, 321–328, 1981.
8. **Singh, S. V. and Rahman, Q.,** Interrelationship between hemolysis and lipid peroxidation of human erythrocytes induced by silicic acid and silicate dusts, *J. Appl. Toxicol.*, 7, 91–96, 1987.
9. **Merchant, R. K., Peterson, M. W., and Hunninghake, G. W.,** Silica directly increases permeability of alveolar epithelial cells, *J. Appl. Physiol.*, 68, 1354–1359, 1990.
10. **Zou, C. Q., Lu, X. R., and Li, Y. R.,** Research on the therapeutic effect of tetrandrine on silicosis: cooperative group of therapeutic study of tetrandrine on silicosis (personal communications).
11. **Weiss, S. J. and LoBuglio, A. F.,** Biology of disease: phagocyte-generated oxygen metabolites and cellular injury, *Lab. Invest.*, 47, 5–18, 1982.
12. **Castranova, V., Pailes, W. H., and Li, C.,** Effects of silica exposure on alveolar macrophages: action of tetrandrine, in *Proc. Int. Symp. Pneumoconioses,* Li, Y., Yao, P., Schlipköter, H. W., Idel, H., and Rosenbruch, M., Eds., Stefan Walbers Velag, Düsseldorf, 1990, 256–260.
13. **Kang, J. H., Van Dyke, K., Pailes, W. H., and Castranova, V.,** Potential role of platelet-activating factor in development of occupational lung disease: action as an activator or potentiator of pulmonary phagocytes, in *Proc. of the 3rd Symp. on Respir. Dust in the Mineral Industry,* Frantz, R. L. and Ramani, R. V., Eds., Society for Mining, Metallurgy, and Exploration, Littleton, CO, 1991, 183–190.
14. **Deuel, T. F., Senior, R. M., Huang, J. S., and Griffin, G. L.,** Chemotaxis of monocytes and neutrophils to platelet-derived growth factors, *J. Clin. Invest.*, 69, 1046–1049, 1982.
15. **Englen, M. D., Taylor, S. M., Laegreid, W. W., Liggitt, H. D., Silflow, R. M., Breeze, R. G., and Leid, R. W.,** Stimulation of arachidonic acid metabolism in silica-exposed alveolar macrophages, *Exp. Lung Res.*, 15, 511–526, 1989.
16. **Teh, B. S., Seow, W. K., Li, S. Y., and Thong, Y. H.,** Inhibition of prostaglandin and leukotriene generation by the plant alkaloids tetrandrine and berbamine, *Int. J. Immunopharm.*, 12, 321–326, 1990.
17. **Hashizume, T., Yamaguchi, H., Sato, T., and Fujii, T.,** Suppressive effect of biscoclaurine alkaloids on agonist-induced activation of phospholipase A_2 in rabbit platelets, *Biochem. Pharmacol.*, 41, 419–423, 1991.
18. **Seow, W. K., Li, S. Y., and Thong, Y. H.,** Inhibitory effects of tetrandrine on human neutrophil and monocyte adherence, *Immunol. Lett.*, 13, 83–88, 1986.
19. **Seow, W. K., Ferrante, A., Li, S. Y., and Thong, Y. H.,** Antiphagocytic and antioxidant properties of plant alkaloid tetrandrine, *Int. Arch. Allergy Appl. Immunol.*, 85, 404–409, 1988.
20. **Dubois, C. M., Bissonnette, E. J., and Rola-Pleszczynski, M.,** Asbestos fibers and silica particles stimulate rat alveolar macrophages to release tumor necrosis factor: autoregulatory role of leukotriene B_4, *Am. Rev. Respir. Dis.*, 139, 1257–1264, 1989.
21. **Kang, J. H., Lewis, D. M., Castranova, V., Rojanasakul, Y., Banks, D. E., Ma, J. Y. C., and Ma, J. K. H.,** Inhibitory action of tetrandrine on macrophage production of interleukin-1 (IL-1)-like activity and thymocyte proliferation, *Exp. Lung Res.*, 18, 719–733, 1992.
22. **Matsuno, T., Orita, K., Sato, E., Nabori, K., Inoue, B., and Utsumi, K.,** Inhibition of metabolic response of polymorphonuclear leukocyte by biscoclaurine alkaloids, *Biochem. Pharmacol.*, 36, 1613–1618, 1987.
23. **Seow, W. K., Ferrante, A., Goh, D. B. H., Chalmers, A. H., Li, S. Y., and Thong, Y. H.,** *In vitro* immunosuppressive properties of the plant alkaloid tetrandrine, *Int. Arch. Allergy Appl. Immunol.*, 85, 410–415, 1988.
24. **Schmidt, J. A., Oliver, C. N., Lepe-Zuniga, J. L., Green, I., and Gery, I.,** Silica-stimulated monocytes release fibroblast proliferative factors identical to interleukin 1: a potential role for interleukin 1 in the pathogenesis of silicosis, *J. Clin. Invest.*, 73, 1462–1472, 1984.
25. **Goldring, M. B. and Krane, S. M.,** Modulation of collagen synthesis in human chondrocyte cultures by interleukin 1, *J. Bone Miner. Res. I* (Suppl. 1), 56, 1986.

26. **Cai, G., Lim, C., Chen, N., Li, C., and Li, Y.,** Studies on the inhibition effect of tetrandrine on silica-induced fibrogenesis *in vitro, J. Inst. Health (China),* 13, 5–11, 1984.
27. **Huang, T., Liu, Y., Zhao, S., and Li, Y.,** Changes of acid-soluble collagen from lungs of silicotic rats and tetrandrine-treated silicotic rats, *Shing Wu Hua Hsueh Yu Shen Wu Li Hsueh Pao,* 13, 61–67, 1981.
28. **Liu, B., Zou, C., and Li, Y.,** Studies of the content of glycosaminoglycans from lungs of silicotic rats and tetrandrine-treated silicotic rats, *Ecotoxicol. Environ. Safety,* 7, 323–329, 1983.
29. **Yu, Y., Zou, C., and Lih, M.,** Observations of the effect of tetrandrine on experimental silicosis of rats, *Ecotoxicol. Environ. Safety,* 7, 306–312, 1983.
30. **Mo, C. G., Yu, X. F., and Zou, C. Q.,** Studies on the relationship between structure and bioactivity of bisbenzylisoquinoline alkaloids, *Wei Sheng Yan Jiu,* 4, 118–125, 1982.
31. **Castranova, V., Kang, J. H., Moore, M. D., Pailes, W. H., Frazer, D. G., and Schwegler-Berry, D.,** Inhibition of stimulant-induced activation of phagocytic cells with tetrandrine, *J. Leuk. Biol.,* 50, 412–422, 1991.
32. **Reist, R. H.,** Cytokine and Pharmacological Regulation of Lung Fibroblast Proliferation, Dissertation, West Virginia University, Morgantown, WV, 1992.
33. **Ma, J. Y. C., Barger, M. W., Ma, J. K. H., and Castranova, V.,** Inhibition of respiratory burst activity in alveolar macrophages by bisbenzylisoquinoline alkaloids: characterization of drug-cell interaction, *Exp. Lung Res.,* 18, 829–843, 1992.
34. **Castranova, V., Kang, J. H., Ma, J. K. H., Mo, C. G., Malanga, C. J., Moore, M. D., Schwegler-Berry, D., and Ma, J. Y. C.,** Effects of bisbenzylisoquinoline alkaloids on alveolar macrophages: correlation between binding affinity, inhibitory potency, and antifibrotic potential, *Toxicol. Appl. Pharmacol.,* 108, 242–252, 1991.
35. **Ma, J. K. H., Mo, C. G., Malanga, C. J., Ma, J. Y. C., and Castranova, V.,** Binding of bisbenzylisoquinoline alkaloids to phosphatidylcholine vesicles and alveolar macrophages: relationship between binding affinity and antifibrogenic potential of these drugs, *Exp. Lung Res.,* 17, 1061–1077, 1991.
36. **Liu, L., Chen, N., Cai, G., Li, Z., Yang, J., and Li, Y.,** Studies on the effect of tetrandrine on microtubules. I. Biochemical observation and electron microscopy, *Ecotoxicol. Environ. Safety,* 15, 142–148, 1988.
37. **Chen, N., Liu, L., Cai, G., Yang, J., and Li, Y.,** Studies of the effects of tetrandrine on microtubules. II. Observation with immunofluorescence techniques, *Ecotoxicol. Environ. Safety,* 15, 149–152, 1988.
38. **Shiraishi, N., Arima, T., Aono, K., Inoue, B., Morimoto, Y., and Utsumi, K.,** Inhibition by biscoclaurine alkaloid of lipid peroxidation in biological membranes, *Physiol. Chem. Phys.,* 12, 299–305, 1980.
39. **Marks, J.,** The neutralization of silica toxicity *in vitro, Br. J. Ind. Med.,* 14, 81–84, 1957.
40. **Wallace, W. E., Vallyathan, V., Keane, M. J., and Robinson, V.,** *In vitro* biologic toxicity of native and surface-modified silica and kaolin, *J. Toxicol. Environ. Health,* 16, 415–424, 1985.

Section IV
Chapter 6

BISBENZYLISOQUINOLINE ALKALOIDS: EXPERIENCE FROM CHINA

Changqi Zou, Xirong Lu, and Shixuan Lu

CONTENTS

I. INTRODUCTION

Tetrandrine is one of the bisbenzylisoquinoline alkaloids extracted from the root of Hanfangji *(Stephania tetrandra S. moore),* a medicinal herb which had been used for centuries in China. Its molecular formula is $C_{38}H_{42}O_6N_2$–R with the following structure:[2]

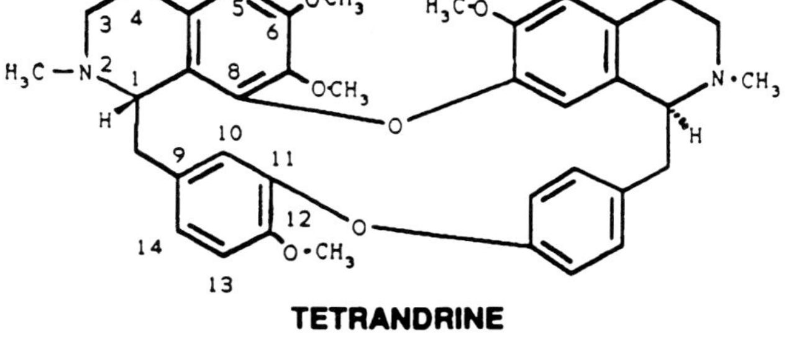

H₃C–N, N·CH₃, O-CH₃, H₃C-O, O·CH₃ (positions 1–14)

Str. A

TETRANDRINE

0-8493-4709-2/96/$0.00+$.50

In 1935, this drug was studied in the light of modern botany and pharmacology and was found to exhibit analgesic and antihypertensive activity. It has since been used to treat hypertension and rheumatism.

In 1975, the Institute of Occupational Medicine of the Chinese Academy of Preventive Medicine in Beijing and the Institutes of Pharmaceutical Industry, of the Occupational Health and Occupational Diseases in Tianjin engaged in a joint research program to screen Chinese herbs for their medical properties. They simultaneously found that tetrandrine might be a treatment for pneumoconiosis.[1] In 1976, The Institute of Occupational Medicine of the Chinese Academy of Preventive Medicine in Beijing organized a task force which included more than 30 institutes and clinics to study tetrandrine. This investigation included: animal studies,[2,3] structure-activity relationships of bisbenzylisoquinoline alkaloids,[2,4] and investigation of the therapeutical effects of tetrandrine on silicosis when used alone or in combination with other drugs.[5,9,16] In 1982, on the basis of results of these studies, a National Committee for Appraisement of the Collaborative Study on Tetrandrine concluded that tetrandrine was a drug of quick action for treatment as well as for prevention of all stages of pneumoconiosis (silicosis). With adequate dosages and well-arranged courses of treatment, even a long-term (3–6 months) medication was believed to be safe and without any untoward deleterious or toxic effects. Therefore, it was recommended as the drug of choice for treatment of pneumoconiosis (silicosis).

II. CLINICAL EXPERIENCE

Since 1970, the Institute of Occupational Health and Occupational Diseases of the Chinese Academy of Medical Sciences has screened a variety of traditional Chinese herbal medicines for the effective treatment of pneumoconiosis. The results with tetrandrine proved promising. It was one of five alkaloids of the bisbenzylisoquinoline group isolated from the root of *S. tetrandra* which had been used for centuries to treat headache, dizziness, and high blood pressure in China.

The indices used for screening as an effective agent were T/C values (ratio of wet weight or total collagen content of lungs from drug-treated silicotic rats to that for nontreated silicotic rats). T/C values less than 0.75 were considered effective, and these drugs then would be evaluated further. For tetrandrine, T/C values of both wet weight and collagen content of lungs were 0.48, much less than 0.75. Lung specimens of tetrandrine-treated silicotic rats showed fibrosis of Grade 2 using King's classification, compared with Grade 4 or 5 in nontreated silicotic rats.[2,3] The treated animals (rats, rabbits, and monkeys)[6,7] also appeared much healthier after tetrandrine (less cough and greater weight gain) than the nontreated silicotic controls. No toxic, mutagenic, or teratogenic reactions were observed in animals after oral ingestion of tetrandrine. Biochemical studies suggested that tetrandrine altered the progression of fibrosis rather than protecting alveolar macrophages from silica-induced cell injury.[8] It was therefore decided that a clinical trial of tetrandrine in silicotic patients was warranted.

From March 1977 until March 1982, 24 clinics participated in a trial of 240 cases with simple silicosis.[13] Of these patients, 236 were male, while 4 were female. Average age was 51.2 years (26 to 67 years). Average duration of dust exposure was 13.2 years (10 months to 37 years). Among 240 cases, there were 30 cases of Stage I (1/1, International Labour Office [ILO]), 122 cases of Stage II (2/2–3/3, ILO), and 88 cases of Stage III (large opacities A and B, ILO). All of the subjects had yearly chest X-ray films taken over the past 3 to 5 years which showed progression of lesions. Before treatment with tetrandrine, the following physical parameters were determined: symptoms and signs, electrocardiogram (EKG), ventilatory pulmonary functions, serum ceruloplasmine, serum lysosome, urine hydroxyproline, serum proteins, liver function (Glutamic pryrunic transaminase [GPT], Thymol turbidity [TT], and Thymol flocculation [TF] tests), erythrocyte sedimentation rate, routine examination of blood and urine, antirheumatic factor, TB in sputum, and in some cases IgA, IgG, IgM, and blood urea nitrogen.

Tetrandrine was administered orally as tablets, each tablet being 20 mg. In order to find an appropriate dose, tetrandrine was given at random to the cases according to three regimes:

1. 300 mg (Group A): 100 mg — three times daily except Sundays for three months; 2 to 3 months free from tetrandrine; and then begin tetrandrine again
2. 200 mg (Group B): 100 mg — twice daily except Sundays, for three months; 2 to 3 months without tetrandrine; and then begin tetrandrine again
3. 100 mg (Group C): 100 mg — once daily except Sundays for six months; 2 to 3 months without tetrandrine; and then begin tetrandrine again

TABLE 1
Chest X-ray Changes over the Course of Tetrandrine Treatment

Group	Number of cases	X-Ray appearance[a]		
		Improvement	Stationary	Progression
100 mg	52	0 (0%)	24 (46.2%)	28 (53.8%)
200 mg	117	29 (24.8%)	73 (62.3%)	15 (12.5%)
300 mg	71	24 (33.8%)	44 (62.0%)	3 (4.2%)
Total	240	53 (22.1%)	141 (58.5%)	46 (19.2%)

[a] Data given as number of cases (percentage of cases tested in that group).

Physical examinations were repeated after *in vivo* treatment with tetrandrine. Symptoms were recorded regularly, throughout the course of treatment, and were finally assessed at the conclusion of the treatment.

Among the 240 cases, 13 cases had one course of treatment and 227 cases had more than two courses (94.5%), of which 62 cases had more than seven courses (3 to 3.5 years). The total amount of tetrandrine for each case varied with the length (course) of treatment. The average amount of oral tetrandrine for each patient was 77 g.

A. RESULTS

Results observed in 240 cases could be summarized as follows:

1. Symptomatic Improvement

Since patients were hospitalized during the course of treatment, improvement or deterioration of symptoms was recorded by attending doctors who knew the patients for a long time. Therefore, the assessment of symptomatic improvement was reliable even though symptoms are subjective and very difficult to quantify. Symptoms evaluated included chest pain, chest tightness, shortness of breath, cough, sputum production, and frequency of attacks of upper respiratory infection. Cases in Group A (300 mg), Group B (200 mg), and Group C (100 mg) showed improvement of 47.4, 68.4, and 26.8%, respectively.

2. Chest X-Ray Changes after Treatment

X-ray appearance was recorded according to the following:

a. Improvement — definite decrease in profusion and extent of the small opacities; decrease in the size of large opacities
b. Stationary — no definite change observed
c. Progression — definite increase in profusion and extent of the small opacities and occurrence of any complication during the course of treatment.

Films of good and comparable quality made before and after treatment were read side by side. The results are shown in Table 1.

Among the 53 cases showing improvement, the small opacities appeared thinner and smaller, bronchial shadows became less diffuse and more clear, and the large opacities appeared thinner and smaller than before.

There were 37 patients in Group A (300 mg) and Group B (200 mg) who were treated with more than two courses of tetrandrine and were followed for 30 months. Of these, 29 (78.3%) began to show improvement after 15 to 18 months of treatment. Improvement in these cases was not enough to change the original category of the X-ray images. When tetrandrine was discontinued for three months, no further improvement was observed and in some cases progression of lesions would be observed again.

3. Laboratory Examinations

In Group A (300 mg) and Group B (200 mg), there were 37 patients showing X-ray improvement who also exhibited a significant decrease in serum ceruloplasmine content during this improvement. No significant changes were observed in other lab tests.

4. Side Effects of Tetrandrine

The following side effects of tetrandrine treatment were noted in this clinical trial:

a. Gastrointestinal tract: anorexia, mild abdominal pain, abdominal distention, and loose stools may develop on the second to third days of treatment. These discomforts can be controlled by means of usual measures and usually subsided per se as tetrandrine treatment continued. In a few exceptional cases, these discomforts became so obstinate that tetrandrine had to be discontinued.
b. Skin: brownish black pigmentation may be seen around the nipples and over the exposed parts of the body (face and hands) 2 to 3 months after the start of tetrandrine treatment. This reaction was dose dependent, i.e., the higher the dosage, the more the pigmentation. Pigmentation receded gradually when tetrandrine therapy was discontinued. No change of 17-hydroxycorticoids or 17-ketosteroids was noted in cases with pigmentation.
c. Transient enlargement of liver and elevation of serum transaminase (SGPT) may be seen in some cases.

B. SUMMARY

The clinical trial of tetrandrine on silicosis could be summarized as follows:

1. On the basis that tetrandrine could reduce the fibrogenicity of silica in experimental animals (rats, rabbits, and monkeys), tetrandrine was used in patients with simple silicosis. The clinical trial lasted for five years (April 1977 to April 1982) and evaluated 240 cases with complete records.
2. The optimal dosage was either 100 mg three times a day/6 d every week for three months or 100 mg twice a day/6 d every week for three months. Each course was followed by 2 to 3 months without tetrandrine in order to avoid accumulation of the drug. Side effects from the drug were very mild.
3. After tetrandrine, there was subjective improvement of general condition and of symptoms pertaining to silicosis. Improvement persisted through the course of treatment in about 60% of the cases.
4. There was X-ray improvement in films of comparable quality made before and after treatment in about 27.4% of the cases. Improvement consisted of a decrease in profusion and extent of small opacities (both rounded and irregular) with thinning and shrinkage of large opacities. X-ray changes usually occurred after the second course of treatment and persisted for about three months after discontinuation of tetrandrine therapy. Progression of the lesions would occur after discontinuation of drug therapy, sometimes more insidiously than before treatment.

C. COMMENTS

It was too early to draw a conclusion on the effect of tetrandrine on silicosis because of the following three points:

1. Without matched control groups, the reliability of this trial is jeopardized. Due to various reasons, the original scheme of setting up a control group could not be followed. Nontechnical factors peculiar to the period of trial were some of the reasons.
2. No standard chest films were used for comparison, and the X-ray techniques were not standardized. Chinese Standard Chest Films for Pneumoconiosis were issued in 1986, and standard X-ray techniques (120 kV) have not been set up until very recently. Comparison of films made before and after treatment was not standardized.
3. Cases were hospitalized during treatment. Hospital life and food might have improved general condition and reduced symptoms. This might explain the recurrence of symptoms afterwards. Nevertheless, tetrandrine in our experience is believed to be a very hopeful remedy for silicosis. For the benefit of 300,000 patients with pneumoconiosis in China, a renewed clinical trial of tetrandrine will be conducted soon.

TABLE 2
Results of Preventive Treatment of Tetrandrine on Rat Silicosis

Period of tetrandrine treatment (month)	Rat (No.)	Dry weight of whole lung		Collagen count of whole lung		Pathological grade
		X (g)	T/C	X (mg)	T/C	
1	7	0.41	0.59[b]	46.93	0.51[a]	I grade
3	6	0.50	0.48[a]	77.30	0.41[b]	I grade
6	5	0.74	0.69[a]	98.31	0.43[b]	Few I grade
9	7	0.81	0.73[a]	123.98	0.53[b]	Few I grade

[a] $p < 0.01$.
[b] $p < 0.001$.

III. ANIMAL STUDIES

A. STUDIES OF THERAPEUTIC EFFECTS

1. On Experimental Silicosis in Rats[2,3,5,10,14]

Male rats of Wistar strain, each about 200 g in weight, were used in this experiment. Normal saline suspension of silica dusts (40 or 50 mg/ml) was administered as a single intratracheal dose. Silica content of the dust was 99%. More than 95% of the silica particles were less than 5 μm in diameter.

Tetrandrine was administered through a small gastric tube, and the dosage was 120–150 mg/kg/week. Tetrandrine treatment was started at different times in accordance with the purpose of observation as follows:

a. "For prevention" — tetrandrine was started 3–5 d after silica exposure. Each experimental group of rats received tetrandrine through a gastric tube. The experimental animals were sacrificed 1, 2, 3, 6, and 9 months after silica exposure and compared with the corresponding controls (silica-exposed rats without tetrandrine).
b. "For treatment" — tetrandrine was started 1 or 2 months after silica exposure. Experimental groups received tetrandrine through a gastric tube every week and were sacrificed 2, 3, and 5 months after silica exposure and compared with the corresponding controls (silicotic rats without tetrandrine).

Results of the "prevention" groups are given in Table 2. The ratio (T/C) of dry weight of lungs of tetrandrine-treated (T) rats to that of control (C) rats was significantly less than one. T/C values for total collagen content of lungs was also significantly decreased by tetrandrine treatment. Pathological studies of lung specimens from drug-treated rats showed significantly milder changes than those of controls. Instead of the firm, fibrotic nodules of silicosis seen in untreated rats, tetrandrine treatment resulted in lesions exhibiting only cellular nodules of macrophages with foamy and abundant cytoplasm. If graded according to King's classification, the fibrosis occurring 6 to 9 months after silica dust exposure was Grade III in controls and was only Grade I in tetrandrine-treated rats.

Results of the "treatment" groups were also significant. Even though tetrandrine was started 1 to 2 months after silica exposure, the results were quite similar in nature to the "prevention" group. In the "treatment" group, T/C ratio for dry weight of lungs varied from 0.55–0.71, while T/C ratio for total collagen content of lungs ranged from 0.33–0.48. Pathologically, the tetrandrine-treated specimens showed much milder changes of silicosis and fewer silicotic nodules with degeneration of collagen fibers and infiltration of macrophages than the silica-exposed control group.

When rabbits were used instead of rats, 120 mg silica dust suspended in normal saline was instilled intratracheally to induce silicosis. Tetrandrine animals received 120–150 mg of drug per kilogram of body weight orally. The results for rabbits were similar in nature to those of rats.

Based upon animal studies, the most effective therapeutic dosage of tetrandrine was 90–120 mg/kg body weight per week. Therapeutic activity was lost at doses below 30 mg/kg body weight per week.

2. On Experimental Silicosis in Monkeys[6,7]

Fourteen monkeys (nine male, five female) *(Macacus mulatt)* of 6.4–10.4 kg body weight were rendered silicotic by means of intratracheal administration of silica dust (4–4.5 g) in a manner similar to that described for rats and rabbits. Tetrandrine therapy was started 6 months after exposure. Tetrandrine was administered into the stomach through a nasal tube twice a week. One group received 60 mg of tetrandrine per kilogram body weight per week, while the other group received 24 mg/kg body weight per week. Both drug groups showed significant improvement of cough and shortness of breath after treatment. Serum ceruloplasmine decreased significantly. Chest films of monkeys sacrificed six months after treatment showed shrinkage of nodular shadows. The T/C ratio for dry weight of lungs was 0.67. The T/C ratio for total collagen content of lungs was 0.57. During autopsy, hilar lymph nodes of treated monkeys were much smaller than those of controls. Microscopic examination of hilar lymph nodes showed significantly less silicotic changes in the tetrandrine-treated group. Degeneration of collagen fibers and infiltration of macrophages were also observed in the tetrandrine-treated groups.

B. TOXICOLOGICAL STUDIES[4–7,12]

1. Acute and Chronic Toxicities

For mice, the LD_{50} for oral administration of tetrandrine was 1064–1478 mg/kg. The main symptoms of intoxication were dull and sluggish response to stimuli, anorexia, tremor, loss of coordination, syncope, and finally death due to respiratory failure. Intragastric administration of tetrandrine to monkeys and dogs for 6 to 9 months in dosage of 24–30 mg/kg/week, i.e., the dosage used clinically, did not cause any adverse changes detectable by routine examination of blood, liver, or kidneys. If tetrandrine was increased to 60 mg/kg/week for monkeys or 120 mg/kg/week for dogs or rats and administered for six months, increases of erythrocyte sedimentation rate and serum transaminases were observed in dogs but not in monkeys. Pathological examination of treated rats revealed fatty degeneration and necrosis of liver cells and of renal epithelial cells of the convoluted tubules.

2. Teratogenicity and Mutagenicity of Tetrandrine

Different dosages of tetrandrine were administered to pregnant rats, i.e., 1/15, 1/25, or 1/50 of LD_{50} for tetrandrine (1478 mg/kg) on the sixth day of pregnancy, once daily for 10 d. Animals were sacrificed on the 20th day of their pregnancy, and the findings were compared with the positive controls. No teratogenic effects were noted.

Ames' tests, micronuclear tests, and chromosome aberration tests were conducted and revealed no *in vitro* mutagenic activity for tetrandrine.

IV. METABOLISM OF TETRANDRINE

The distribution, excretion, and metabolism of tetrandrine has been studied in mice, rats, dogs, monkeys, and humans by means of chemical methods or tracer studies with radiolabeled ^3H-tetrandrine.

After ingestion, the biological half-life of tetrandrine in the blood was 30 h for mice and 52–55 h for rats. After being absorbed, tetrandrine was distributed widely in the body with the greatest accumulation occurring in the liver, lungs, kidneys, and adrenal glands. It did not pass through the blood-brain barrier. The clearance of tetrandrine from the lungs was slow, thus potentiating the therapeutic action of the drug. Accumulation of tetrandrine in viscera paralleled the intake of this drug and decreased gradually after discontinuation of medication, i.e., two months after cessation of drug treatment tetrandrine levels in the viscera would fall to 1/10 of their original level. Tetrandrine was excreted through urine and feces. In the mouse, 90% of the ingested drug would be excreted within 7 d. Within 30–40 d all the clearance was complete in the mouse. It took 60 d for rats to completely clear the drug.

In the rats, most of the ingested tetrandrine remained in the unmetabolized form. Oxidation and demethylization of tetrandrine was relatively slow. Oxidized and demethylated forms represented 9% (in liver and lungs) and 7% (in liver) of the total tetrandrine content, respectively. In the urine, oxidized tetrandrine reached 26% of the total drug content.

V. MECHANISM OF THERAPEUTIC ACTION

The *in vitro*[8] effect of tetrandrine on the survival rate of pulmonary macrophages, the release of lactic acid dehydrogenase and acid phosphatase, and glycolysis after silica exposure indicated that unlike PVNO (poly-2-vinyl-pyridine-N-oxide) or Al (derivatives of aluminum compounds), which act to coat SiO_2 particles,[9] tetrandrine did not prevent silica-induced cell injury. Tetrandrine directly affected intracellular DNA, collagen, and other proteins such as plasma proteins and procollagen. It inhibited the proliferation of fibroblasts and the intracellular synthesis and secretion of procollagen until no extracellular formation of collagen fibers would occur. Furthermore, tetrandrine inhibited the silica-induced increase of glycosaminoglycans and lipids in the lung.[15] These data suggest that tetrandrine may act by retarding the cascade of cellular events which results in the development of silicosis.

VI. STRUCTURE-ACTIVITY RELATIONSHIPS

Screening of a number of bisbenzylisoquinoline (BIQ) alkaloids indicates that a relationship exists between chemical structure and biological activity. The potency of several bisbenzylisoquinoline alkaloids has been investigated by Mo et al.[11] The following structure-activity relationships have been noted:

1. There was a close relationship between biological activity and substituents at the C-7 and C-12 positions in the ring structure. Among the nine BIQ studied, the therapeutic efficacy of tetrandrine against silicosis in experimental animals was significantly higher than that of fangchinoline. Cycleanine was also effective against animal silicosis, yet isochondrodendrine was not efficacious. Different substituents at C-7 and C-12 might throw light on the differences. The chemical group at sites C-7 and C-12 for tetrandrine and cycleanine was $-OCH_3$ while there was –OH substitution at these sites for fangchinoline and isochondrodendrine. It was possible that the H atom of the OH group might react with adjacent $-OCH_3$ groups of the O of the oxygen bridge to form an intramolecular H-chain, which might sterically hinder interaction of the drug with receptors.
2. There was a relationship between the spatial structure at sites C-1 and C-1′ and the biological activity of the drug. Combination of receptors with compounds of SS (Sinister-Sinister) configuration was much stronger than with compounds of RS (Rectus-Sinister) or SR (Sinister-Rectus) configuration, thus resulting in higher efficacy. The spatial structure of tetrandrine or cycleanine was of the SS isomer, while that of isotetrandrine or 7.1-methoxylhomoaromoline were RS or SR, respectively. The former two compounds were efficacious in treating silicosis, while the latter two were not.[10]
3. Benzylisoquinolines, which contain a double oxygen bridge to form cyclic hydrocarbon compounds, exhibited biological activity. Tetrandrine and cycleanine contain two oxygen bridges and are dioxide octodeca cyclic hydrocarbons. These drugs reacted strongly with plasma proteins and were efficacious in treating silicosis in rats. L-Curine and 7,12-dimetheoxycurine contain a double oxygen bridge but are dioxide eicosunic cyclic hydrocarbons and were not effective. Dauricine had only one oxygen bridge and had no effect on pneumoconiosis. Therefore, the double oxygen bridge is important for activity, and the dioxide octodeca cyclic structure seems to be preferred over the dioxide eicosunic cyclic structure for the oxygen double bridge.

REFERENCES

1. **Zou, C. Li, T., et al.,** Observation of therapeutic effects of 12 kinds of traditional Chinese medicine and herbs on experimental silicosis, Proc. of Symp. of Silicosis at 5 Provinces of Middle-South of China, 1975.
2. **Yu, X. Zou, C., et al.,** Observation of therapeutic effects of 5 kinds of bisbenzylisoquinoline alkaloids on experimental silicosis of rats, *J. Hyg. Res.*, 6(2), 92–98, 1977.

3. **Zou, C. Lin, M., et al.,** Observation of therapeutic effects of tetrandrine on the experimental silicosis of rats, *J. Hyg. Res.,* 8(1), 1–11, 1979.
4. **Zou, C. Lin, M., et al.,** Studies of chronic toxicity of tetrandrine and 12-ethoxy berbamine on dogs, *J. Hyg. Res.,* 8(4), 227–235, 1979.
5. **Yu, X. Zou, C., et al.,** Studies of the therapeutic effects of combined use of tetrandrine and anti-silicotic drugs on experimental silicosis of rats, *J. Hyg. Res.,* 10(4), 61–67, 1981.
6. **Yin, R. Zou, C., et al.,** Observation of the therapeutic effect and toxicity of tetrandrine on monkeys, *J. Hyg. Res.,* 11(4), 55–65, 1982.
7. **Zou, C. Liu, J., et al.,** E.M. observation of the toxicity of tetrandrine on the liver and kidney of experimental silicosis of monkeys, *J. Hyg. Res.,* 11(4), 65–69, 1982.
8. **Chen, N. Zou, C., et al.,** Observation of inhibitory effect of tetrandrine on silica-induced fibrogenesis by culture system *in vitro, J. Hyg. Res.,* 11(4), 79–86, 1982.
9. **Zou, C. Yu, X., et al.,** Observation of the therapeutic effect of combined use of tetrandrine and PVNO or kangxi-1 on experimental silicosis of rats, *J. Hyg. Res.,* 11(4), 86–89, 1982.
10. **Yu, X. Zou, C., et al.,** Studies of the therapeutic effect of n-2′-oxide-tetrandrine on experimental silicosis of rats, *J. Hyg. Res.,* 11(4), 94–98, 1982.
11. **Mo, C., Yu, X., Zou, C., et al.,** Study on the relationship between chemical structure and biochemical action of bisbenzylisoquinoline alkaloids, *J. Hyg. Res.,* 11(4), 118–130, 1982.
12. **Li, T. Hu, T., Zou, C., et al.,** Studies of the chronic toxicity of tetrandrine in dogs, *Ecotoxicol. Environ. Safety,* 6, 528–534, 1983.
13. **Zou, C. Lu, X., et al.,** Research on the therapeutic effect of tetrandrine on silicosis, VI International Conf., Bochom, FRG, Vol (1), 467, 1983.
14. **Yu, X., Zou, C., Lim, M. et al.,** Observation of the effect of tetrandrine on experimental silicosis of rat, *Ecotoxicol. Environ. Safety,* 7, 306–312, 1983.
15. **Liu, B., Zou, C., and Li, Y.,** Studies on the contents of glycosaminoglycans from lungs of silicotic rats and tetrandrine-treated silicotic rats, *Ecotoxicol. Environ. Safety,* 7, 323–329, 1983.
16. **Zou, C. and Idel, H.,** Studies of the therapeutic effect of combined use of tetrandrine and PVNO on the experimental silicosis of rats, *Umwelthygiene,* 19, 91, 1986–1987.
17. **Lin, M., Zhang, W., et al.,** *In vivo* studies on the metabolism and conversion of tetrandrine, *J. Hyg. Res.,* 10(4), 93–98, 1981.

Section IV
Chapter 7

PHARMACEUTICAL CONSIDERATIONS IN THE USE OF TETRANDRINE TO TREAT SILICOSIS

Joseph K. H. Ma, De-Hwa Chao, Jane Y. C. Ma, Ann Hubbs, and Vincent Castranova

CONTENTS

I. INTRODUCTION: AN OVERVIEW OF THE ACTION OF TETRANDRINE ON SILICOSIS

Because of the persistent presence of silica dust in the lungs, silicosis is a progressive and irreversible disease. At present, there is no proven effective therapy for silicosis. Limited choices of therapeutic intervention with corticosteroids and other immunosuppressive regimens[1,2] have been accepted for some forms of pulmonary fibrosis. These treatments are only minimally effective, and the results provide little understanding of the disease state due to the lack of correlation between drug activity and the mechanism of fibrosis. Thus, continuing effort must be made in the search for effective antifibrotic agents, which may be used to provide a sequential analysis of the fibrotic process and to open the door for further research and clinical development.

Tetrandrine is one of hundreds of drugs screened for antifibrotic activity by Chinese scientists. It has been used in China as a treatment for silicosis in open clinical trials[3] and in laboratory animals[4–6] The action of tetrandrine on pulmonary fibrosis has been attributed to its ability to inhibit particle stimulation of alveolar macrophages, a key cell type central to the fibrotic process, to release oxygen radicals and inflammatory cytokines. Alveolar macrophages (AM), residing on the alveolar wall, are the predominant phagocytic cells of the lungs responsible for pulmonary defense against inhaled microorganisms and other particles, and thus play an important role in maintaining the homeostasis of the lungs.[7] Ample evidence suggests that cells of the monocyte-macrophage series play an important role in the immunopathogenesis of pulmonary fibrosis. When upregulated by silica, alveolar macrophages generate reactive oxygen metabolites[8,9] which can damage lung parenchyma and release fibrogenic growth factors and cytokines,[10,11] such as interleukin 1 (IL-1), which can induce fibroblast proliferation and collagen synthesis. The cytokine-mediated fibroblast proliferation and collagen synthesis are key steps in the development and progression of pulmonary fibrosis.[12] Previous studies by our group have shown that tetrandrine exhibits strong binding affinity to AM and inhibits particle-stimulated respiratory burst

0-8493-4709-2/96/$0.00+$.50

activity (oxygen consumption, superoxide anion release, and hydrogen peroxide secretion) in these cells.[13] In addition, studies by Kang et al.[14] have reported that tetrandrine inhibits silica-induced release of fibrogenic factors such as IL-1 which are capable of inducing fibroblast proliferation and collagen synthesis. Reist et al.[15] further suggested that the antifibrotic action of tetrandrine may be mediated in part by the direct effect of this drug on the ability of fibroblasts to respond to proliferative agents. These results indicate that the mechanism of silicosis involves activation of AM and fibroblasts by silica, resulting in abnormal collagen production due to miscommunications between the cell types. Tetrandrine may interrupt this process by direct interaction with the lung cells.

II. DISADVANTAGES OF CONVENTIONAL TETRANDRINE THERAPY IN THE TREATMENT OF SILICOSIS

The *in vivo* activity of tetrandrine has been studied primarily via oral administration of the drug. Tetrandrine is a bisbenzylisoquinoline alkaloid with two methyl-substituted amino groups. Although the lung has a well-established capacity to sequester certain basic amines, oral administration of this lipophilic drug is subject to significant first-pass hepatic extraction. In addition, tetrandrine has been shown to exhibit long biological half-life in experimental animals (30 h in mice and 52–55 h in rats),[4–6] suggesting that chronic use of tetrandrine may result in an accumulation and redistribution of the drug in various tissue and blood compartments. Indeed, the pharmacokinetic behavior of tetrandrine is well reflected by the adverse effects of the drug. Oral delivery of tetrandrine in the treatment of silicosis has been associated with diverse side effects including skin darkening, diarrhea, elevated levels of serum alanine transferase activity, and liver dysfunction, which are reversible following the cessation of drug administration.[3] Hence, the oral tetrandrine therapy requires the insertion of frequent resting periods (2 to 3 months) of no drug treatment to alleviate potential drug toxicity.[3] Despite *in vitro* and *in vivo* data indicating the antifibrogenic activity of the drug, tetrandrine has not been proven clinically effective for the treatment of silicosis. This may be in part due to its low therapeutic index under the oral regimen, which may have limited its safe use as a therapeutic agent. It is also possible that the lack of sound pharmaceutical approaches in drug delivery strategies may have also obscured the observation of the pharmacological effect of the drug.

Both the pharmacological action and the pharmacokinetic behavior of tetrandrine suggest that targeted delivery of tetrandrine to the lungs can enhance the efficacy of the drug in the treatment of silicosis. Targeted drug delivery has the advantage of achieving effective drug concentrations at the site of action with a dose which is significantly lower than that of a conventional therapy. This would in turn lower the systemic drug toxicity and allow for long-term use of the drug for chronic diseases such as silicosis. The fact that tetrandrine has a low therapeutic index and long biological half-life due to high tissue distribution suggests that this drug is an ideal candidate for developing a strategy for targeted drug delivery. Recently, studies carried out in our laboratory have demonstrated that pharmaceutical emulsions may be an effective delivery system to target tetrandrine to AM.[16,17] The emulsion system, which will be discussed in the following section, was shown to enhance the pharmacological action of tetrandrine *in vivo* and allow one to determine the antifibrotic activity of the drug at the cellular level.

III. PHARMACEUTICAL STRATEGY FOR IMPROVED THERAPEUTIC EFFECT OF TETRANDRINE

A. MULTIPLE EMULSION AS A DRUG DELIVERY SYSTEM

Selective delivery of therapeutic agents via carrier to appropriate sites in the body has the potential to improve the successful treatment of diseases. Multiple emulsions of the w/o/w (water-in-oil-in-water) type have emerged as an attractive system for controlled drug delivery in contemporary biomedical research.[18,19] These emulsions are characterized by the encapsulation of water-in-oil droplets in an external aqueous phase which may be prepared by a two-step emulsification method first reported by Matsumoto et al.[20,21] Although the emulsion system has been known for quite some time, it is only recently that the w/o/w emulsions have been produced with consistency and stability and have become applicable to various fields of study, including microencapsulation,[22] enzyme immobilization and blood detoxification,[23,24] sustained drug release,[25] treatment of wastewater,[26] and separation of hydrocarbons.[27] For pharmaceutical use, the w/o/w multiple emulsions may be developed into injection or inhalation dosage forms. Although the pulmonary route of drug delivery is most appropriate for drug intervention of lung diseases, aerosol technology for delivery of consistent drug doses to the lower airway remains to be developed. The emulsion system, however, does exhibit liposomal characteristics which may be administered intravenously for drug targeting to the lungs. Similar to other microparticulate carriers, the emulsion systems are biologically recognized as foreign by the mononuclear phagocyte system, i.e., they can be rapidly removed from the circulation following intravenous administration and accumulated in particular tissues such as the lungs, liver, spleen, and bone marrow.[28] Multiple emulsions with desirable particle size distribution may be sequestered by the lung through filtration mechanisms, and the intravenous route offers further advantage over oral dosage form for improved pulmonary drug delivery by eliminating the first-pass hepatic extraction.

B. TETRANDRINE EMULSION

A multiple emulsion system containing tetrandrine (5.5 μm in mean droplet diameter) was developed by Chao[29] using a blend of peanut oil and hydrogenated soybean oil (7:3) as the lipid membrane. In this formulation, the primary w/o emulsion was stabilized by Tween® 80 and Span 80 with a combined HLB (hydrophile-lipophile balance) of 5.5, whereas the external aqueous phase was stabilized using Tween® 80 and trace amount of Triton® X-100. This emulsion system was shown to be stable at 4°C with no changes in particle number or size distribution and drug release rate when monitored for eight weeks. Furthermore, the blank emulsion (without drug) was shown to have no effect on the viability of AM over 4 h incubation, indicating that the emulsion system is nontoxic to these lung cells.

C. EFFECT OF EMULSION ON DRUG-CELL INTERACTIONS

The respiratory burst activity of AM is a convenient marker for the assessment of the pharmacological and toxicological effects of drugs and dosage forms intended for pulmonary drug delivery. Chao et al.[16] have studied the effect of the emulsion system on macrophage respiratory burst and the potential of the emulsion system to alter drug-cell interactions by measurement of resting and zymosan-induced oxygen consumption by AM in response to emulsion treatment. Zymosan is a particulate stimulant isolated from the cell wall of *Saccharomyces cerevisiae* yeast which stimulates a macrophage respiratory burst. Studies have shown that, in short-term incubations when cell viability is not affected, tetrandrine has no effect on the resting level of oxygen consumption by AM but inhibits the stimulatory effect of zymosan.[13] Thus, by monitoring the oxygen consumption of AM, one can assess the emulsion-cell interaction as well as the effect of the emulsion system on drug activity. In addition, measurement of oxygen consumption also yields information on cell viability or drug toxicity. For example, Table 1 shows the effect of tetrandrine on the resting and zymosan-induced oxygen consumption by AM measured after 1-h incubation. The drug

TABLE 1
Effect of Tetrandrine on the Oxygen Consumption of AM at Rest and in Response to Zymosan Stimulation Following 1-h Incubation

	Oxygen consumption (% control)[a]	
Tetrandrine (μg/ml)	**Resting level**	**Zymosan-induced level**
Control	100	100
6	101 ± 2	99 ± 3
12	108 ± 1	106 ± 4
24	75 ± 2*	59 ± 2*
36	69 ± 2*	33 ± 2*
48	71 ± 2*	29 ± 1*
60	68 ± 3*	19 ± 2*

[a] Measurements were carried out in samples containing 4×10^6 AM, at 37°C. The control values for the resting and zymosan-induced oxygen consumption are 1.1 ± 0.6 and 2.8 ± 1.1 nmol O_2/min/10^6 cells, respectively. Asterisks indicate significant difference from control ($p \leq 0.05$).

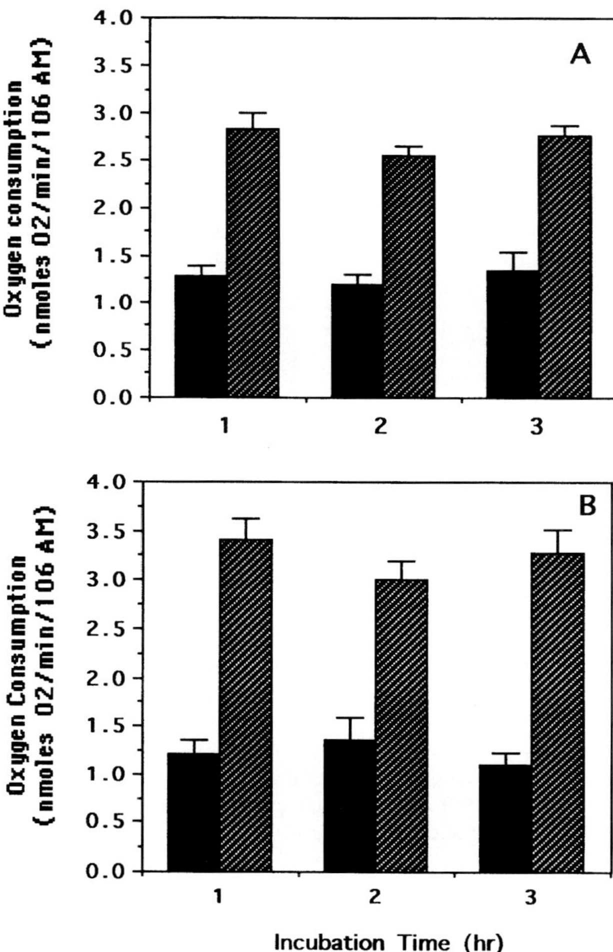

FIGURE 1 Effect of the blank multiple emulsion on the oxygen consumption of AM at rest (dark bar) and in response to zymosan stimulation (light bar): (A) control; (B) treatment with blank emulsion (11.5 μl/ml cell suspension).

is seen to have a strong, dose-dependent inhibitory effect on zymosan-induced oxygen consumption. However, a decrease in the resting level of oxygen consumption by AM occurs at high drug doses. This reduction is consistent with measured decreases in cell viability, indicating that tetrandrine is toxic to AM in prolonged incubations.

Figures 1 and 2 show the effect of the emulsion system on tetrandrine activity and cytotoxicity via measurement of macrophage oxygen consumption. Neither the resting nor zymosan-stimulated levels of oxygen consumption by AM measured at various time periods was affected by the treatment of cells with blank emulsion (Figure 1), suggesting that the emulsion system does not alter cell surface-mediated response to zymosan stimulation over the time period studied and has no effect on cell viability. In Figure 2, data on oxygen consumption were obtained from AM treated with either free tetrandrine (in solution) or the tetrandrine emulsion. Both the solution and emulsion dosage forms of tetrandrine are shown to completely inhibit the zymosan-induced oxygen consumption by AM. Treatment of cells with free tetrandrine is associated with a time-dependent reduction of resting oxygen consumption by AM, indicating decreased cell viability. In contrast, the emulsion system containing the same concentration of tetrandrine has little or no effect on the resting level of oxygen consumption. These results indicate that the multiple emulsion system, which is nontoxic to AM, reduces drug cytotoxicity but retains the pharmacological effect of the drug. The emulsion-mediated activity may be attributed to the ability of the emulsion droplets to deliver the drug intracellularly, thus preventing cell membrane damage associated with prolonged drug-cell interactions at the plasma membrane.

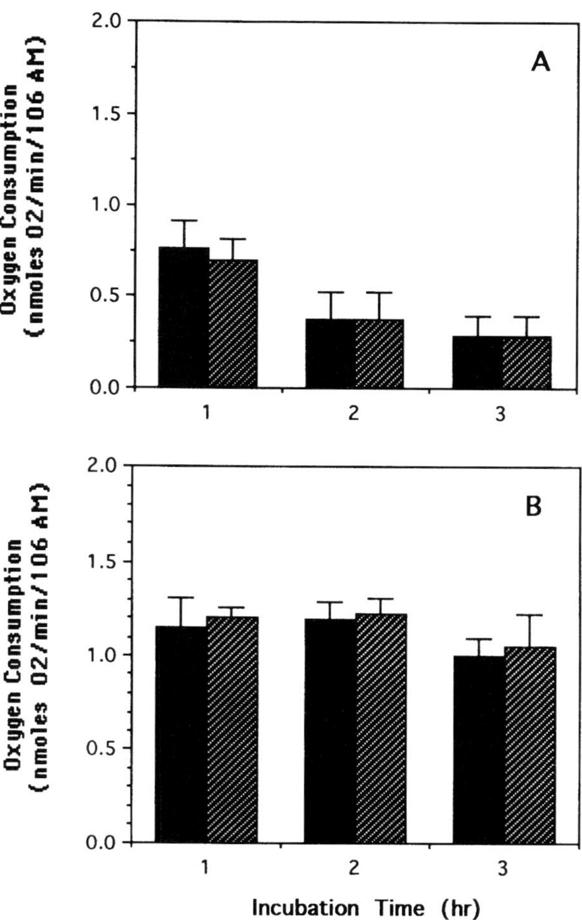

FIGURE 2 The formulation-dependent effect of tetrandrine (60 μg/ml) on the oxygen consumption of AM at rest (dark bar) and in response to zymosan stimulation (light bar): (A) effect from tetrandrine solution; (B) effect from tetrandrine emulsion (contains 5.25 mg/ml drug).

D. EMULSION-MEDIATED TETRANDRINE ACTIVITY *IN VIVO*

Despite several studies indicating the use of tetrandrine to treat silicosis in experimental animals, evidence of direct *in vivo* interaction of tetrandrine with lung cells has not been clearly demonstrated. With the aid of the emulsion system, which has been shown to alter the pharmacokinetics of tetrandrine in rats in favor of increased lung distribution,[17] studies have been carried out to provide *in vivo* evidence of direct tetrandrine effect on AM respiratory burst. These studies and selected results are described as follows.

Male Sprague-Dawley rats (180–200 g) were anesthetized with sodium brevital and silica (Min-U-Sil; 98.5% purity; specific surface area: 3.97 m^2/g), 40 mg/0.5 ml of saline, or saline (nonsilicotic control) was instilled into the lungs via the trachea. Following dust exposure, a daily single dose of tetrandrine either in solution or in emulsion (13 mg/kg) was administered through the tail vein for 4 d. Animals were maintained under normal care for two or four weeks before sacrifice. AM were then harvested by bronchoalveolar lavage (BAL) and lungs isolated. The left and right lungs were used for measurements of lung weight and collagen content (as hydroxyproline), respectively. Lung specimens were also prepared for histological examination. AM from nonsilicotic and silicotic control or drug-treated rats were obtained and subjected to measurements of resting and zymosan-challenged respiratory burst activity.

TABLE 2
Effects of *in Vivo* Silica and Tetrandrine on AM Activity and Lung Hydroxyproline Content in Rats at Two Weeks Post-Silica Exposure

Treatment	AM oxygen consumption ($nmol\ O_2/min/10^6$ cells) Resting	Zymosan-stimulated	Hydroxyproline (mg/lung)
Saline (control)	0.66 ± 0.05	1.35 ± 0.19	1.60 ± 0.08
Saline + drug solution	0.72 ± 0.08	1.44 ± 0.22	1.69 ± 0.01
Saline + drug emulsion	0.61 ± 0.04	1.21 ± 0.11	1.62 ± 0.09
Silica (silicotic control)	0.29 ± 0.07[a]	0.44 ± 0.16[a]	3.96 ± 0.18[a]
Silica + drug solution	0.35 ± 0.08[a]	0.56 ± 0.23[a]	2.80 ± 0.18[a,b]
Silica + drug emulsion	0.50 ± 0.15[b]	1.02 ± 0.19[b]	2.00 ± 0.05[a]

[a] Indicates significant difference from saline control.
[b] Indicates significant difference from silicotic control.

Table 2 shows the results on oxygen consumption using AM harvested two weeks post-silica exposure. In the nonsilicotic groups, both the resting and zymosan-induced oxygen consumptions were unaffected by the tetrandrine treatment, suggesting that the drug did not change the normal function of the cell *in vivo*. This is expected since tetrandrine does not affect the resting cell activity when present and is probably completely eliminated from the lungs at two weeks postexposure. The estimated pulmonary half-life for tetrandrine in the solution and emulsion dosage forms are 23 and 36 h, respectively.[17] In silicotic rats, AM are shown to exhibit reduced levels of resting and zymosan-stimulated oxygen consumption when compared to the nonsilicotic control. This suggests that silica alters normal cell activity or cell differentials due to silica-mediated cell death or epithelial lung damage. The *in vivo* effect of tetrandrine on silica-mediated cell activity is of interest. Tetrandrine appears to restore the normal function of AM as indicated by the increased levels of both resting and zymosan-induced oxygen consumption in comparison to the silicotic control. This effect is especially clear in the case of treatment with tetrandrine emulsion, where the oxygen consumption levels approach normal values.

At necropsy, the lungs of silica-exposed rats receiving no drug treatment were extremely heavy, firm, and gray. In contrast, treatment of silicotic rats with tetrandrine in solution or in emulsion diminished gross lesions. The silica effect is associated with an increase in the dry weight and collagen content of the lungs. The lung collagen synthesis was assessed by measurement of total tissue hydroxyproline. Table 2 shows that lungs from the silicotic controls exhibit a 2.5-fold increase in hydroxyproline content in comparison to the nonsilicotic control. This silica effect was inhibited by tetrandrine, and the inhibition was more effectively achieved by treatment using the tetrandrine emulsion. These results are very consistent with those of the oxygen consumption studies, indicating that silica-induced collagen synthesis in the lung may be related to abnormal macrophage activity. The increase in lung collagen formation resulting from silica exposure indicates an on-going fibrotic process.

Histological examination of alveolar cell types and lung tissue also demonstrates the emulsion-mediated enhancement of tetrandrine activity. Ultrastructurally, AM harvested from nonsilicotic rats exhibit normal cell characteristics (Figure 3) with typical organelles and numerous phagocytic vacuoles shown in the cytoplasm. AM obtained from silicotic control rats four weeks postexposure contained phagocytized material resembling surfactant and crystal-like material morphologically consistent with cholesterol (Figure 4). Heppleston[30] had described the material accumulated within alveoli in alveolar lipoproteinosis as having biochemical features similar to surfactant but lacking surface-reduction properties. The mechanism of accumulation of this material is unknown, but could be related either to a decrease in the degradation of lung surfactant or to an increase in its production. Hallmark to the acute outcome of the silica-lung interaction is the development of lipidosis, involving abnormal production of phospholipids in Type II cells. Miller et al.[31] have shown that Type II cells isolated from the lungs of rats receiving intratracheal silica consist of a bimodal population of Type II cells: one population that resembled Type II cells from control animals, and one that had an increased cell volume with an increased number of lamellar bodies per cell. In addition, the average volume of lamellar bodies was also increased in those hypertrophic Type II pneumocytes. Indeed, Figure 5 shows one isolated Type II cell obtained from the BAL of a rat receiving silica, where, in a serendipitic moment, the surfactant-like content is seen

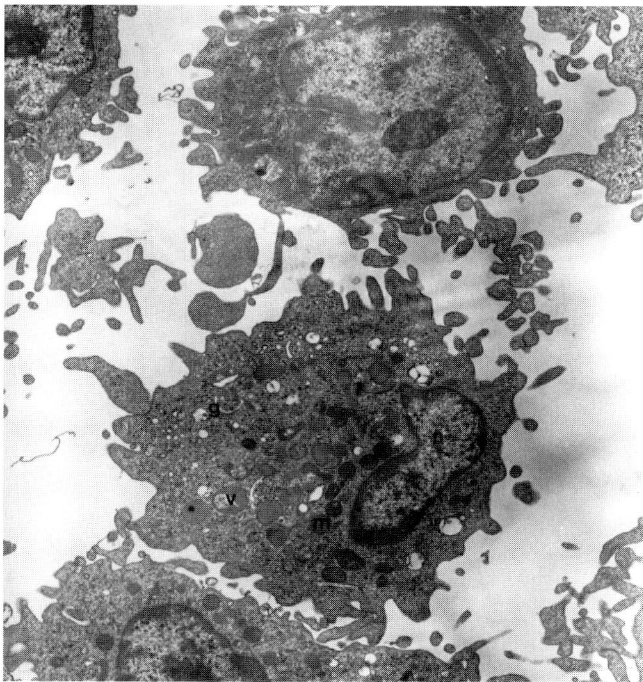

FIGURE 3 Transmission electron micrograph (TEM) of alveolar macrophages from a nonsilicotic rat illustrating the appearance of several organelles: nucleus (n), mitochondrion (m), golgi apparatus (g), and numerous vacuoles (v) in the cytoplasm. (Original magnification × 10,000.)

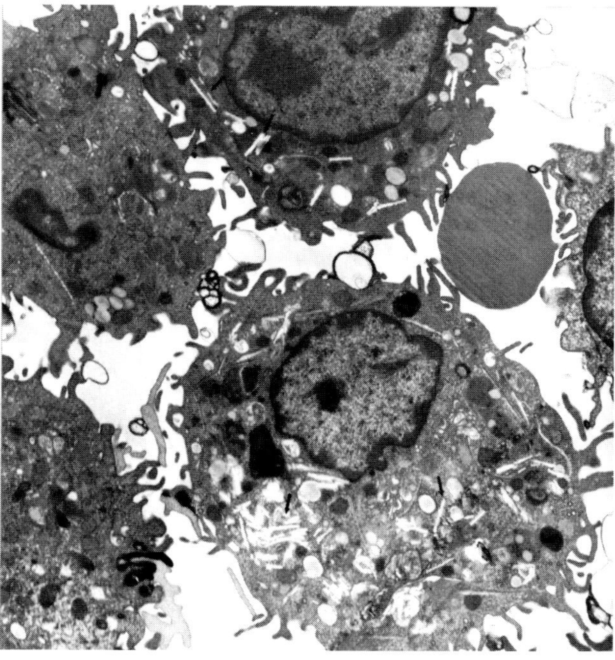

FIGURE 4 Electron micrograph of alveolar macrophages from a rat exposed to 40 mg silica at four weeks post-intratracheal instillation. Increased numbers of macrophages are seen within the alveolar space which are shown to contain phagocytized debris and cytoplasmic crystalline structure (arrows) consistent with cholesterol. (Original magnification × 10,000.)

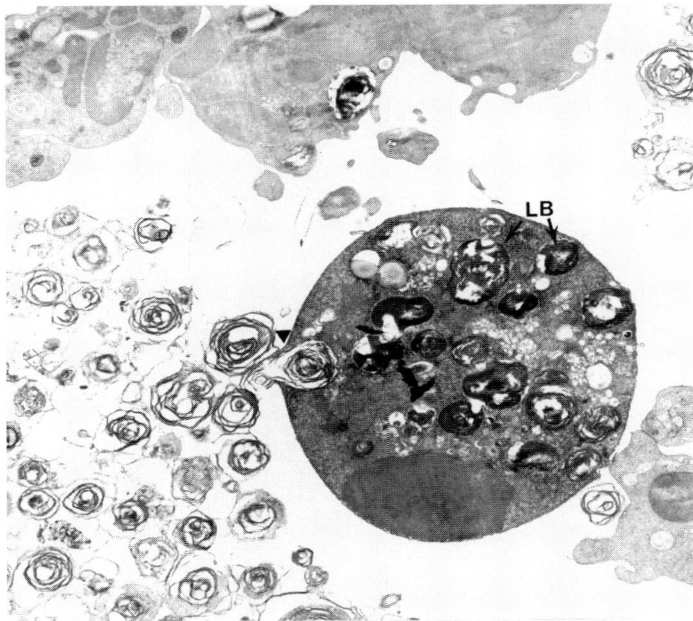

FIGURE 5 TEM morphometry of an alveolar Type II cell obtained from BAL of a rat exposed to 40 mg silica at four weeks postexposure. This Type II cell contains numerous lamellar bodies (LB) and is caught in the act of exocytosis of a lamellar body at the cell surface (arrowhead). It has been busy for quite some time as indicated by the secreted surfactant-like material near the site of exocytosis. (Original magnification × 10,000.)

exocytozed from the lamellar bodies. With transmission electron micrograph morphometry, collagen deposition was also found in the lungs of rats exposed to silica for four weeks (Figure 6), indicating early development of fibrotic lesions.

The therapeutic effect of tetrandrine on silica-induced lung lesions can be readily seen from light microscopic alterations observed in the rat lung. Rats that received saline display normal lungs. For the silicotic control, at four weeks postexposure, lesions were characterized by granulomatous pneumonia varying from moderate, multifocal to severe, multifocal and coalescent, and by alveolar lipoproteinosis varying from mild, multifocal to multifocal and coalescent, consistent with acute silicosis (Figure 7A). This is in line with observations of increased cellular production of lung surfactant shown in Figures 4 and 5, which is likely responsible for the light microscopic evidence of lipoproteinosis. Treatment with tetrandrine emulsion dramatically decreased light microscopic lesions in silicotic rat lungs. Figure 7B, which shows no significant lesions in a rat lung treated with tetrandrine emulsion taken at four weeks post-silica exposure, is representative of the results found in this experimental group. Treatment of silicotic rats with the tetrandrine solution also diminished lesions of acute silicosis but was found to be less effective than using the tetrandrine emulsion. Mild multifocal granulomatous pneumonia and foci comprised of epithelioid macrophages were found in some rat lungs.

The consistent observation of a greater drug effect from the emulsion system than from free tetrandrine in all of the described studies may be attributed to the ability of the emulsion system to enhance drug delivery to the pulmonary region. This observation is supported by pharmacokinetic data which showed that the same emulsion system can result in more than a twofold increase in lung distribution of tetrandrine with a concurrent decrease in systemic drug circulation when compared to tetrandrine solution.[17]

IV. SUMMARY

Current evidence suggests that tetrandrine effectively inhibits the macrophage-orchestrated inflammatory process in response to silica exposure and the subsequent fibrotic development. Data presented in

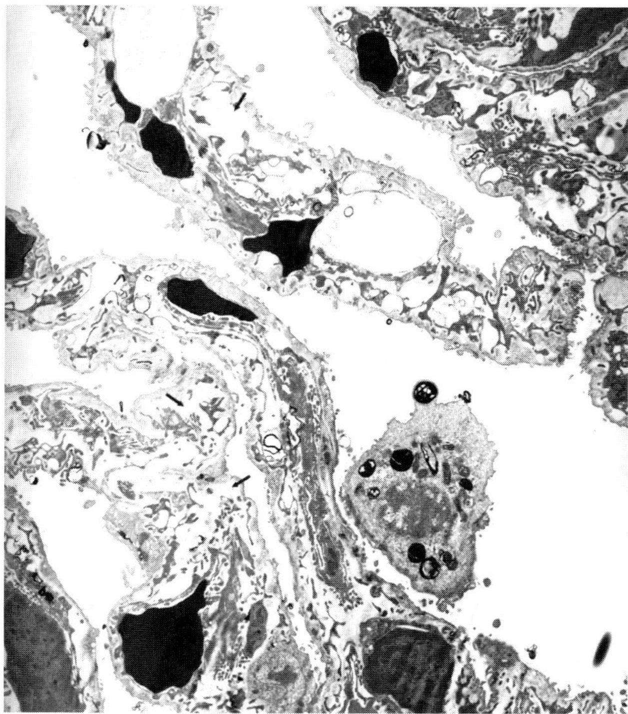

FIGURE 6 Transmission electron micrograph of lung interstitium from a rat exposed to 40 mg silica at four weeks post-intratracheal instillation. Arrows indicate increased collagen fibrils in the interstitium. (Original magnification × 6000.)

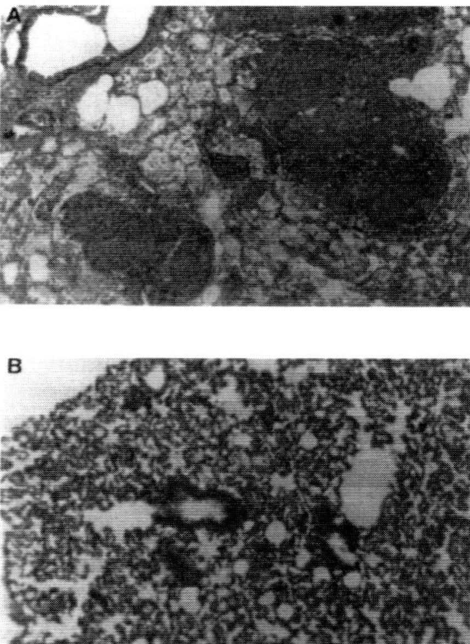

FIGURE 7 Light micrographs of hematoxylin-stained lung sections from (A) silicotic control and (B) silicotic rat treated with tetrandrine emulsion, at four weeks post-silica exposure. Panel A indicates marked granuloma and alveolar lipoproteinosis; panel B shows no significant lesion. (Original magnification × 1000.)

this chapter show that tetrandrine protects lung cells from silica toxicity and stimulation and restores healthy AM populations even after the drug has been eliminated from the pulmonary region. The premise that a multiple emulsion is an effective delivery system for pulmonary drug targeting is demonstrated. Tetrandrine emulsion was consistently more efficacious than the solution dosage form in the treatment of silica-induced granulomatous pneumonia and alveolar lipoproteinosis in rats. Fibrosis is a slow chronic disease which is considered "irreversible," but the disease development may be delayed or stopped if treated with an effective antifibrotic agent. The emulsion studies presented here demonstrate that early drug treatment following silica exposure may delay the fibrotic process by inhibiting abnormal cellular activity prior to the fibrotic event and restoring normal cell functions, thus allowing time for the lung to clear its dust problem. Given the long time required for the development of silicosis in humans, a delay or inhibition of the fibrotic process could have a very significant effect on disease development.

ACKNOWLEDGMENT

This work was supported in part by a grant from the U.S. Bureau of Mines through the Generic Mineral Technology Center for Respirable Dust (BOM1195142–5430) and by a cooperative grant from the National Institute for Occupational Safety and Health (U60/OCU306149).

REFERENCES

1. **Sharma, S. K., Pande, J. N., and Verma, K.,** Effect of prednisolone treatment in chronic silicosis, *Am. Rev. Respir. Dis.,* 143, 814–821, 1991.
2. **Goodman, G. B., Kaplan, P. D., Stachura, I., Castranova, V., Pailes, W. H., and Lapp, N. L.,** Acute silicosis responding to corticosteroid therapy, *Chest,* 101, 366–370, 1992.
3. **Lu, X. R. and Li, Q. R.,** Clinical studies of the therapeutic effect of tetrandrine on silicosis, *Chin. J. Ind. Hyg. Occup. Med.,* 2, 106–110, 1983.
4. **Li, Q., Xu, Y., Zhow, Z., Chen, X., Huang, X., Chen, S., and Zhun, C.,** The therapeutic effect of tetrandrine on silicosis, *Chin. J. Tuberc. Respir. Dis.,* 4, 321–328, 1981.
5. **Huang, T., Liu, Y., Zhao, S., and Li, Y.,** Changes of acid-soluble collagen from lungs of silicotic rats and tetrandrine-treated silicotic rats, *Acta Biochem. Biophys. Sintca,* 13, 61–68, 1981.
6. **Yu, X. F., Zou, C. Q., and Lim, M. B.,** Observations of the effect of tetrandrine on experimental silicosis of rats, *Ecotoxicol. Environ. Safety,* 7, 306–312, 1983.
7. **Holian, A. and Scheule, R.,** Alveolar macrophage biology, *Hosp. Pract.,* 25, 53–62, 1990.
8. **Heppleston, A. G.,** Silicotic fibrogenesis: a concept of pulmonary fibrosis, *Ann. Occup. Hyg.,* 26, 449–452, 1982.
9. **Davis, G. S.,** The pathogenesis of silicosis, *Chest,* 89, 166S–169S, 1986.
10. **Leibovich, S. J. and Rose, R.,** A macrophage-dependent factor that stimulates the proliferation of fibroblasts in vitro, *Am. J. Pathol.,* 84, 501–513, 1976.
11. **Bitterman, P. B., Adelberg, S., and Crystal, R. G.,** Mechanisms of pulmonary fibrosis: spontaneous release of alveolar macrophage derived growth factor in the interstitial lung disorders, *J. Clin. Invest.,* 72, 1801–1813, 1983.
12. **Goldstein, R. H. and Fine, A.,** Fibrotic reactions in the lung: the activation of the lung fibroblast, *Exp. Lung Res.,* 11, 245–261, 1986.
13. **Ma, J. Y. C., Barger, M. W., Ma, J. K. H., and Castranova, V.,** Inhibition of respiratory burst activity in alveolar macrophages by bisbenzylisoquinoline alkaloids: characterization of drug-cell interaction, *Exp. Lung Res.,* 18, 829–843, 1992.
14. **Kang, J. H., Lewis, D. M., Castranova, V., Rojanasakul, Y., Banks, D. E., Ma, J. Y. C., and Ma, J. K. H.,** Inhibitory action of tetrandrine on macrophage production of interleukin-1 and thymocyte proliferation, *Exp. Lung Res.,* 18, 715–729, 1992.
15. **Reist, R. H., Dey, R. D., Durham, J. P., Rojanasakul, Y., and Castranova, V.,** Inhibition of proliferative activity of pulmonary fibroblasts by tetrandrine, *Toxicol. App. Pharmacol.,* 122, 70–76, 1993.
16. **Chao, D. H., Peng, X. S., Rojanasakul, Y., Malanga, C. J., Castranova, V., and Ma, J. K. H.,** Evaluation of a multiple emulsion system for delivery of tetrandrine to the lungs. I. Formulation stability, drug release, and cellular activity. Manuscript in preparation, abstract published in *Pharm. Res.,* 7, S-150, 1990.
17. **Chao, D. H., Pan, W. F., Rojanasakul, Y., and Ma, J. K. H.,** Evaluation of a multiple emulsion system for delivery of tetrandrine to the lungs. II. Emulsion mediated drug distribution and activity in rat lungs, Manuscript in preparation, abstract published in *Pharm. Res.,* 9, S-201, 1992.

18. **Brodin, A. F., Kavaliunas, D. R., and Frank, S. G.,** Prolonged drug release from multiple emulsions, *Acta Pharm. Suec.,* 15, 1–12, 1978.
19. **Miyakawa, T., Zhang, W., Uchida, T., Kim, N. S., and Goto, S.,** *In vivo* release of water-soluble drug from stabilized w/o/w type multiple emulsions following intravenous administrations using rats, *Biol. Pharm. Bull.,* 16, 268–272, 1993.
20. **Matsumoto, S., Kita, Y., and Yonezawa, D.,** An attempt at preparing water-in-oil-in-water multiple-phase emulsions, *J. Colloid Interface Sci.,* 57, 353–361, 1976.
21. **Matsumoto, S., Khoda, M., and Murata, S.,** Preparation of liquid vesicles on the basis of a technique for providing w/o/w emulsions, *J. Colloid Interface Sci.,* 62, 149–157, 1977.
22. **Iso, M., Shirahase, T., Haramura, S., Urushiyama, S., and Omi, S.,** Application of encapsulated enzyme as a continuous packed-bed reactor, *J. Microencapsul.,* 6, 285–299, 1989.
23. **Volkel, W., Poppe, W., Halwachs, W., and Schugerl, K.,** Extraction of free phenols from blood by a liquid membrane enzyme reactor, *J. Membr. Sci.,* 11, 333–347, 1982.
24. **Volkel, W., Bosse, J., Poppe, W., Halwachs, W., and Schugerl, K.,** Development and design of a liquid membrane enzyme reactor for the detoxification of blood, *Chem. Eng. Commun.,* 22, 801–818, 1984.
25. **Omotosho, J. A., Whateley, T. L., and Florence, A. T.,** Methotrexate transport from the internal phase of multiple w/o/w emulsions, *J. Microencapsul.,* 6, 183–192, 1989.
26. **Yan, N., Huang, S., and Shi, Y. J.,** Removal of acetic acid from wastewater with liquid surfactant membranes: an external boundary layer and membrane diffusion controlled model, *Sep. Sci. Technol.,* 22, 801–818, 1987.
27. **Goswami, A. N., Rawat, B. S., and Krishna, R.,** Studies on permeation of hydrocarbons through liquid membrane in a continuous contactor, *J. Membr. Sci.,* 25, 101–108, 1985.
28. **Juliano, R. L.,** Factors affecting the clearance kinetics and tissue distribution of liposomes, microspheres and emulsions, *Adv. Drug Deliv. Rev.,* 2, 31–54, 1988.
29. **Chao, D. H.,** Multiple Emulsion-Mediated Therapeutic Enhancement of Tetrandrine Against Silicosis, Ph.D. dissertation, West Virginia University, Morgantown, WV, 1994.
30. **Heppleston, A. G.,** Atypical reaction to inhaled silica, *Nature,* 213, 199, 1967.
31. **Miller, K., Dethloff, L. A., and Hook, G. E. R.,** Silica-induced hypertrophy of type II cells in the lungs of rats, *Lab. Invest.,* 55, 153–163, 1986.

Section V
Silica and Cancer—A Current Issue

Section V
Chapter 1

CARCINOGENESIS BY CRYSTALLINE SILICA: ANIMAL, CELLULAR, AND MOLECULAR STUDIES

Umberto Saffiotti, A. Olufemi Williams, Lambert, N. Daniel, M. Edward Kaighn, Yan Mao, and Xianglin Shi

CONTENTS

I. INTRODUCTION

In the last decade, research on silica-induced lung disease has acquired a new focus, extending from the study of silicosis to that of associated lung cancer. Strong evidence has been obtained for carcinogenesis by crystalline silica in rats, and an increasing number of epidemiologic studies have reported an excess risk for lung cancer in human subjects with silicosis. There is another side to this story, however, because other experimental animal species, namely mice and hamsters, appear resistant to silica-induced lung carcinogenesis and because some of the epidemiologic studies have failed to reveal an increased cancer risk associated with silicosis. Our research interest was stimulated, rather than discouraged, by these discrepancies, and we set out to investigate what pathogenetic mechanisms or susceptibility factors may be involved in cancer induction by crystalline silica.

II. ANIMAL CARCINOGENESIS STUDIES

A. REVIEW OF *IN VIVO* CARCINOGENESIS DATA

The first experimental indication of the carcinogenic activity of crystalline silica was provided by a series of experiments by Wagner et al.[1–3] in which different samples of quartz, cristobalite, and tridymite were injected intrapleurally in rats and resulted in the induction of malignant histiocytic lymphomas.

The main experimental evidence of the carcinogenicity of crystalline silica for the lung is based on the induction of lung cancer in rats by quartz particles, administered either by inhalation or by intratracheal instillation. Reports on the carcinogenic effects of crystalline silica in rat lungs were presented at the meeting on "Silica, Silicosis and Cancer" in 1984[4] by Holland et al.,[5] Dagle et al.,[6] and Groth et al.[7] They presented results of long-term (2-year) experiments in rats, following exposure to dust samples of quartz (Min-U-Sil <5) or novaculite (a microcrystalline variety of quartz), or mixed dusts containing 8–12% quartz (raw shale or spent shale). Induction of lung cancer was demonstrated in all these experiments, including both male and female rats. These and some other limited experiments in other species or by other routes of administration were described in the comprehensive monograph on silica carcinogenesis, prepared by a Working Group of the International Agency for Research on Cancer in 1986.[8] Additional experiments of lung carcinogenesis by quartz in rats were subsequently reported by Muhle et al.[9,10] and by Spiethoff et al.[11] The results of these lung carcinogenesis tests are summarized in Table 1.

The initial group of experiments[5–8] did not describe the progressive development of histopathological changes resulting in lung cancer in the rats treated with quartz. However, at the 1984 meeting, Saffiotti[12] presented a pathology study of histological slides from his previous experiments in rats exposed to various silica dusts and sacrificed at intervals up to six months; hyperplastic reactions of the alveolar epithelium, adjacent to silicotic granulomas, were detected as early as 10 d after instillation of crystalline silica and were found to persist for several months. These slides were derived from experiments conducted in the late 1950s on rats maintained in pathogen-contaminated (non-specific-pathogen-free or non-SPF) facilities. At the 1984 meeting, Saffiotti[12] suggested, as a working hypothesis for further

TABLE 1
Summary of Data on Lung Tumors Induced in Rats by Crystalline Silica

Treatment sample	Exposure conditions	Rat strain	Sex	Incidence of lung tumors* Treated	Controls	Ref.
Quartz (Min-U-Sil <5)	Intratracheal instillation 7 mg weekly for 10 weeks	Sprague-Dawley	?	6/36[a]	0/58	Holland et al. 1983
	Inhalation (nose only) 12 ± 5 mg/m³ for up to two years	Fischer 344	F	20/60[b]	0/54	Holland et al. 1986
	Inhalation of 51.6 mg/m³ for various durations; sacrificed at 24 months	Fischer 344	F	10/53[c]	0/47	Dagle et al. 1986
		Fischer 344	M	1/47[d]	0/42	
	Intratracheal instillation 20 mg in left lung, sacrificed at 12, 18, and 22 months, or found dead	Fischer 344	M	30/67[e]	1/75[f]	Groth et al. 1986
Novaculite	Intratracheal instillation 20 mg in left lung, sacrificed at 12, 18, and 22 months, or found dead	Fischer 344	M	21/72[g]	Same as above	Same as above
Raw shale dust	Inhalation (nose only) of 152 ± 51 mg/m³ (average quartz content: 8–12%)	Fischer 344	F	17/59[h]	0/54 1/15[i]	Holland et al. 1986
Spent shale dust	Inhalation (nose only) of 176 ± 75 mg/m³ (average quartz content: 8–12%)	Fischer 344	F	11/59[j]	Same as above	Same as above
Quartz (DQ12)	Inhalation of 1 mg/m³ for 24 months	Fischer 344	F	12/50[k]	3/100[l] (M + F)	Muhle et al. 1989
		Fischer 344	M	6/50[m]		
	Inhalation (nose only) of 6 mg/m³ for 29 d, followed by lifetime observation	Wistar	F	62/82[n]	0/85	Spiethoff et al. 1992
	Inhalation (nose only) of 30 mg/m³ for 29 d, followed by lifetime observation	Wistar	F	69/82[o]	Same as above	Same as above

* Number of lung tumors per number of rats observed.
[a] 1 adenoma and 5 carcinomas;
[b] 6 adenomas, 11 adenocarcinomas, and 3 epidermoid carcinomas;
[c] All epidermoid carcinomas;
[d] 1 epidermoid carcinoma;
[e] All adenocarcinomas;
[f] 1 adenocarcinoma;
[g] 20 adenocarcinomas and 1 epidermoid carcinoma;
[h] 2 adenomas, 8 adenocarcinomas, and 7 epidermoid carcinomas;
[i] 1 adenoma;
[j] 2 adenomas, 8 adenocarcinomas, and 1 epidermoid carcinoma;
[k] 2 keratinizing cystic squamous cell tumors, 2 adenomas, and 8 adenocarcinomas;
[l] 2 adenomas and 1 adenocarcinoma;
[m] 2 keratinizing cystic squamous cell tumors, 2 adenocarcinomas, 1 adenosquamous carcinoma, and 1 epidermoid carcinoma;
[n] 8 adenomas, 17 bronchioloalveolar carcinomas, and 37 epidermoid carcinomas;
[o] 13 adenomas, 26 bronchioloalveolar carcinomas, and 20 epidermoid carcinomas.

studies, that the early epithelial hyperplasia was the precursor of lung cancers observed in long-term studies and that cellular mediators released by the cells of the granulomatous reaction were a significant factor in the pathogenesis of lung cancers associated with silicosis.

With this background, animal pathology studies were undertaken in our laboratory to investigate the sequence of events leading to silica-induced lung carcinogenesis.

B. ANIMAL EXPERIMENTS ON LUNG CARCINOGENESIS BY CRYSTALLINE SILICA IN THE LABORATORY OF EXPERIMENTAL PATHOLOGY, NCI: A REPORT

Beginning in 1984, our laboratory performed a series of animal experiments to investigate, by serial sacrifices and lifetime observations, the effects of a single intratracheal administration of crystalline silica on lung histopathology and/or carcinogenesis, with the following goals: (1) to study the histopathogenesis of quartz-induced lesions in the lungs of susceptible and resistant rodent species (rats, mice, and hamsters) in order to observe the development of granulomatous fibrogenic reactions and the associated development of epithelial hyperplasia and carcinogenesis; (2) to evaluate the incidence and types of quartz-induced benign and malignant lung tumors; (3) to characterize the animal model of fibrosis-associated lung cancer by studies on pathogenetic mechanisms; (4) to compare the pathology observed in the animal models with the pathology in human subjects with silicosis and associated lung cancer, as a basis for investigating human susceptibility factors and mechanisms.

The animal experiments were designed primarily for serial sacrifice observations. The histological changes in the lungs of crystalline silica-treated rodents of both sexes, using different species, were studied to ascertain the nature and progression of the cellular reactions to dusts at frequent time intervals in the first six months after treatment. Groups of F344 rats, each of approximately 18 males and 18 females, were also sacrificed at 11 months and at 17 months, in order to assess the progression of hyperplastic lesions and tumor yield. Rats that died (or were sacrificed as moribund) between 17 and 26 months were evaluated for cumulative tumor development. Summary reports of these studies were previously published.[13–16] A detailed pathology report is presented here.

1. Methods

a. Animals

Animals of three species and both sexes were obtained, at four to five weeks of age, from the Animal Production Branch, NCI/Frederick Cancer Research Facility, in 1985–86. They included F344/NCr rats, 15:16/EHS:Cr Syrian golden hamsters, and three strains of mice: BALB/cAnNCr, A/JCr, and NCr/NU athymic nude. They were housed in a barrier facility and maintained in SPF conditions, with *ad libitum* access to food and water. The following methods, described here for the rat studies, were also used for studies in mice and hamsters with minor modifications.

b. Route of Administration and Experimental Procedures

Single intratracheal instillation was chosen as the mode of administration for several reasons. We had extensive experience with this method of administration for particulate materials, both in serial sacrifice studies and in long-term studies. A moderate dose of dust (e.g., 10–15 mg suspended in saline) becomes well distributed in the lung parenchyma, readily penetrates into the interstitium, and induces discrete lesions. The main advantage of this method is that, following a single instillation, the development of pathological reactions can be studied by serial sacrifices, observing the progression of the reactions starting from a single time point. The dose of dust is easily defined and the technique is very simple.

At the age of eight weeks, the rats were anesthetized in a chamber with a mixture of oxygen and methoxyflurane and placed hanging with their backs on a $8^1/_2'' \times 5''$ metal board slanted at a 60° angle, with their mouth kept open by retaining the upper incisor teeth with a tight rubber band attached to the top of the board and hooking the lower incisor teeth to a semicircular wire loop (3.5 cm radius) attached with two screws near the top of the slanted board. This board was adapted from the design used for hamsters.[17] As soon as the rats were positioned on the board, they were given a single intratracheal instillation through a 7-cm-long, 19-gauge stainless steel blunt cannula, bent at a 140° angle near the top, connected to a 0.25-ml tuberculin syringe. A direct-focusing headlight, worn by the operator, provided a clear view of the pharynx, after the tongue was pulled laterally with a forceps. The cannula was inserted under the epiglottis to uncover the vocal cords, and gently pushed between these into the tracheal lumen. Preferably at the end of an expiration, the suspension was gently instilled and the cannula withdrawn. During the following inspiration, the dust suspension penetrated rapidly into the distal pulmonary airways. Inspection of the pharynx after the instillation showed no regurgitation. The apparatus used in preparing and instilling the suspensions was previously sterilized.

The rats were sacrificed by exsanguination under anesthesia. The trachea was exposed by dissection and ligated between the first and second cartilage rings, during maximal inspiration. The larynx, trachea, bronchi, lungs, lymph nodes, and heart were removed *en bloc* and fixed in 4% formaldehyde in a 300-

milliosmolar phosphate buffer. Necropsies were performed and other tissues were removed and fixed. The larynx, the trachea, each lung lobe (sectioned along its main bronchial axis), the mediastinal lymph nodes, and all grossly abnormal tissues were embedded in paraffin, sectioned, and routinely stained with hematoxylin and eosin. Selected special stains were used. Dust localization was detected by polarized light microscopy. Immunoperoxidase staining, with specific antibodies against rat surfactant apoprotein or against Clara cell antigen, was also performed in selected cases, through the courtesy of Dr. Gurmukh Singh, Veterans Administration Medical Center, Pittsburgh, PA.[18]

c. *Dust Samples and Treatments*

The α-quartz samples were Min-U-Sil <5 (MQZ), obtained from the Pennsylvania Glass Sand Co., Pittsburgh, PA, and hydrofluoric acid-etched MQZ (HFMQZ), prepared as described.[19] The particle size distribution of both samples was very similar, mostly between 0.5 and 2.0 μm, and their surface areas were, respectively, 3.15 and 2.98 m^2/g, as previously reported.[20] Both samples were 99% pure quartz; a small iron peak (<0.1%) was detected in MQZ, but not in HFMQZ, by X-ray fluorescence analysis, performed at the Illinois Institute of Technology Research Institute (IITRI), Chicago. Samples of the two crystalline silica polymorphs, cristobalite and tridymite, were synthesized and purified at IITRI; their surface areas[20] were, respectively, 3.93 and 5.24 m^2/g. Just before use, the dusts were autoclaved, suspended in neutral buffered saline in a small flask, and briefly sonicated in a water bath to provide full dispersion. Aliquots of 0.3 ml saline containing 12 mg dust, or 0.5 ml saline with 20 mg dust, were instilled in rats; 0.1 ml saline with 10 mg dust in mice; and 0.3 ml saline with 20 mg dust in hamsters. For comparison, the nonfibrogenic dust, hematite (ferric oxide, Fe_2O_3), was used. Rats of both sexes were assigned to experimental groups that received a single instillation, respectively, of 12 mg MQZ, 20 mg MQZ, 12 mg HFMQZ, or 20 mg Fe_2O_3. Untreated controls were also observed. The number of animals in each group and the number of animals observed at sacrifice or after unscheduled death are given in Table 2.

From the MQZ (12 mg), MQZ (20 mg), and HFMQZ (12 mg) groups, two male and two female rats were sacrificed at 1, 3, 5, 7, 10, 15, 21, 30, and 45 d and at 2, 3, 4, 5, and 6 months after treatment. Sacrifices of approximately 18 males and 18 females each were made at 11 months and at 17 months, for groups MQZ (12 mg) and HFQMZ. The remaining animals were kept until spontaneous death or sacrificed when moribund, up to 26 months.

Additional short-term pilot experiments were conducted on groups of 25 male and 25 female rats that were sacrificed at intervals up to two months after receiving a single instillation of crystalline silica, including cristobalite (20 mg) and tridymite (20 mg).

2. Results

a. *Rat Studies*

i. Tissue Reactions to Quartz Dust (12 mg MQZ) in Rats at Serial Sacrifices (Figures 1–9)

On day 1, the dust was detected in the lung parenchyma of all lobes, located in alveolar spaces and occasionally in alveolar septa. Sites of dust deposition showed aggregates of macrophages, some with ruptured cell membrane, pyknotic nuclei and cell debris, occasional polymorphonuclear leukocytes (PMN), and perivascular eosinophils; edema was present in focal areas. On day three, in addition to dust in the alveolar spaces, more dust was observed in alveolar septa. In addition to macrophages and some perivascular eosinophils, fibroblasts and initial fibrosis were seen in the areas of reaction to dust; the peribronchial lymphoid tissue was enlarged, with clusters of reactive histiocytic cells. On day five, the granulomas showed mainly macrophages with phagocytosed dust but also more fibroblasts and fibrosis with thin collagen bundles. On day seven, the granulomas showed a more distinct nodular pattern, composed of alveolar and interstitial macrophages, fibroblasts, some lymphocytes, and occasional eosinophils, with cell debris and collagen bundles; the alveolar epithelium showed focal areas of Type II cell hypertrophy and hyperplasia. On days 10 and 15 (Figures 1 and 2), the granulomas showed increased numbers of necrotic cells, with dust scattered among cell debris and focal areas of Type II cell hypertrophy and hyperplasia; the peribronchial lymphoid tissue was moderately hyperplastic; focal areas of alveolar proteinosis were seen.

On days 21 and 30, most silicotic granulomas were discrete, and some were larger; they showed collagen deposition and a cellular reaction with macrophages, necrotic macrophages, fibroblasts, and some lymphocytes; areas of alveolar Type II hypertrophy and hyperplasia were observed (Figure 3); the

TABLE 2
Lung Tumors Induced in Fischer 344 Rats by a Single Intratracheal Instillation of Quartz

Treatment sample	Treatment dose[a]	Sex	Observation time	Incidence of lung tumors[b]	Total no. of lung tumors[c]	Histological types
Untreated	None	M	Died, after 17 months	0/32	0	
	None	F	Died, after 17 months	1/20 (5%)	1	(1 adenoma)
Quartz (Min-U-Sil <5)	12 mg	M	Sacrificed, 11 months	3/18 (17%)		
			Sacrificed, 17 months	6/19 (32%)	37	(6 adenomas, 25 adenocarcinomas, 1 undifferentiated carcinoma, 2 mixed carcinomas, and 3 epidermoid carcinomas)
			Died, after 17 months	12/14 (86%)		
	12 mg	F	Sacrificed, 11 months	8/19 (42%)		
			Sacrificed, 17 months	10/17 (59%)	59	(2 adenomas, 46 adenocarcinomas, 3 undifferentiated carcinomas, 5 mixed carcinomas, and 3 epidermoid carcinomas)
			Died, after 17 months	8/9 (89%)		
	20 mg	F	Died, after 17 months	6/8 (75%)	13	(1 adenoma, 10 adenocarcinomas, 1 mixed carcinoma, and 1 epidermoid carcinoma)
Quartz (HF-etched Min-U-Sil <5)	12 mg	M	Sacrificed, 11 months	2/18 (11%)		
			Sacrificed, 17 months	7/19 (37%)	20	(5 adenomas, 14 adenocarcinomas, and 1 mixed carcinoma)
			Died, after 17 months	7/9 (78%)		
	12 mg	F	Sacrificed, 11 months	7/18 (39%)		
			Sacrificed, 17 months	13/16 (81%)	45	(1 adenoma, 36 adenocarcinomas, 3 mixed carcinomas, and 5 epidermoid carcinomas)
			Died, after 17 months	8/8 (100%)		

[a] As mg quartz suspended in 0.3 ml saline.
[b] Number of rats with lung tumors per number of rats observed.
[c] At all observation times.

Data from the Laboratory of Experimental Pathology, National Cancer Institute (Saffiotti et al., 1993).

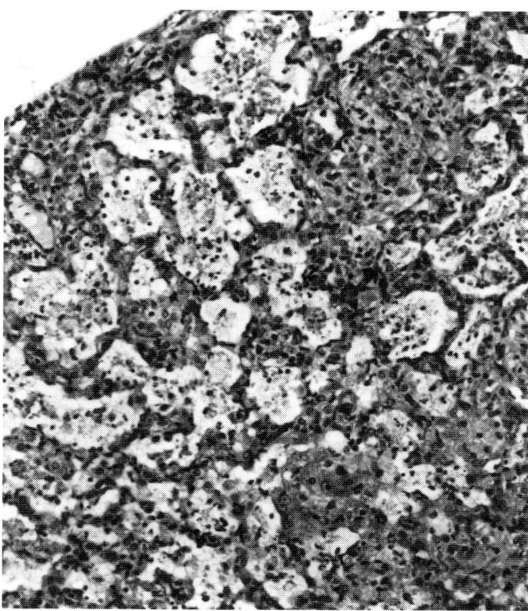

FIGURE 1 Rat lung 10 d after instillation of 12 mg MQZ. Alveolar spaces contain macrophages and some cellular debris; early macrophagic granuloma at upper right; alveolar walls show some hyperplastic Type II cells. (H&E stain; × 145.)

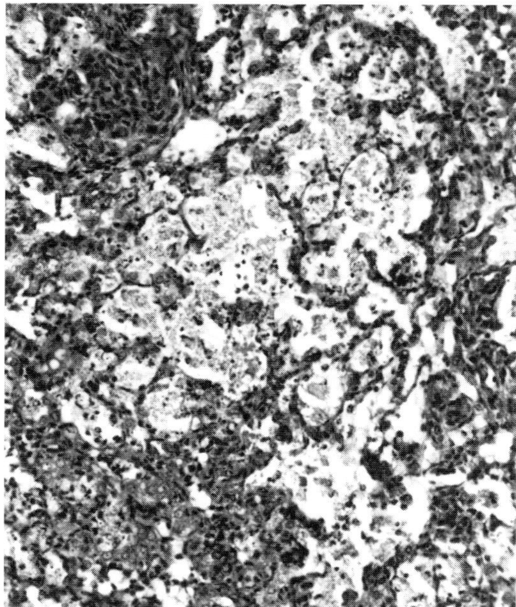

FIGURE 2 Rat lung 15 d after instillation of 12 mg MQZ. Alveolar spaces contain macrophages, cell debris, and pyknotic nuclei; early granuloma composed of macrophages and fibroblasts at upper left, and some hyperplastic alveolar Type II cells near it (center top). (H&E stain; × 145.)

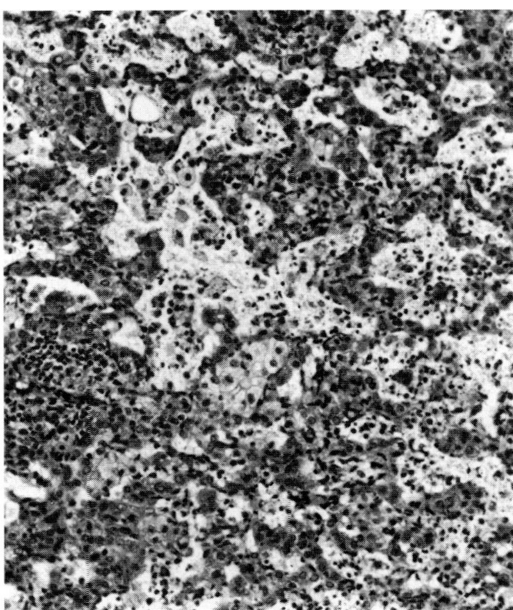

FIGURE 3 Rat lung 30 d after instillation of 12 mg MQZ. Alveolar walls show more extensive hyperplasia of Type II cells than at previous times. Note alveolar and interstitial macrophages, some fibroblasts, and a small lymphocytic infiltrate at lower left. (H&E stain; × 145.)

lymphoid tissue showed marked reactive centers. On days 45 and 60, the granulomas were larger; some of them showed fibrotic centers, and, in several instances, several granulomas appeared confluent; foci of alveolar epithelial hyperplasia were present.

At three and four months, the granulomas, mostly discrete but sometimes confluent, showed increasing fibrosis; in focal areas adjacent to granulomas, there was marked alveolar epithelial hyperplasia (Figures 4–6), including the first observed instance of nodular hyperplasia (Figure 4); focal alveolar proteinosis was present, often together with epithelial hyperplasia.

At five and six months, the alveolar epithelial hyperplasia, often adjacent to nodular fibrotic granulomas, was more prominent and showed areas with varying morphology (Figure 7), sometimes including adenomatoid patterns with cords of epithelial cells. The peribronchial lymphoid tissue and the mediastinal lymph nodes showed reactive hyperplasia. In the lungs observed up to this time, the parenchymal areas, in which dust was not detected, showed no pathological changes, except for occasional thickening of alveolar walls by edema and a slight increase in interstitial macrophages.

Groups of rats were sacrificed at 11 and 17 months, and the remaining rats were observed at the time of unscheduled deaths up to 26 months. These rats showed further progression in the silicotic granulomas, which were larger and more fibrotic, although they retained a cellular component of macrophages and fibroblasts. The alveolar epithelial hyperplastic reaction became even more conspicuous and included areas of adenomatoid proliferation (Figure 8). Occasionally, large alveolar spaces were observed, lined by hyperplastic epithelium and showing thick fibrous septa. Throughout the experiment, mast cells were also observed (Figure 9); these cells, frequent in control rat lungs, appeared with moderately increased frequency in the lung granulomas. Plasma cells were rarely seen in the granulomas.

ii. Lung Adenomas and Carcinomas (Figures 10–18)

Rats, observed at 11- and 17-month sacrifices or thereafter, were found to have developed increasing numbers of epithelial tumors, most of which were adenocarcinomas, arising in the vicinity of silicotic granulomas. The frequencies of lung tumors, observed at 11- and 17-month sacrifices and at subsequent times of death, and their histological diagnoses are reported in Table 2.

These results show that a significant incidence of lung tumors was already induced by the 11th month, more in females (42%) than in males (17%). The incidence of lung tumors increased at the 17-month sacrifice (59% in females and 32% in males). In the rats that died after 17 months, the incidence of lung

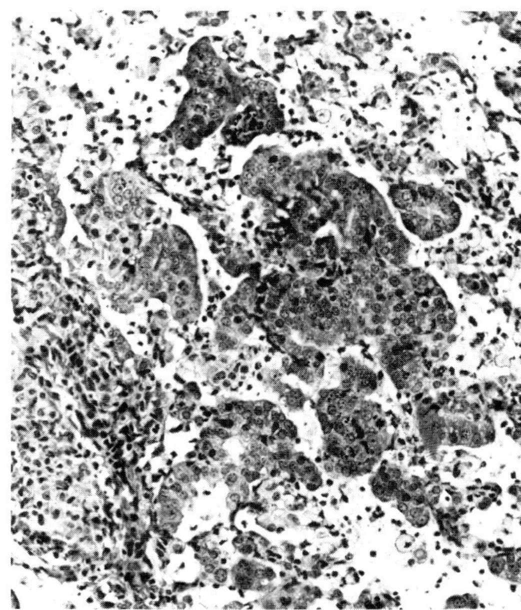

FIGURE 4 Rat lung three months after instillation of 12 mg MQZ. Nodular hyperplasia of alveolar epithelial cells. Note adjacent granuloma at lower left. (H&E stain; × 145.)

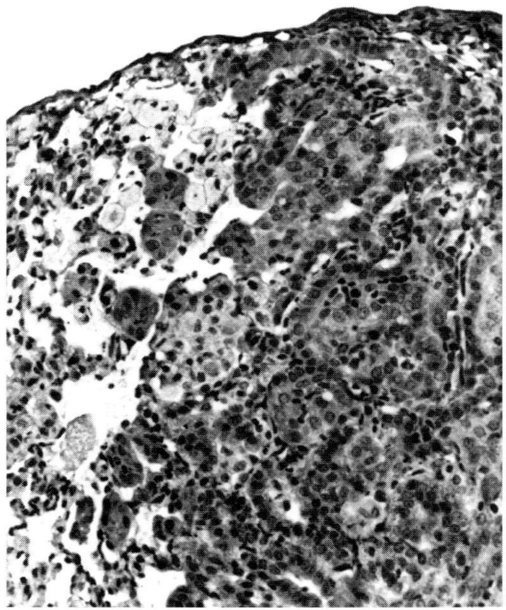

FIGURE 5 Rat lung four months after instillation of 12 mg MQZ. Adenomatoid hyperplasia composed of alveolar Type II cells, near pleural surface. (H&E stain; × 145.)

tumors was very high in both males (86%) and females (89%). Many animals had more than one primary tumor, often in different lobes. When tumor multiplicity was considered, females showed a higher number of tumors per tumor-bearing animal than did the males. In addition, the males had a higher ratio of adenomas to adenocarcinomas (6:25) than did the females (2:46), suggesting that a higher proportion of tumors with this glandular differentiation had become malignant in females than in males. In

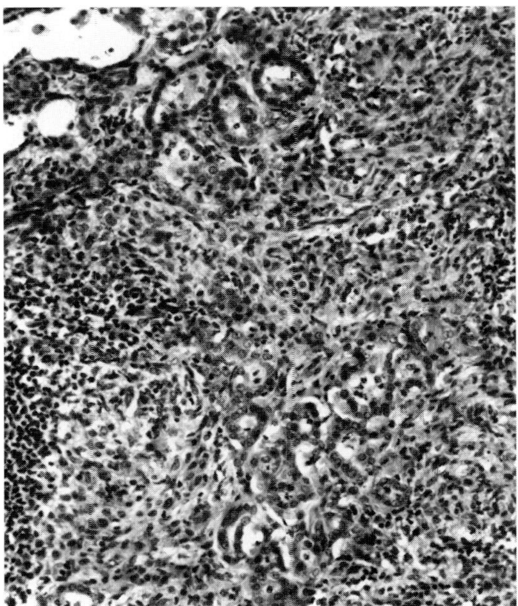

FIGURE 6 Rat lung four months after instillation of 12 mg MQZ. Focal area with acini of hyperplastic alveolar Type II cells in silicotic fibrous tissue. Note lymphocytic infiltrate at left. (H&E stain; × 145.)

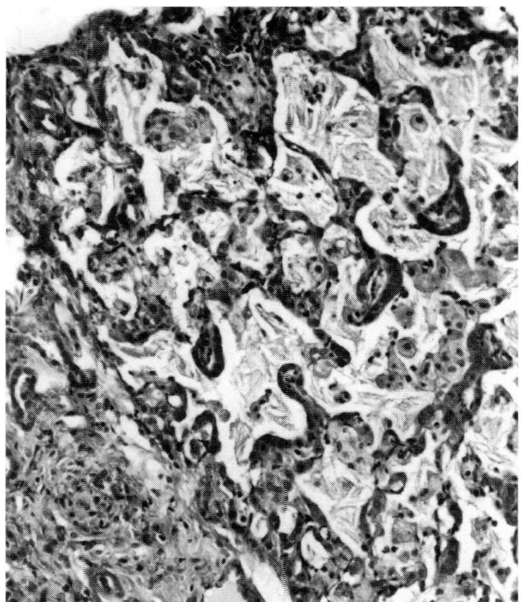

FIGURE 7 Rat lung five months after instillation of 12 mg MQZ. Hyperplasia of alveolar Type II cells. Note proteinaceous material and macrophages in alveolar spaces; granuloma at lower left. (H&E stain; × 145.)

conclusion, female rats responded to quartz treatment with an earlier onset of tumors, a higher tumor multiplicity, and a higher proportion of malignant vs. benign tumors than the males.

Adenocarcinomas were the most frequently observed tumor type in both sexes (Figures 10–15). Most adenocarcinomas had an acinar or alveolar pattern, others a papillary pattern, and showed varying degrees of differentiation. About a third of the adenocarcinomas had a fibrous center, in which doubly refractile

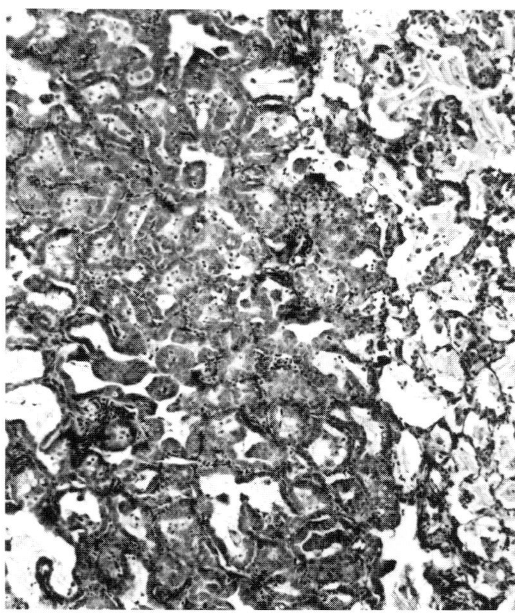

FIGURE 8 Rat lung 11 months after instillation of 12 mg MQZ. Hyperplastic alveolar Type II cells forming adenomatoid lesion. (H&E stain; × 73.)

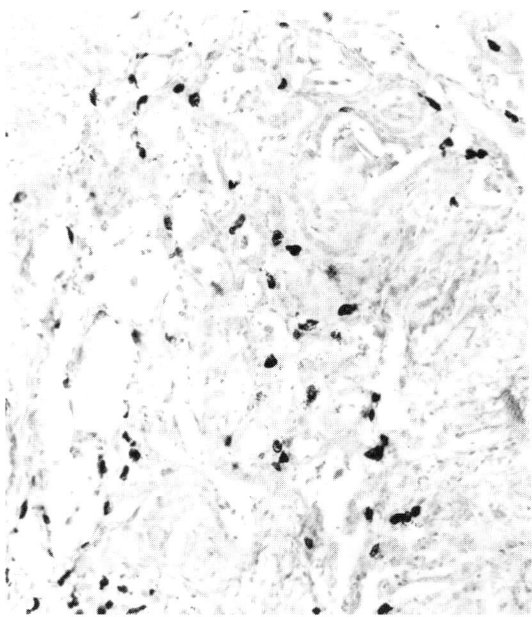

FIGURE 9 Rat lung 11 months after instillation of 12 mg MQZ. Numerous mast cells (dark) in the stroma of alveolar walls with hyperplastic alveolar Type II cells. (Toluidine blue stain; × 145.)

particles could be detected under polarized light, and showed a centrifugal invasive pattern of the carcinoma into the surrounding lung parenchyma (Figures 10 and 11). These adenocarcinomas resembled the morphology of human lung cancers surrounding fibrotic lesions and described as "scar cancers."[21]

Other types of carcinoma, observed in much lower frequencies, were keratinizing epidermoid carcinomas; undifferentiated carcinomas of the large or intermediate cell types (Figure 16); and mixed

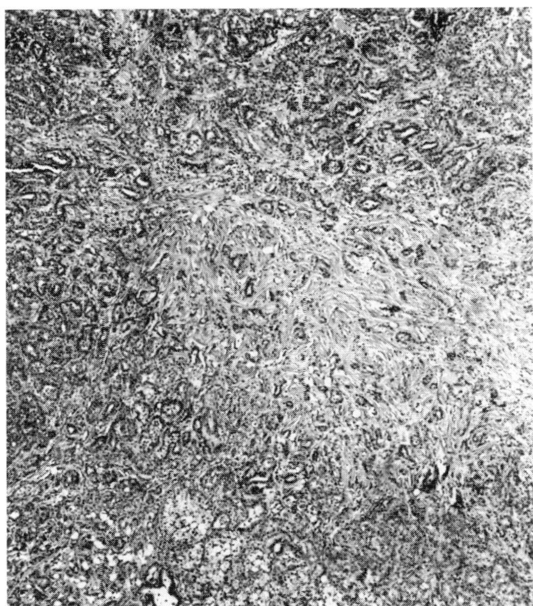

FIGURE 10 Rat lung 24 months after instillation of 12 mg MQZ. Adenocarcinoma with fibrous core. The tumor extends peripherally from a fibrous center that contains doubly refractile silica particles (detectable by polarized light, not shown). (H&E stain; × 36.)

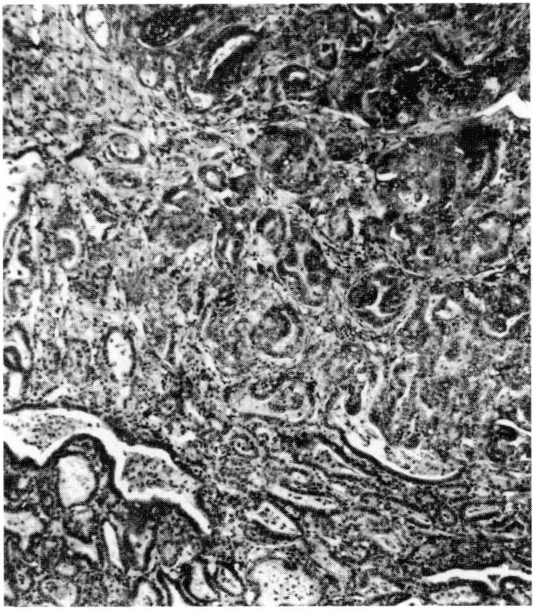

FIGURE 11 Rat lung 17 months after instillation of 12 mg MQZ. Different patterns of glandular and tubular differentiation in an adenocarcinoma that had a fibrous core similar to that in Figure 9. (H&E stain; × 73.)

carcinomas, mostly composed of areas of adenocarcinoma combined with undifferentiated or epidermoid areas (Figure 17).

The adenomas showed well-differentiated cuboidal epithelial cells in acinar or tubular patterns (Figure 18). None of the sections of tumors examined showed transition from adenoma to carcinoma, even on serial sections.

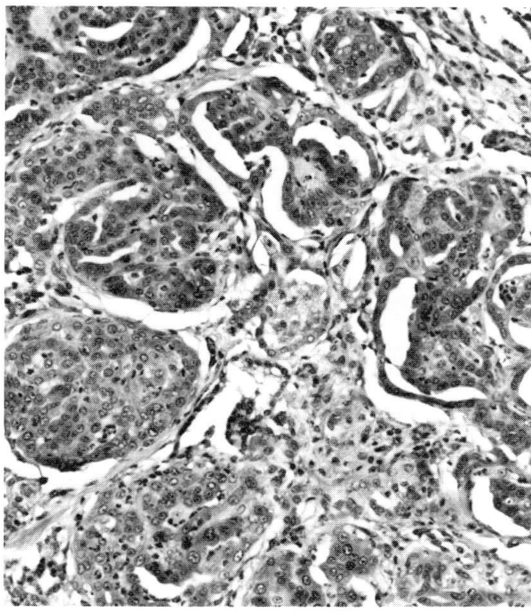

FIGURE 12 Rat lung 24 months after instillation of 12 mg MQZ. Adenocarcinoma (with fibrous core) showing formation of tubular structures and solid areas of poorly differentiated cells. (H&E stain; × 145.)

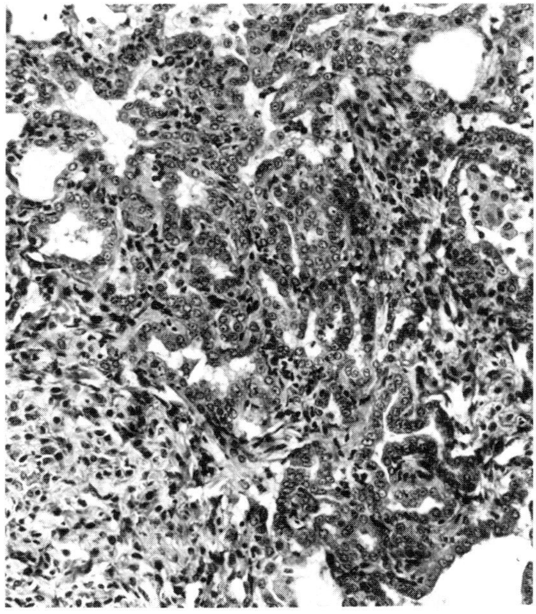

FIGURE 13 Rat lung 17 months after instillation of 12 mg MQZ. Adenocarcinoma adjacent to silicotic granuloma at lower left. (H&E stain; × 145.)

iii. Other Dust Treatments in Rats

The pattern of reaction was essentially the same for the 12-mg dose of MQZ and for the other two experimental protocols (a 20-mg dose of MQZ and a 12-mg dose of HFMQZ), and the description given above applies to all three protocols. The sequential pattern of histopathological changes, up to six months, observed in the 20-mg MQZ treatment group, showed little difference from the pattern described above

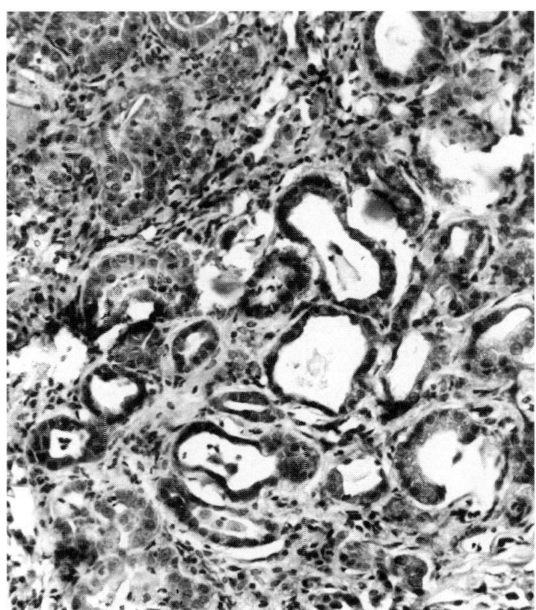

FIGURE 14 Rat lung 17 months after instillation of 12 mg MQZ. Adenocarcinoma with varying patterns of differentiation. (H&E stain; × 145.)

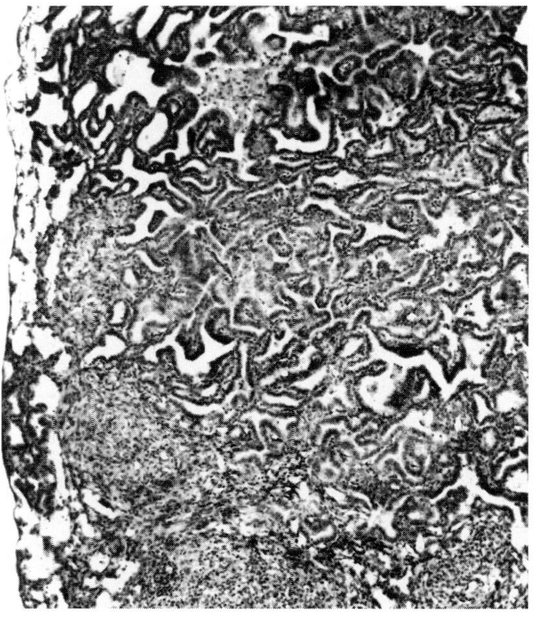

FIGURE 15 Rat lung 11 months after instillation of 12 mg MQZ. Adenocarcinoma with papillary differentiation, adjacent to granulomas (lower left) near pleura (left). (H&E stain; × 73.)

for the 12-mg MQZ group. For the 20-mg MQZ group, longer-term observations were only available for female rats after 17 months; their tumor incidence was not higher than that in the corresponding 12-mg MQZ groups (Table 2). The 12-mg HFMQZ treatment group also showed a sequential response pattern and tumor incidence analogous to those observed for the 12-mg MQZ group. The frequencies and types of lung tumors, observed at 11 and 17 months and at subsequent times in the HFMQZ group, were very similar to those observed in the MQZ group (Table 2).

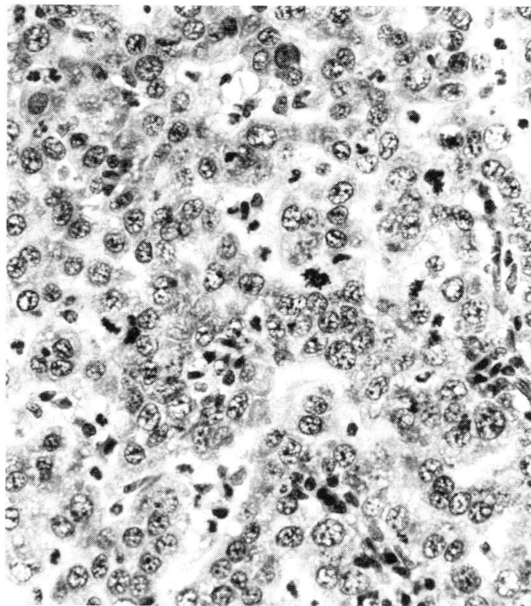

FIGURE 16 Rat lung 17 months after instillation of 12 mg MQZ. Undifferentiated carcinoma with numerous mitotic cells. (H&E stain; × 73.)

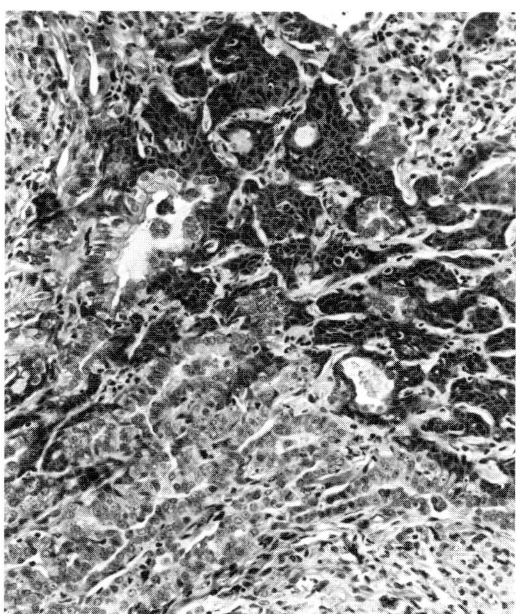

FIGURE 17 Rat lung 11 months after instillation of 12 mg HFMQZ. Mixed type carcinoma, composed of squamous cell carcinoma adjacent to poorly differentiated adenocarcinoma. (H&E stain; × 145.)

Cristobalite and tridymite were instilled in pilot tests in rats, at a 20-mg dose, and the rats were examined only up to two months. The histological changes in the lungs were similar to those described for MQZ at the corresponding times.

For comparison, rat groups were treated with hematite (20 mg); for each sex, 55 rats were sacrificed at intervals up to six months, five were sacrificed at 11 months and five at 17 months; five males and eight

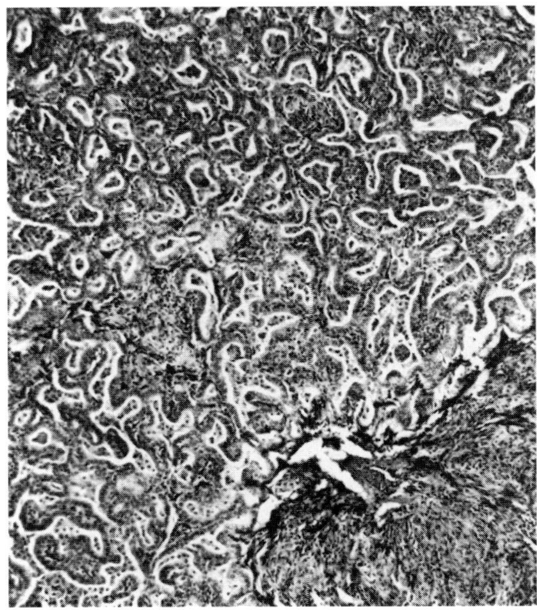

FIGURE 18 Rat lung 11 months after instillation of 12 mg HFMQZ. Adenoma adjacent to silicotic granuloma at lower right. (H&E stain; × 73.)

females were observed at unscheduled death after 17 months. Hematite gave rise to pulmonary macrophagic storage lesions with minimal fibroblastic reaction and minimal fibrosis; no alveolar epithelial hyperplasia was found, except for a single isolated focus, and no tumors were observed.

The untreated rat groups (32 male and 20 female rats), observed at unscheduled death, showed normal lung morphology and no lung tumors, except for one small adenoma in an untreated female.

b. Mouse Studies

To study lung reactions in mice, following a single intratracheal instillation of 10 mg of either quartz (MQZ) or tridymite in 0.1 ml saline, groups of 50 male mice were used from each of three strains: A/JCr, BALB/cAnNCr, and NCr-NU (athymic nude). Three mice of each strain were sacrificed at 1, 3, 7, 15, and 30 d and at two, three, and six months. The remaining mice were kept until unscheduled death.

The histopathological changes in mice (Figures 19 and 20) differed from those described in rats. The silicotic nodules in mice showed large necrotic centers. No persistent alveolar epithelial hyperplasia, no epithelial proliferative lesions, and no induction of lung carcinomas were observed, in contrast with the epithelial reaction so conspicuously observed in rats.

i. Strains A/J and BALB/c

The following description summarizes the histopathological changes in the lungs of mice, observed after a single instillation of 10 mg of either MQZ or tridymite. The findings were analogous for both strains and for both silica samples.

On day three, the dust appeared well distributed throughout the lungs, with considerable amounts of free silica dust still present in the alveolar spaces and some dust in the septal interstitium; diffuse interstitial edema and areas of alveolar proteinosis were seen; around dust deposits, foci of cell reaction were composed of macrophages, pyknotic nuclei with cell debris, and PMN; the alveolar epithelium showed some scattered hypertrophic Type II cells, occasionally focally clustered near dust deposits; moderate bronchiolar hyperplasia was observed. On day seven, larger granulomatous areas, some of them confluent, were observed. They contained macrophages, cell debris, some PMN, and fibroblasts, sometimes forming initial nodular patterns. The alveolar epithelium showed only occasional Type II cells, rarely forming small hyperplastic areas in the alveolar lining; areas of hyperplasia were more frequently seen in the epithelium of segmental bronchi and bronchioles. The perivascular lymphoid tissue showed small reactive areas. On day 15, silicotic granulomas were often nodular and discrete; the extent of

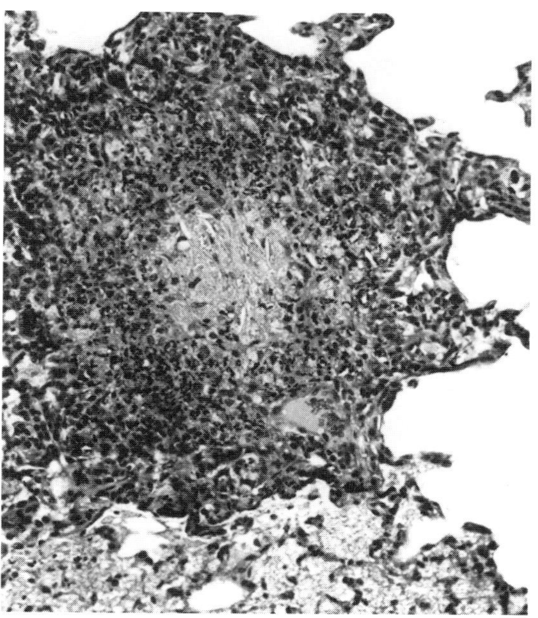

FIGURE 19 Mouse (A/J) six months after instillation of 10 mg MQZ. Silicotic granuloma with central necrotic area. Note lack of fibrosis and of alveolar Type II hyperplasia. (H&E stain; × 73.)

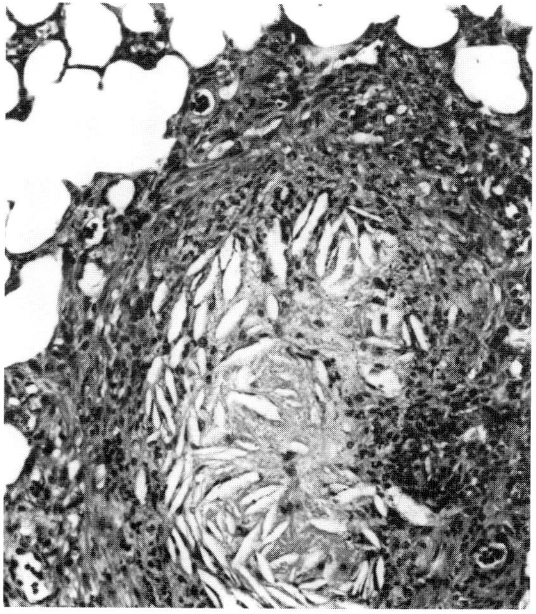

FIGURE 20 Mouse (athymic nude) six months after instillation of 10 mg MQZ. Silicotic granuloma with central necrotic area with typical lipid clefts. Note moderate fibrosis and lack of alveolar Type II hyperplasia. (H&E stain; × 145.)

epithelial hyperplasia had decreased; the alveolar and bronchial epithelia appeared mostly normal, but the bronchiolar epithelium showed areas of moderate hyperplasia. On day 30, silicotic nodules were more prominent, composed of macrophages and fibroblasts, and showed central areas with dust deposits, cellular debris, and some fibrosis. Epithelial hyperplasia was observed only in bronchiolar areas.

TABLE 3
Lung Tumors Observed in Mice Treated with a Single Instillation of 10 mg of Either MQZ or Tridymite and Observed at Unscheduled Death More Than Six Months After Treatment

Strain	Silica sample	Number of mice autopsied	Tumor-bearing mice	Total tumors	Adenoma	Adenocarcinoma
A/J						
	MQZ	15	2	2	1	1[a]
	TRID	16	4	4	4[b]	
BALB/C						
	MQZ	26	2	2	1	1
	TRID	22	2	2	2	
NCr/NU						
	MQZ	4	1	1	1	
	TRID	5	0			

[a] Not in a silicotic area.
[b] One adenoma not in silicotic area.

At two months, many discrete silicotic nodules, rarely confluent, showed macrophages, fibroblasts, and collagen fibers; their central areas had high concentrations of dust, cell debris, and few collagen fibers. Perivascular lymphocytic tissue reaction remained slight to moderate. Some areas showed moderate bronchiolar hyperplasia. The parenchyma between silicotic nodules was normal in several areas, but in other areas it showed alveolar proteinosis, thickened septa with interstitial macrophages, and groups of macrophages and necrotic macrophages in alveolar spaces. At three months, many silicotic nodules were seen; they were mostly discrete, but some were confluent; they showed large acellular centers with high dust concentration; the lymphoid reaction was more marked; the other features were similar to those at two months. At six months, in addition to the features previously described, there were some lipid clefts in the central acellular areas of the nodules. The epithelium was mostly normal at all airway levels. Alveolar proteinosis and lymphoid tissue reactions were more marked.

In mice observed at unscheduled deaths from 7 to 24 months, the silicotic lesions remained similar to those observed above. In some mice, subpleural fibrous lesions were observed. The incidence of observed lung tumors is reported in Table 3. In strain A/J mice, the only adenocarcinoma and one adenoma (4 mm in diameter) were located in lung areas without silicotic lesions; the other four adenomas were small (1–1.5 mm in diameter). In view of the spontaneous incidence of lung adenomas in strain A mice, these findings were not attributed to silica treatment. In strain BALB/c mice, the low incidence of lung tumors (2/26 for MQZ and 2/22 for tridymite) was not attributed to the treatment. This conclusion is supported by our serial observations, which showed that the hyperplasia of the alveolar epithelium was only sporadic and transient.

ii. Nude Mice (NCr/Nu)

The nude mice were used for a comparative study of the histogenesis of silicotic lesions; too few of these mice survived long enough for an evaluation of tumor incidence. The pulmonary changes were mostly similar to those observed in the immunocompetent strains, although some silicotic nodules showed fibrosis with only few cells.

iii. Summary of Mouse Studies

In the observed three strains of this species, crystalline silica induced granulomas with minimal to moderate fibrosis and extensive necrosis but no persistent alveolar epithelial hyperplasia and no tumors.

c. *Hamster Studies*

The experiments in hamsters were set up only for histogenesis studies up to one year. Long-term results of experiments by inhalation and by intratracheal instillation of quartz in hamsters were previously published and showed a lack of carcinogenic response at the end of two years.[8,22–24]

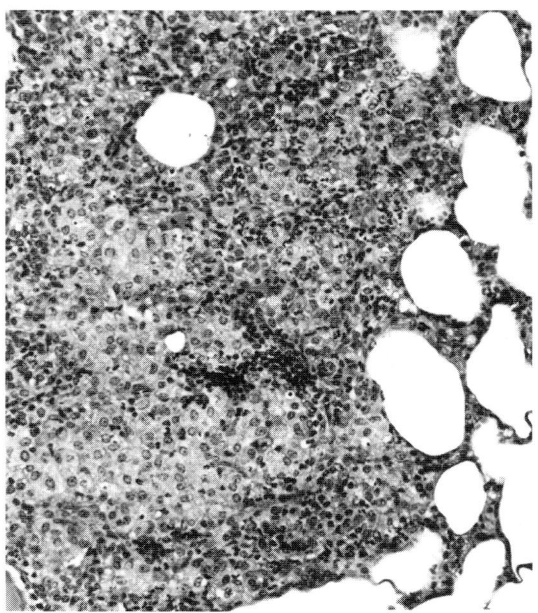

FIGURE 21 Hamster 30 d after instillation of 20 mg MQZ. Silicotic granuloma showing aggregates of macrophages and lymphocytic infiltrates. Note loss of alveolar architecture, lack of fibrosis and lack of alveolar Type II hyperplasia. (H&E stain; × 145.)

In the present study, two silica samples, MQZ and tridymite, were tested in hamsters by single intratracheal instillation of 20 mg in 0.3 ml saline. For each sample, three male and three female hamsters were sacrificed at each of the following time points: 3, 7, 15, and 30 d and 2, 3, 6, and 12 months.

On days three and seven, the dust appeared well distributed in hamster lungs; the early cellular reaction was composed predominantly of macrophages, many with foamy appearance, with silica particles in the cytoplasm, but with minimal evidence of necrosis; in addition, there were some PMN and a slight perivascular lymphocytic reaction; no epithelial hyperplasia was observed; the remaining large areas of pulmonary parenchyma were normal.

From day 15 to 6 months, the cellular lesions around silica deposits in the lungs remained composed predominantly of macrophages, with only occasional fibroblasts; the lymphocytic reaction remained slight and sometimes was found at the periphery of macrophagic clusters; no epithelial hyperplasia was observed (Figure 21).

At one year, the hamsters showed more consolidated areas of cellular reaction around silica deposits, still composed predominantly of macrophages; scattered among these cells, there were clusters of larger macrophages with clearer cytoplasm containing silica particles and small foci of lymphocytes; the fibrotic reaction was minimal; no epithelial hyperplasia was observed (Figure 22).

i. Summary of Hamster Studies

The results of the observations in hamsters showed that, in this species, quartz and tridymite elicited a macrophagic storage reaction but no fibrogenic and no epithelial reactions.

d. Discussion of Results in Rats, Mice, and Hamsters

The rat studies show sequential progression of pathological changes induced by a single dose of crystalline silica in this species and demonstrate, at sequential times of observation, the induction of progressively higher incidences of lung tumors, mostly adenocarcinomas, associated with silicotic fibrosis. The silicotic reaction in rats was accompanied by progressive hyperplasia of the alveolar Type II epithelial cells. These cells proliferated to form adenomatoid lesions, adjacent to the fibrous granulomas. The evidence for the alveolar Type II origin of the adenomatoid lesions and of adenocarcinomas was confirmed by positive immunohistochemical staining, using antibodies to rat surfactant apoprotein, whereas staining for antibodies to the Clara cell antigen was consistently negative (courtesy of Dr. Gurmukh Singh).[18]

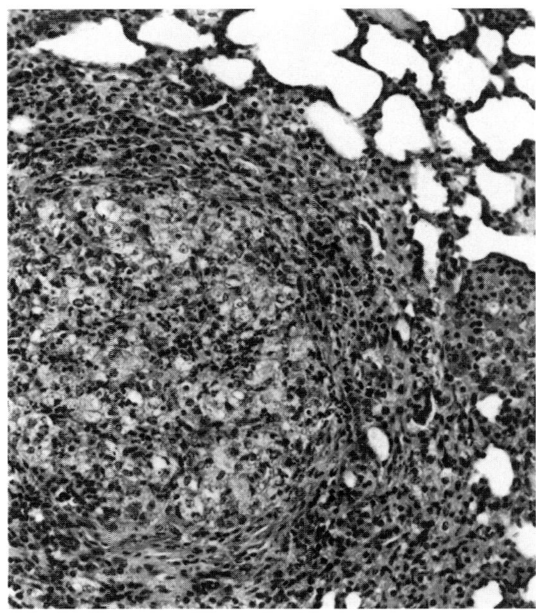

FIGURE 22 Hamster 12 months after instillation of 20 mg MQZ. Silicotic granuloma composed of macrophages and few fibroblasts and lymphocytes. Note loss of alveolar architecture, minimal fibrosis, and lack of alveolar Type II hyperplasia. (H&E stain; × 145.)

The distribution of histological lung tumor types induced by quartz in rats (Tables 1 and 2) shows that the predominant type of differentiation is adenomatous, as represented by adenomas, adenocarcinomas (the most frequent tumor type), and mixed carcinomas with an adenocarcinomatous component. Adenomas were more frequently observed in males than in females, but adenocarcinomas were more frequent in females than in males. Undifferentiated carcinomas of the large or intermediate cell type were infrequent, and no small cell carcinomas were reported in any of the studies. Epidermoid carcinomas were found at lower frequencies in our experiments, but they were the prevalent type in two experiments from other laboratories.[6,11] The reasons for this discrepancy are not clear and may be due to strain differences, dietary factors (e.g., vitamin A levels, not reported in these studies), or other factors.[16]

Electron microscopic evidence of the alveolar Type II origin of quartz-induced lung cancers in rats was reported by Johnson et al.,[25] who examined the tissues from the long-term experiments in rats conducted at the Los Alamos National Laboratory. A recent electron microscopic study of selected areas of paraffin-embedded lung tissues from the MQZ-treated rats in our laboratory revealed the presence of particles in both alveolar and interstitial macrophages, examined up to 11 months after quartz instillation. Collagen fibrils were abundant in the alveolar walls adjacent to the macrophages and epithelial cells, particularly in lesions older than six months.[26] In addition, electron microscopic examination of rat lung tissues, obtained within 30 min of a single intrabronchial instillation of 1.25 mg of quartz (Min-U-Sil <2 μm) in 0.1 ml saline, revealed the presence of quartz particles in alveolar Type II cells and in the interstitium of alveolar walls.[26]

The constant association of alveolar epithelial proliferative lesions and lung tumors with silicotic lesions, in this rat model, makes it a unique animal model for the study of human fibrosis-associated lung cancers or scar cancers.

The previously published data on quartz carcinogenesis (Table 1) do not include dose-response studies. In our experiments, the rat groups treated with 12 mg MQZ showed a high level of induction of lung carcinomas, and no further increases were observed in the only group of female rats treated with 20 mg MQZ. This limited observation suggests that the single 12-mg dose already achieved a level of effect in the maximal range. It remains to be determined what doses would induce lower response levels in this model.

The comparison of results obtained in parallel studies with MQZ and HFMQZ, in the rat model, is interesting because HF etching removed iron as impurity from the MQZ sample, as shown by X-ray fluorescence analysis. In tests for surface reactivity and for DNA damage *in vitro* (see section VI in this chapter), the MQZ sample always appeared more active than HFMQZ. The results of the long-term tests in rats, however, showed similar levels of fibrogenesis and carcinogenesis induced by the two samples, suggesting that the differences in short-term reactivity were not critical in altering the long-term fibrogenic and carcinogenic activities. Treatment protocols that would result in a lower level of carcinogenic response (e.g., lower single doses) or protocols that would modulate the response (e.g., concurrent treatment with inhibitors of fibrogenesis) might reveal differences in the degree of carcinogenic activity shown by different quartz samples and clarify whether surface impurities play a role in the resulting carcinogenic activity.

The studies in mice were of interest for several reasons. Strain A is well known for its high susceptibility to the induction of lung adenomas and adenocarcinomas by a wide variety of carcinogens, and therefore it was chosen to determine if early epithelial reactions and tumors would be induced by instillation of crystalline silica; interestingly, i.v. injection of silica (type not specified) in strain A mice did not induce lung adenomas.[27] Strain BALB/c was selected as a strain of average sensitivity to carcinogens, and also as the strain of origin of the BALB/3T3 cell line used in cell transformation assays. Athymic nude mice were selected because T lymphocyte-mediated mechanisms had been suggested in the pathogenesis of silicotic fibrosis by Pernis and Vigliani.[28] It was therefore of interest to observe if the pathology of silicosis in athymic nude mice would differ from that in the immunocompetent strains and to observe possible differences in susceptibility to tumor induction by crystalline silica.

The detailed cellular reaction in tissues from these mice requires further study. The finding of a comparable level of silicotic reaction, at the histological level, in immunosuppressed and immunocompetent mice suggests that fibrogenesis may be independent of the role of T lymphocytes, which had been hypothesized as a cell mediator in the pathogenesis of silicosis.[28] It would be interesting to investigate the susceptibility to quartz-induced fibrogenesis and carcinogenesis in totally immunosuppressed mice as well as in mouse strains known to be susceptible to bleomycin-induced pulmonary fibrosis.[29]

The hamster studies showed that this species responded to quartz instillation in the lungs only with granulomas that remained predominantly macrophagic, without progressive development of fibrosis or epithelial hyperplasia, as reported above, and without lung tumor induction, as reported in long-term experiments.[8,22–24] Hamster embryo cells, however, were found susceptible to quartz-induced neoplastic transformation,[30] as discussed later. The mechanisms of hamster lung resistance to the fibrogenic and carcinogenic effects of quartz need to be investigated and could provide critical clues to elucidate the pathogenesis of silica-induced reactions.

In older studies, Saffiotti and co-workers[19,31] examined the cellular reactions to crystalline silica in conventional rats, following a single intratracheal instillation of 50 mg quartz, HF-etched quartz, or tridymite. In contrast to the lung reactions described above for rats in SPF conditions, semiquantitative observations in conventional rats showed a prominent reaction of mast cells and plasma cells in the silicotic lung lesions, which also developed massive fibrosis with hyaline deposits of gamma globulins.[19,31] The more intense fibrogenic reactions to crystalline silica in conventional vs. SPF rats have been well documented by a comparative study by Chiappino and Vigliani.[32] These authors, however, did not describe the epithelial reaction.

The role of mast cells in the pathogenesis of silica-induced lung lesions should be further investigated. Their number and their degranulation rate markedly increased in silicotic rat lungs as compared with controls, including hematite-treated rat lungs.[19,31,33] Mast cell products include histamine and serotonin-like substances and several cytokines: their effects on the epithelial cell reaction in experimental silicosis have not been examined so far. In our present studies, mast cells were found in much higher numbers in the lungs of untreated rats than in the lungs of untreated mice (of strains A, BALB/c, or nude) or hamsters; quartz treatment increased the number of mast cells in rat lungs but not in those of mice and hamsters. A recent study[34] investigated the role of mast cells in silica-induced pulmonary inflammation in mice (silica type unspecified). This study compared the C57BL/6 strain, known for its susceptibility to bleomycin-induced lung fibrosis, with the mast cell-deficient strain WBB6F$_1$-W/W^v and their mast cell-intact littermates WBB6F$_1$-+/+. Cultured mast cells were also injected intravenously in mast cell-deficient mice. The results showed that mast cell-deficient mice had a significantly lower degree of lung inflammation, measured by various parameters and especially by the number of neutrophils. The mice in this study were observed only for 28 d, and no information is available on later effects, including epithelial reactions.

TABLE 4
Species Differences in the Lung Reactions to Silica[a]

Species	Fibrogenesis	Carcinogenesis
Rat	+++++	+++++
Mouse	++	–
Hamster	–	–

[a] Relative intensities: +++++ = strong; ++ = moderate; – = absent

The histological appearance of silicotic granulomas differed considerably in the three species studied in our experiments, as reported above. In rats, the granulomas showed intense cellular reactions with heavy collagen deposition; in mice, they showed large necrotic centers and relatively little collagen; and in hamsters, they were limited to macrophagic storage lesions. The overall conclusion, drawn from our studies, comparing rats, mice, and hamsters for their histopathological reaction to crystalline silica, is that these species provide evidence of strikingly different host responses, both for fibrogenesis and for carcinogenesis, as summarized in Table 4.

These species and organ differences provide a basis for further investigating pathogenetic mechanisms, especially those linking fibrogenesis with the accompanying epithelial hyperplasia and carcinogenesis.

III. PATHOGENESIS OF QUARTZ-INDUCED LUNG CANCER: FIBROSIS-ASSOCIATED ALVEOLAR EPITHELIAL HYPERPLASIA AND NEOPLASIA

A. HISTOGENESIS AND PATHOGENETIC HYPOTHESIS

The pattern of epithelial reactions to quartz, demonstrated in the serial sacrifice experiments in rats (Section II.B of this Chapter), started with foci of hyperplasia of the alveolar Type II cells adjacent to silicotic granulomas, which were observed as early as 5–10 d after single intratracheal instillation of quartz. At subsequent times of observation, the hyperplastic epithelial lesions became more frequent and sometimes nodular and eventually included areas of adenomatoid proliferation, adjacent to silicotic granulomas. Increasing tumor incidences were found at the three successive observation times of 11- and 17-month sacrifices and 17- to 24-month deaths. Thus the epithelial proliferative lesions became more frequent and advanced, in parallel with the development of the fibrogenic reaction.

As a working hypothesis for carcinogenesis by crystalline silica, Saffiotti[12] proposed, at the 1984 meeting on "Silica, Silicosis and Cancer," that cell mediators, produced in silicotic granulomas on a chronic basis, would act upon alveolar epithelial cells and combine their effects, on a chronic basis, with those due to direct genetic damage induced by crystalline silica in target alveolar epithelial cells, to account for crystalline silica-induced carcinogenesis in pulmonary epithelia of susceptible hosts. The consistent finding of a close association of silicotic granulomas with alveolar epithelial hyperplasia, in our rat experiments, provides further support for the suggested role of cell-cell interactions between the cells of mesenchymal origin (macrophages, fibroblasts, lymphocytes, mast cells) and adjacent epithelial cells (alveolar Type II cells). This working hypothesis, recently updated and illustrated,[16,35] stimulated a new coordinated research effort in our laboratory that included several lines of investigation discussed below.

B. THE ROLE OF CELL MEDIATORS IN QUARTZ-INDUCED TISSUE AND CELL REACTIONS

The role of cytokines was first described in studies on the interactions of different cell types in the immune system, but recent studies showed their importance also for epithelial cells.[36]

Several cytokines have been studied for their involvement in silicotic lesions. Previous histogenesis studies on the development of cellular reactions in experimental silicosis in non-SPF rats, following a single intratracheal instillation of a large dose (50 mg) of crystalline silica (quartz, cristobalite, and tridymite),[19,31] had shown a pattern of cellular reactions involving: macrophages; necrosis of macrophages; a modest and transient increase in granulocytes (eosinophils and rare neutrophils); progressive increase of fibroblasts, plasma cells, mast cells, and lymphocytes; and progressive development of fibrosis with hyalinization. The present histogenesis studies in SPF rats, following instillation of 12 mg of quartz, showed a more moderate lung reaction, mostly involving macrophages, necrosis of macrophages, and progressive increase of fibroblasts, lymphocytes, mast cells, and fibrosis. Alveolar epithelial hyperplastic reactions to crystalline silica were found both in the old studies in non-SPF rats[12] and in the present SPF rats.

Production of cytokines in silicotic lesions has been reported, so far in a few experimental conditions, for interleukin 1 (IL-1), IL-6, tumor necrosis factor α (TNF-α), and transforming growth factor β1 (TGF-β1). IL-1 was found to be released *in vitro* by human macrophages stimulated by crystalline silica, resulting in fibroblast proliferation.[37] Crystalline silica induced the release of increased levels of IL-1 from alveolar macrophages in rats, following inhalation exposure[38] or intratracheal instillation.[39] Rabbit macrophages stimulated by endotoxin were found to release increased amounts of IL-1 when incubated with silica.[40] In contrast, studies by Piguet et al.[41] showed that IL-1 was not overproduced in the lung tissues of (CBAxC57BL/10)F1 mice treated with an intratracheal instillation of 2 mg of a fibrogenic crystalline silica sample in 0.1 ml saline. In the same study, IL-6 was reported to be detectable in most cells of the silicotic nodule, the expression of TNF-α mRNA was increased in silicotic mouse lungs, and, in addition, TNF-α administration for 15 d through an osmotic minipump significantly increased collagen content of the lungs in crystalline silica-treated mice but not in control mice. In this study,[41] TNF-α was detected in cells interspersed in the silicotic nodules by *in situ* hybridization and by immunohistochemical staining, but TGF-β mRNA levels were not significantly altered in mice after crystalline silica treatment. In rats, after intratracheal instillation of crystalline silica, TNF-α was found to be released in increased amounts from alveolar macrophages.[41] Our studies with TGF-β1 are discussed later.

As we previously pointed out,[16] the frequency of pulmonary mast cells in different species and their reaction to crystalline silica suggest an analogy with species susceptibility to crystalline silica-induced lung cancer. The role of mast cell mediators in the carcinogenesis mechanisms induced by crystalline silica should be further investigated.

Recent methods have made it possible to study the cellular localization of specific markers for cell mediators and certain gene products in animal and human tissues that were fixed in formalin and embedded in paraffin. Such archival tissue sources can thus be used to investigate specific factors of interest. Our laboratory has used this approach, at the tissue level, to study the pathogenesis of crystalline silica-induced fibrogenesis and associated carcinogenesis.

C. TGF-β1 IN QUARTZ-INDUCED RAT LUNG LESIONS: EPITHELIAL-MESENCHYMAL INTERACTIONS

TGF-β is a family of polypeptides with multifunctional regulatory activity, which has been shown to play a major role in various physiological and pathological processes, including inflammation and repair.[36,42,43] Different isoforms of this peptide (TGF-β1, β2, β3) have shown similar biological activities but differ in their regulatory functions and tissue specificity of expression.[36,44] TGF-β1 controls cell growth and differentiation, induces production of extracellular matrix, stimulates formation of collagen and production of granulation tissue, and thus is a critical factor in the repair process.[36,45] Increased production of TGF-β1, accompanied by elevated levels of TGF-β1 mRNA, has been associated with chronic inflammatory and fibrotic diseases in humans[46–50] and rodents.[51,52]

The localization of TGF-β1 in the pathogenesis of experimental silicosis and associated carcinogenesis was studied in our laboratory, using immunohistochemical methods applied to paraffin sections of lung tissues from the animals treated by a single intratracheal instillation of quartz, described in section II.B of this chapter. For immunostaining, three polyclonal antibodies were raised in rabbits to the NH_2 terminal 1–30 amino acids of mature TGF-β1 (antibody LC [1–30] staining for intracellular TGF-β1 and antibody CC [1–30] staining for extracellular TGF-β1) and to amino acids 266–278 of the TGF-β1 precursor latency-associated peptide (LAP), staining for intracellular sites of TGF-β1 production.[35]

In quartz-treated rats, LC(1–30), for intracellular mature TGF-β1, was localized, in all observed lung sections, in fibroblasts and mononuclear cells, particularly those around hyperplastic alveolar Type II cells and at the periphery of granulomas, as well as in a few interstitial macrophages. This immunoreactivity to LC(1–30) was first observed in macrophages by day 15 and became more intense in fibroblasts and macrophages with the development of progressive fibrosis. CC(1–30), for extracellular TGF-β1, was detected in the connective tissue matrix adjacent to hyperplastic alveolar cells and in the granulomas, beginning 10–15 d after treatment and increasing with the progression of fibrosis of the silicotic nodules. Immunolocalization of TGF-β1/LAP was first observed in the hyperplastic alveolar Type II cells of quartz-treated rats at 10–15 d from treatment. By one month, these cells, particularly those adjacent to the silicotic granulomas, showed strong immunostaining, which persisted up to 24 months of observation. Immunoreactivity to this antibody for TGF-β1 precursor was also intense in the cells forming the adenomas, but it was negative in the cells forming the carcinomas. No immunoreactivity to any of the forms of TGF-β1 was observed in any of the examined controls, which included lungs of hematite-treated rats with multifocal deposits of dust in alveolar and interstitial macrophages and in lungs of untreated rats. The immunostaining reaction was controlled using normal rabbit immunoglobulin (IgG). The results of these studies were recently reported in detail.[26,35]

In contrast, minimal immunoreactivity to TGF-β1/LAP was detected in quartz-treated A/J mice, starting around 30 d, without further progression. In hamster lungs (treated and controls), this immunoreactivity was not detected.[116]

The close relationship of the hyperplastic alveolar Type II cells, stained for TGF-β1/LAP, to the cells of the periphery of silicotic granulomas and the stroma, where mature TGF-β1 was localized, suggests an active role of the proliferating epithelial cells in the process of silicotic fibrogenesis. The role of TGF-β1 in fibrogenesis and carcinogenesis has been widely documented.[36,53,54]

We investigated, at the protein level, the possible role of the *ras* family of oncogenes and of the tumor suppressor gene, p53. These genes are currently of major interest for the study of carcinogenesis mechanisms and were chosen because of their frequent activation in lung cancer.[55] Immunohistochemical investigations, in the same quartz-treated rat lung tissues described above, revealed that the localization of antibodies to pan-reactive p21 *ras* protein was strongly positive in the hyperplastic alveolar Type II cells adjacent to silicotic granulomas, the same cells that showed a strong localization of TGF-β1/LAP. The cells of the adenomas, that also showed localization of TGF-β1/LAP, however, were not immunoreactive to the p21 *ras* protein. The carcinomas showed no immunostaining for either TGF-β1/LAP or for p21 *ras* protein.[56] The lack of detectable p21 *ras* protein in the adenomas, that are positive for TGF-β1/LAP, suggests that the negative regulatory control by TGF-β1 is still maintained after the *ras* protein was downregulated. These findings suggest a diagnostic criterion for lung adenomas, based on molecular markers, namely TGF-β1/LAP (positive) and p21 *ras* protein (negative). Further studies are planned on mRNA expression of these molecular markers in quartz-induced lung adenomas. Foci of nuclear immunostaining to p53 protein were observed in the malignant cells of two out of eight of the silica-associated lung carcinomas examined, which were undifferentiated carcinomas.[56]

In related studies on the FRLE cell line (see Section IV.C), cytoplasmic and membranous immunostaining to pan-reactive p21 *ras* protein was moderate in foci of untreated FRLE cells and negative in other foci, but it was strong in *ras*-transformed FRLE cells. The solid carcinomas, obtained in nude mice from these transformed FRLE cell lines, were negative for p21 *ras* protein. Nuclear reactivity to *p53* antibody was seen in foci of transformed FRLE cells and in two out of eight tested solid tumors derived from these cells in nude mice.[56]

We hypothesize that, in the carcinomas, when both TGF-β1 and p21 *ras* genes were downregulated, the p53 gene was activated. This hypothesis may be supported by studies which show that TGF-β1 regulates c-*myc*, pRB, and cell cycle progression with resultant increase in mutant *p53*.[54,57,58] Initial studies on TGF-β1 mechanisms in cultured cells are discussed below.

IV. CELLULAR MODELS FOR CRYSTALLINE SILICA-INDUCED NEOPLASTIC TRANSFORMATION AND FOR MECHANISM STUDIES

A. TRANSFORMATION OF SYRIAN HAMSTER EMBRYO CELLS

The mechanisms of carcinogenesis by crystalline silica dust can be studied directly at the cellular level in cell culture systems susceptible to silica-induced neoplastic transformation. The first demonstration of transforming activity by quartz was obtained using the Syrian hamster embryo cell system.[30,59] This assay system is based on the induction of altered colony morphology in primary cultures; treatment with carcinogens gives rise to morphological changes in a fraction of the colonies, recognizable by piling up of the cells and by an intersecting pattern of spindle-shaped cells at the outgrowth margins of the colonies (criss-cross pattern). Colonies characterized by such altered morphology correspond to malignant phenotypes when tested for anchorage independence (growth in soft agar) and for tumorigenicity in immunosuppressed athymic nude mice.[60] Transformation assays were carried out in this system with two samples of α-quartz.[30,59] Both samples (one was a Min-U-Sil sample, the second was not defined) induced morphological transformation in a dose-dependent manner, when tested at doses of 2.5, 5, and 10 $\mu g/cm^2$ for Min-U-Sil and of 10–80 $\mu g/cm^2$ for the other quartz sample. The induced transformation frequency was relatively low for the second quartz sample (which was practically nontoxic in this cell system), higher for the more toxic Min-U-Sil sample, and much higher for samples of chrysotile and crocidolite asbestos (which were highly cytotoxic). The morphologically transformed colonies were not reported to have been further tested for tumorigenicity in nude mice. These studies showed that morphological transformation was induced by quartz and that different quartz samples showed different levels of activity. The second sample was notable for inducing transformation at doses that were not cytotoxic.

B. TRANSFORMATION OF BALB/3T3/A31–1-1 CELLS

A series of experiments in our laboratory studied the cytotoxicity and transforming activity of several quartz samples, using the mouse embryo cell line, BALB/3T3/A31–1-1. This cell line was established from the BALB/3T3/A31 line by selection of sublines susceptible to transformation by ultraviolet light and a chemical carcinogen[61] and characterized in our laboratory as susceptible to transformation by a range of organic and inorganic carcinogens.[62–64] BALB/3T3/A31–1-1 cells, maintained in MEM medium with 10% fetal bovine serum (FBS), were plated in plastic dishes (culture area of 50 mm diameter, or 20 cm^2) at the density of 200 cells per dish for cytotoxicity assays measuring colony forming efficiency (CFE) or at the density of 10^4 cells per dish for transformation assays. The medium was changed 1 d after plating to the experimental medium in which the test particles had been suspended and sonicated in a water bath for 2 min, immediately prior to use, at dust concentrations measured as $\mu g/cm^2$ (since the dust rapidly settles from the medium on the dish surface and the attached cells). The CFE was measured by counting surviving colonies per dish after one week, and transformation frequency was determined, after five weeks, by the number of morphologically transformed foci in at least 15 dishes, divided by the number of cells at risk (calculated from the CFE). In the transformation assay, the cells grow to confluence in a monolayer and then may develop morphologically altered foci growing on top of the monolayer. The foci that show an altered morphology, characterized by piling up and darker staining spindle cells forming criss-cross patterns at the margins, are classified as Type III foci and are considered as malignant transformants. When injected subcutaneously in nude mice, the cells of such foci give rise to invasive malignant tumors (sarcomas).[60]

We tested[65] five samples of α-quartz: MQZ, HFMQZ, Chinese standard quartz (CSQZ),[66] DQ12,[67] and F600. The samples were characterized for surface area and surface charge.[20] They were tested at doses from 6 to 100 $\mu g/cm^2$. F600 had very low cytotoxicity and MQZ the highest cytotoxicity. All samples showed an analogous dose-response pattern for transformation, with dose-dependent increases of transformation frequencies at the lower doses, reaching a plateau level at higher doses. The MQZ sample was tested repeatedly in five independent experiments and consistently showed maximal transformation frequency at 25 $\mu g/cm^2$ and no further significant increases at 50 and 100 $\mu g/cm^2$. The F600 sample showed a transforming activity comparable to the other samples, in spite of its very low cytotoxicity. Morphologically transformed foci from several quartz-treated experimental groups were subcultured and cryopreserved as transformed lines. When injected subcutaneously in nude mice, all these transformed lines showed rapid growth as sarcomas with invasion of surrounding tissues, whereas untreated monolayers and the parent cell line were negative in the tumorigenicity test.[65]

The BALB/3T3/A31–1-1 cell line is subtetraploid with four marker chromosomes.[68] Nine quartz-induced transformed sublines were examined and showed a similar karyotype pattern, but all had one or more additional marker chromosomes showing translocations and amplifications, not seen in the untreated cell line.[65] This finding suggests that quartz-induced transformation involves chromosomal damage.

C. TRANSFORMATION OF THE FETAL RAT LUNG EPITHELIAL CELL LINE, FRLE

The target cell for quartz-induced rat lung carcinogenesis *in vivo* is the alveolar Type II cell. Therefore it was desirable to investigate mechanisms of neoplastic transformation in a cellular model derived from such a cell type. Extensive studies have been reported on the characterization of alveolar Type II pneumocytes by methods that use primary cultures of these cells obtained from bronchoalveolar lavage.[69]

Type II pneumocytes in primary cultures were shown to retain morphological and biochemical markers of specific differentiation, namely large lamellar bodies and specific molecular markers for surfactant proteins (SP), such as SP-A and SP-C, as well as biochemical evidence of a high content level of surfactant-specific phospholipids, especially disaturated phosphatidylcholine.[69] Primary cultures of adult rat Type II cells, however, may not be suitable for the development of quantitative assays for neoplastic transformation, which require large numbers of source cells with identical characteristics. Quantitative assay systems for the induction of cell transformation by chemical or physical factors, currently in use, are based on the use of fetal rodent cells (Syrian hamster embryo cells in primary culture and the mouse embryo cell lines BALB/3T3/A31–1-1 and C3H/10T$^{1}/_{2}$).[60] For our studies on neoplastic transformation of lung alveolar epithelial cells, we chose the FRLE cell line that was established by Leheup et al.[70] by double clonal selection from lung epithelial cells explanted from Sprague-Dawley fetal rats at day 20 of gestation, using medium RPMI 1640 with 16% fetal bovine serum (FBS). The cells, at early passage, were shown to retain markers of specific alveolar Type II differentiation, such as electron microscopic evidence of lamellar bodies.[70] We obtained the FRLE cell line at passage 35, through the courtesy of Dr. M.A. Haralson, Department of Pathology, Vanderbilt University, Nashville, TN, and used it as a model for the development of methods for the induction of neoplastic transformation.

The FRLE cell line, at passage 38, was further characterized in our laboratory.[71] The cells grew well in several media. The medium we routinely used was MEM with 10% FBS. The karyotype was found to be in the hypotetraploid range, with all normal chromosomes represented by two to four copies, with two normal X and two normal Y chromosomes. A large metacentric chromosome was present in all 30 metaphases examined.[71a] The cells showed characteristics compatible with those of fetal pre-Type II alveolar cells in primary cultures.[72] The cells show lamellar body-like structures with osmiophilic concentrical membranes. The cells were found to lack expression of SP-C mRNA, as expected in cells grown on plastic surfaces but, on electron microscopy, immunogold localization of SP-C was observed in their lamellar body-like structures.[72a]

The FRLE cells were exposed to MQZ quartz at concentrations from 6 to 100 $\mu g/cm^2$ in MEM medium without serum or with 1 or 10% FBS, for 24 h, after which the cultures were fed with MEM/10% FBS. Uptake of quartz particles by FRLE cells was observed under these test conditions.[73] The ultrastructural localization of quartz particles is described below. Dose-dependent cytotoxicity was induced by quartz, and it was particularly evident when the cells were kept in serum-free MEM medium during the first 24 h.[73] FRLE cells showed marked dose-dependent toxicity for quartz and low toxicity for the nonfibrogenic titanium dioxide polymorph, anatase. The antioxidants, poly(2-vinyl-pyridine-*N*-oxide) (2-PVPNO) and 4-PVPNO, were shown to inhibit quartz cytotoxicity in this cell line.[73]

In order to study a model of neoplastic transformation in this cell line, FRLE cells were transfected by lipofection with the pZIP · Neo shuttle vector containing a codon-12 Gly → Cys mutated c-K-*ras* insert (pZip·K12·Cys). Colonies were selected for Genticin resistance and tested for tumorigenicity by subcutaneous injection in nude mice and nude rats. Abnormal colony morphology, showing irregular cell sizes, discontinuous borders, and outward migration, multilayering, and criss-crossing of cells, was observed in 15 out of 18 *ras*-transfected lines, all of which were tumorigenic in nude mice, growing as predominantly undifferentiated carcinomas.[71]

Methods are currently being developed in our laboratory for the neoplastic transformation of FRLE cells by crystalline silica and other carcinogens. Three recent experiments, still unpublished, showed that quartz-treated FRLE cells developed morphological changes indicative of transformation, as demonstrated by their growth as carcinomas in nude mice.[73a] The development of a cellular model for neoplastic transformation of alveolar epithelial cells by crystalline silica will be important for studies on cellular mechanisms of silica-induced lung carcinogenesis.

D. ELECTRON MICROSCOPIC LOCALIZATION OF QUARTZ IN TARGET CELLS

The uptake and localization of quartz particles was investigated by scanning and transmission electron microscopy in two cell culture systems used for studies on quartz-induced transformation, namely the BALB/3T3/A31–1-1 and FRLE cell lines.[72a] Following exposure of the respective cultures to MQZ particles suspended in medium, the particles were internalized by both cell types and were commonly found in the cytoplasm within single membrane-bound vacuoles. Quartz particles were examined in FRLE cells undergoing mitosis and were found in mitotic spindles, although not in intrachromatinic locations. A thorough search for silica particles in the nuclei of FRLE cells, exposed to quartz in culture, revealed the presence of small particles, usually <0.5 μm, inside the nuclei of several cells, and the intranuclear particles were confirmed as quartz by energy dispersive X-ray spectrometry.[26,74] Similar intranuclear localization of small quartz particles was observed in the BALB/3T3/A31–1-1 cells. The finding of quartz particles in the cell nuclei, as well as in the mitotic spindles of dividing cells, is suggestive of a mechanism involving direct contact of the quartz particles with chromatin.

E. STUDIES ON CELLULAR MECHANISMS RELATED TO TRANSFORMATION BY QUARTZ

Mechanism studies in cellular systems have recently explored, in our laboratory, the relationship between quartz-induced cytotoxicity and its transforming activity, as well as the effects of modifiers of these activities, including inhibitors of quartz toxicity and fibrogenicity. Since *in vivo* studies had shown that several cytokines are produced in silicotic lesions, as discussed above, we also undertook to examine the role of TGF-β1 and of TNF-α in the cellular models discussed above.

1. TGF-β1 Studies in FRLE Cells

Mechanisms involving TGF-β1 were investigated in the FRLE cell line of fetal rat alveolar origin, discussed above, as a counterpart to the findings obtained in alveolar Type II cells in rat tissue sections.[35] As recently reported,[26] untreated FRLE cells showed no detectable immunostaining with antibodies for mature TGF-β1, LC(1–30) and CC(1–30), or to TGF-β1/LAP. FRLE-derived neoplastic cell lines, transformed by transfection with a mutated K-*ras* plasmid,[71] showed intracellular immunoreactivity for TGF-β1/LAP, but no intracellular reactivity to LC(1–30).

The secretion of TGF-β1 was measured for FRLE cells (passage 43), exposed to 25 μg/cm^2 quartz (Min-U-Sil 5) for 24 h in serum-free MEM medium, using the conditioned media for ELISA sandwich assays, as described by Danielpour et al.[75] Such quartz treatment of FRLE cells increased the secreted amount of TGF-β1 approximately threefold compared with untreated control cells.[26]

2. The Role of TNF-α in BALB/3T3/A31-1-1 Cell Transformation by Quartz

TNF-α has been implicated as a promoting factor for transformation initiated by 3-methylcholanthrene (MCA) in the BALB/3T3/A31–1-1 cell line.[76] We examined the possible role of TNF-α in quartz-induced transformation of BALB/3T3/A31–1-1 cells.[77] When human TNF-α was applied for two weeks, following treatment of the cells with either MCA or MQZ, the following results were obtained: (a) TNF-α alone resulted in moderate transformation levels, possibly by enhancement of spontaneous background levels; (b) TNF-α markedly enhanced MCA-induced transformation; (c) in contrast, TNF-α consistently decreased the transformation frequency induced by quartz (confirmed in a duplicate experiment); (d) heat-inactivated TNF-α (95°C for 30 min), however, increased the transformation frequency of quartz. These results confirm the enhancing effect of TNF-α on MCA-initiated transformation but demonstrate an opposite effect on quartz-induced transformation, suggesting that the underlying mechanisms of transformation by quartz are different from those due to MCA.[77]

3. Relationship Between Toxic and Carcinogenic Mechanisms of Quartz

It was noted above that some quartz samples induced very low cytotoxicity but significant transforming activity. The reasons for this discrepancy need to be identified, because they may help to clarify possibly different specific pathways responsible, respectively, for toxic and transforming effects.

Samples of hematite (Fe_2O_3) and of two titanium dioxide (TiO_2) polymorphs, anatase and rutile, were tested in the BALB/3T3/A31–1-1 cell line, alone or in a 1:1 mixture by weight with MQZ. Hematite and anatase alone showed minimal toxicity, whereas rutile showed higher toxicity than MQZ. When combined with MQZ, hematite and anatase markedly inhibited the toxicity of quartz and also markedly inhibited its transforming activity. The rutile sample, in contrast, markedly enhanced the toxicity of MQZ, but it did not increase its transforming activity.[65,71a]

These observations point to the important fact that other minerals, associated with quartz, can strongly modify its biological effects in opposite directions. Exposure to quartz dust in the work environment is usually accompanied by exposure to other mineral dusts. Quartz samples used for experimental studies may also contain other minerals as impurities. The role of associated minerals is an important issue that needs to be further investigated.

Other inhibitors of quartz toxicity have been identified using different biological endpoints. PVPNO is a polymer that binds to silanol groups on the crystalline silica surface. Its binding is proportional to the surface area of the sample and occurs independently of the binding of an agent such as the dye Janus Green B, that reacts with the ionized groups on the silica surface.[20] PVPNO was found to inhibit biological activities of quartz, including hemolysis[78] and cytotoxicity.[73] 2-PVPNO and 4-PVPNO were found to bind to the quartz surface at approximately the same level and to inhibit quartz toxicity in FRLE cells also at the same level; in contrast, PVPNO did not bind to the surface of the nontoxic titanium dioxide polymorph, anatase, which lacks surface hydroxyl groups.[73] The effects of PVPNO on quartz-induced transformation require further investigation.

4. Studies on Tetrandrine

While at present there is no established method for the pharmacological prevention or treatment of silicosis, tetrandrine, a benzylisoquinoline plant alkaloid, was reported to retard and reverse the fibrotic lesions of silicosis in humans.[79–81] The mechanism of action of tetrandrine is not clear. Tetrandrine was reported to be a possible superoxide radical ($O_2^{\cdot-}$) scavenger, as measured by superoxide dismutase-inhibitable ferricytochrome C reduction.[82] Tetrandrine did not affect hydrogen peroxide (H_2O_2)-induced chemiluminescence in a cell-free system or the resting rate of oxygen consumption, $O_2^{\cdot-}$ release, or H_2O_2 secretion by alveolar macrophages.[83]

Shi et al.[84] recently investigated the antioxidant properties of tetrandrine, using electron spin resonance (ESR) spin trapping with the spin trap 5,5-dimethyl-1-pyrroline-*N*-oxide. Tetrandrine efficiently reacted with hydroxyl radicals ($^{\cdot}OH$) generated by the Fenton reaction [Fe(II) + H_2O_2], as well as by reaction of chromium(V) with H_2O_2. Similar results were obtained using $^{\cdot}OH$ radicals generated by reaction of freshly fractured quartz particles with aqueous medium. Tetrandrine also scavenged superoxide (O_2^-) radical produced from xanthine/xanthine oxidase. The effect of tetrandrine on lipid peroxidation induced by freshly fractured quartz particles was evaluated using linoleic acid as a model lipid. The results showed that tetrandrine caused 37.6% inhibition on lipid peroxidation induced by freshly fractured quartz. Since tetrandrine is able to bind to the cell membrane of macrophages,[85] it may scavenge oxygen free radicals at this site of generation. The antioxidant property of tetrandrine may be important for the inhibition of silicosis and may provide a basis for designing more active antioxidant alkaloids for the prevention and treatment of silicosis. No data are available on the effects of tetrandrine on quartz-induced neoplastic transformation.

V. DNA DAMAGE BY QUARTZ

A. QUARTZ-INDUCED DNA DAMAGE *IN VITRO*

The evidence that quartz particles are carcinogenic *in vivo* and induce neoplastic transformation in cultured cells points to a mechanism involving DNA damage. In addition, cell systems used for quartz-induced transformation also showed other evidence of genetic damage. In Syrian hamster embryo cells, MQZ (20 $\mu g/cm^2$) induced a significant increase in the percent of cells with micronuclei.[59] In BALB/3T3/A31–1-1 cells, quartz samples were found to induce chromosomal alterations (translocations and amplifications) not seen in the control cells.[65]

Our laboratory investigated the induction of DNA strand breakage by direct interaction with particles of crystalline silica in aqueous medium at physiological pH.[86] DNA (phage λ Hind III digest) in phosphate buffer was exposed to quartz particles alone or in the presence of hydrogen peroxide, with or without modifiers of reactive oxygen pathways, such as superoxide dismutase (SOD), catalase, chelating agents, and oxygen radical scavengers. DNA double strand breakage was assessed after agarose gel electrophoresis and ethidium bromide staining by evidence of degradation of discretely sized bands. The results showed that DNA double strand breaks were induced by quartz alone but only after extended time periods (up to three weeks). Control DNA was stable in buffer, and no DNA damage was detected with H_2O_2 alone. The combination of quartz and H_2O_2 resulted in rapid DNA strand breakage after only a few hours. The reactions obtained with various modifiers of reactive oxygen pathways concurred in demonstrating that the DNA damaging activity of quartz was produced by oxygen radicals and that iron impurities acted as Fenton reaction catalysts in the generation of hydroxyl radicals. Replacing atmospheric oxygen with argon inhibited the DNA damage.[86]

Infrared spectroscopy of silica-DNA complexes provided evidence that DNA binds to the surface of quartz.[87,88] Attenuated total reflectance Fourier-transform infrared spectra were obtained, in phosphate buffer under a nitrogen atmosphere, for quartz alone (using two samples, Min-U-Sil <5 and CSQZ), calf thymus DNA alone, and the coincubation of quartz with DNA. The results showed that both samples of quartz induced modifications of the DNA spectrum, indicative of structural changes in the DNA phosphate backbone due to reorientation of the phosphate groups and their involvement in the DNA-quartz interaction. Conversely, DNA-quartz interaction was found to modify the quartz spectra in the band corresponding to the ≡Si–O stretch in the ≡Si–OH group on the quartz surface. The changes in the infrared spectra of quartz and of DNA, following their interaction, indicate involvement of the DNA phosphate backbone and of the silanol groups and suggest that hydrogen bonds are formed between silanol groups and the DNA phosphate backbone, according to the following pathway.[87–89]

$$=\mathrm{Si}\overset{\mathrm{O}}{\diagup\;\diagdown}\mathrm{Si}= \;(=\mathrm{Si{-}O{-}Si}=)\xrightarrow{+H_2O} =\underset{}{\overset{\mathrm{OH}}{\mathrm{Si}}}-\mathrm{O}-\overset{\mathrm{OH}}{\mathrm{Si}}= \xrightarrow{+\mathrm{DNA}\ +H_2O} =\overset{\mathrm{OH\cdots H_2O}}{\mathrm{Si}}-\mathrm{O}-\overset{\mathrm{OH\cdots DNA}}{\mathrm{Si}}=$$

Further support for this pathway was provided by the finding that pretreatment of quartz with PVPNO, the agent discussed above as blocking silanol groups and inhibiting quartz cytotoxicity, almost completely abolished the ability of quartz to induce specific alterations of the DNA spectrum.[87] The spectra of quartz, obtained by transmission Fourier-transform infrared spectroscopy for both MQZ and CSQZ, were significantly altered by coincubation with DNA, consistent with alteration of the silicon-oxygen bond. In addition, increasing concentrations of quartz were shown to induce increasingly marked alterations of the specific peaks of the DNA spectra, using D_2O instead of H_2O in order to avoid interference from water absorbance.[87,89]

The evidence for DNA binding to the quartz surface suggested a mechanism for the effective induction of DNA damage.[88] The production of reactive oxygen species on the quartz surface and the evidence that DNA damage is mediated by reactions yielding hydroxyl radical need to be considered in relation to the very short half-life of the hydroxyl radical, which has a reaction distance of approximately 15 Å, less than the width of the DNA helix. We suggested that binding of quartz to the DNA phosphate backbone provides a mechanism that anchors DNA strands close to the sites of oxygen radical production on the quartz surface, so that oxygen radicals are generated within a few angstroms from their target nucleotides.[88]

Evidence was obtained that crystalline silica (different samples of quartz, cristobalite, and tridymite) induced increased production of the oxidized base, thymine glycol, from DNA incubations, determined *in vitro* by chromatography/mass spectrometry.[90] This evidence suggests that direct damage to DNA bases is a likely mechanism for crystalline silica-induced carcinogenesis.

VI. MINERALOGICAL CHARACTERIZATION, SURFACE REACTIVITY, AND GENERATION OF FREE RADICALS

A. MINERALOGICAL CHARACTERIZATION OF SAMPLES FOR BIOLOGICAL STUDIES

The results of studies on the mechanisms of biological effects of mineral particles can be adequately interpreted only if the mineral samples used are sufficiently well characterized in terms of mineralogical identification, presence of impurities, and physical characteristics such as particle size distribution, surface area, and a measure of surface charge or reactivity. Collaboration between biological investigators and experts in mineralogy and physicochemical analysis of minerals is essential and has been recently reviewed in an interdisciplinary course.[91]

The role of mineral impurities, especially iron and other metals, that can act as catalists in Fenton-like reactions yielding free radicals, needs to be evaluated. The role of associated minerals, mixed with quartz at the time of exposure, has been pointed out above as a possible major modifier of quartz toxicity and/or transformation. The role of such factors in modifying the carcinogenic activity of quartz *in vivo,* in laboratory animals or in humans, needs to be investigated. Quantitative studies on the biological activity of minerals, especially as it involves carcinogenesis, require the use of well-characterized samples of reproducible activity. Samples representing major categories of mineralogical and physicochemical properties of crystalline silica and related minerals (including control samples of amorphous silica and of several crystalline metal oxides) are needed for comparative studies on biological effects, especially now that models for the induction of neoplastic transformation by silica are becoming established.

Exposure doses to particulate minerals, especially at the target cell level, need to be defined for comparative studies. Studies on dose-response relationships are lacking for *in vivo* quartz carcinogenesis and are still very limited for cell transformation.

One important variable has been identified as playing an important role in quartz toxicity by comparing the effects of freshly fractured quartz particles with those of aged quartz particles derived from the same sample.[92] These studies show that freshly fractured quartz exhibits a greater cytotoxic effect on cell membrane integrity than quartz that was aged for 4 d after fracturing, as demonstrated by a 1.5-fold increase in lactic dehydrogenase release from macrophages and a 3-fold increase in the induction of lipid peroxidation. The samples that were used for *in vivo* carcinogenesis and for cell transformation experiments, described in sections II.B, IV.B, and IV.C, were not freshly fractured; these results therefore indicate that aged quartz retained carcinogenic activity. The effect of fresh fracturing remains to be investigated in relation to the induction of neoplastic cell transformation and *in vivo* carcinogenesis.

B. GENERATION OF FREE RADICALS

Surface reactivity of quartz and other mineral particles needs to be investigated in relation to the induction of biological interactions leading to neoplastic transformation, *in vivo* or in cultured cells. Different agents bind to silanol groups, ≡Si–OH, or to ionized groups, $\equiv Si–O^-$, as shown by the independent binding of PVPNO and Janus Green B, respectively.[20] The studies on DNA damage by crystalline silica *in vitro* (section V) indicate that the underlying mechanism is dependent on the formation of reactive oxygen radicals.

Recent studies in our laboratory have further investigated the mechanisms of free radical generation by crystalline silica.[93,94]

While earlier ESR studies have shown that aqueous suspension of freshly fractured quartz particles generate ˙OH radicals,[92,95,96] recent results demonstrate that freshly fractured quartz in aqueous suspension is also capable of generating H_2O_2, $O_2^{\bar{\cdot}}$ radicals, and singlet oxygen ($^1O_2$).[93] These reactive oxygen species are capable of causing lipid peroxidation, DNA double strand breaks, and deoxyguanine (dG) hydroxylation.[94]

It has been reported that the breakage of quartz lattice, when quartz is fractured, implies the breaking of ≡Si–O–Si≡ bonds and the generation of silicon-based free radicals (≡Si˙, ≡SiO˙, and ≡SiOO˙).[97–100] For ≡SiO˙ radicals, the bonding between Si and O atoms is quite strong ($\Delta H = 108$ kcal/mol) and will not be easily broken upon hydrolysis.[101] Upon reaction with H_2O, the following reactions involving ≡SiO˙ take place:

$$\equiv SiO^{\cdot} + H_2O \rightarrow \equiv SiOH + {}^{\cdot}OH \tag{1}$$

$$\equiv SiO^{\cdot} + {}^{\cdot}OH \rightarrow \equiv SiOOH \tag{2}$$

$$\equiv SiOOH + H_2O \rightarrow \equiv SiOH + H_2O_2 \tag{3}$$

The inhibition by catalase of quartz-induced cellular damage, reported in a number of studies,[92,96,102–104] supports the generation of H_2O_2 by quartz particles in aqueous media.

Spin trapping measurements show that ˙OH generation was inhibited in the presence of SOD, suggesting that $O_2^{\bar{\cdot}}$ was not only generated, but also involved in the mechanism of ˙OH radical generation.[93] $O_2^{\bar{\cdot}}$ may function as a reductant to reduce metal ions or reactive centers on the surface of silica particles. These redox reactions may facilitate silica-mediated ˙OH generation from H_2O_2 according to Equations (4) and (5) and the overall equation (6):

$$O_2^{\bar{\cdot}} + M^{n+} \rightarrow M^{(n-1)+} + O_2 \tag{4}$$

$$M^{(n-1)+} + H_2O_2 \rightarrow M^{n+} + {}^{\cdot}OH + OH^- \tag{5}$$

$$O_2^{\bar{\cdot}} + H_2O_2 \xrightarrow{M^{n+}/M^{(n-1)+}} {}^{\cdot}OH + O_2 + OH^- \tag{6}$$

where M^{n+} represents metal ions or certain reactive centers on the surface of silica particles. The reactions described in Equations (4) to (6) are Haber-Weiss type reactions. The inhibitory effect of deferoxamine on ·OH generation provides additional support for the presence of metal ions or reactive centers on the surface of silica particles.[105]

Evidence for the generation of $^1O_2$ from aqueous suspension of freshly fractured quartz, in the presence of H_2O_2, was obtained using ESR spin trapping. $^1O_2$ is very reactive and can cause DNA damage. For example, it has been reported that $^1O_2$ causes hydroxylation of dG residue in DNA to generate 8-hydroxydeoxyguanosine (OHdG).[106] It may be noted that $^1O_2$ generation, in reactions mediated by Cr(VI), Ni(II), and Co(II), was suggested to play an important role in causing DNA damage.[107–109] Similarly, $^1O_2$ generated by silica particles may also play a significant role in DNA damage and possibly in silica-induced carcinogenesis.

Electrophoretic assays demonstrate that freshly fractured quartz can cause DNA double strand breaks.[86,93,94] DNA damage by freshly fractured quartz is dependent on the presence of molecular oxygen.[93,94] Oxygen radicals may therefore play an important role in the mechanism of quartz-mediated DNA damage, which may significantly contribute to our understanding of the mechanism of silica-induced carcinogenesis.

Recent studies also demonstrate that quartz particles can cause lipid peroxidation.[93,94] SOD, catalase, and the ·OH radical scavenger, sodium benzoate, all efficiently inhibit lipid peroxidation, supporting the role of oxygen radicals in quartz-induced lipid peroxidation. This finding supports the earlier hypothesis that membrane damage via quartz-induced lipid peroxidation is a primary step in the pathogenetic mechanism of silicosis[110] and may be relevant to quartz carcinogenesis.

Using high performance liquid chromatography (HPLC) with electrochemical detection, it was shown that reactive oxygen species generated from quartz particles in suspension cause dG hydroxylation to produce 8-OHdG.[94] 8-OHdG was chosen as a model for reactive oxygen species-induced DNA damage, because DNA damage by these species is important in mutagenesis and carcinogenesis. Among DNA base modifications, 8-OHdG is one of the most representative and most specific for damage induced by reactive oxygen species.[105,111–113] In addition, 8-OHdG is mutagenic in DNA replication, and levels of 8-OHdG are directly correlated with carcinogenic effects *in vivo*. Thus it is possible that quartz particles may cause carcinogenesis via hydroxylation of dG residue in DNA, mediated by reactive oxygen species.

VII. CONCLUSIONS

The questions raised at the 1984 conference on "Silica, Silicosis and Cancer"[4] have stimulated new research that, in the past decade, resulted in a new body of knowledge about the biological effects of crystalline silica, especially quartz, that now provides a plausible basis for the carcinogenicity of quartz. Much research work remains to be done to gain a more detailed understanding of mechanisms involved in quartz-induced carcinogenesis and to relate them to the biological effects of quartz exposure in humans.

Carcinogenesis by quartz has been clearly demonstrated by strong experimental evidence, based on numerous experiments in rats of both sexes, by different routes and modes of administration. Inhalation and intratracheal instillation of various quartz preparations resulted in the induction of lung adenomas and carcinomas, with a prevalence of adenocarcinomas.

The histopathogenesis of lung epithelial reactions and epithelial tumors in rats, following a single intratracheal instillation of quartz, is described here in detail. It is characterized by alveolar Type II cell hyperplasia adjacent to granulomas with fibrosis, development of alveolar Type II hyperplastic areas and adenomatoid foci, and eventually adenomas and carcinomas, predominantly adenocarcinomas, many of which show a central area of fibrosis.

In mice, a single intratracheal instillation of quartz gave rise to lung granulomas with minimal or moderate fibrosis, with no persistent alveolar epithelial hyperplasia and no significant tumor induction. Comparable quartz treatment in hamsters induced macrophagic storage granulomas without progressive fibrosis, no epithelial proliferation, and no tumors. These species differences indicate the important role of host factors in the pathogenesis of silicosis and of quartz-induced lung cancers.

The histopathological progression of epithelial hyperplastic and neoplastic lesions associated with the development of silicosis in the rat model, illustrated here, and the identification of specific patterns of localization of molecular markers, in the different stages of these epithelial reactions, indicate the important role of alveolar Type II cells in pulmonary reactions to quartz and in the pathogenesis of quartz-induced lung tumors in susceptible species. The evidence that the lungs of certain species or strains do not develop an alveolar epithelial proliferative reaction to quartz (mice) or even a fibrogenic reaction (hamsters), suggests host-dependent pathogenetic factors. To identify such factors and to investigate their relevance for human subjects are major goals of present research.

The rat model for lung cancer induction by quartz, leading to fibrosis-associated carcinomas, is a unique experimental model for studying the pathogenesis of human adenocarcinomas of peripheral lung origin. These types of lung cancer, now becoming more prevalent in humans, are often associated with fibrosis. Even the presence of multiple lung carcinomas in individual silicotic rats, frequently observed in our experiments (Table 2), is not without a counterpart in human subjects: a recent case report described the occurrence of three separate lung cancers in different lobes of the same silicotic patient (a moderately differentiated squamous cell carcinoma, a bronchioloalveolar carcinoma, and a bronchial squamous carcinoma *in situ*).[114]

We examined histological sections from cases of human silicosis that showed foci of alveolar hyperplastic Type II lesions similar to those illustrated here for the rat model.[15,26] We hope to extend our studies of lung pathology in human pneumoconioses and their associated lung cancers and especially to investigate the frequency and significance of alveolar Type II epithelial hyperplasia and dysplasia in human fibrosis-associated lung carcinogenesis.

Molecular markers for cellular mediators and specific gene products, demonstrated in the animal models, such as TGF-β1, p21 *ras* protein, and p53 protein, discussed previously, will be studied in human lungs to compare the reactivity of individuals with different types or stages of silicosis and/or lung cancer. It is hoped that studies on the association of lung cancer with human silicosis will be focused on specific histological types of lung cancer. Other associated conditions, such as silicotuberculosis, and associated exposures, such as radioactive materials, cigarette smoke, and other minerals that may modify the biological effects of silica, need to be evaluated in relation to pulmonary lesions. The use of molecular markers may provide clues for early diagnosis of preneoplastic lesions and identify individuals at risk for the development of lung cancer.

Long-term animal carcinogenesis experiments would be needed to learn whether known inhibitors of quartz toxicity or reactivity are effective in preventing cancer induction *in vivo*. Before undertaking long-term animal experiments, which are expensive and time consuming, preliminary studies are needed using effective cellular and molecular models.

Cellular models for neoplastic transformation by quartz and other minerals are becoming available, including models using lung alveolar cells. Quartz-induced neoplastic transformation can be obtained in cultures derived from alveolar cells of the susceptible species, the rat, as shown by the results of our studies on the FRLE cell line. Establishing optimal and possibly quantitative methods for the transformation of lung alveolar cells by quartz and other particulate minerals will make it possible to investigate cellular and molecular events critically involved in the transformation of these target cells. Future studies may determine the feasibility of replacing the fetal cell line, FRLE, with adult alveolar cells for quartz-induced transformation. In this context, it is interesting that rat lung epithelial cells, isolated and cultured from silica-treated rats 15 months after dust instillation and tested for *hprt* mutants, showed a dose-related increase in mutations when compared with nonexposed controls.[115]

The relationship between cytotoxicity and transformation, induced by crystalline silica samples, needs to be further investigated, especially in relation to the effects of toxicity inhibitors. The fact that the transformation frequencies, induced by several different quartz samples in the BALB/3T3/A31–1-1 cell line, all show a dose-dependent increase followed by a plateau suggests that there may be rate-limiting factors in the expression of quartz-induced transformed foci. The inhibitory effect of TNF-α on quartz-induced transformation, in contrast with the promoting effect of TNF-α on MCA-induced transformation, suggests that the "initiating" pathways for quartz differ from those induced by the polycyclic aromatic hydrocarbon.

Studies on quartz-DNA interactions revealed two important steps. Quartz was found to bind to DNA *in vitro,* as shown by altered DNA spectra (at wavelengths corresponding to the phosphate backbone and base stacking) and by altered silica spectra corresponding to silanol groups, confirmed by the inhibition of DNA spectral changes by pretreatment of quartz with the silanol blocking agent, PVPNO. Quartz was also found to induce DNA strand breakage *in vitro* by a mechanism dependent on the generation of oxygen free radicals, especially hydroxyl radical. Quartz-DNA interaction *in vitro* was also found to produce the oxidized base, thymine glycol. We hypothesized that the hydrogen bonding between DNA and the silanol groups anchors DNA within a few angstroms from the sites of oxygen radical production on the crystalline surface and thus enables the short-lived toxic radicals, such as the hydroxyl radical, to reach DNA bases and induce its critical DNA damage.

ACKNOWLEDGMENTS

The authors gratefully acknowledge the collaboration of Dr. Sherman F. Stinson, NCI/FCRDC, for the animal treatments and early sacrifices and of Mr. Alan D. Knapton and Mrs. Nadera Ahmed of our laboratory for their excellent assistance. The authors wish to thank Dr. Friedrich Pott, Düsseldorf, Germany, for the samples of DQ12 and F600 quartz; Dr. Kathleen C. Flanders, NCI, for the antibodies to TGF-β1; Dr. David Danielpour, NCI, for antibodies for ELISA; Dr. Gurmukh Singh, Pittsburgh, PA, for providing immunostaining for surfactant apoprotein and Clara cell antigen; Mrs. Shirley Hale and Mr. Kunio Nagashima, NCI/FCRDC, for excellent technical support, respectively, for histotechnology and electron microscopy; and Mr. Ricardo Dreyfuss, NIH, for microphotography.

REFERENCES

1. **Wagner, M. M. F. and Wagner, J. C.,** Lymphomas in the Wistar rat after intrapleural inoculation of silica, *J. Natl. Cancer Inst.,* 49, 81–91, 1972.
2. **Wagner, M. M. F.,** Pathogenesis of malignant histiocytic lymphoma induced by silica in a colony of specific-pathogen-free Wistar rats, *J. Natl. Cancer Inst.,* 57, 509–518, 1976.
3. **Wagner, M. M. F., Wagner, J. C., Davies, R., and Griffiths, D. M.,** Silica-induced malignant hystiocytic lymphoma: incidence linked with strain of rat and type of silica, *Br. J. Cancer,* 41, 908–917, 1980.
4. **Goldsmith, D. F., Winn, D. M., and Shy, C. M., Eds.,** *Silica, Silicosis, and Cancer,* Praeger, New York, 1986.
5. **Holland, L. M., Wilson, J. S., Tillery, M. I., and Smith, D. M.,** Lung cancer in rats exposed to fibrogenic dusts, in *Silica, Silicosis, and Cancer,* Goldsmith, D. F., Winn, D. M., and Shy, C. M., Eds., Praeger, New York, 1986, 267–279.
6. **Dagle, G. E., Wehner, A. P., Clark, M. L., and Buschbom, R. L.,** Chronic inhalation exposure of rats to quartz, in *Silica, Silicosis, and Cancer,* Goldsmith, D. F., Winn, D. M., and Shy, C. M., Eds., Praeger, New York, 1986, 255–266.
7. **Groth, D. H., Stettler, L. E., Platek, S. F., Lal, J. B., and Burg, J. R.,** Lung tumors in rats treated with quartz by intratracheal instillation, in *Silica, Silicosis, and Cancer,* Goldsmith, D. F., Winn, D. M., and Shy, C. M., Eds., Praeger, New York, 1986, 243–253.
8. International Agency for Research on Cancer, Silica, in *IARC Monographs on the Evaluation of the Carcinogenic Risk of Chemicals to Humans,* International Agency for Research on Cancer, Lyon, 42, 39–143, 1987.
9. **Muhle, H., Takenaka, S., Mohr, U., Dasenbrock, C., and Mermelstein, R.,** Lung tumor induction upon long-term low-level inhalation of crystalline silica, *Am. J. Ind. Med.,* 15, 343–346, 1989.
10. **Muhle, H., Bellmann, B., Creutzenberg, O., Dasenbrock, C., Ernst, H., Kilpper, R., MacKenzie, J. C., Morrow, P., Mohr, U., Takenaka, S., and Mermelstein, R.,** Pulmonary response to toner upon chronic inhalation exposure in rats, *Fund. Appl. Toxicol.,* 17, 280–299, 1991.
11. **Spiethoff, A., Wesch, H., Wegener, K., and Klimisch, H.-J.,** The effects of thorotrast and quartz on the induction of lung tumors in rats, *Health Phys.,* 63, 101–110, 1992.
12. **Saffiotti, U.,** The pathology induced by silica in relation to fibrogenesis and carcinogenesis, in *Silica, Silicosis, and Cancer,* Goldsmith, D. F., Winn, D. M., and Shy, C. M., Eds., Praeger, New York, 1986, 287–307.
13. **Saffiotti, U. and Stinson, S. F.,** Lung cancer induction by crystalline silica: relationships to granulomatous reactions, *Environ. Carcino. Rev. (J. Environ. Sci. Health),* C6(2), 197–222, 1988.
14. **Saffiotti, U.,** Lung cancer induction by silica in rats, but not in mice and hamsters: species differences in epithelial and granulomatous reactions, in *Environmental Hygiene II,* Seemayer, N. H. and Hadnagy, W., Eds., Springer-Verlag, New York, 1990, 235–238.
15. **Saffiotti, U.,** Lung cancer induction by crystalline silica, in *Relevance of Animal Studies to the Evaluation of Human Cancer Risk,* D'Amato, R., Slaga, T. J., Farland, W. H., and Henry, C., Eds., (*Progr. Clin. Biol. Res.,* 374), Wiley-Liss, New York, 1992, 51–69.
16. **Saffiotti, U., Daniel, L. N., Mao, Y., Williams, A. O., Kaighn, M. E., Ahmed, N., and Knapton, A. D.,** Biological studies on the carcinogenic mechanisms of quartz, *Rev. Mineral.,* 28, 523–544, 1993.
17. **Saffiotti, U., Cefis, F., and Kolb, L.,** A method for the experimental induction of bronchogenic carcinoma, *Cancer Res.,* 28, 104–124, 1968.
18. **Singh, G., Katyal, S. L., and Torikata, C.,** Carcinoma of type II pneumocytes. Immunodiagnosis of a subtype of "brochoalveolar carcinomas," *Am. J. Pathol.,* 102, 195–2008, 1981.

19. **Saffiotti, U.,** The histogenesis of experimental silicosis. III. Early cellular reactions and the role of necrosis, *Med. Lavoro,* 53, 5–18, 1962.
20. **Daniel, L. N., Mao, Y., Vallyathan, V., and Saffiotti, U.,** Binding of the cationic dye, Janus Green B, as a measure of the specific surface area of crystalline silica in aqueous suspension, *Toxicol. Appl. Pharmacol.,* 123, 62–67, 1993.
21. **Spencer, H.,** Scar cancer of the lung, in *Pathology of the Lung,* 4th ed., Spencer, H., Ed., Pergamon Press, Oxford, 1985, 885–892.
22. **Holland, L. M., Gonzales, M., Wilson, J. S., and Tillery, M. I.,** Pulmonary effects of shale dusts in experimental animals, in *Health Issues Related to Metal and Nonmetallic Mining,* Wagner, W. L., Rom, W. N., and Merchant, J. A., Eds., Butterworths, Boston, 1983, 485–496.
23. **Niemeier, R. W., Mulligan, L. T., and Rowland, J.,** Cocarcinogenicity of foundry silica sand in hamsters, in *Silica, Silicosis, and Cancer,* Goldsmith, D. F., Winn, D. M., and Shy, C. M., Eds., Praeger, New York, 1986, 215–227.
24. **Renne, R. A., Eldridge, S. R., Lewis, T. R., and Stevens, D. L.,** Fibrogenic potential of intratracheally instilled quartz, ferric oxide, fibrous glass, and hydrated alumina in hamsters, *Toxicol. Pathol.,* 13, 306–314, 1985.
25. **Johnson, N. F., Smith, D. M., Sebring, R., and Holland, L. M.,** Silica-induced alveolar cell tumors in rats, *Am. J. Ind. Med.,* 11, 93–107, 1987.
26. **Williams, A. O., Knapton, A. D., and Saffiotti, U.,** Growth factors and gene expression in silica-induced fibrogenesis and carcinogenesis, *Appl. Occup. Environ. Hyg.,* in press.
27. **Shimkin, M. B. and Leiter, J.,** Induced pulmonary tumors in mice. III. The role of chronic irritation in the production of pulmonary tumors in strain A mice, *J. Natl. Cancer Inst.,* 1, 241–254, 1940.
28. **Pernis, B. and Vigliani, E. C.,** The role of macrophages and immunocytes in the pathogenesis of pulmonary diseases due to mineral dusts, *Am. J. Ind. Med.,* 3, 133–137, 1982.
29. **Adamson, I. Y. R., Hedgecock, C., and Bowden, D. H.,** Epithelial cell-fibroblast interactions in lung injury and repair, *Am. J. Pathol.,* 137, 385–392, 1990.
30. **Hesterberg, T. W. and Barrett, J. C.,** Dependence of asbestos- and mineral dust-induced transformation of mammalian cells in culture on fiber dimension, *Cancer Res.,* 44, 2170–2180, 1984.
31. **Saffiotti, U., Tommasini Degna, A., and Mayer, L.,** The histogenesis of experimental silicosis. II. Cellular and tissue reactions in the histogenesis of pulmonary lesions, *Med. Lavoro,* 51, 518–552, 1960.
32. **Chiappino, G. and Vigliani, E. C.,** Role of infective, immunological and chronic irritative factors in the development of silicosis, *Br. J. Ind. Med.,* 39, 253–258, 1982.
33. **Pernis, B., Saffiotti, U., and Tommasini Degna, A.,** Il comportamento delle mastcellule polmonari nel corso della silicosi del ratto, *Med. Lavoro,* 49, 405–418, 1958.
34. **Suzuki, N., Horiuchi, T., Ohta, K., Yamaguchi, M., Ueda, T., Takizawa, H., Hirai, K., Shiga, J., Ito, K., and Miyamoto, T.,** Mast cells are essential for the full development of silica-induced pulmonary inflammation: a study with mast cell-deficient mice, *Am. J. Respir. Cell Mol. Biol.,* 9, 475–483, 1993.
35. **Williams, A. O., Flanders, K. C., and Saffiotti, U.,** Immunohistochemical localization of transforming growth factor-β1 in rats with experimental silicosis, alveolar type II hyperplasia, and lung cancer, *Am. J. Pathol.,* 142, 1831–1840, 1993.
36. **Roberts, A. B. and Sporn, M. B.,** The transforming growth factor-βs, in *Peptide Growth Factors and their Receptors,* Sporn, M. B. and Roberts, A. B., Eds., Springer-Verlag, New York, 1990, 419–472.
37. **Schmidt, J. A., Oliver, C. N., Lepe-Zuniga, J. L., Green, I., and Grey, I.,** Silica-stimulated monocytes release fibroblast proliferation factors identical to interleukin-1. A potential role for interleukin-1 in the pathogenesis of silicosis, *J. Clin. Invest.,* 73, 1462–1472, 1984.
38. **Oghiso, Y. and Kubota, Y.,** Enhanced interleukin 1 production by alveolar macrophages and increase in IA-positive lung cells in silica-exposed rats, *Microbiol. Immunol.,* 30, 1189–1198, 1986.
39. **Driscoll, K. E., Lindenschmidt, R. C., Maurer, J. K., Higgins, J. M., and Ridder, G.,** Pulmonary response to silica or titanium dioxide: inflammatory cells, alveolar macrophage-derived cytokines, and histopathology, *Am. J. Respir. Cell Mol. Biol.,* 2, 381–390, 1990.
40. **Kampschmidt, R. F., Worthington, M. L., and Mesecher, M. I.,** Release of interleukin 1 (IL-1) and IL-1-like factors from rabbit macrophages with silica, *J. Leucocyte Biol.,* 2, 39–123, 1986.
41. **Piguet, P. F., Collart, M. A., Grau, G. E., Sappino, A.-P., and Vassalli, P.,** Requirement of tumor necrosis factor for development of silica-induced pulmonary fibrosis, *Nature,* 344, 245–247, 1990.
42. **Roberts, A. B., Heine, U. I., Flanders, K. C., and Sporn, M. B.,** Transforming growth factor β: major role in regulation of extracellular matrix, *Ann. N.Y. Acad. Sci.,* 580, 225–232, 1990.
43. **Roberts, A. B., Sporn, M. B., Assoian, R. K., Smith, J. M., Roche, N. S., Wakefield, L. M., Heine, U. I., Liotta, L. A., Falanga, V., Kehrl, J. H., and Fauci, A. S.,** Transforming growth factor type β: rapid induction of fibrosis and angiogenesis *in vivo* and stimulation of collagen formation *in vitro, Proc. Natl. Acad. Sci. U.S.A.,* 83, 4167–417, 1986.
44. **Sporn, M. B. and Roberts, A. B.,** Peptide growth factors are multifunctional, *Nature,* 332, 217–219, 1988.
45. **Roberts, A. B., Flanders, K. C., Kondaiah, P., Thompson, N. I., Van Obberghen-Schilling, E., Wakefield, L., de Crombrugghe, R. P., Heine, U. I., and Sporn, M. B.,** Transforming growth factor β — biochemistry and roles in embryogenesis, tissue repair and remodelling, and carcinogenesis, *Recent Prog. Horm. Res.,* 44, 157–197, 1988.

46. **Khalil, N., O'Connor, R. N., Unruh, H. W., Warren, P. W., Flanders, K. C., and Kemp, A.,** Increased production and immunohistochemical localization of transforming growth factor-β in idiopathic pulmonary fibrosis, *Am. J. Respir. Cell Mol. Biol.*, 5, 155–162, 1991.
47. **Braun, L., Mead, M., Panzica, R., Mikumo, G., Bell, G. T., and Fausto, N.,** Transforming growth factor β mRNA increases during liver regeneration: a possible paracrine mechanism of growth regulation, *Proc. Natl. Acad. Sci. U.S.A.*, 85, 1539–1543, 1988.
48. **Connor, T. B., Roberts, A. B., Sporn, M. B., Danielpour, D., Dart, L. L., Michels, R. G., de Bustros, S., Enger, C., Kato, H., Lansing, M., Hayashi, H., and Glaser, B. M.,** Correlation of fibrosis and transforming growth factor β type 2 levels in the eye, *J. Clin. Invest.*, 83, 1661–1666, 1989.
49. **Castilla, A., Prieto, J., and Fausto, N.,** Transforming growth factors β1 and α in chronic liver disease — effects of interferon alfa therapy, *N. Engl. J. Med.*, 324, 933–940, 1991.
50. **McCune, B. K., Mullin, B. R., Flanders, K. C., and Sporn, M. B.,** Localization of transforming growth factor-β isotypes in lesions of the human breast, *Hum. Pathol.*, 23, 13–20, 1992.
51. **Laurent, G. J., Harrison, N. K., and McAnulty, R. F.,** The regulation of collagen production in normal lung and during interstitial lung disease, *Postgrad. Med. J.*, 64, 26–34, 1988.
52. **Khalil, N., Bereznay, M., Sporn, M. B., and Greenberg, A. H.,** Macrophage production of transforming growth factor β and fibroblast collagen synthesis in chronic pulmonary inflammation, *J. Exp. Med.*, 170, 727–737, 1989.
53. **Roberts, A. B., Frolik, C. A., Anzano, M. A., and Sporn, M. B.,** Transforming growth factors from neoplastic and non-neoplastic tissues, *Fed. Proc.*, 42, 2621–2626, 1983.
54. **Munger, K., Pietenpohl, J. A., Pittelkow, M. R., Holt, J. T., and Moses, H. L.,** Transforming growth factor beta 1 regulation of c-myc expression, pRB phosphorylation, and cell cycle progression in keratinocytes, *Cell Growth Differ.*, 3, 291–298, 1992.
55. **Carbone, D. P. and Minna, J. D.,** Molecular biology of lung cancer, in *Foundations of Oncology*, Broder, S., Ed., Williams & Wilkins, Baltimore, 1991, 339–366.
56. **Williams, A. O. and Saffiotti, U.,** TGF-β1, *ras* and *p53* in silica-induced fibrogenesis and carcinogenesis, *Scand. J. Work Environ. Health*, in press.
57. **Reiss, M., Vellucci, V. F., and Zhou, Z. L.,** Mutant p53 tumor suppressor gene causes resistance to transforming growth factor beta-1 in murine keratinocytes, *Cancer Res.*, 53, 899–904, 1993.
58. **Gerwin, B. I., Spillare, E., Forrester, K., and Lehman, T. A.,** Mutant p53 can induce conversion of human bronchial epithelial cells and reduce their responsiveness to a negative growth factor, transforming growth factor beta 1, *Proc. Natl. Acad. Sci. U.S.A.*, 89, 2759–63, 1992.
59. **Hesterberg, T. W., Oshimura, M., Brody, A. R., and Barrett, J. C.,** Asbestos and silica induce morphological transformation of mammalian cells in culture: a possible mechanism, in *Silica, Silicosis, and Cancer*, Goldsmith, D. F., Winn, D. M., and Shy, C. M., Eds., Praeger, New York, 1986, 177–190.
60. **Kakunaga, T. and Yamasaki, H., Eds.,** Transformation assay of established cell lines: mechanisms and application, IARC Scientific Publications No. 67, International Agency for Research on Cancer, Lyon, 1985, 221 pp.
61. **Kakunaga, T. and Crow, J. D.,** Cell variants showing different susceptibility to ultraviolet light-induced transformation, *Science*, 209, 505–507, 1980.
62. **Cortesi, E., Saffiotti, U., Donovan, P. J., Rice, J. M., and Kakunaga, T.,** Dose-response studies on neoplastic transformation of BALB/3T3 clone A31–1-1 cells by aflatoxin B_1, benzidine, benzo[*a*]pyrene, 3-methylcholanthrene and *N*-methyl-*N'*-nitro-*N*-nitrosoguanidine, *Teratogenesis, Carcinog. Mutagen.*, 3, 101–110, 1983.
63. **Bignami, M., Ficorella, C., Dogliotti, E., Norman, R. L., Kaighn, M. E., and Saffiotti, U.,** Temporal dissociation in the exposure times required for maximal induction of cytotoxicity, mutation and transformation by *N*-methyl-*N'*-nitro-*N*-nitrosoguanidine in the BALB/3T3 Cl A31–1-1 cell line, *Cancer Res.*, 44, 2452–2457, 1984.
64. **Bertolero, F., Pozzi, G., Sabbioni, E., and Saffiotti, U.,** Cellular uptake and metabolic reduction of pentavalent to trivalent arsenic as determinants of cytotoxicity and morphological transformation, *Carcinogenesis*, 8, 803–808, 1987.
65. **Ahmed, N. and Saffiotti, U.,** Crystalline silica-induced cytotoxicity, transformation, tumorigenicity, chromosomal translocations and oncogene expression (Abstr.), *Proc. Am. Assoc. Cancer Res.*, 33, 119, 1992.
66. **Fu, S. C., Yang, G. C., Shong, M. Z., and Du, Q. Z.,** Characterization of a new standard quartz and its effects in animals (in Chinese), *Chin. J. Ind. Hyg. Occup. Dis.*, 2, 134–137, 1984.
67. **Robock, K.,** Standard quartz DQ-12 <12 μm for experimental pneumoconiosis research projects in the Federal Republic of Germany, *Ann. Occup. Hyg.*, 16, 63–66, 1973.
68. **Saffiotti, U., Bignami, M., and Kaighn, M. E.,** Parameters affecting the relationships among cytotoxic, genotoxic, mutational and transformational responses in BALB/3T3 cells, in *Mammalian Cell Transformation*, Barrett, J. C. and Tennant, R. W., Eds., Raven Press, New York, 1985, 139–151.
69. **Voelker, D. R. and Mason, R. J.,** Alveolar type II epithelial cells, in *Lung Cell Biology*, Massaro, D., Ed., Marcel Dekker, New York, 1989, 487–538.
70. **Leheup, B. P., Federspiel, S. J., Guerry-Force, M. L., Wetherall, N. T., Commers, P. A., DiMari, S. J., and Haralson, M. A.,** Extracellular matrix biosynthesis by cultured fetal rat epithelial cells. I. Characterization of the clone and the major genetic types of collagen produced, *Lab. Invest.*, 60, 791–807, 1989.

71. **Saffiotti, U., Kaighn, M. E., Knapton, A. D., and Williams, A. O.,** Transformation of the fetal rat alveolar type II cell line, FRLE, by lipofection with a mutated K-*ras* gene (Abstr.), *Proc. Am. Assoc. Cancer Res.,* 34, 102, 1993.
71a. **Williams, A. O. et al.,** unpublished observations.
72. **Mallampalli, R. K., Floerchinger, C. S., and Hunninghake, G. H.,** Isolation and immortalization of rat pre-type II cell lines, *In Vitro Cell Dev. Biol.,* 28A, 181–187, 1992.
72a. **Saffiotti, V. et al.,** unpublished observations.
73. **Mao, Y., Daniel, L. N., Knapton, A. D., Shi, X., and Saffiotti, U.,** Protective effects of silanol group binding agents on quartz toxicity to rat lung alveolar cells, *Appl. Occup. Environ. Hyg.,* in press.
73a. **Williams, A. O., Knapton, A. D., Mao, Y., and Saffiotti, U.,** unpublished observations.
74. **Daniel, L. N., Mao, Y., Williams, A. O., and Saffiotti, U.,** Direct interaction of crystalline silica and DNA: a proposed model for silica carcinogenesis, *Scand. J. Work Environ. Health,* in press.
75. **Danielpour, D., Kim, K.-Y., Dart, L. L., Watanabe, S., Roberts, A. B., and Sporn, M. B.,** Sandwich enzyme-linked immunosorbent assays (SELISAs) quantitate and distinguish two forms of transforming growth factor-beta (TGF-β1 and TGF-β2) in complex biological fluids, *Growth Factors,* 2, 61–71, 1989.
76. **Komori, A., Yatsunami, J., Suganuma, M., Okabe, S., Abe, S., Sakai, A., Sasaki, K., and Fujiki, H.,** Tumor necrosis factor acts as a tumor promoter in BALB/3T3 cell transformation, *Cancer Res.,* 53, 1982–85, 1993.
77. **Mao, Y., Saffiotti, U., Daniel, L. N., Shi, X., and Ahmed, N.,** Tumor necrosis factor-α (TNF-α) inhibits neoplastic transformation (Tf) induced by quartz in BALB/3T3/A31-1-1 cells, *Proc. Am. Assoc. Cancer Res.,* 36, 177, 1995.
78. **Nolan, R. P., Langer, A. M., Harington, J. S., Oster, G., and Selikoff, I. J.,** Quartz hemolysis as related to its surface functionalities, *Environ. Res.,* 26, 503–520, 1981.
79. **Li, Q., Xu, Y., Zhon, Z., Chen, X., Huang, X., Chen, S., and Zhan, C.,** The therapeutic effect of tetrandrine on silicosis, *Chin. J. Tuberc. Respir. Dis.,* 4, 321–328, 1981.
80. **Liu, B., Zou, C., and Li, Y.,** Studies of the contents of glycosaminoglycans from lungs of silicotic rats, *Ecotoxicol. Environ. Safety,* 7, 323–329, 1983.
81. **Yu, V., Zou, C., and Lih, M.,** Observation of the effect of tetrandrine on experimental silicosis of rats, *Ecotoxicol. Environ. Safety,* 7, 306–312, 1983.
82. **Seow, W. K., Ferrante, A., Li, S., and Thong, Y. H.,** Antiphagocytic and antioxidant properties of plant alkaloid tetrandrine, *Int. Arch. Allergy Appl. Immunol.,* 85, 404–409, 1988.
83. **Castranova, V., Kang, J., Moore, M. D., Pailes, W. H., Frazer, D. G., and Schwegler-Berry, D.,** Inhibition of stimulant-induced activity of phagocytic cells with tetrandrine, *J. Leukocyte Biol.,* 50, 412–422, 1991.
84. **Shi, X., Mao, Y., Daniel, L. N., Saffiotti, U., Wang, L., Rojanasakul, Y., Leonard, S. S., and Vallyathan, V.,** Antioxidant activity of tetrandrine and its inhibition of quartz-induced lipid peroxidation, *J. Toxicol. Environ. Health,* 46, 101–116, 1995.
85. **Ma, J. K. H., Mo, C., Malanga, C. J., Ma, J. Y. C., and Castranova, V.,** Binding of bisbenzylisoquinoline alkaloids to phosphatidylcholine vesicles and alveolar macrophages: relationship between binding affinity and antifibrogenic potential of those drugs, *Exp. Lung Res.,* 17, 1061–1077, 1991.
86. **Daniel, L. N., Mao, Y., and Saffiotti, U.,** Oxidative DNA damage by crystalline silica, *Free Radical Biol. Med.,* 14, 463–472, 1993.
87. **Mao, Y., Daniel, L. N., Whittaker, N. F., and Saffiotti, U.,** DNA binding to crystalline silica characterized by Fourier-transform infrared spectroscopy, *Environ. Health Perspect.,* 102, Suppl. 10, 165–171, 1994.
88. **Saffiotti, U., Daniel, L. N., Mao, Y., Shi, X., Williams, A. O., and Kaighn, M. E.,** Mechanisms of carcinogenesis by crystalline silica in relation to oxygen radicals, *Environ. Health Perspect.,* 102, Suppl. 10, 159–163, 1994.
89. **Daniel, L. N., Mao, Y., Williams, A. O., and Saffiotti, U.,** Direct interaction of crystalline silica and DNA: a proposed model for silica carcinogenesis, *Scand. J. Work Environ. Health,* in press.
90. **Daniel, L. N., Mao, Y., Markey, S. P., Markey, C. J., Wang, T.-C. L., and Saffiotti, U.,** DNA strand breakage and base oxidation produced by crystalline silica (Abstr.), Oxygen Radicals and Lung Injury Conference, Morgantown, WV, 1993.
91. **Guthrie, G. D. and Mossman, B. T., Eds.,** Health effects of mineral dusts, *Rev. Mineral.,* 28, 1993.
92. **Vallyathan, V., Shi, X., Irr, W., and Castranova, V.,** Generation of free radicals from freshly fractured silica dust: potential role in acute silica-induced lung injury, *Am. Rev. Respir. Dis.,* 138, 1213–1219, 1988.
93. **Shi, X., Mao, Y., Daniel, L. N., Saffiotti, U., and Vallyathan, V.,** Freshly fractured crystalline silica particles generate hydroxyl and superoxide radicals and singlet oxygen, and cause molecular oxygen dependent DNA damage and lipid peroxidation, *Environ. Health Perspect.,* 102, Suppl. 10, 149–154, 1994.
94. **Shi, X., Mao, Y., Daniel, L. N., Saffiotti, U., Dalal, N. S., and Vallyathan, V.,** Generation of reactive oxygen species by quartz particles and its implication for cellular damage, *Appl. Occup. Environ. Hyg.,* in press.
95. **Shi, X., Dalal, N. S., and Vallyathan, V.,** ESR evidence for hydroxyl formation in aqueous suspension of quartz particles and its possible significance to lipid peroxidation in silicosis, *J. Toxicol. Environ. Health,* 25, 237–245, 1988.
96. **Dalal, N. S., Shi, X., and Vallyathan, V.,** Potentional role of silicon-oxygen radicals in acute lung injury, *NATO ASI Series,* H30, 265–772, 1989.
97. **Hochstrasser, G. and Antonini, J. F.,** Surface states of pristine silica surface, *Surf. Sci.,* 32, 644–664, 1972.

98. **Fubini, B., Bolis, V., and Giamello, E.,** The surface chemistry of crushed quartz dust in relation to its pathogenicity, *Inorg. Chim. Acta,* 138, 193–197, 1987.
99. **Kolbanev, I. V., Berestetskaya, I. Z., and Butyagin, P. Y.,** Mechanochemistry of quartz surface. VI. Properties of peroxide ≡SiOOOSi≡, *Kinet. Katal.,* 21, 1154–1158, 1980.
100. **Fubini, B., Giamello, E., Volante, M., and Bolis, V.,** Chemical functionalities at the silica surface determining its reactivity when inhaled. Formation and reactivity of surface radicals, *Toxicol. Ind. Health,* 6, 571–598, 1990.
101. **Durrent, P. J.,** Sub-group IV N. Carbon, silicon, germanium, tin, and lead, in *Introduction to Advanced Inorganic Chemistry,* John Wiley & Sons, New York, 1970, 633–644.
102. **Daniel, L. N., Mao, Y., and Saffiotti, U.,** Oxidative DNA damage by crystalline silica, *Free Radical Biol. Med.,* 14, 463–472, 1992.
103. **Vallyathan, V., Mega, J. F., Shi, X., and Dalal, N. S.,** Enhanced generation of free radicals from phagocytes induced by mineral dust, *Am. J. Respir. Cell Mol. Biol.,* 6, 404–413, 1992.
104. **Kennedy, T. P., Doson, R., Rao, N., Ky, H., Hopkins, C., Baser, M., Tolley, E., and Hoidal, J. R.,** Dusts causing pneumoconiosis generate ˙OH and produce hemolysis by acting as Fenton catalysts, *Arch. Biochem. Biophys.,* 269, 359–364, 1989.
105. **Shi, X. and Dalal, N. S.,** ESR spin trapping detection of hydroxyl radicals in the reactions of Cr(V) complexes with hydrogen peroxide, *Free Radical Res. Commun.,* 10, 17–26, 1990.
106. **Kohda, K., Nakashi, T., and Kawazoe, Y.,** Singlet oxygen takes part in 8-hydroxydeoxyguanosine formation in deoxyribonucleic acid treated with the horeseradish peroxidase-H_2O_2 system, *Chem. Pharm. Bull.,* 38, 3072–3075, 1990.
107. **Inoue, S. and Kawanishi, S.,** ESR evidence for superoxide, hydroxyl radical and singlet produced from hydrogen peroxide and nickel(II) complex of glydylglycyl-I-histidine. *Biochem. Biophys. Res. Commun.,* 159, 445–451, 1989.
108. **Kawanishi, S. K., Inoue, S., and Sano, S.,** Mechanism of DNA cleavage induced by sodium chromate(VI) in the presence of hydrogen peroxide, *J. Biol. Chem.,* 261, 5952–5958, 1986.
109. **Yamamoto, K., Inoue, S., Yamazaki, A., Yoshinaga, T., and Kawanishi, S.,** Site-specific DNA damage induced by cobalt(II) ion and hydrogen peroxide: role of singlet oxygen, *Chem. Res. Toxicol.,* 2, 234–239, 1989.
110. **Shi, X., Dalal, N. S., Vallyathan, V., and Hu, X.,** The chemical properties of silica particle surface in relation to silica-cell interactions, *J. Toxicol. Environ. Health,* 27, 434–454, 1989.
111. **Kasai, H. and Nishimura, S.,** Hydroxylation of deoxyguanosine at the C-8 position by ascorbate and other reducing agents, *Nucleic Acids Res.,* 12, 2137–2144, 1984.
112. **Dizdaroglu, M.,** Chemical determination of free radical-induced damage to DNA, *Free Radical Biol. Med.,* 10, 225–242, 1991.
113. **Floyd, R. A.,** The role of 8-hydroxyguanine in carcinogenesis, *Carcinogenesis,* 11, 1447–1450, 1987.
114. **Honma, K., Shida, H., Mishina, M., and Chiyotani, K.,** Triple lung cancers in a patient with silicosis, *Wien. Klin. Wochenschr.,* 105/10, 289–293, 1993.
115. **Driscoll, K. E., Carter, J. M., Howard, B. W., and Hassenbein, D. G.,** An *in vivo* model to investigate the mutagenicity of mineral dust exposure for rat lung epithelial cells (Abstr.), *FASEB J.,* 8, A805, 1994.

Section V
Chapter 2

SILICA AND LUNG CANCER

J. Corbett McDonald

CONTENTS

I. INTRODUCTION

Only in the past decade has the hypothesis been seriously advanced that the inhalation of crystalline silica dust might cause lung cancer. Previously, it was generally believed that workers exposed to silica had, if anything, less risk of the disease than expected.[1] It appears anomalous therefore that, as silica exposures and silicosis have declined, this suspicion should have gained ground; however, smoking habits have changed and less severe silicosis may permit survival to an age and era of higher lung cancer risk. The hypothesis allows two possibilities: first, that the risks of lung cancer and silicosis which result from exposure are separate and independent; alternatively, that the risk of lung cancer is confined to those persons who develop silicosis. Either way, the nature of any exposure-related risk could well be affected by some form of smoking-silica interaction.

Millions of working men and women throughout the world — particularly those employed in mining and quarrying; steel, iron, and other metal foundries; granite, stone, glass, and ceramic industries; transport and construction — together with an even larger number of consumers and the general public have been and continue to be exposed to crystalline silica dust. Neither national nor international control measures presently take account of carcinogenic as opposed to fibrogenic risks. The far-reaching implications of the lung cancer hypothesis led the International Agency for Research on Cancer (IARC) to call together, in 1986, an expert working group in Lyon to evaluate the published evidence then available. After lengthy discussion, the group concluded that, although evidence for carcinogenicity in experimental animals was sufficient, in man it was *limited*.[2] This implied that a causal interpretation was credible but that chance, bias, and confounding factors could not be excluded. This cautious conclusion stemmed largely from the fact that occupational exposure to silica has nearly always included other carcinogens, such as asbestos, radon, metals, and polycyclic hydrocarbons, and that evidence from studies of persons compensated for silicosis was highly susceptible to various sources of bias, in particular to

0-8493-4709-2/96/$0.00+$.50

unrepresentative case selection. Nonetheless, the IARC subsequently assigned the overall classification of 2A — probably carcinogenic to humans — to crystalline silica.[3]

This chapter will review in detail the main epidemiological studies which bear on these issues, focusing first on the information available to the expert working group in 1986, then turning back to reasons why the question had not been raised earlier. Finally, results of research published since 1986 will be considered. Animal studies cannot prove or disprove the capacity of silica to cause lung cancer in man; those studies already reported, though few, appeared sufficient to establish plausibility for the hypothesis, so resolution of the controversy now lies primarily with epidemiology.

The considerably larger body of information on the biological effects of the fibrous minerals has shown that much depends on particle size and specific physical and chemical characteristics. Attention has focused on crystalline silica, but amorphous silica has been scarcely investigated; just as the three main types of asbestos fiber differ in their biological behavior, the same could be true of quartz, cristobalite, and tridymite. The persistence of mineral particles in lung tissue is likely to be an important determining factor in carcinogenicity. There has been little study of this phenomenon and no epidemiological findings based on tissue analysis for silica.

A major source of difficulty in the interpretation of evidence based on occupational exposure to crystalline silica has been the potentially confounding effect of known carcinogens also present in the workplace. The most important of these are ionizing radiation (mainly due to radon), asbestiform mineral fibers (including fibrous hematite and talc), and some heavy metals (notably arsenic, nickel, and chromium). This problem is not simply one of simultaneous exposure to these agents as impurities or contaminants but that employees in mining, quarrying, and other dusty trades may also have worked for substantial periods of time with other materials. Cohort surveys seldom take account of lifetime occupational histories and even case-referent studies commonly do not do so. In practice, cigarette smoking is less important as a confounder, because prevailing levels of smoking seldom differ sufficiently between occupations and the general population for this to exert much effect.[4] There can be no such assurance, however, when studies are based on subjects with respiratory complaints where smoking may well be the main cause of their disability.

Reference has been made to two possible aspects of the silica hypothesis, depending on the extent to which the suspected cancer risk is or is not mediated by silica-related pulmonary fibrosis (silicosis). This issue is not only important scientifically but also for occupational hygiene standards in that it could imply that the control of the latter might also prevent the former. On the other hand, it does not follow that even if silicosis were demonstrably a risk factor for lung cancer that silica would necessarily be the cause. Silicosis might conceivably do no more than identify persons with below average ability to clear toxic or carcinogenic dust and fume from the respiratory tract. It is important therefore to determine not only whether silica-induced fibrosis carries an increased cancer risk but also whether silica exposure per se carries this risk regardless of the mechanism.

II. EVIDENCE REVIEWED IN 1986

It may be useful to examine critically the results of published surveys considered by the IARC working group in 1986, or at least those with greatest weight. These included, first, cohort and case-referent studies on the effects of occupational exposure to crystalline silica in various industries and, then, studies with silicosis as the risk factor. We shall adopt the same sequence.

A. SILICA EXPOSURE

1. Mining and Quarrying

Large cohort mortality studies have been made in several major mining industries — gold mining in Australia,[5] Canada,[6] South Africa,[7] and the U.S.,[8–10] and other metal mining in Canada[6] and the U.S.[11,12] One of the latter, by Lawler et al.,[11] was a well-conducted survey of 10,403 Minnesota hematite miners, but, although the ore body was said to have an average content of 8%, there lacked objective evidence of exposure to significant levels of respirable silica. The number of deaths from all causes (4699) was less than expected in underground miners (standard mortality ratio [SMR] 90) and overground miners (SMR 98). Essentially the same applied to most specific causes, except accidents and suicide, including cancers and respiratory disease. Deaths from pneumoconiosis were not mentioned, and SMR for respiratory cancer were 94 and 100, respectively. Whereas native born miners had an even more favorable mortality than the total cohort, the reverse was true of the foreign born. Men from Finland and especially from Yugoslavia had raised SMR from lung cancer, whether compared to U.S. rates (108 and 208) or St. Louis County rates (113 and 211). Finnish born, but not Yugoslav, also had increased SMR from nonmalignant respiratory disease. This pattern of nonmalignant respiratory disease mortality suggests that silica exposure was probably low. While this survey makes little contribution one way or the other to the silica cancer question, the substantial variation in lung cancer mortality by country of birth underlines the potentially important confounding effect of social factors apparently unrelated to occupation.

The other study of American metal miners reported by Costello[12] is also difficult to interpret. The cohort comprised 12,258 white nonuranium miners from 50 mines in 16 states. The men had voluntarily participated in a national silicosis survey in 1958–61 and were followed through 1975 with only 23 losses. Comparisons made state by state against average mortality for the three years, 1968–70, gave an SMR for lung cancer of 127 (163 cases observed). The excess was statistically significant in miners of lead, zinc, mercury, and chrome but not gold, silver, copper, iron, or molybdenum. There was no apparent correlation between the SMR for lung cancer and pneumoconiosis mortality or radiographic evidence of silicosis. Various important aspects of methodology were not adequately described, and results from a cohort of currently employed volunteers, analyzed against reference mortality rates for only three years, are inevitably inconclusive.

Arising out of the same national silicosis survey in the U.S., 1958–61, was a mortality study by Gillam et al.[8] of a cohort of 440 men employed underground for five years or more in a South Dakota gold mine where silicosis was known to have been a serious problem. Both this and a larger study by McDonald et al.[9] of 1321 men with at least 21 years of employment in this mine were undertaken, not because of the silica, but to assess the effect of exposure to the host rock, cummingtonite-grunerite, which, in fibrous habit, is amosite asbestos. In the former study, 10 deaths from lung cancer were observed against 2.7 expected, but only 7 against 2.2 for those with more than 19 years from first employment. In the latter study[9] there was no overall excess (17 observed, 16.5 expected), although in the period before 1955 there were 6 deaths observed against 3.4 expected. Whereas, remarkably, Gillam et al.[8] found no excess mortality from nonmalignant respiratory disease, the larger cohort of McDonald et al.[9] experienced substantial excess overall mortality (SMR 1.15), entirely explained by silica-related diseases — pneumoconiosis, tuberculosis, silico-tuberculosis, and heart disease — shown to be linearly related to estimated silica concentrations.[13] Other causes of death, including malignant neoplasms (93 observed, 90.5 expected) were close to expectation. The substantial number of silica-related deaths (about 100) implies that some degree of nonfatal silicosis must have been widely prevalent in the cohort and that any resulting lung cancer could hardly have been obscured by competing risks. The weaknesses of the study are mainly associated with any possible selection bias due to 21 years of continuous employment with the company. So far as malignancies are concerned this seems quite unlikely, unless perhaps related to smoking habit. The exposure estimates were approximate but internally validated by exposure response.

A further study of the same workforce was later reported by Brown et al.[10] Their cohort comprised all 3328 white males employed full time underground for one year or more, 1940 through 1964, excluding 64 men known to have worked in uranium mines. Information on exposure was based on various surveys in the mine reported in 1960, 1973, 1974, and 1981. These studies established that exposure to radon daughters and arsenic had been measurable but on average within the occupational standards at that time. Airborne samples collected in 1981 indicated that 69% of "fibers" were of cummingtonite-grunerite, 15% tremolite-actinolite, and 16% hornblende. Weighted average exposures to fibers ≥5 μm in length ranged from less than 0.44/cm^3 for underground work to 1.16/cm^3 for some surface workers. Before the 1950s, the free silica content of respirable dust was estimated at 13.1%. At that time total dust levels were above the threshold limit value (TLV) for silica but were reduced to well below that level thereafter. The cohort as a whole suffered excess mortality from all causes (SMR 112), explained almost entirely by respiratory tuberculosis (SMR 364), other respiratory disease (SMR 279), and accidents (SMR 300). There were 43 deaths from lung cancer compared with 42.9 expected, and more detailed analyses gave little indication of risk in specific subcategories, although a nonsignificant excess was noted after 30 years from first employment — 29 deaths compared with 22.5 expected. In contrast, the substantial excess mortality from nonmalignant respiratory diseases was related fairly systematically to duration of underground employment and to exposure measured in dust days, with some differences in pattern exhibited by tuberculosis. This study thus provided close and independent confirmation for the findings of McDonald et al.[9] despite the possible confounding effect of arsenic and radon daughters.

A study of 1974 gold miners and 213 coal miners in Western Australia by Armstrong et al.[5] was based on records of men in a health survey of current employees conducted in 1961–62. The way in which these men were selected was not described, and the records of a further 318 could not be found. At the time of the original survey, men ranged in age from 24 to 79 years, almost all had 10 years or more mining experience, mostly underground, and about two thirds were cigarette smokers. By the end of 1975, 500 of the gold mining cohort were dead, 59 from respiratory cancer (SMR 140) and 15 from pneumoconiosis or tuberculosis (SMR 455). Mortality from respiratory cancer was about 40% higher in those who had worked underground but was not related to the number of years they had done so. Overall, the respiratory cancer mortality was 13% higher in men with radiographic evidence of silicosis than in those without.

Mortality in the large population of metal miners in Ontario has been under investigation over many years. Analysis of 6757 deaths, 1955–77, among 50,201 men was reported in 1983 by Muller et al.[6] As compared with provincial rates, significant excess mortality from silicosis, silico-tuberculosis, and cancer of the respiratory tract was observed in miners of gold, uranium, and mixed ore but not nickel, copper, or iron. The authors concluded that in nonuranium miners, the difference between observed and expected deaths from malignant and nonmalignant respiratory disease was entirely attributable to gold mining. Although these differences were substantial, no information was then available on exposure levels in the gold mines to silica, radon, or arsenic, so the cause of the lung cancer remained in doubt. This study will be discussed further in section B in the light of further data.

A cohort of 3971 white South African gold miners studied by Wyndham et al.[7] gave an SMR for lung cancer of 1.61, but more detailed analysis led the authors to conclude that smoking and neither radon nor silica were responsible for the increase. Further evidence on silica exposure in gold mining was later obtained from a case-control study by Hessel et al.[14] Records of the gold miners' pension fund, 1979–83, showed 133 deaths from primary lung cancer, each of the 133 with two deaths from other causes matched for age and smoking habit. Cause of death was reliably determined, with autopsy rates of just more than 86% in both sexes. Comparison of cases and controls for cumulative silica exposure, average intensity, and shifts at high dust levels showed very close similarity. The average cigarette consumption per day was only slightly lower in the case series. This study, although of relatively small size and therefore of limited power, made full allowance for smoking habit and found no link between lung cancer and silica dust exposure. Association with pathological and radiographic signs of pulmonary fibrosis, which were rather less negative, will be discussed in section B with other evidence on silicosis.

2. Granite and Stone Industry

Of six reports considered by the IARC working group on occupational exposure in this industry, none could be considered wholly satisfactory — two because of probable exposure to radon or asbestos and one where choice of controls was questionable. The remaining three were studies of cohorts, certainly exposed to substantial concentrations of silica, but in two[15,16] the analyses were confined to proportionate mortality, and in one[17] the followup was probably incomplete. Two of the cohorts were based on employees in the large Vermont granite industry, voluntarily enrolled in a medical surveillance scheme and therefore liable to selection bias. The first of these studies, reported in 1983 by Davis et al.,[15] found a proportional ratio for lung cancer of 1.2. Ratios calculated against Vermont mortality rates after exclusion of silicosis and tuberculosis appeared to be unrelated to dust exposure. A later study reported in 1986 by Costello and Graham[16] gave suggestive evidence of excess mortality from both silicosis and lung cancer in men first employed before but not after 1940, a pattern compatible with the application at that time of dust control.

Although not strictly a cohort study, an analysis was made by Steenland and Beaumont[17] of 2274 deaths recorded in the U.S. Granite Cutters Union, 1949 through 1982. The certified cause was obtained for 1911 (84%) deaths, and, after recoding by a nosologist, the percentage distribution by cause was compared with that expected from national rates. As some 36% of deaths had occurred in Vermont, these would probably have been included in the two previously mentioned studies of American granite workers, and, overall, the results from all three studies were similar. That of Steenland and Beaumont[17] confirmed the large excess mortality from silicosis and silico-tuberculosis, but gave only slight nonsignificant excess from lung cancer (97 observed, 81.1 expected, proportional mortality ratio [PMR] = 1.19). The lung cancer mortality was unrelated to duration of employment, but there was evidence from a case-control analysis of an association between lung cancer and silicosis recorded on death certificates. No account was taken of cigarette consumption.

3. Ceramics and Glass

Evidence from this industry was mainly derived from a study of proportional mortality in the U.S. Potters and Allied Workers Union, reported in 1982 by Thomas,[18] and a case-referent study by Forastiere et al.[19] in Italian pottery workers, published in 1986. Tuberculosis as a cause of death in Union members was grossly excessive (62 observed, 18.3 expected) but less so for nonmalignant respiratory disease (268 observed, 173.7 expected). There was some excess of lung cancer (178 observed, 146.6 expected, PMR = 1.21), almost entirely explained by work in the sanitary ware divisions (62 observed, 34.4 expected) where exposure was also to talc. The case-referent study[19] was conducted among the male residents of a small town in central Italy where pottery was the predominant industry and sanitary ware and crockery the main product. Silica exposure was known to be heavy, but talc and chromates were also used. The case series comprised 84 subjects certified to have died from carcinoma of the lung in the period 1968–84. A total of 334 referents, four for each case, were selected from the same source from persons who died from other causes, matched for age and year of death; 35 subjects whose underlying cause of death was pneumoconiosis or chronic bronchitis were replaced by an equal number of subjects with other diagnoses. The latter exclusion was justified on the grounds that the two diseases in question might also have been caused by silica exposure and thus have biased the comparison. A detailed work history and record of smoking habits were sought for each subject by three nurses blind to the study hypothesis and causes of death. In addition, names of cases and referents were checked against the official register of persons with a disability pension for silicosis, with dates and degree of disability, etc., up to December 31, 1984. All compensated silicotics had been ceramic workers. The ratio of cases to referents was the basis of the analysis which considered exposure in terms of (a) quarry work and (b) ceramic work, for cases with and without silicosis. The crude rate ratio for ceramic work was 1.8 (1.3 without silicosis and 3.4 with silicosis). Standardized for the age, smoking, and period of death, these ratios became 2.0 (95% CI = 1.1–3.5), 1.4 (95% CI = 0.7–2.8), and 3.9 (95% CI = 1.8–8.3). The corrected ratio for quarry work was 1.0. A feature of this otherwise well-designed study was the subject of some controversy, namely the exclusion from the referent series of 35 deaths from pneumoconiosis or chronic bronchitis.[20] Had these cases not been removed,[21] the standardized rate ratio for ceramic work would have been reduced to 1.5 (95% CI = 0.9–2.6), and only that for silicosis would have remained significant (2.1, 95% CI = 1.0–4.4).

4. Foundries

The probability of exposure to polycyclic hydrocarbons and asbestos makes the interpretation of studies of foundry workers particularly difficult. As stated by Fletcher,[22] "Foundries are not a good choice of industry for identifying any single carcinogenic substance." There have been many cohort and proportionate mortality studies in iron and steel foundry workers in North America and Europe during the last 20 years, only some of which were reviewed by the IARC working group in 1986. Virtually all these studies found evidence of an increased risk of lung cancer, often of gastric cancer and usually of nonmalignant respiratory disease, in a wide range of foundry occupations. There seems little doubt that during the second half of this century levels of respirable silica in foundries have fallen, while occupational risks from lung cancer have risen; this suggests that silica has not been the most important etiological factor.[22] A summary of the main studies reviewed in this section is given in Table 1.

B. SILICOSIS

Studies of the association between silicosis and lung cancer, whether conducted in cohort or case-referent mode, provide evidence at two levels. Most reliable are studies in which the cases of silicosis were ascertained by some objective screening procedure; much less reliable were studies in which the identification of cases was subject to self-selection or to potentially biased judgment. In the latter category are all studies based on compensated silicotics. There are many reasons why a person may or may not be compensated for an occupational disease, and case series derived from compensation registers can seldom, if ever, be considered representative of all cases to have occurred as a result of a given exposure. Of 13 epidemiological surveys of silicotics reviewed by the IARC Working Group in 1986, only two[14,19] were relatively free from this type of ascertainment bias. A third study in Japan was based on patients admitted to a specialist hospital for silicosis,[23] and the methods by which they were selected and graded for severity were unclear. The findings from all 13 reports are summarized in Table 2 where it can be seen that, with the exception of one of the two more satisfactory studies mentioned, the risk estimates for lung cancer were generally substantial.

TABLE 1
Studies Published Before 1987 on Silica Exposure and Lung Cancer

Reference	Authors	Country	Study design	Industry	Lung cancer risk	Comments
5	Armstrong et al., 1979	Australia	Cohort	Gold mining	SMR 140	Unrelated to duration of exposure
6	Muller et al., 1983	Canada	Cohort	Metal mining	SMR 145	Excess in gold, uranium, and mixed ore; not in nickel, copper, or iron
7	Wyndham et al., 1986	RSA	Cohort	Gold mining	SMR 161	In case-referent analysis smoking identified as main factor
9	McDonald et al., 1978	U.S.	Cohort	Gold mining	SMR 103	Same mine; substantial mortality from silica-related diseases
10	Brown et al., 1986	U.S.	Cohort	Gold mining	SMR 100	
11	Lawler et al., 1983	U.S.	Cohort	Iron mining	SMR 90	Silica exposure probably low
12	Costello, 1982	U.S.	Cohort	Metal mining	SMR 127	Several methodological questions
14	Hessel et al., 1986	RSA	Case-referent	Gold mining	No increase	Limited power
15	Davis et al., 1983	U.S.	Proportional mortality	Granite	PMR 120	Cohort of volunteers
16	Costello and Graham, 1986	U.S.	Proportional mortality	Granite	SMR 105	SMR all causes 80; proportion traced not stated
17	Steenland and Beaumont, 1986	U.S.	Proportional mortality	Granite	PMR 119	Unrelated to duration of employment
18	Thomas, 1982	U.S.	Proportional mortality	Potteries	PMR 121	Excess almost all in sanitary ware
19	Forastiere et al., 1986	Italy	Case-referent	Ceramics	RR 2.0	With silicosis 3.9; without silicosis 1.4

TABLE 2
Studies of the Association Between Silicosis and Lung Cancer Published Before 1987

Reference	Authors	Country	Silicosis ascertainment	Lung cancer risk[a]
		Cohort surveys		
24	Westerholm, 1980	Sweden	Pneumoconiosis register	SMR 2.2–5.9
25	Finkelstein et al., 1982	Canada	Compensated cases	SMR 2.0–7.4
26	Gudbergsson et al., 1984	Finland	National registers	SMR 3.0
23	Chiyotani, 1984	Japan	Pneumoconiosis hospital	SMR 2.7–6.6
27	Zambon et al., 1985	Italy	Compensated cases	SMR 2.5
28	Westerholm et al., 1986	Sweden	Silicosis register	SMR 1.8–4.1
29	Finkelstein et al., 1986	Canada	Compensated cases	SMR 1.8–3.6
30	Kurppa et al., 1986	Finland	Compensated cases	SMR 1.8–4.4
31	Zambon et al., 1986	Italy	Compensated cases	SMR 2.3
		Proportionate mortality analyses		
32	Rubino et al., 1985	Italy	Compensated cases	PMR 1.4
33	Neuberger et al., 1986	Austria	Compensated cases	PMR 1.3–1.4
		Case-referent studies		
14	Hessel et al., 1986	RSA	Death certificates	RR 1.0–1.1
19, 21	Forastiere et al., 1986, 1987	Italy	Death certificates	RR 2.1–3.9

[a] Range of values shown for specific subgroups.

III. EARLIER EVIDENCE

It is somewhat remarkable that until 1982 when Goldsmith et al.[34] first brought the question into prominence, a link between silica exposure and lung cancer was generally considered improbable. Even in 1986, experimental evidence on the carcinogenic activity of crystalline silica, although considered *sufficient* by the working group,[2] was both recent and scanty. Experimental scientists working on mineral dusts had perhaps come to believe that particle length and diameter were the important determinants of carcinogenicity. Bearing in mind the uncertain evidence even today on the risk of lung cancer in silica-exposed cohorts, compared with the more pressing problems of silicosis and silico-tuberculosis, it is understandable that, in the past, few epidemiologists pursued the question. Surveys based on compensation registries or similarly selected case series have not enjoyed a high reputation scientifically or been readily funded. Even with asbestos, where the relationship of lung cancer to pulmonary fibrosis is also unsettled, studies have been few. A comprehensive review of published data on the silica question made by Heppleston[35] in 1984 concluded that the weight of evidence then available was against the carcinogenic hypothesis. His views were based mainly on the experience of South African gold miners, coal miners in several countries, and on iron ore miners in Britain, France, and Sweden. Also cited were data on large necropsy series from various silica-exposed occupations which showed no association between the presence or severity of silicotic lesions and bronchial carcinoma. The quality of some of these studies, mainly undertaken during the 1950s and 1960s, is open to question, but the findings seemed consistent and without obvious bias. Serial analyses based on more than 10,000 autopsies in white South African gold miners from about 1920 to 1960 showed no evidence that lung cancer was more frequent in miners than in nonminers or in those with silicosis than those without silicosis. Age was taken into account in these analyses, which covered a period when primary lung cancer increased in prevalence from about 1% to more than 7%, presumably as a result of cigarette smoking. Equally consistent and over much the same period were many reports of lower mortality from lung cancer in coal miners, with or without pneumoconiosis, than in the general population. Much the same pattern of mortality was noted in collieries from various parts of the U.K., from Germany, and, with some exceptions, from the U.S. However, the quartz content of respirable dust to which these miners were exposed averaged only about

3% to 6%. In iron ore miners, smelter employees, and foundry workers, a considerable variation in lung cancer risk was thought by Heppleston[35] to better reflect the varying distribution of arsenic, radon, and polycyclic hydrocarbons than of the silica to which they were all exposed.

IV. EVIDENCE SINCE 1986

Relevant publications after the Lyon meeting in 1986 can again be considered in two categories: those primarily aimed at the effects of exposure to crystalline silica and those aimed at the association between lung cancer and silicosis. The main findings reported, all but two based on longitudinal studies, are summarized chronologically in Tables 3 and 4.

The paper by Kusiak et al.[36] extended the earlier reported studies of Ontario gold miners[6] which, it will be recalled, identified excess mortality from lung cancer, but left open the cause of the increase. Further data and analyses led to the conclusion, mainly because of dose-response relationships, that exposures to arsenic and radon decay products were probably to blame, rather than asbestiform mineral fiber or crystalline silica. The report by Koskela et al.[37] was the most recent in a series by these authors on the health of 1026 employees of granite quarries and yards in three regions of Finland where, by the end of 1985, 296 had died. Of 40 deaths from respiratory disease (SMR 255), 13 were from silicosis; of 31 deaths from lung cancer (SMR 156), the excess was entirely in men ≥20 years from entry (SMR 225). On the other hand, gastrointestinal cancers were also in excess (18 deaths; SMR 156) and there was a large and unexplained deficiency of deaths attributed to tumors at other sites (10 observed, 22.9 expected).

A deficiency of this kind was also present in two other studies with some evidence of excess lung cancer, both in pottery workers.[39,40] In the first of these from the U.S., the SMR for nonmalignant respiratory disease was raised (64 observed, SMR 1.73), as was that for lung cancer (52 observed, SMR 1.43), but at other anatomic sites there were 72 deaths from malignant neoplasms against 85.7 expected. In the second study, from the U.K., there were 39 deaths from respiratory disease against 38.5 expected from locally adjusted rates; 60 deaths from lung cancer (SMR 1.32), a small excess of gastrointestinal cancer (30 observed, SMR 1.14), and some deficiency at all other sites (28 observed, 35.8 expected). Five of the other studies listed in Table 3 were essentially negative,[36,38,43,45,46] but two were clearly positive[42,47] and others suggestively so.[37,39,40,41,44] Of the negative studies, that by Carta et al.[45] in two cohorts of Sardinian metal miners was the most convincing. In one mine where exposure to quartz was high, but low to radon, there was no lung cancer excess, whereas in the other mine with the exposure pattern reversed the SMR was raised, although not significantly so. However, in neither cohort were the numbers at risk very large. Two of the three positive studies were difficult to interpret. A small excess of lung cancer (SMR 1.28) among metal miners in the U.S. largely concentrated among those with silicosis was reported by Amandus and Costello,[43] but no data were given on other causes of death. A statistically significant relationship between death from lung cancer and silica dust particle-years standardized for smoking, year of birth, and age was found in a study of South African gold miners by Hnizdo and Sluis-Cremer.[42] At face value this is strong evidence, but there are several reasons for regarding this with some caution. First, it is not clear that overall there was any excess risk of lung cancer in this cohort, although an SMR of 1.61 had been previously reported for an earlier period.[7] Second, no link was found between dust exposure and parenchymal silicosis, which is hard to explain if silica was the cause of the lung cancer excess. Third, two carefully controlled case-control studies in the same working population[14,36] had shown no increase in risk; the writers speculated that this might have resulted from overmatching. Finally, the possible contribution of radon exposure had yet to be assessed. No similar reservations can be expressed about the third positive study, very recently reported by Checkoway et al.[47] Their cohort comprised 2570 white males employed for one year or more in the mining and processing of diatomaceous earth in California, including at least one day during the period 1942–87. The type of crystalline silica to which these men were exposed was predominantly cristobalite; 104 employees with past evidence of asbestos exposure were excluded from the analysis. In a followup to the end of 1987, 628 deaths were observed from all causes (SMR 1.12), 59 from lung cancer (SMR 1.43) and 77 from nonmalignant respiratory disease (NMRD) (SMR 2.27); cancer deaths at other sites were close to the expectation at 73 (SMR 0.92). Radiographic surveys conducted by the U.S. Public Health Service in 1957 had shown that a very high prevalence of pneumoconiosis in this industry had been reduced to a very low level by 1984. A rather complex index of cumulative exposure was calculated from measures of duration, nonquantitative estimates of intensity, and opinions as to the effectiveness of respirator use. Clear and parallel trends in

TABLE 3
Studies Published Since 1986 on Silica Exposure and Lung Cancer

Reference	Authors	Country	Study design	Industry	Lung cancer risk	Comments
36	Kusiak et al., 1991	Canada	Cohort	Gold mining	SMR 1.29	Attributed to arsenic and radon exposure
37	Koskela et al., 1990	Finland	Cohort	Granite quarries	SMR 1.56	Substantial deficiency of cancer at other sites
38	Mehnert et al., 1990	GDR	Cohort	Slate quarry	SMR 1.09	Silicotics 2.03, ns; nonsilicotics 1.04, ns
39	Thomas, 1990	U.S.	Cohort	Potteries	SMR 1.43	Deficiency of cancer at other sites
40	Winter et al., 1990	U.K.	Cohort	Potteries	SMR 1.32	SMR = 1.32 against local rates; some deficiency of cancer at other sites
41	Hessel et al., 1990	RSA	Case-referent	Gold mining	RR 1.1	No association with either silicosis at necropsy or cumulative silica exposure
42	Hnizdo and Sluis-Cremer, 1991	RSA	Cohort	Gold mining	RR 1.02	Per 1000 particle years
43	Amandus and Costello, 1991	U.S.	Cohort	Metal mining	SMR 1.23	Silicotics 1.73; nonsilicotics 1.18; other causes of death not reported
44	Siemiatycki et al., 1990	Canada	Case-referent	Any	RR 1.07	Substantial exposure, RR 1.38
45	Carta et al., 1992	Italy	Cohort	Metal mining	SMR 1.12	ns; risk higher in those with lower silica, but higher radon exposures
46	Benn et al., 1992	U.K.	Cohort	Silica sand	SMR 1.20	ns; silica exposure levels around 0.1 mg/m^3
47	Checkoway et al., 1993	U.S.	Cohort	Diatomaceous earth	SMR 1.43	RR increased steadily with exposure to silica (mainly cristobalite)

TABLE 4
Studies Published Since 1986 on the Association Between Silicosis and Lung Cancer

Reference	Authors	Country	Silicosis ascertainment	Industry	Lung cancer risk	Comments
48	Finkelstein et al., 1987	Canada	Compensated cases	Metal mining	SMR 2.42	Excess in all occupational groups
49	Tornling et al., 1990	Sweden	Compensated cases	Ceramics	SMR 1.88	Obs 9; Exp 4.8; ns
50	Merlo et al., 1990	Italy	Hospitalized cases	Various	SMR 6.85	SMR all other cancers = 2.73
51	Carta et al., 1991	Italy	Hospitalized cases	Mines and quarries	SMR 1.29	ns; no relation to radiographic severity
52	Chiyotani et al., 1990	Japan	Hospitalized cases	Various	SMR 6.03	Compensated cases in hospital
53	Infante-Rivard et al., 1989	Canada	Compensated cases	Various	SMR 3.47	Excess in all types of industry
54	Amandus et al., 1991	U.S.	Routine medical examination	Dusty trades	SMR 2.56	SMR = 2.29 — silica exposure only
55	Amandus et al., 1992	U.S.	Routine medical examination	Dusty trades	SMR 2.11	Reevaluation of previous study[54]

relative risk against this index were found for lung cancer and NMRD. These findings provide strong support for the conclusion that cristobalite exposure was causally related to the lung cancer excess, but rather less convincing evidence for the gradients in exposure-response, which could conceivably have resulted from artefactual errors in exposure estimation. It seems unlikely, however, that either cigarette smoking, asbestos, or other work-related exposures were important confounders in this study. It is also clear that even after allowance for excess deaths attributed to lung cancer (17.6) and NMRD (43) there was no deficiency in deaths from all other causes (567, SMR 1.01).

The seven more recent studies (listed in Table 4) of lung cancer in compensated or hospitalized cases of silicosis were in general as strongly positive as those reported earlier (Table 1), but remain subject to the same kinds of bias outlined previously. The study by Amandus et al.[54,55] may be less vulnerable than others in that their cases of silicosis were ascertained radiographically among silica-exposed workers routinely examined by the Industrial Commission for North Carolina. The authors set out four criteria which should be met if studies of silicotics are to make a useful contribution to knowledge, including the definition of cases on radiographic evidence. However, the Industrial Commission for North Carolina also had a questionnaire available, which included work history, medical symptoms, and smoking habits. It is to be hoped that this additional information was not used in making a diagnosis, but this was not explicitly stated. The effects of selection bias inherent in studies of compensated silicotics were discussed in the paper by Infante-Rivard et al.,[53] in particular the increased cancer risk if compensation were associated with cigarette smoking. It was suggested that allowance could be made for such differences by use of the known size of risk of lung cancer due to smoking. However, the problem is not simply a matter of smoking level, but that men whose smoking has led to respiratory symptoms may be more likely to seek or be granted compensation. Other mechanisms which might possibly link lung cancer, silicosis, and smoking have been reviewed by Swaen and Meijers,[56] who presented evidence that heavy smoking increased considerably the risk of silicosis in Dutch ceramic workers. On the other hand, this association did not appear sufficient to cause a lung cancer excess of the magnitude recorded in Tables 2 and 4.

V. CONCLUSION

As explained at the outset, the fundamental question concerns the ability of exposure to crystalline silica to induce lung cancer in man and not whether silicosis, compensated or not, increases the risk of the disease. In fact, virtually all the evidence which appears to incriminate silicosis as a risk factor could as well be explained by various types of selection bias as by cause and effect. A small number of studies are less easily dismissed, but whereas two of these showed evidence of an association,[19,54] two did not.[14,36] There remains the question of whether silicosis should be considered a marker of silica exposure or an indicator, directly or indirectly, of impaired capacity to deal with inhaled dust.

On the basic issue of silica exposure and lung cancer, some 25 reports, summarized in Tables 1 and 3, appear relevant, but in few of these were the findings entirely clear. Of those which provide the strongest evidence, six were positive[19,39–41,43,47] and six were negative,[8,9,14,36,45,46] but the latter were based on only four population groups, so the balance of evidence may perhaps support a causal association. It is sometimes stated that SMR of about 1.2 to 1.5 do not represent a high level of risk, but it must be remembered that these estimates are for whole cohorts, most members of which had probably short or light exposure. The two positive studies with information on exposure-response, both in mining populations,[42,47] point to a range of dust-related risk quite similar to that for miners and millers of chrysotile asbestos.

What overall conclusion can be drawn from the considerable amount of conflicting information now available? It no longer seems reasonable to dismiss all the positive results as attributable to chance, bias, or confounding, but it is equally clear that other studies were quite negative. The explanation could well be that, in some circumstances, exposure to airborne silica is carcinogenic, but not in others. Experience with asbestos has shown the importance of fiber type, particle size, and durability and of co-carcinogens. Epidemiologists have hardly begun to explore the analogous aspects of crystalline silica, which also varies mineralogically. Until we have a consensus or understandable pattern of results from a larger number of well-conducted surveys, with adequate characterization of exposure and other relevant factors, room for substantial doubt will remain.

REFERENCES

1. **Parkes, W. R.,** *Occupational Lung Disorders,* 2nd ed., Butterworths, London, 1982, 157.
2. International Agency for Research on Cancer, Monographs on the evaluation of the carcinogenic risk of chemicals to humans, in *Silica and Some Silicates,* IARC, Lyon, Vol. 42, 1987.
3. IARC Working Group on the Evaluation of Carcinogenic Risks to Humans, Overall evaluations of carcinogenicity: an updating of IARC monographs, Supplement 7, World Health Organization, Lyon, Vol. 1–42, 1987.
4. **Axelson, O.,** Aspects of confounding in occupational health epidemiology, *Scand. J. Work Environ. Health,* 4, 85, 1978.
5. **Armstrong, B. K., McNulty, J. C., Levitt, L. J., Williams, K. A., and Hobbs, M. S. T.,** Mortality in gold and coal miners in Western Australia with special reference to lung cancer, *Br. J. Ind. Med.,* 36, 199, 1979.
6. **Muller, J., Wheeler, W. C., Gentleman, J. F., Suranyi, G., and Kusiak, R. A.,** Study of Mortality of Ontario Miners, 1955–1977, Part 1, Toronto: Ministry of Labour/Ontario Workers' Compensation Board/Atomic Energy Control Board of Canada, 1983.
7. **Wyndham, C. H., Benzuidenhout, B. N., Greenacre, M. J., and Sluis-Cremer, G. K.,** Mortality of middle-aged white South African gold miners, *Br. J. Ind. Med.,* 43, 677, 1986.
8. **Gillam, J. D., Dement, J. M., Lemen, R. A., Wagoner, J. K., Archer, V. E., and Blejer, H. P.,** Mortality patterns among hard rock gold miners exposed to an asbestiform mineral, *Ann. N.Y. Acad. Sci.,* 271, 336, 1976.
9. **McDonald, J. C., Gibbs, G. W., Liddell, F. D. K., and McDonald, A. D.,** Mortality after long exposure to cummingtonite-grunerite, *Am. Rev. Respir. Dis.,* 118, 271, 1978.
10. **Brown, D. P., Kalplan, S. D., Zumwalde, R. D., Kaplowitz, M., and Archer, V. E.,** Retrospective cohort mortality study of underground gold mine workers, in *Silica, Silicosis, and Cancer. Controversy in Occupational Medicine,* Goldsmith, D. F., Winn, D. M., and Shy, C. M., Eds., Praeger, New York, 1986, 335.
11. **Lawler, A. B., Mandel, J. S., Schuman, L. M., and Lubin, J. H.,** Mortality study of Minnesota iron ore miners: preliminary results, in *Health Issues Related to Metal and Non-metallic Mining,* Wagner, W. L., Rom, W. N., and Merchant, J. A., Eds., Butterworths, Boston, 1983, 211.
12. **Costello, J.,** Mortality of metal miners. A retrospective cohort and case-control study, in *Proceedings of an Environmental Health Conference, Park City, UT, 6–9 April 1982,* National Institute for Occupational Safety and Health, Morgantown, WV, 1982.
13. **McDonald, J. C. and Oakes, D.,** Exposure-response in miners exposed to silica, in *VIth International Pneumoconiosis Conference, Bochum, 1983,* International Labour Office, Geneva, Vol. 1, 1984, 114.
14. **Hessel, P. A., Sluis-Cremer, G. K., and Hnizdo, E.,** Case-control study of silicosis, silica exposure and lung cancer in white South African gold miners, *Am. J. Ind. Med.,* 10, 57, 1986.
15. **Davis, L. K., Wegman, D. H., Monson, R. R., and Froines, J.,** Mortality experience of Vermont granite miners, *Am. J. Ind. Med.,* 4, 705, 1983.
16. **Costello, J. and Graham, W. G. B.,** Vermont granite workers' mortality study, in *Silica, Silicosis and Cancer. Controversy in Occupational Medicine,* Goldsmith, D. F., Winn, D. M., and Shy, C. M., Eds., Praeger, New York, 1986, 437.
17. **Steenland, K. and Beaumont, J.,** A proportionate mortality study of granite cutters, *Am. J. Ind. Med.,* 9, 189, 1986.
18. **Thomas, T. L.,** A preliminary investigation of mortality among workers in the pottery industry, *Int. J. Epidemiol.,* 11, 175, 1982.
19. **Forastiere, F., Lagorio, S., Michelozzi, P. et al.,** Silica, silicosis and lung cancer among ceramic workers: a case-referent study, *Am. J. Ind. Med.,* 10, 363, 1986.
20. **Hessel, P. A. and Sluis-Cremer, G. K.,** Letter to Editor, *Am. J. Ind. Med.,* 12, 219, 1987.
21. **Forastiere, F., Lagorio, S., Michelozzi, P. et al.,** Letter to Editor, *Am. J. Ind. Med.,* 12, 221, 1987.
22. **Fletcher, A. C.,** The mortality of foundry workers in the United Kingdom, in *Silica, Silicosis and Cancer. Controversy in Occupational Medicine,* Goldsmith, D. F., Winn, D. M., and Shy, C. M., Eds., Praeger, New York, 1986, 385.
23. **Chiyotani, K.,** Excess risk of lung cancer deaths in hospitalized pneumoconiotic patients, in *Proceedings of the VIth International Conference on Pneumoconiosis, Bochum, 1983,* International Labour Office, Geneva, 1984, 228.
24. **Westerholm, P.,** Silicosis. Observations on a case register, *Scand. J. Work Environ. Health,* 6 (Suppl. 2), 1, 1980.
25. **Finkelstein, M., Kusiak, R., and Suranyi, G.,** Mortality among miners receiving workmen's compensation for silicosis in Ontario: 1940–1975, *J. Occup. Med.,* 24, 663, 1982.
26. **Gudbergsson, H., Kurppa, K., Koskinen, H., and Vasama, M.,** An association between silicosis and lung cancer. A register approach, in *Proceedings of the VIth International Conference on Pneumoconiosis, Bochum, 1983,* International Labour Office, Geneva, 1984, 212.
27. **Zambon, P., Simonato, L., Mastrangelo, G., Winkelmann, R., Rizzi, P., Comiati, D., Saia, B., and Crepet, M.,** Epidemiological cohort study on the silicosis-pulmonary cancer association in the Veneto region (Ital.), in *Silice, Silicosi e Cancro (Silica, Silicosis and Cancer),* Deutsch, E. I. and Marcato, A., Eds., University of Padua, Padua, 1985, 103.

28. **Westerholm, P., Ahlmark, A., Maasing, R., and Segelberg, I.,** Silicosis and lung cancer — a cohort study, in *Silica, Silicosis and Cancer. Controversy in Occupational Medicine,* Goldsmith, D. F., Winn, D. M., and Shy, C. M., Eds., Praeger, New York, 1986, 327.
29. **Finkelstein, M. M., Liss, G. M., Krammer, F., and Kusiak, R. A.,** Mortality among surface-industry workers receiving workers' compensation awards for silicosis in Ontario: 1940–1984. A preliminary report, Toronto, Ontario Workers' Compensation Board, 1986.
30. **Kurppa, K., Gudbergsson, H., Hannunkari, I., Koskinen, H., Hernberg, S., Koskela, R. S., and Ahlman, K.,** Lung cancer among silicotics in Finland, in *Silica, Silicosis and Cancer. Controversy in Occupational Medicine,* Goldsmith, D. F., Winn, D. M., and Shy, C. M., Eds., Praeger, New York, 1986, 311.
31. **Zambon, P., Simonato, L., Mastrangelo, G., Winkelmann, R., Saia, B., and Crepet, M.,** A mortality study of workers compensated for silicosis during 1959 to 1963 in the Veneto region of Italy, in *Silica, Silicosis and Cancer. Controversy in Occupational Medicine,* Goldsmith, D. F., Winn, D. M., and Shy, C. M., Eds., Praeger, New York, 1986, 367.
32. **Rubino, G. F., Scansetti, G., Coggiola, M., Pira, E., Piolatto, G., and Coscia, G. C.,** Epidemiologic study of the mortality of a cohort of silicotics in Piedmont (Ital.), in *Silice, Silicosi e Cancro (Silica, Silicosis and Cancer),* Deutsch, E. I. and Marcato, A., Eds., University of Padua, Padua, 1985, 121.
33. **Neuberger, M., Kundi, M., Westphal, G., and Gründorfer, W.,** The Viennese dusty worker study, in *Silica, Silicosis and Cancer. Controversy in Occupational Medicine,* Goldsmith, D. F., Winn, D. M., and Shy, C. M., Eds., Praeger, New York, 1986, 415.
34. **Goldsmith, D. F., Guidotti, T. L., and Johnston, D. R.,** Does occupational exposure to silica cause lung cancer? *Am. J. Ind. Med.,* 3, 423, 1982.
35. **Heppleston, A. G.,** Silica, pneumoconiosis, and carcinoma of the lung, *Am. J. Ind. Med.,* 7, 285, 1985.
36. **Kusiak, R. A., Springer, J., Ritchie, A. C., and Muller, J.,** Carcinoma of the lung in Ontario gold miners, *Br. J. Ind. Med.,* 48, 828, 1991.
37. **Koskela, R. S., Klockars, M., Järvinen, E., Rossi, A., and Kolari, P. J.,** Cancer mortality of granite workers, 1940–1985, in *Occupational Exposure to Silica and Cancer Risk,* Simonato, L., Fletcher, A. C., Saracci, R., and Thomas, T. L., Eds., IARC Scientific Publications, Lyon, No. 97, 1990, 43.
38. **Mehnert, W. H., Staneczek, W., Möhner, M., Konetzke, G., Müller, W., Ahlendorf, W., Beck, B., Winkelmann, R., and Simonato, L.,** A mortality study of a cohort of slate quarry workers in the German Democratic Republic, in *Occupational Exposure to Silica and Cancer Risk,* Simonato, L., Fletcher, A. C., Saracci, R., and Thomas, T. L., Eds., IARC Scientific Publications, Lyon, No. 97, 1990, 55.
39. **Thomas, T. L.,** Lung cancer mortality among pottery workers in the United States, in *Occupational Exposure to Silica and Cancer Risk,* Simonato, L., Fletcher, A. C., Saracci, R., and Thomas, T. L., Eds., IARC Scientific Publications, Lyon, No. 97, 1990, 75.
40. **Winter, P. D., Gardner, M. J., Fletcher, A. C., and Jones, R. D.,** A mortality follow-up study of pottery workers: preliminary findings on lung cancer, in *Occupational Exposure to Silica and Cancer Risk,* Simonato, L., Fletcher, A. C., Saracci, R., and Thomas, T. L., Eds., IARC Scientific Publications, Lyon, No. 97, 1990, 83.
41. **Hessel, P. A., Sluis-Cremer, G. K., and Hnizdo, E.,** Silica exposure, silicosis, and lung cancer: a necropsy study, *Br. J. Ind. Med.,* 47, 4, 1990.
42. **Hnizdo, E. and Sluis-Cremer, G. K.,** Silica exposure, silicosis and lung cancer, *Br. J. Ind. Med.,* 48, 53, 1991.
43. **Amandus, H. and Costello, J.,** Silicosis and lung cancer in United States metal miners, *Arch. Environ. Health,* 46, 82, 1991.
44. **Siemiatycki, J., Gérin, M., Dewar, R., Lakhani, R., Begin, D., and Richardson, L.,** Silica and cancer associations from a multicancer occupational exposure case-referent study, in *Occupational Exposure to Silica and Cancer Risk,* Simonato, L., Fletcher, A. C., Saracci, R., and Thomas, T. L., Eds., IARC Scientific Publications, Lyon, No. 97, 1990, 29.
45. **Carta, P., Cocco, P. L., and Picchiri, G.,** Lung cancer and airways obstruction among metal miners exposed to silica and low levels of radon daughters, Presented at 9th International Symposium on Epidemiology in Occupational Health, Cincinnati, September 1992.
46. **Benn, R. T., Hutchings, S. J., Thomas, P. G., Elliott, R. C., Osman, J., and Jones, R. D.,** Lung cancer in a silica-exposed population, Presented at meeting of British Thoracic Society, London, December 1992.
47. **Checkoway, H., Heyer, N. J., Demers, P. A., and Breslow, N. E.,** Mortality among workers in the diatomaceous earth industry, *Br. J. Ind. Med.,* 50, 586, 1993.
48. **Finkelstein, M., Liss, G. M., Krammer, F., and Kusiak, R. A.,** Mortality among workers receiving compensation awards for silicosis in Ontario 1940–1985, *Br. J. Ind. Med.,* 44, 588, 1987.
49. **Tornling, G., Hogstedt, C., and Westerholm, P.,** Lung cancer incidence among Swedish ceramic workers with silicosis, in *Occupational Exposure to Silica and Cancer Risk,* Simonato, L., Fletcher, A. C., Saracci, R., and Thomas, T. L., Eds., IARC Scientific Publications, Lyon, No. 97, 1990, 113.
50. **Merlo, F., Doria, M., Fontana, L., Ceppi, M., Chesi, E., and Santi, L.,** Mortality from specific causes among silicotic subjects: a historical prospective study, in *Occupational Exposure to Silica and Cancer Risk,* Simonato, L., Fletcher, A. C., Saracci, R., and Thomas, T. L., Eds., IARC Scientific Publications, Lyon, No. 97, 1990, 105.

51. **Carta, P., Cocco, P. L., and Casula, D.,** Mortality from lung cancer among Sardinian patients with silicosis, *Br. J. Ind. Med.*, 48, 122, 1991.
52. **Chiyotani, K., Saito, K., Okubo, T., and Takahashi, K.,** Lung cancer risk among pneumoconiosis patients in Japan, with special reference to silicotics, in *Occupational Exposure to Silica and Cancer Risk*, Simonato, L., Fletcher, A. C., Saracci, R., and Thomas, T. L., Eds., IARC Scientific Publications, Lyon, No. 97, 1990, 95.
53. **Infante-Rivard, C., Armstrong, B., Petitclerc, M., Cloutier, L. G., and Theriault, G.,** Lung cancer mortality and silicosis in Quebec, 1938–85, *Lancet*, 2, 1504, 1989.
54. **Amandus, H. E., Shy, C. M., Wing, S., Blair, A., and Heineman, E. F.,** Silicosis and lung cancer in North Carolina dusty trades workers, *Am. J. Ind. Med.*, 20, 57, 1991.
55. **Amandus, H. E., Castellan, R. M., Shy, C. M., Heineman, E. F., and Blair, A.,** Re-evaluation of silicosis and lung cancer in North Carolina dusty trades workers, *Am. J. Ind. Med.*, 22, 147, 1992.
56. **Swaen, M. H. and Meijers, J. M. M.,** Lung cancer risk among workers with silicosis: potential confounding by smoking habits, *Am. J. Ind. Med.*, 12, 223, 1987.

Section V
Chapter 3

POTENTIAL MECHANISMS OF SILICA-INDUCED CANCER

Zu-Wei Gu and Tong-man Ong

CONTENTS

I. INTRODUCTION

Although the last 20 years have led to considerable advances in cancer research, a complete understanding of the mechanism of action for any given carcinogen, including silica, as a lung cancer inducer is still lacking. Currently, the generally accepted concept is that carcinogenesis is a long-lasting, multistage, multigenic, and multicausal process. As such, both genetic and epigenetic factors are probably important. In other words, cancer is regarded as the end point of a connected series of changes and/or actions. A three-stage theory of initiation, promotion, and progression has been proposed on the basis of experimental induction of mouse skin cancer by the application of a polycyclic aromatic hydrocarbon (PAH).[1] More recently, the multistage nature of carcinogenesis has been demonstrated with various chemical compounds for other tissues such as liver, urinary bladder, thyroid, mammary gland, and lung.[1] Further experiments have shown that initiation is an irreversible process, while promotion is reversible and can be further divided into several substages.[1] It is now believed that initiation is related to DNA damage, or genotoxic effects, but promotion is considered to be an epigenetic process. During the promotion stage, initiated cells expand clonally over surrounding normal cells. Recent studies suggest that the activation of cellular proto-oncogenes or the deactivation of tumor suppressor genes may be responsible for certain cancers, and that the crucial targets for chemical carcinogens inside cells are specific proto-oncogenes.[2] The normal physiological role of some cellular proto-oncogenes is in the control of cell proliferation and cell differentiation. Alteration of their normal function by chemical carcinogens may therefore change the differentiation pathway and lead to tumor formation.[2]

Silica, a group of minerals including many occupationally important dusts, is polymorphic. Various forms of silica, including α- and β-quartz, display diverse physical properties such as particle size, surface properties, and crystallinity. Different varieties also contain different impurities, some of which are thought to reduce the biological activity of "free silica."[3] The differences in physical and chemical properties of silica varieties do influence their pathogenic effects, including carcinogenicity.[4] This makes the carcinogenesis of silica more complex. Moreover, it is believed that the multistage process of carcinogenesis can be influenced by a variety of exogenous and endogenous factors. Human beings are surrounded by chemical, physical, and biological factors which may be mutagenic and/or carcinogenic. Simultaneous or sequential combinations of these factors may modify the reaction of the exposed human body, resulting in a response different from the response that any single factor could induce. It is especially important to note that, in addition to silica dust, workers often are simultaneously exposed to many chemical compounds in their living environment and workplaces; therefore, combination effects in silica carcinogenesis should be considered.

Here, we review the genotoxic and epigenetic activities of silica and the combination effects of known carcinogens with silica dust. To some extent, the reason that our understanding of the mechanisms of chemical carcinogenesis in general, and of silica carcinogenesis in particular, is rather limited is that there is no obvious approach to such mechanistic studies. Therefore, based on recent developments in understanding the role of oncogene activation in chemical carcinogenesis, some possible mechanisms of silica carcinogenesis are discussed.

II. SILICA AS A GENOTOXICANT

The term genotoxicant is a general description, distinguishing chemicals that have an affinity for direct DNA/chromosome interaction from those that do not. Genotoxicants produce alterations or damage in the genetic material at subtoxic exposure levels. Silica has not been studied extensively as a genotoxicant. The genotoxicity data for silica from available literature and some results from our laboratory are summarized below.

A. GENE MUTATION

The Ames Salmonella/microsome assay measures mutation in histidine-requiring auxotrophs of *Salmonella typhimurium*. Mutant strains are used to detect agents which cause base pair substitution or frameshift mutations. One study has shown that silica is not mutagenic in tester strains TA98, TA100, TA1535, TA1537, and TA1538.[5] The rec-assay in *Bacillus subtilis* is also negative.[6] Data are not available for mutagenesis assays using mammalian cells.

B. CLASTOGENICITY

Min-U-Sil, a type of α-quartz, at the concentration of 1 $\mu g/cm^2$ caused no change in the number of binucleated and micronucleated Syrian hamster embryo (SHE) cells, nor was there evidence of a change in the percentage of tetraploid or near-tetraploid cells compared to untreated controls. However, when cells were treated with a dose of Min-U-Sil (20 $\mu g/cm^2$) similar in transforming potency to 1 $\mu g/cm^2$ of chrysotile asbestos, an increase in the incidence of cells with micronuclei was observed.[7] Micronuclei are formed either by acentric chromosomal fragments due to chromosomal breakage or by centric chromosomes lagging behind in mitosis due to spindle damage. Therefore, the increase in the incidence of micronuclei following treatment of cells is an indication of clastogenic and/or aneuploidogenic activity of silica. The number of binucleated cells also increased relative to controls, but not to the same degree as in asbestos-treated cells. The incidence of tetraploid cells was not significantly increased in the Min-U-Sil-treated cells. This contrasts with the effects observed following chrysotile asbestos treatment.

A nonfibrous mineral dust, α-quartz, at the concentration of 2 $\mu g/cm^2$ did not induce chromosomal aberrations, micronucleus formation, or binucleated cells in SHE cells following 48-h exposure.[8] Positive results were found in other experiments.[9] The *in vivo* studies of Vanchugova et al.[10] demonstrated that quartz did not induce micronuclei in mice following one intraperitoneal injection at a dose of 500 mg/kg b.w. Price-Jones et al.[11] found no increase in the number of aneuploidies and polyploidies or in the frequency of sister chromatid exchanges (SCE) in Chinese hamster lung fibroblasts (V79) cells treated with Min-U-Sil at concentrations ranging from 1 to 15 μg/ml.

Recently, Pairon et al.[12] tested samples of Min-U-Sil <5 and tridymite 118 using the SCE assay in human monocytes and lymphocytes. The results showed that the level of SCE was increased after combined cultures of lymphocytes and monocytes were treated with tridymite and Min-U-Sil <5 separately at a concentration of 100 μg/ml. The increase, however, was not observed in purified lymphocytes. There was no increase in the SCE levels with tridymite filtrates. These tests indicate that the induction of SCE in lymphocytes results from an interaction of lymphocytes and monocytes with tridymite particles, not from soluble compounds released in the culture medium by tridymite.

C. DNA DAMAGE AND REPAIR

Silicic acid leached from silica is considered to be responsible for some of the pathological alterations associated with silica toxicity. DNA strand breaks, after exposure of cells to silicic acid, have been detected by the alkaline unwinding assay, which is considered to be a sensitive technique for the quantitation of strand breaks in cellular DNA induced by various chemical and physical agents. This effect is temperature dependent. Relative to room temperature, higher temperatures cause the formation of a larger number of strand breaks, indicating an increased rate of reaction of silicic acid with DNA.[13] Silicic acid has also been shown to cause a disruption of the secondary structure of DNA *in vitro*.[14] Such disruption may be due to single-strand breaks.[13]

D. CELL TRANSFORMATION

Unlike other short-term assays, *in vitro* cell transformation systems have been developed to simulate the *in vivo* process of carcinogenesis. Under normal conditions, the mammalian cells used for *in vitro* transformation assays will grow in a monolayer until they reach confluency. However, due to genetic and/or epigenetic changes induced by carcinogens, some of the cells may lose control and continue to divide. The dividing cells will pile up and form transformed foci. Thus, these systems have been used to detect potential carcinogens regardless of their mechanisms of action, i.e., genotoxic or nongenotoxic.[15]

Using SHE cells, Hesterberg and Barrett[9] have shown that at concentrations comparable to transforming concentrations of chrysotile asbestos (0.25–1 μg/cm^2), Min-U-Sil and another α-quartz sample were neither cytotoxic nor transforming in SHE cells. However, at 10 μg/cm^2, both quartz dusts reproducibly enhanced the colony-forming efficiency of cells, although further increases in concentration resulted in decreases in relative survival. Both types of dust induced a dose-dependent increase in transformation frequency at concentrations greater than 2 and 10 μg/cm^2, respectively. Min-U-Sil was more potent than the other α-quartz at all concentrations tested. The slopes of the dose-response curves for these quartz dusts were 0.7 and 0.5, respectively. Electron microscopic examination of both quartz dusts revealed the presence of only nonfibrous particulates in these samples. However, Oshimura et al.[8] reported that nonfibrous α-quartz induced neither cell transformation nor cytogenetic effects in SHE cells at the concentration of 2 μg/cm^2.

Saffiotti and co-workers[15a] have found that four silica dust samples including Min-U-Sil <5 induced cell transformation in BALB/c-3T3 cells. The response was dose dependent up to 25–50 μg/cm^2 followed by plateau. In our laboratory, Min-U-Sil <5 silica dust particles were examined using the BALB/c-3T3 cell transformation system. Positive results were found for concentrations of 90 μg/cm^2 and higher. The data are presented in Table 1.

E. CONCLUDING REMARKS

Studies of Hesterberg and co-workers[7] have shown that silica can be taken up by mammalian cells and can accumulate in the perinuclear region. These findings, as indicated by the authors, suggest that mineral particulates might indeed gain access to the genetic material of the cell, especially during mitosis when the nuclear membrane disappears. It is not known, however, whether silica per se, chemicals associated with silica, or mediators and free radicals generated directly or indirectly by silica are responsible for the genotoxicity described in the previous sections.

It should be noted that some of the results in genotoxicity studies are conflicting. It is not known whether the nongenotoxic response in some reports is due to the low concentration of silica, the different

TABLE 1
Induction of Cell Transformation in BALB/c-3T3 Cells Treated with Min-U-Sil <5 for 72 h

Treatment	Concentration	Relative cloning efficiency (%)	Transformation frequency[a] No. foci per total flasks	Foci per flask (mean ± S.D.)
DMSO	2 μl/ml	100	5/19	0.26 ± 0.10
Min-U-Sil <5	23 μg/cm²	69.7	18/19	0.95 ± 0.24
	45 μg/cm²	36.4	21/20	1.05 ± 0.24
	90 μg/cm²	20.5	23/20	1.15 ± 0.24*
	180 μg/cm²	14.2	22/20	1.10 ± 0.28**
Benzo(a)-pyrene	2 μg/ml	—	38/20	1.90 ± 0.31

[a] Only Type III foci scored.
* $p < 0.05$,
** $p < 0.01$.

assay systems, or the different test protocols used. The concentration of silica used in the experiments varies highly from study to study.

An hypothesis has been formulated to explain the role of monocytes in the induction of SCE in lymphocytes by silica particles. Phagocytosis of silica particles by monocytes could be followed by release of mediators from monocytes, some of which may be responsible for inducing SCE in lymphocytes.[12] Monocytes are known to release interleukin 1, prostaglandins, leukotrienes, oxygen derivatives, arachidonic acid, and growth factors after stimulation.[16,17]

Grinding of silica produces $\dot{S}i$ and $Si\dot{O}$ radicals. These silicon and silicon-oxygen-based radicals react with metal ions in silica-containing aqueous media to produce highly reactive species such as the hydroxyl radical, $\dot{O}H$.[18] Hydroxyl radicals react with DNA and generate a series of modified purine and pyrimidine bases which could lead to gene mutations and other genetic damage.[19] Daniel et al.[20] found that freshly ground crystalline silica caused detectable changes in phage λ DNA due to formation of crystalline silica-derived superoxide free radicals in aqueous solution. Silica also has been found to affect lipid peroxidation. Peroxy radicals, cytotoxic aldehydes, and alkoxy radicals, generated by decomposition of lipid peroxides, may also cause DNA damage.[19]

III. EPIGENETIC ACTIVITIES

Any activities which influence the phenotype without damaging and/or altering DNA/chromosomes are epigenetic activities. Induction of cell proliferation, for instance, is considered to be an epigenetic activity. It is known that macrophages release substances that stimulate fibroblasts and induce fibrosis.[21] Several studies have suggested that silica interacts with macrophages, leading to production of a factor or factors that, in turn, alter fibroblast proliferation. *In vitro* studies have also shown that silica has a direct effect on fibroblasts. Absher and Sylvester[22] found a variable proliferative response to silica that appeared to be related to the age and type of fibroblast cultures. Thus, some fibroblast cultures are stimulated to proliferate in the presence of silica, while others are not. Pathological studies indicate that epithelial proliferative lesions in rats exposed to dusts appear to be located near fibrotic reactions.[17] In mice, silica was reported to penetrate Type 1 alveolar epithelial cells, causing cell injury and cell death, but this was rapidly repaired by induced proliferation of Type 2 alveolar epithelial cells.[17] Mediators such as interleukins, prostaglandins, and tumor necrosis factor released by monocytes after phagocytosis of silica particles are related to the inflammatory process, cell proliferation, and differentiation.[23]

IV. SYNERGISTIC OR COMBINATIONAL EFFECTS

In addition to silica, workers may also be exposed, intentionally or unintentionally, to other agents such as cigarette smoke, other chemicals, and radiation. Limited evidence indicates that there are synergistic or combinational effects.

A. CIGARETTE SMOKE

The available information indicates that dusty trade workers who smoke are at greater risk of lung cancer than either smokers unexposed to silica or nonsmokers exposed to silica. As indicated by Goldsmith and Guidotti[24] in their review of the literature, cigarette smoking plays a prominent role in the development of lung cancer in dusty trade workers and in silicotics.

It has been reported that smoking underground gold miners[25] and smoking silicotics[26] have a high relative risk for lung cancer compared to nonsmoking miners, dust-exposed nonsmokers without fibrosis, or unexposed nonsmokers. These reports support the synergistic effects of the combination of silica exposure and smoking.[24–26] However, in most epidemiological studies, cigarette smoking, though a major confounding factor, was not adjusted for in the findings. This factor must be included in future risk assessment studies of silica-exposed workers, and the synergistic or combinational effect of silica exposure and cigarette smoke needs further investigation.

B. CHEMICALS

PAH include hundreds of compounds which have attracted much attention because many of them are carcinogenic, especially those containing four to six aromatic rings. PAH are formed by pyrolysis or incomplete combustion of organic materials containing carbon and hydrogen. In the air, PAH are emitted as vapors from the zone of burning. Due to their low vapor pressures, most PAH will immediately condense as particles on soot or form very small particulates themselves. Those entering the atmosphere as vapor will be adsorbed by existing particles, including silica dusts. The most important source of PAH in the occupational environment is coal tar, formed by pyrolysis of coal in gas and coke works where emission of fumes from the hot tar occurs. Tar preparations are used in furnaces and ingot molds.[27] Many steel and foundry workers who are chronically exposed to silica also inhale carcinogenic pyrolysis products of hydrocarbons such as PAH adsorbed by silica dusts.

Stenbäck and Rowland[28] showed that intratracheal instillation of benzo(a)pyrene (BaP), a PAH, in combination with silica results in a high incidence of lung tumors. When instilled alone, the silica dusts induced nonspecific bronchial epithelial alterations, interstitial cell proliferation, and a few granulomatous changes in the lung. No respiratory tract tumors were seen. BaP alone induced only tracheal epithelial alterations, desquamation and metaplasia, and a few papillomas or squamous cell carcinomas. Silica with BaP was highly effective in inducing papillomas; squamous cell carcinomas; adenomas; and adenocarcinomas of the larynx, trachea, and lung. The tumors were preceded by epithelial proliferative dysplastic alterations not seen in animals treated with BaP plus MnO_2 or dibenzanthracene plus Fe_2O_3.[28,29]

Niemeier et al.[30] used Syrian hamsters to test ten silica compounds or silica substitutes and iron oxide administered in saline by intratracheal instillation. The respirable particle dosage was based on surface area standardized to Min-U-Sil 5. Each group receiving silica was matched to a group receiving silica plus BaP. There were no tumors in saline-treated control and very few in silica-treated animals, but silica plus BaP-treated animals showed significantly more tumors than saline plus BaP control animals.[30]

A high incidence of respiratory disease among hematite miners in the northwest of Britain has been noted. Pathological studies suggest that lung cancer is a relatively common cause of death, apparently related to the presence of siderosilicosis.[31] While it is possible that a combination of iron and silica is carcinogenic to the lung, an alternative cause was suggested when a survey of radon in British mines revealed high levels of radiation in these same hematite mines.

C. RADIATION

An excess of lung cancer among underground miners has been observed.[32,33] The question of whether or not silica and radon daughters are both involved in the induction of lung cancer has been investigated. Silica is one of the most abundant minerals in the crust of the earth, and it is found in the air of most underground mines. On the other hand, any hole in the ground will contain higher levels of radon and radon daughters than those which occur on the ground surface, due to the small amounts of uranium and radium occurring in all soils, which are constantly emitting radon. This means that most miners are exposed to both silica dust and higher than normal levels of radon and radon daughters. However, the quantitative relationship between the two agents often differs. This difference has been used to assess the role of the two agents in the development of lung cancer in miners. Archer et al.,[33] in their review paper, indicated that lung cancer incidence is a function of radon daughter exposure in hard rock mines where a variety of ores from iron to uranium have been excavated. A similar relationship between radon daughter exposure and lung cancer has been demonstrated in rat experiments where there was no accompanying silica exposure. In uranium mines, there is no correlation between levels of airborne quartz dust and radon daughters. The rates of silicosis and lung cancer were compared among five mining or milling groups selected on the basis of their exposure to silica dust and radon daughters. When quartz dust levels were high, pneumoconiosis rates were high. However, lung cancer rates were high only when radon daughter levels were also elevated. This comparison demonstrates that the two effects of mine exposures are basically independent, although there may be some minor interaction between the two disease-producing agents. The independent action is supported by the Swedish mining experience with different ventilation rates of the air through old mines to warm the air. Large volumes of air greatly lowered the airborne quartz concentrations, but tended to increase radon daughter levels. As a result, the frequency of silicosis was markedly reduced in the cohorts, whereas lung cancer rates rose or remained unchanged.[33]

In contrast, miners with very low exposures to radon and decay products have had little or no excess of lung cancer (i.e., in coal, potash, and iron mines). It seems therefore that radioactivity rather than other factors in the mine atmosphere is mainly responsible for the lung cancer risk, even if some other agents may be contributors. In some mining situations, other factors such as diesel exhaust or heavy metals in respirable particles may contribute to a carcinogenic hazard. It has become clear in recent years, however, that certain silica dust exposure is associated with lung cancer risk, and some contribution to lung cancer in miners cannot be ruled out.[34]

D. CONCLUDING REMARKS

Occupational exposures to mineral dusts, including silica dusts, are particularly complex. The mineral mixture to which workers are exposed may differ according to geological source. Workers in different processes, such as mining, milling, production, and use, may be exposed to different mineral phases and components. Workers are exposed to additional agents in the occupational environment and in daily life. Therefore, a combinational effect of silica with other known carcinogens or suspected causative agents should be considered when silica-induced lung cancer is investigated. Other agents may potentiate the induction of lung cancer by silica, or may act as confounding factors. In most investigations conducted in an effort to assess the role of silica exposure in the pathogenesis of lung cancer, confounding factors, such as cigarette smoking and nonsiliceous environmental pollutants, have not been considered. It is important to determine the contribution of other factors to the incidence of lung cancer among silica-exposed workers. In addition to epidemiologic studies, animal experiments (for example, the intratracheal instillation of BaP in combination with silica results in a high incidence of lung tumors) and *in vitro* assays may be of great help in solving this problem. The combination and/or synergistic effect of the factors mentioned in this section should be considered with respect to the role of silica in the pathogenesis of bronchogenic carcinoma in humans.

V. POTENTIAL MECHANISM OF CARCINOGENESIS

As described in the other chapters and according to the International Agency for Research on Cancer, there is sufficient and limited evidence for the carcinogenicity of crystalline silica in experimental animals and humans, respectively.[4] However, the mechanism of cancer induction by silica in either animals or humans has not been elucidated. Based on a knowledge of chemical carcinogenesis in general and genotoxic as well as epigenetic activities, it may be construed that silica may act as initiator and/or promotor in multistage carcinogenesis and/or may act as a cocarcinogen.

A. AS AN INITIATOR

The somatic mutation theory for the etiology of cancer was proposed in the 1920s. This theory receives support from the observations that

1. Cancer originates from a single cell or a clone.
2. Cancer cells possess heritable phenotypes.
3. There is a correlation between mutagenicity and carcinogenicity of certain groups of chemicals.
4. Certain chromosomal aberrations and gene mutations are related to cancer incidence.
5. Defective DNA repair increases cancer risk.

Researchers generally agree that alteration of genetic material plays an important role in the initiation and progression of chemical carcinogenesis.

Recent studies in the area of molecular biology have found that more than 50 and possibly as many as 100 genes in the eukaryotic organism are involved in the governance of cell growth and/or differentiation.[35] These genes generally are referred to as proto-oncogenes and tumor suppressor genes. Indeed, genetic alteration or damage in these genes, the *ras* proto-oncogene and p53 tumor suppressor gene in particular, has been shown to be present in a variety of human cancers. Proto-oncogenes can be activated and tumor suppressor genes can be deactivated by gene amplification, gene rearrangement, or point mutation.[35]

The mechanism of gene amplification is not yet clear. Different models including replication, unequal exchange, episome excision, double rolling circle, and chromosome breakage have been proposed as possible mechanisms for mammalian gene amplification. A recent review regarding these models has been provided by Windle and Wahl.[36] Using SV40 as a model, Aladjem and Lavi[37] have shown that amplification of viral sequences may be induced by chemical carcinogens in a replication-dependent manner which involves overactivation of the origin region and the generation of inverted repeats. In a variety of tumors, one or another proto-oncogene is known to be expressed abundantly because it resides within an amplified region of DNA.[38] Chromosomal translocation, inversion, and deletion can lead to gene rearrangement.[39] If the rearrangement moves a proto-oncogene from where it is usually dormant or suppressed to a location adjacent to an active region of chromosome, the proto-oncogene may be activated. Deletion of certain chromosomal fragments may result in loss of tumor suppressor genes and result in deregulation of cell division and differentiation. Chromosomal translocations and inversions have been reported to be the most common and diverse of the karyotypic abnormalities found in human cancer cells.[40] A point mutation such as a change of a single base at specific sites has been shown to result in expression of the transforming activity of proto-oncogenes. Different point mutations have been associated with different cancer types.[41,42]

Induction of micronuclei in mammalian cells by silica indicates that silica is clastogenic and/or aneuploidogenic. Induction of chromosomal or DNA breaks may lead to translocation, deletion, or inversion. Free radicals generated directly or indirectly by silica dusts may induce point mutations. Therefore, silica may act as an initiator in multistep carcinogenesis. Genetic alteration or damage caused by silica may also be involved in the progression stage of carcinogenesis. A recent study reported by Ahmed and Saffiotti[43] shows that the transformed BALB/3T3 cells induced by quartz are tumorigenic in nude mice and have new chromosomal translocations as well as elevated expression of several proto-oncogenes including *ras* and p53.

B. AS A PROMOTER

Chemical carcinogens can be broadly grouped into genotoxic carcinogens and nongenotoxic or epigenetic carcinogens. An epigenetic carcinogen is operationally defined by the absence of genotoxicity as demonstrated by short-term assays. The carcinogenic mechanism of epigenetic carcinogens is not well understood. They are believed, however, to act by altering gene expression without permanent damage to the genetic material, leading to cell proliferation. Epigenetic carcinogens therefore may act as promoters. For instance, the phorbol ester 12-O-tetradecanoylphorbol-13-acetate (TPA), an epigenetic carcinogen, is a known promoter. Its promoting action is accompanied by inhibition of cell differentiation and enhancement of proliferation and by alteration of enzymes and cell surface properties. Induction of cell proliferation by chemical agents, either by direct mitogenesis of the target cell population or by cytotoxicity and consequent regenerative proliferation, has been suggested to play an important role in chemical carcinogenesis.[44] It may be involved in the fixation and/or expression of oncogenic changes.

Epidemiological studies show that the incidence of lung cancer is higher in silicotics than in exposed workers without silicosis.[45] A mortality study of South African gold miners showed no association between lung cancer and silicosis of the parenchyma or pleura, but a positive association existed between silicosis of the hilary glands and lung cancer.[46] Experimental foreign body tumorigenesis has demonstrated a role of chronic fibrosis in the induction of tumors.[21] Hepatitis B virus can cause chronic hepatitis and cirrhosis, characterized by persistent necrosis and regenerative hyperplasia, and is also associated with an increased incidence of hepatoma.[47] The common element in these observations is the presence of chronic fibrosis. Fibrosis is causally linked to preneoplastic promotion. This role appears plausible in view of the structural disorder inflicted on tissues and organs. Intercellular communication and, consequently, homeostatic growth regulation are impaired as evidenced by the frequent development of epithelial dysplasias adjacent to fibrotic areas.[20]

Concerning the relationship of cell proliferation to silica-induced lung cancer, the following hypothesis has been proposed: one or more of the cell mediators released by macrophages and other reticuloendothelial cells during the complex process of fibrogenesis acts upon the adjacent epithelial cells of the distal airways throughout the duration of the fibrogenic response to induce cell damage and/or stimulate cell proliferation. These effects act in combination with direct genetic damage, possibly at the chromosomal level, induced by silica particles upon the epithelial cells in the early phases of the pulmonary response. In so doing, they provide a combined mechanism sufficient to account for the full carcinogenic activity of silica on the epithelia of susceptible species.[17]

The role of silica in the synergistic or combinational effects on carcinogenesis is not known. Radiation, many PAH, and chemicals associated with cigarette smoke are known to be genotoxic and carcinogenic. These agents are capable of altering or damaging genes, including proto-oncogenes and tumor suppressor genes. It is possible therefore that silica may act as a promoter, causing the damaged cells to proliferate and leading to cancer development. This may account for the results discussed above in the section on Synergistic or Combinational Effects.

C. AS A COCARCINOGEN

Silica may act as a cocarcinogen by functioning as a vehicle for an adsorbed carcinogen such as BaP, and also may act as a carcinogen through specific physiological and biochemical activities and through interference with respiratory function.[48] One of the main effects of the vehicle is to increase the retention time of BaP in the lungs. Chemicals which are adsorbed by particles, such as silica, are more rapidly transported to target cells. In addition, silica has been shown to facilitate membrane uptake of BaP.[49]

D. CONCLUDING REMARKS

The possible mechanisms regarding the carcinogenesis of silica discussed in this section are based on conjecture. More studies such as that reported by Ahmed and Saffiotti[43] on the molecular aspects of functional and structural changes caused by silica need to be pursued to more clearly understand the mechanism of silica carcinogenesis.

VI. SUMMARY

Results of animal and epidemiological studies indicate that silica, at least in the crystalline form, may be carcinogenic. The process and mechanism by which silica may induce carcinogenesis are not known. It is known, however, that silica is genotoxic and can cause fibroblast proliferation. Genotoxic and mitogenic effects of silica, its metabolites, free radicals produced, or the mediators released by damaged macrophages and other reticuloendothelial cells may lead to the activation of proto-oncogenes or inactivation of tumor suppressor genes. Such activation and/or inactivation may play an important role in the initiation, promotion, and/or progression of cancer in silica-exposed animal and human populations. More work is needed to better understand the mechanism of silica carcinogenesis.

REFERENCES

1. **Roberfroid, M. B.,** From normal cell to cancer: an overview introducing the concept of modulation of carcinogenesis, in *Concepts and Theories in Carcinogenesis,* Maskens, A. P. et al., Eds., Elsevier Science Publishers, Amsterdam, 1987, 157.
2. **Yamasaki, H.,** Aberrant control of intercellular communication and cell differentiation during carcinogenesis, in *Concepts and Theories in Carcinogenesis,* Maskens, A. P. et al., Eds., Elsevier Science Publishers, Amsterdam, 1987, 117.
3. IARC Monographs on the Evaluation of Carcinogenic Risks to Humans, Silica and some silicates, Vol. 42, Lyon, France, 1987.
4. IARC Monographs on the Evaluation of Carcinogenic Risks to Humans, Overall evaluation of carcinogenicity: an updating of IARC Monographs Vol. 1–42, Suppl. 7, p. 341, Lyon, France, 1987.

5. **Mortelmans, K. E. and Griffin, A. F.,** Microbial Mutagenesis Testing of Substances, Compound Report: F76–037, Silica-Silcron G-910, SCM Glidden Pigments, Lot. No. 14-J-2, CAS No. 7631869, Government Printing Office, Washington, D.C., 1981.
6. **Kada, T., Hirano, K., and Shirasu, Y.,** Screening of environmental chemical mutagens by the rec-assay system with *Bacillus subtilis,* in de Serres, F. J. and Hollaender, A., Eds., *Chemical Mutagens: Principles and Methods for Their Detection,* Vol. 6, Plenum Press, New York, 1980, 149.
7. **Hesterberg, T. W., Oshimura, M., Brody, A. R., and Barrett, J. C.,** Asbestos and silica induce morphological transformation of mammalian cells in culture: a possible mechanism, in *Silica, Silicosis, and Cancer: Controversy in Occupational Medicine,* Goldsmith, D. F. et al., Eds., Praeger Publishers, New York, 1986, 177.
8. **Oshimura, M., Hesterberg, T. W., Tsutsui, T., and Barrett, J. C.,** Correlation of asbestos-induced cytogenetic effects with cell transformation of Syrian hamster embryo cells in culture, *Cancer Res.,* 44, 5017, 1984.
9. **Hesterberg, T. W. and Barrett, J. C.,** Dependence of asbestos- and mineral dust-induced transformation of mammalian cells in culture on fiber dimension, *Cancer Res.,* 44, 2170, 1984.
10. **Vanchugova, N. N., Frash, V. N., and Kogan, F. M.,** The use of a micronuclear test as a short-term method in detecting potential blastomogenicity of asbestos-containing and other mineral fibers, *Gig. Tr. Prof. Zabol.,* 6, 45, 1985.
11. **Price-Jones, M. J., Gubbings, G., and Chamberlain, M.,** The genetic effects of crocidolite asbestos: comparison of chromosome abnormalities and sister-chromatid exchanges, *Mutat. Res.,* 79, 331, 1980.
12. **Pairon, J. C., Jaurand, M. C., Kheuang, L., Janson, X., Brochard, P., and Bignon, J.,** Sister chromatid exchanges in human lymphocytes treated with silica, *Br. J. Ind. Med.,* 47, 110, 1990.
13. **Sikandar, G. K., Rizvi, R. Y., Hadi, S. M., and Rahman, Q.,** Strand breakage in DNA by silicic acid, *Mutat. Res.,* 208, 27, 1988.
14. **Rohman, Q., Alvi, N. K., Rizvi, R. Y., and Hadi, S. M.,** Degradation of DNA by silicic acid, *Mutat. Res.,* 141, 1, 1984.
15. **Fitzgerald, D. J., Piccoli, C., and Yamasaki, H.,** Detection of nongenotoxic carcinogens in the BALB/c-3T3 cell transformation/mutation assay system, *Mutagenesis,* 4, 286, 1989.

15a. **Ahmed, N. and Saffiotti, U.,** personal communication.

16. **Schmidt, J. A., Oliver, C. N., Lepe-Zumiga, J. L., Green, J., and Gery, I.,** Silica-stimulated monocytes release fibroblast proliferation factors identical to interleukin 1, *J. Clin. Invest.,* 73, 1462, 1984.
17. **Saffiotti, U.,** The pathology induced by silica in relation to fibrogenesis and carcinogenesis, in *Silica, Silicosis, and Cancer: Controversy in Occupational Medicine,* Goldsmith D. F. et al., Eds., Praeger Publishers, New York, 1986, 287.
18. **Shi, X., Dalal, N. S., Hu, X. N., and Vallyathan, V.,** The chemical properties of silica particle surface in relation to silica-cell interactions, *J. Toxicol. Environ. Health,* 27, 435, 1989.
19. **Halliwell, B. and Gutteridge, J. M. C.,** *Free Radicals in Biology and Medicine,* 2nd ed., Clarendon Press, Oxford, 1989, 466.
20. **Daniel, L. N., Mao, Y., and Saffiotti, U.,** Toxic free radical production by crystalline silica, *Carcinogenesis,* 33, 176, 1992.
21. **Brand, K. G.,** Fibrotic scar cancer in the light of foreign body tumorigenesis, in *Silica, Silicosis, and Cancer: Controversy in Occupational Medicine,* Goldsmith D. F. et al., Eds., Praeger Publishers, New York, 1986, 281.
22. **Absher, M. and Sylvester, D.,** Effects of silica on human lung fibroblasts: survival data analysis of time-lapse cinematography data, *Environ. Res.,* 26, 438, 1981.
23. **Brown, G. M., Li, X. Y., and Donaldson, K.,** Secretion of interleukin 1 and tumour necrosis factor by alveolar macrophages following exposure to particulate and fibrous dusts, in *Mechanisms in Fibre Carcinogenesis,* Broun, R. C. et al., Eds., Plenum Press, New York, 1991, 499.
24. **Goldsmith, D. F. and Guidotti, T. L.,** Combined silica exposure and cigarette smoking: a likely synergistic effect, in *Silica, Silicosis, and Cancer: Controversy in Occupational Medicine,* Goldsmith, D. F. et al., Eds., Praeger Publishers, New York, 1986, 451.
25. **Armstong, B. K., McNulty, J. C., Levitt, L. J., Williams, K. A., and Hobbs, M. S. T.,** Mortality in gold and coal miners in Western Australia with special reference to lung cancer, *Br. J. Ind. Med.,* 36, 199, 1979.
26. **Mastrangelo, G., Zambon, P., Saia, B., Braga, M., and Crepet, M.,** Exposure to silica and lung cancer: a case-referent study, *Scand. J. Work Environ. Health,* 9, 70, 1982.
27. **Sollenberg, J.,** Polycyclic aromatic hydrocarbons, in *Encyclopaedia of Occupational Health and Safety,* Parmeggiani, L., Ed., International Labour Office, Geneva, 1989, 1755.
28. **Stenbäck, F. and Rowland, J.,** Experimental respiratory carcinogenesis in hamsters: environmental, physicochemical and biological aspects, *Oncology,* 36, 63, 1979.
29. **Stenbäck, F., Rowland, J., and SellaKumar, A.,** Carcinogenicity of benzo(a)pyrene and dusts in the hamster lung (instilled intratracheally with titanium oxide, aluminum oxide, carbon and ferric oxide), *Oncology,* 33, 29, 1976.
30. **Niemeier, R. W., Mulligan, L. T., and Rowland, J.,** Cocarcinogenicity of Foundry Particulates. Third National Cancer Institute/Environmental Protection Agency/NIOSH Collaborative Workshop: Progress on Joint Environmental and Occupational Cancer Studies, Bethesda, MD, 1984.
31. **Faulds, J. S. and Stewart, M. J.,** Carcinoma of the lung in hematite miners, *J. Pathol. Bacteriol.,* 72, 353, 1956.

32. **Radford, E. P. and Renard, K. G. S.,** Lung cancer in Swedish iron miners exposed to low doses of radon daughters, *N. Engl. J. Med.*, 310, 1485, 1984.
33. **Archer, V. E., Rascoe, J. R., and Brown, D.,** Is silica or radon daughters the important factor in the excess lung cancer among underground miners? in *Silica, Silicosis, and Cancer: Controversy in Occupational Medicine,* Goldsmith, D. F. et al., Eds., Praeger Publishers, New York, 1986, 287.
34. **Axelson, O.,** Cancer risks from exposure to radon progeny in mines and dwellings, in *Occupational Cancer Epidemiology,* Band, P., Ed., Springer-Verlag, Berlin, 1990, 148.
35. **Weinberg, R. A., Ed.,** *Oncogenes and the Molecular Origins of Cancer,* Cold Spring Harbor Laboratory, Cold Spring Harbor, NY, 1989, 4.
36. **Windle, B. E. and Wahl, G. M.,** Molecular dissection of mammalian gene amplification: new mechanistic insights revealed by analyses of very early events, *Mutat. Res.*, 276, 199, 1992.
37. **Aladjem, M. I. and Lavi, S.,** The mechanism of carcinogen-induced DNA amplification: in vivo and in vitro studies, *Mutat. Res.*, 276, 339, 1992.
38. **Alitalo, K. and Schwab, M.,** Oncogene amplification in tumor cells, *Adv. Cancer Res.*, 47, 235, 1986.
39. **Hall, E. J.,** From chimney sweeps to oncogenes: the quest for the causes of cancer, *Radiology,* 179, 297, 1991.
40. **Yunis, J. J.,** Chromosomal rearrangements, genes, and fragile sites in cancer: clinical and biologic implications, in *Important Advances in Oncology,* De Vita, V. T. et al., Eds., J.B. Lippincott, Philadelphia, 1986, 93.
41. **Nigro, J. M., Baker, S. J., Preisinger, A. C., Jessup, J. M., Hostetter, R., Cleary, K., Bigner, S. H., Davidson, N., Baylin, S., Devilee, P., Glover, T., Collins, F. S., Weston, A., Modali, R., Harris, C. C., and Vogelstein, B.,** Mutations in the p53 gene occur in diverse human tumour types, *Nature,* 342, 705, 1989.
42. **Hollstein, M., Sidransky, D., Vogelstein, B., and Harris, C. C.,** p53 mutations in human cancers, *Science,* 253, 49, 1991.
43. **Ahmed, N. and Saffiotti, U.,** Crystalline silica-induced cytotoxicity, transformation, tumorigenicity, chromosomal translocations and oncogene expression, *Proc. Am. Assoc. Cancer Res.* 33, 119, 1992.
44. **Cohen, S. M. and Ellwein, L. B.,** Cell proliferation in carcinogenesis, *Science,* 249, 1007, 1990.
45. **Amandus, H. E., Shy, C., Wing, S., Blair, A., and Heineman, E. F.,** Silicosis and lung cancer in North Carolina dusty trades workers, *Am. J. Ind. Med.*, 20, 57, 1991.
46. **Hnizdo, E. and Sluis-Cremer, G. K.,** Silica exposure, silicosis, and lung cancer: a mortality study of South African gold miners, *Br. J. Ind. Med.*, 48, 53, 1991.
47. **Beasly, R. P.,** Hepatitis B virus, the major etiology of hepatocellular carcinoma, *Cancer,* 61, 1942, 1988.
48. **Gibson, E. S., McCalla, D. R., Kaiser-Farrell, C., Kerr, A. A., Lockington, J. N., Hertzman, C., and Rosenfeld, J. M.,** Industrial mutagenicity testing: assessing silica's role in lung cancer among foundry workers, in *Silica, Silicosis, and Cancer: Controversy in Occupational Medicine,* Goldsmith, D. F. et al., Eds., Praeger Publishers, New York, 1986, 167.
49. **Lakowicz, J. R., Hylden, J. L., Englund, F., Hidmark, A., and McNamara, M.,** Asbestos-facilitated membrane uptake of polynuclear aromatic hydrocarbons studied by fluorescence spectroscopy: a possible explanation of the cocarcinogenic effects of particulates and PAH, in Jones, P. W. and Leber, P., Eds., *Polynuclear Aromatic Hydrocarbons,* Ann Arbor Science Publishers, Ann Arbor, MI, 1979, 835.

INDEX

A

B

C

D

J

K

L

M

N

Q

T

U

V

W

X

Z